CARE
OF THE
YOUNG
ATHLETE

SECOND EDITION

AMERICAN ACADEMY OF PEDIATRICS
AMERICAN ACADEMY OF ORTHOPAEDIC SURGEONS

STEVEN J. ANDERSON, MD, FAAP
SALLY S. HARRIS, MD, MPH, FAAP
EDITORS

ANDREW J. M. GREGORY, MD, FAAP, FACSM
EDITOR, PATIENT EDUCATION HANDOUTS

American Academy
of Pediatrics

DEDICATED TO THE HEALTH OF ALL CHILDREN™

AAOS
AMERICAN ACADEMY OF
ORTHOPAEDIC SURGEONS

AAP STAFF

Maureen DeRosa, MPA, *Director, Department of Marketing and Publications*

Mark Grimes, *Director, Division of Product Development*

Martha Cook, *Senior Product Development Editor*

Tracey Douglas, *Developmental Editor*

Sandi King, MS, *Director, Division of Publishing and Production Services*

Theresa Wiener, *Manager, Editorial Production*

Leesa Levin-Doroba, *Manager, Print Production Services*

Peg Mulcahy, *Manager, Graphic Design and Production*

Jill Ferguson, *Director, Division of Marketing*

Linda Smessaert, *Manager, Clinical and Professional Publications Marketing*

Robert Herling, *Director, Division of Sales*

David Roberts, *Graphic Design*

Graphic World Inc., *Editorial Services and Composition*

AAOS STAFF

Mark W. Wieting, *Chief Education Officer*

Marilyn L. Fox, PhD, *Director, Department of Publications*

Library of Congress Control Number 2008941469
ISBN: 978-1-58110-304-5
MA0448

The recommendations in this publication do not indicate an exclusive course of treatment or serve as a standard of care. Variations, taking into account individual circumstances, may be appropriate.

Brand names are furnished for identifying purposes only. No endorsement of the manufacturers or products listed is implied.

Suggested Citation: Anderson SJ and Harris SS, eds. *Care of the Young Athlete,* 2nd ed. Elk Grove Village, IL: American Academy of Pediatrics; 2010.

3-207/0909

1   2   3   4   5   6   7   8   9

CONTRIBUTORS

Steven J. Anderson, MD, FAAP
Clinical Professor
Department of Pediatrics
University of Washington
Seattle, Washington

Rodney S.W. Basler, MD
Adjunct Assistant Professor of Internal Medicine
University of Nebraska Medical Center
Lincoln, Nebraska

David T. Bernhardt, MD, FAAP
Professor of Pediatrics, Orthopedics, and Rehabilitation
University of Wisconsin School of Medicine and Public
 Health
Madison, Wisconsin

Joel S. Brenner, MD, MPH, FAAP
Associate Professor of Pediatrics
Eastern Virginia Medical School
Medical Director, Children's Hospital of the King's
 Daughters Sports Medical Program
Norfolk, Virginia

Cora Colette Bruener, MD, MPH
Associate Professor of Pediatrics
University of Washington
Children's Hospital and Regional Medical Center
Seattle, Washington

Frank M. Chang, MD, FAAP
The Children's Hospital Disabled Sports Program
Co-Medical Director, Center for Gait and Movement
 Analysis
Associate Professor of Orthopedic Surgery, Rehabilitation
 Medicine and Pediatrics
University of Colorado at Denver and Health Sciences
 Center
Denver, Colorado

Joseph A. Congeni, MD, FAAP
Associate Professor of Pediatrics
Northeastern Ohio University Colleges of Medicine and
 Pharmacy
Medical Director, Sports Medicine Center
Akron Children's Hospital
Akron, Ohio

Ronald A. Feinstein, MD, FAAP
Professor of Clinical Pediatrics
Louisiana State University School of Medicine
Louisiana State University Health Sciences Center–New
 Orleans
New Orleans, Louisiana

Jorge E. Gómez, MS, MD
Clinical Professor, Sports Medicine and Pediatrics
University of Texas Health Science Center at San Antonio
San Antonio, Texas

Daniel R. Gould, PhD
Director, Institute for the Study of Youth Sports
Michigan State University
East Lansing, Michigan

Andrew J. M. Gregory, MD, FAAP, FACSM
Assistant Professor of Orthopedics and Pediatrics
Program Director, Pediatric Sports Medicine Fellowship
Vanderbilt University School of Medicine
Nashville, Tennessee

Bernad A. Griesemer, MD, FAAP
Director, HealthTracks Center
St. John's HealthTracks Center
Springfield, Missouri

Sally S. Harris, MD, MPH, FAAP
Department of Pediatrics and Sports Medicine
Palo Alto Medical Clinic
Palo Alto, California

**Kristin M. Houghton, MD, MSc, FRCPC, FAAP, Dip Sports
Med**
Clinical Assistant Professor
Division of Rheumatology
Department of Pediatrics, University of British Columbia
Vancouver, British Columbia
Canada

John B. Jeffers, DVM, MD
Director, Emergency Department
Director of Resident Education
Department of Ophthalmology
Wills Eye Hospital
Philadelphia, Pennsylvania

Mimi D. Johnson, MD, FAAP, FACSM
Private Practice, Pediatric and Young Adult Sports Medicine
Clinical Associate Professor
Department of Pediatrics
University of Washington
Seattle, Washington

Amanda Kay Weiss Kelly, MD, FAAP
Assistant Professor of Pediatrics
Case Western Reserve University
Rainbow Babies & Children's Hospital
Cleveland, Ohio

Michael C. Koester, MD, ATC
Slocum Center for Orthopedics & Sports Medicine
Eugene, Oregon

Daniel E. Kraft, MD, FAAP
Youth Sports Medicine Institute
Methodist Sports Medicine
Indiana University
Indianapolis, Indiana

Michele LaBotz, MD, FAAP
Physician, Sports Medicine Clinic
Intermed, Physician Associates
South Portland, Maine

Gregory L. Landry, MD, FAAP
University of Wisconsin School of Medicine and Public Health
Team Physician, University of Wisconsin Athletic Teams
Madison, Wisconsin

Claire M. A. Le Blanc, MD, FRCPC, FAAP, Dip Sports Med
Associate Professor of Pediatrics
University of Alberta
Edmonton, Alberta
Canada

Barbara J. Long, MD, MPH
Associate Clinical Professor
Division of Adolescent Medicine
University of California–San Francisco
San Francisco, California

P. Cameron Mantor, MD, FAAP
Professor of Surgery
University of Oklahoma College of Medicine
Section of Pediatric Surgery
Children's Hospital
Oklahoma City, Oklahoma

Teri M. McCambridge, MD, FAAP
Assistant Professor of Pediatrics
Johns Hopkins School of Medicine
Baltimore, Maryland

Larry G. McLain, MD, MBA, FAAP
Chief Medical Coordinator, Illinois Department of Financial and Professional Regulation
Associate Professor of Clinical Pediatrics
University of Illinois College of Medicine
Chicago, Illinois

Russel Medbery, MS, PhD
Assistant Professor, Exercise and Sports Science
Colby Sawyer College
New London, New Hampshire

David M. Orenstein, MD
Professor of Pediatrics
University of Pittsburgh School of Medicine
Pittsburgh, Pennsylvania

Stephen G. Rice, MD, PhD, MPH, FAAP
Director, Sports Medicine
Jersey Shore University Medical Center
Clinical Associate Professor of Pediatrics
University of Medicine and Dentistry of New Jersey–Robert Wood Johnson Medical School
Neptune, New Jersey

William L. Risser, MD, PhD, FAAP
Professor of Pediatrics
Director, Division of Adolescent Medicine
University of Texas–Houston Medical School
Houston, Texas

Thomas W. Rowland, MD, FAAP
Pediatric Cardiologist
Baystate Medical Center
Springfield, Massachusetts

Eric Small, MD, FAAP
Assistant Clinical Professor of Pediatrics, Orthopedics, Rehabilitation Medicine
Department of Pediatrics
Mount Sinai School of Medicine
New York, New York

Bryan W. Smith, MD, PhD, FAAP
Medical Consultant
Atlantic Coast Conference
Greensboro, North Carolina

Paul R. Stricker, MD, FAAP
Sports Medicine Specialist
Scripps Clinic
La Jolla, California

Steven M. Sullivan, DDS
Professor and Chairman
Department of Oral and Maxillofacial Surgery
University of Oklahoma
Oklahoma City, Oklahoma

Weyton W. Tam, MD
Medical Imaging Director
Northwest Surgical Hospital
Oklahoma City, Oklahoma

David W. Tuggle, MD, FAAP
Professor and Chief, University of Oklahoma College of
  Medicine
Section of Pediatric Surgery
Children's Hospital of Oklahoma
Oklahoma City, Oklahoma

Reginald L. Washington, MD, FAAP, FACC, FAHA
Chief Medical Officer
Rocky Mountain Hospital For Children
Denver, Colorado

REVIEWERS

AMERICAN ACADEMY OF PEDIATRICS

Committee on Adolescence

Committee on Injury, Violence, and Poison Prevention

Committee on Nutrition

Committee on Practice and Ambulatory Medicine

Council on Children with Disabilities

Division of State Government Affairs

Section on Allergy and Immunology

Section on Cardiology and Cardiac Surgery

Section on Clinical Pharmacology & Therapeutics

Section on Complementary and Integrative Medicine

Section on Early Education and Child Care

Section on Endocrinology

Section on Hematology/Oncology

Section on Infectious Diseases

Section on Nephrology

Section on Ophthalmology

Section on Orthopaedics

Section on Rheumatology

Section on Urology

AMERICAN ACADEMY OF ORTHOPAEDIC SURGEONS

Daniel J. Downey, MD
Orthopaedic Surgeon, Dillon, Montana
Member, AAOS Publications Committee

Theodore J. Ganby, MD
Children's Hospital of Philadelphia
Philadelphia, Pennsylvania
Member, AAOS Publications Committee

CONTENTS

SECTION 3

Basic Management Concepts

41 Overuse Injuries of the Knee

David T. Bernhardt, MD

42 Lower Leg

Michael C. Koester, MD

43 Acute Foot and Ankle Injuries

Steven J. Anderson, MD

44 Chronic Foot and Ankle Injuries

Daniel E. Kraft, MD

45 Nontraumatic Causes of Musculoskeletal Pain

Claire M. A. LeBlanc, MD; Kristin Houghton, MD; and Eric Small, MD

46 Sport-Specific Injury Prevention Strategies

Sally S. Harris, MD, MPH, and Steven J. Anderson, MD

APPENDIX

INTRODUCTION

The foundation for *Care of the Young Athlete (COYA)* can be traced to important historical developments in youth sports and the field of sports medicine over the past half century. During the 1950s and 1960s, organized sports for children emerged as a popular alternative to informal games, recreational activities, and free play. This growth took place largely without medical input on issues such as proper training, injury treatment, or injury prevention. Sports injuries were generally treated in a similar manner to accidents or other traumatic injuries—return to the activity that caused the injury was discouraged rather than facilitated.

Shortly after the emergence of organized youth sports, reports on adverse medical consequences began to appear. Sudden cardiac death from strenuous exercise raised questions about whether or not organized sports were safe. Many thought that children were better off regulating their own physical activity. In Little League baseball, reports of shoulder and arm problems—including permanent effects on developing bones—also raised questions about the safety of organized youth sports. Medical professionals were confronted with the possibility that a young person playing sports for enjoyment may actually die or become disabled.

The preparticipation sports evaluation was one of the first formal responses of the medical community to these concerns. The preparticipation evaluation (PPE) was intended to screen individuals at risk for injury or sudden death and to protect at-risk individuals by restricting their participation. In Little League baseball, limits on pitching were instituted as a way to reduce arm injuries. As other sports-related risks were identified, the standard medical response during the 1960s and 1970s was to advise against participation. Early policy statements from the Committee on Sports Medicine and Fitness (COSMF) of the American Academy of Pediatrics (AAP) focused on identifying risks and discouraging the risky activity or participation of the at-risk individual. Children were discouraged from lifting weights, running marathons, boxing, and starting organized sports too early. Children with hypertension or mitral valve prolapse were discouraged from exercising. These policy statements were an important first step in addressing the risks of sports participation and providing medical guidance on issues related to safety. Unfortunately, when restricting participation is the only tool used to enhance sports safety, risk reduction may ultimately reduce the number of acceptably safe sports and participants.

Health care providers for young athletes were challenged to eliminate risk without eliminating sports.

In the 1980s and 1990s, a philosophical shift was reflected in the medical response to health and safety issues in youth sports. Treating injuries like accidents fails to recognize that, in sports settings, the patient wants to return to the very activity that caused the injury. Physicians are understandably uncomfortable in clearing a patient to return to an activity that has already proved to be risky. However, when proven and effective treatments are known to be available, prescribing rest could result in patients either ignoring the advice or seeking care elsewhere. Increasingly, advances in sports medicine during this era identified options for safe return to play following injury. Components of a safe and appropriate return-to-play decision include establishing an accurate diagnosis, recognizing injury risk factors, understanding the demands of training, understanding the impact of the injury or condition on performance, carrying out treatment programs that ensure full functional recovery from the injury, and reducing risk factors that contributed to the primary injury.

As the specialty of sports medicine has evolved, pediatricians have had access to more resources on sports-related issues in children. Sports medicine practitioners with pediatric or general medical backgrounds have emerged from a field that was dominated by orthopedic surgeons. Policy statements from the COSMF have continued to identify risks but have begun to emphasize a more proactive approach to safety and injury prevention. "Finding a safe way for all individuals to participate" recognizes the positive aspects of sports and physical activity. When the focus is entirely on avoiding risk, the benefits of participation are less apparent.

During the 1980s and 1990s, participation in organized sports continued to grow. Children started sports at an earlier age, played longer seasons, participated on multiple teams, and played at higher levels of intensity. Concerns about physical and psychological effects of sports resurfaced. Ironically, during this growth period for organized sports, children overall became less active and less fit. More children are overweight and inactive than ever before. Epidemic levels of obesity and related health problems have prompted medical professionals to examine how physical activity levels can be increased for children. Depending on one's perspective regarding activity levels in children, it could be argued that they either did too much or too little.

Pediatricians and other healthcare professionals caring for children now face a number of challenges related to physical activity and sports in children. Children need to be safeguarded from the risks of excessive or inappropriate activity. At the same time, healthy levels of physical activity need to be promoted for children who are not active enough. Pediatricians face additional pressures from patients and families who demand immediate treatment of injuries and a speedy return to play. Premature clearance to return to play carries a risk of further injury to the patient and liability for the doctor. Delayed clearance to return to play may send patients shopping for more favorable opinions. Extended delays in returning to play may lead to adverse health effects associated with inactivity. Consulting a sports medicine specialist can be helpful when handling complex injuries or difficult medical problems. However, referral to a specialist is not necessary or practical for most patients. Furthermore, many specialists do not share the pediatricians' familiarity with the patient's long-term health history or the impact of growth and development on injury risk and recovery.

The second edition of *COYA* is designed to help pediatricians and other primary care practitioners better address the challenge of optimizing the benefits of physical activity and sport while minimizing the risks. *COYA* is the first sports medicine text of this magnitude that is written by pediatricians for pediatricians. The authors who are not pediatricians by training have been selected because their subspecialties and clinical practices deal primarily with children. In addition, *COYA* was written to help the many other specialists in sports medicine and related fields to better appreciate the unique aspects of the child athlete. For certified athletic trainers, physical therapists, chiropractors, podiatrists, nurses, nurse practitioners, physican assistants, and personal trainers, *COYA* provides insights to the young athlete that can enhance the level of care administered by specialists whose primary training is in a field other than pediatrics.

The first section of *COYA* reviews the health benefits and risks associated with sports participation. Background information on growth and maturational issues, effects of training, and guidelines for determining readiness to participate are discussed. Sports nutrition, weight management, strength training, and performance-enhancing substances are also covered in this section. Injury prevention is discussed in the chapter on the preparticipation sports evaluation and also in a separate chapter on injury prevention. The first section of *COYA*

also reviews medical conditions that affect sports participation, including disorders involving the heart, respiratory system, skin, and immune system. Finally, issues that relate to specific populations, including the female athlete and the disabled athlete, are discussed.

Later sections of *COYA* focus on the diagnosis and treatment of musculoskeletal injuries. Chapter 29 provides an overview that defines common orthopedic terminology and reviews clinical strategies for efficient use of the medical history, physical examination, and radiologic evaluation for both acute and overuse injuries. Chapter 30 provides an outline for optimal use of various imaging modalities as they pertain to accurately diagnosing musculoskeletal problems. Injury treatment principles and methods are covered in Chapter 31. Chapter 18 reviews current concepts on complementary and alternative care. Familiarity with nontraditional care will hopefully expand the number of treatment options that can be considered and can help pediatricians more intelligently evaluate treatments that are proposed or utilized by patients or families. Determining when it is safe for a patient to return to sports following an illness or injury is a vexing challenge that all pediatricians can face. Chapter 14 discusses return-to-play decisions and demonstrates how a systematic process can lead to decisions that are sound, fair, and defensible.

Injuries in each anatomic area are discussed in individual chapters. For the shoulder, knee, and ankle, the subject material has been divided into chapters on acute injuries and overuse injuries. Each chapter reviews relevant anatomy as well as the history, physical examination, diagnostic imaging, treatment, and return-to-play criteria for the common injuries in the respective areas. Each chapter in the musculoskeletal section is written by a practicing pediatric sports medicine specialist. While surgical conditions are addressed, the focus is on problems that can be effectively diagnosed and managed by physicians who do not have orthopedic backgrounds.

Much of the information conveyed to athletes and parents in an office visit might be better understood and retained if supplemental educational materials were provided. *COYA* provides a compendium of patient education materials that can be accessed by purchasers of this book via a password-protected Web site. The materials can be customized, printed, and copied. These materials can be distributed to patients and families who are interested in learning more about their conditions or those who want to explore options for better preparation, training, or injury prevention in their sport. Topics include treatment of common injuries, proper training methods, conditioning exercises, and injury prevention for specific sports, as well as guidelines on general topics such as nutrition, drug use, stretching, weight lifting, use of ice, and when to contact a doctor about an injury or illness.

In the relatively short history of pediatric sports medicine, a few consistent and enduring themes have emerged. First, despite many important advances in the field, sports are still associated with a risk of injury that cannot be entirely eliminated. Second, despite the known risk of injury, organized sports are likely to remain as an entity and young people are likely to continue to participate. Third, it has become increasingly evident that regular physical activity is an important component of health for all children—including those who don't participate in sports. Finally, with all that is known about sports injuries, injury risk, and health-related aspects of physical activity in children and adolescents, pediatricians are in the ideal position to deal with these issues. *COYA* will hopefully provide the necessary academic foundation, pediatric practice perspective, and educational resources to help pediatricians better meet the challenges of promoting safe, healthy sports and physical activity for all of their patients.

Steven J. Anderson, MD, FAAP
Sally S. Harris, MD, MPH, FAAP
Editors

General Health and Fitness

CHAPTER 1

Benefits of Sports Participation

Gregory L. Landry, MD

Like most books on sports medicine, this text is written to assist physicians in managing a variety of problems associated with sports participation. The discussion covers a wide range of medical problems, psychological problems, and various types of injuries. In the United States, large amounts of money and time are spent managing injuries that children sustain during sports participation. According to a United States Consumer Product Safety Commission report, the public cost of injuries in the United States sustained by youth younger than age 15 years during participation in 29 sports was $49 billion in 1997. Sometimes young athletes are encouraged to remain in sports activities even after they have been injured. Despite the risk of injury, record numbers of youngsters are participating in sports. So why are sports so popular? What is it about sports that is so important to our society, and why should physicians encourage young patients to participate in sports?

The benefits of sports participation are discussed in this chapter in an attempt to answer these questions. Physicians and others would not spend so much time caring for athletes if there were not something desirable about participation in sports. This chapter emphasizes the psychosocial benefits of participation in sports; the physical benefits are discussed in other chapters.

DEFINITIONS

Many of the benefits of sports participation accrue because most sports involve physical activity, which is defined as any body movement that results in energy expenditure. Physical fitness is the ability to perform physical activity and is a set of physiologic traits that are related to health, skills, or both.

Sports participation usually involves physical activity, which may improve health and wellness but may not improve physical fitness. Sports are *played*—a word that implies that amusement or recreation is a component of the activity. Play involves behavior that is free, spontaneous, and expressive, in contrast to sports, which are often thought of as competitive and organized. However, this need not be the case. For the purpose of the following discussion, the broadest definition of sports is intended, without implying that the benefits of participation must be realized through competition. Sports participation encompasses both team and individual activities, including activities such as bicycling and martial arts, which can be lifelong physical activities but which often are not thought of as sports.

PSYCHOSOCIAL BENEFITS

Developmental Progression of Play Activity

From early infancy children engage in play, which helps them learn about objects and events. Between the ages of 2 and 7 years, children spend most of their waking hours in play. They experiment with various kinds of social interactions through cooperation, sharing, or competition. They also engage in make-believe play, where they simulate the use of skills that they are unable to perform in the real world, such as driving a car or cooking.

By age 6, most children understand rules, and if a particular activity has no rules they will create them. Children also tend to exert pressure on their peers to follow the rules. This process teaches children that social systems depend on adherence to rules. A child's interest in rules is compatible with the introduction of organized sports.

When children begin elementary school, the number of significant people in their lives expands to include schoolmates and teachers. This is an important time for children as they discover and judge their own abilities and form a stable self-concept and feelings of self-worth. Many children enter organized sports programs at this time.

Self-Concept and Self-Esteem

Self-concept and self-esteem develop as children interpret others' responses to them and as children compare their skills and characteristics with those of others. Comparison and competition in a variety of activities begin at about age 5 years and increase throughout elementary school, which is a good time to test motor skills in sports activities. Because no single sport tests all motor skills, a variety of sports activities should be offered. Children should begin sports at a relatively young age so that they will learn to understand that their physical, cognitive, musical, and artistic talents differ from those of their peers.

However, participation in sports does not offer the same psychosocial benefits for all children. Sports participation tends to attract the most physically talented children. Because they acquire motor skills more easily than other children, participation improves their sense of self-esteem and self-worth. For them, participation in sports activities builds self-confidence. Although physically talented youngsters may acquire new skills faster than those who are less physically talented, virtually all children can acquire motor skills, develop self-esteem, and have fun by participating in sports activities. Successful acquisition of these skills helps children feel competent and proud that they have mastered a skill.

Motivational Factors and Competence

Factors that motivate children to play sports provide some insight into the benefits of sports participation. These are traditionally termed *intrinsic factors* and *extrinsic factors.* Participants who perceive themselves to be competent, in control, and successful will want to play that same game or engage in the same sports activity the next day. This process is known as competence motivation. Competence motivation is a powerful intrinsic factor. As a child acquires new skills, the approval of important adults such as parents and coaches is an important extrinsic factor. Children rely on the comments of important adults to help them judge their competence. Peer approval is another extrinsic factor that gains increasing importance as the child enters adolescence. Ribbons and trophies are also extrinsic motivators, but they are less powerful and not sustained compared with other factors.

Children are attracted to activities that they consider enjoyable. Research confirms that children participate in sports mostly to have fun. Additionally, boys and girls report that they want to improve their skills, achieve physical fitness, spend time with existing friends, and make new friends (**Table 1.1**). As children get older, they report that they like to test their abilities against others and participate for the excitement of the game. Adolescents enjoy being competitive, winning, and achieving goals. Girls tend to be more goal oriented, particularly toward personal goals, while boys tend to be motivated to win. When asked why they try to perform well when they engage in sports, children between ages 9 and 14 years reported that the most important reason was "feeling good about how you played" (**Table 1.2**). Intrinsic rewards appear at the top of the list, and extrinsic rewards appear at the bottom. Intrinsic factors are also more likely to lead to continued participation in older children and adolescents than are extrinsic rewards or pressure from parents and coaches.

Not all children benefit from continued participation in sports. Some children discover that some motor skills are more difficult for them to master compared with their peers. Self-selection begins among school-age children as they participate in a variety of sports. Children who find a particular activity difficult rarely feel competent when participating and often are therefore attracted to other activities. For example, a child who is physically less capable at sports that require cardiopulmonary endurance is not likely to enjoy distance running or swimming. Such children should be encouraged to explore other sports and physical activities that they find enjoyable and that better suit their physical skills; perhaps martial arts or dance, for example, would be more appealing. The goal is for all children to experience early success and to develop habits that lead to lifelong participation in physical activity.

TABLE 1.1

Reasons Children Want to Play Sports

- To have fun
- To improve their skills
- To learn new skills
- To be with their friends
- To make new friends
- To succeed or win
- To become physically fit

TABLE 1.2

Reasons for Trying to Perform Well in Sports

Reason for Trying to Play Well	Order of Importance for Children Aged:	
	9–11 Years	12–14 Years
Feeling good about how you played	1	1
Making sure you won't blame yourself for losing	2	2
Being praised by your parents for playing well	6	4
Making sure your parents won't be displeased with your play	3	8
Making your coach proud of you	4	3
Making sure your coach won't be displeased with you	5	6
Making the other kids like you more	8	7
Making sure that the other kids don't get upset with you	7	5

Reprinted and adapted from *Parents' Complete Guide to Youth Sports* (1989) with permission from the National Association for Sport and Physical Education (NASPE), 1900 Association Drive, Reston, VA 20191-1599.

Many children who want to participate in organized sports in high school are cut from the programs by coaches, who tend to focus their efforts on physically talented athletes. Schools should provide no-cut sports to accomodate all students who want to participate. Ideally, the sports chosen for no-cut status would be those that may lead to lifelong participation, such as cross-country and tennis.

Importance of Adult Involvement

Children benefit from the presence of adults in sports activities, particularly when the involved adults focus on teaching skills and showing children how to be good sports. All adults, especially coaches, should be considered educators, and coaches should have proper qualifications and training. Parents should provide consistent support and encouragement regardless of the child's degree of success, level of skill, or playing time. In older children and adolescents, adults should promote the connections among sports, lifelong learning, and character development, thus promoting their children's mental, social, and emotional development in addition to their physical development.

Adults typically organize games and ensure that the rules are followed. They may also teach children how to choose teams and how to keep score. With the help of adults, children feel a sense of accomplishment when they have learned something new, and they learn the fundamentals of the sport through adult involvement.

Children also benefit from participating in sports activities without adult involvement. When given an opportunity for free play without adult supervision, children learn different skills, such as negotiating and cooperating with their peers. They learn to be creative in choosing teams, and they often modify the rules to make the game more fun. One of the most common modifications is the do-over, in which a ruling is disputed and the play is performed again. Children want the score of games to be close; if a contest becomes dramatically one-sided, they may stop and choose teams again, or they may trade players to make the score closer. They may increase the size of the teams when other children arrive to allow everyone a chance to play. Children may also help one another learn new skills and may modify the rules to give children with less talent a chance to learn. For example, a younger child might get an extra strike in baseball to give him or her a better chance at hitting the ball.

Competition

Older children value competition more than their younger counterparts, but children of all ages enjoy team and individual sports. Team sports offer an opportunity for camaraderie, a chance to be with friends outside of school, and a chance to work with peers toward a common goal. Children may participate to experience competition. This can be achieved through team or individual sport participation. Children aged less than 10 years rarely appreciate competition in the same way that adolescents and adults do. Younger children enjoy participating in sports for fun and to show off their new skills, not to win. When sports and games are set up, they should be designed for the children, not the involved adults, and they should be age-appropriate.

A good example of controlled competition that includes younger children is the Special Olympics program, where the emphasis is on individual effort and the ability to finish a competition. The Special Olympics views everyone who participates as a winner; all participants receive a medal or a ribbon. In this environment, competition results in joy and compassion because personal development and achievement are emphasized. Individuals are judged on their own improvement. This kind of environment should be modeled by adults who manage sports programs for able-bodied and able-minded children. When implemented properly, this type of controlled competition increases the psychosocial benefit of many youth sports.

Other Benefits

Sports participation allows children to experiment with their own physical skills and to experience personal growth, success, and failure in an arena outside school and family. The consequences of successes and failures in sports are often much less significant than in real-life endeavors. For example, failing to learn the rules of a sport carries a lower risk than failing to learn the rules of the road for a young bicyclist, where the results may be catastrophic.

Sports participation offers many other benefits for children as they enter early adolescence and high school. Children can learn the importance of setting goals and making plans to achieve those goals, while also learning how to handle success with grace and failure with dignity. Sports participation also provides an environment where youth can learn core values such as discipline, respect, responsibility, fairness, and trustworthiness. In addition to learning physical skills, youth can learn about teamwork, relationships, and leadership.

Habitual physical activity, such as adolescents' experience in most organized sports, is positively correlated with academic performance. Studies have also shown that school dropout rates, misconduct, anxiety and stress, teen pregnancy rates, and involvement in risky behaviors such as smoking and substance use are reduced in adolescents who participate in sports. Organized basketball programs have reduced unlawful behavior by inner-city boys. With these known benefits, it may be even more important to keep children involved in sports during adolescence.

PHYSICAL BENEFITS

Sports participation helps develop a child's motor skills. Studies have suggested that certain motor skills will not develop well unless they are performed during the appropriate time in childhood. For example, a child may have trouble hitting a ball with a bat if he or she is not encouraged to do so early in the school-age years. If hand-eye coordination is not developed at the right time, the child may struggle to master this skill as an adolescent. Critical periods for learning particular skills are part of normal brain development—the younger the child, the more plastic the brain is at acquiring new skills. However, the importance of a critical learning period in neurologic development does not apply to all motor skills, but only to the most complex motor skills.

Certain skills should not be taught before a child is developmentally ready. Parents must be cautioned that children who are pushed to do too much, too soon, may become frustrated, which may lower their self-esteem. For example, the ability to track the velocity of a ball is rarely developed before age 8, so T-ball is a good way for a 6-year-old child to learn to hit a ball with a bat. Asking a 5-year-old child to hit a thrown ball will not accelerate his or her development and does not offer any long-term advantage to the young athlete.

Physical Growth and Maturation

Many studies have shown that physical activity is important in promoting the growth and development of children. It is difficult to separate the genetic determinants of growth and maturation, but researchers agree that in the presence of good nutrition, exercise is good for growing children. Physical activity cannot alter genetically programmed growth and maturation processes, but the activity helps children develop to their full genetic potential. Studies of school-age children have shown that participants in organized sports had greater total daily energy expenditure than those who did not participate. Sports participation that includes physical activity improves the body composition of young athletes. The most active children are thinner and weigh less than their less-active counterparts. This increase in lean body mass is an important physical characteristic that can be altered by exercise in children, especially if they are overweight. Children who are more active will also improve bone mass.

Training Effects and Fitness

Despite the great interest in determining whether aerobic or anaerobic power is increased in children through training and sports participation, there seems to be too little training effect to give a child a sense of mastery. However, adolescents can achieve significant improvement, which may help motivate them to continue training. Chapter 6 provides detailed information on the effects of training on a child's body.

Despite the long-standing belief that strength training is not beneficial to young athletes and is risky, studies have shown a benefit. Although few young children will enroll in a strength program for the sheer joy of lifting weights, if the program focuses on sport-specific tasks, they may experience improved sports performance as a result. This benefit is most relevant to children who participate in sports that involve power. Weight training is also an excellent form of physical activity for overweight children because they are often stronger than their leaner counterparts, so it provides an environment in which they can experience success and improve self-esteem (see Chapter 7, "Strength Training").

HEALTH-RELATED BENEFITS

The most important benefit of sports participation is the opportunity to teach children of all ages that physical activity is an important part of everyday life. Cardiovascular fitness is the key to preventing or reducing coronary artery disease, hypertension, obesity, and non–insulin-dependent diabetes mellitus. Even less frequent and intense physical activity has been shown to benefit health, including reducing the risk of or managing chronic disease in adulthood and maintaining a healthy body weight. The greatest reduction in the relative risk of all-cause mortality in adults occurs between the lowest level of fitness and the next lowest level. Although the effects of exercise on cardiovascular risk factors in children have not been studied extensively, mounting evidence indicates that increased physical activity in youth improves insulin sensitivity, blood lipid profile, blood pressure, and blood vessel function. More recent studies on all-cause mortality in adults strongly indicate that any physical activity is better than none at all.

Experts agree that exercise-related behaviors and attitudes begin to form early in childhood, when patterns are established that may persist through life. Because habitual exercise begins in childhood, it is imperative to engage children in sports and other physical activities so that they are more likely to be active as adults. Most children prefer to perform physical activities with other people, preferably people their age. Some children will be motivated to exercise if given the opportunity to do so with family members, including their parents. Most sports activities

are good for children because sports motivate them to be physically active. Children and adolescents who are exposed to and encouraged to continue participation in lifelong sports and physical activities will reap the health benefits, now and later in life.

SUMMARY POINTS

- Many of the benefits of sports participation in children and adolescents are psychosocial; children gain increased self-confidence and self-esteem as they master new skills and improve their bodies with increased aerobic capacity and strength.
- Children participate in a specific activity because they like the activity, and they will continue if they have more positive than negative experiences.
- If young athletes continue to participate in sports, they may develop regular exercise habits that stay with them over their lifetime, which will help prevent adult diseases associated with inactivity.
- Children should be asked to perform skills that are developmentally appropriate.
- Schools should be encouraged to create no-cut sports to encourage the participation of students of all abilities.

SUGGESTED READING

2008 Physical Activity Guidelines for Americans. http://www. health.gov/PAGuidelines.

Blair SN, Kohl HW III, Paffenbarger RS Jr, Clark DG, Cooper KH, Gibbons LW. Physical fitness and all-cause mortality: a prospective study of healthy men and women. *JAMA.* 1989;262:2395-2401.

Coakley JJ, ed. *Sports in Society: Issues and Controversies.* 8th ed. Minneapolis, MN: McGraw-Hill; 2004.

Sirard JR, Pfeiffer KA, Pate RR. Motivational factors associated with sports participation in middle school students. *J Adolesc Health.* 2006;38:696-703.

Smith RE, Smoll FL, Smith NJ, eds. *Parents' Complete Guide to Youth Sports.* Costa Mesa, CA: HDL Publishing; 1989.

CHAPTER 2

Readiness to Participate in Sports

Sally S. Harris, MD, MPH

A child's readiness to participate in organized sports or structured training sessions depends on a combination of factors, including neurodevelopmental level (acquisition of motor skills), social development (interaction with coaches and teammates), and cognitive level (ability to understand instructions). Optimal care of young athletes requires health care providers to understand that child athletes are not small adults. They have distinct physiologic, psychological, and developmental responses and needs that affect sports training and participation. Sports activities that require skills beyond the developmental level of the participants are likely to be frustrating to the child. The structure of organized sports may not permit the flexibility of permitting children to play at their own developmental level. Health care providers need to recognize the developmental appropriateness of an individual child's participation in sports so they can advocate appropriate sports activities and appropriately advise parents, coaches, and community sports programs.

THE ROLE OF PHYSICAL AND COGNITIVE GROWTH

The dramatic changes of physical growth are apparent during childhood, but children also develop in other, less obvious ways that have important implications for appropriate sports activities. Children should not be expected to respond to coaching, interact with teammates, or understand strategies in the same way that adults do.

One example of the developmental limitations of children in sports is described by the term *beehive soccer.* This term describes the way children aged 5 and 6 years play soccer. The children follow the ball like a swarm of bees. They do not

necessarily head toward the goal. Coaches and parents often shout directions about players' field positions and the execution of plays, but the children fail to follow the adults' instructions because they lack the social and cognitive skills required for competition, teamwork, rapid decision making, and appropriate positioning. Children at this age do not really understand the fine points of the game. Instead, they rely on physical skills and the ability to imitate. Individuals who coach children at this level should accept the chaos and emphasize learning basic skills, rather than attempting to get the children to play at a level that they are cognitively and socially incapable of understanding. Coaching that attempts to avoid beehive soccer may result in decreased interest and boredom, and it can undermine the spontaneous action and personal involvement that makes the experience fun for children.

MOTOR DEVELOPMENT

Because sports readiness requires that motor development match the demands of the sport, it is important to understand how children acquire motor skills. The fundamental skills include throwing, kicking, running, jumping, catching, striking, hopping, and skipping. By preschool age, children have acquired some of these skills, but it is not until early elementary school age that most children have acquired most of them. For instance, only about 20% to 30% of children aged 4 years are proficient at throwing and catching. Therefore, age 6 years is thought to be appropriate for most children to begin organized sports activities that require performing these fundamental skills in various combinations. Before age 6 years, most children do not have the necessary fundamental motor skills to perform the actions required for organized sports.

Sequence of Development

Like the developmental milestones of infancy, such as rolling over, sitting up, crawling, and walking, the fundamental motor skills required for organized sports develop in a certain sequence. At its most basic level, acquisition of motor skills seems to be an innate process, independent of sex, disability, or stage of physical maturity. Like other childhood developmental milestones, the rate at which children master motor skills varies widely. It cannot be predicted by the age, size, weight, or strength of an individual child. Although it may be possible to accelerate the acquisition and refinement of fundamental motor skills by early instruction and practice, children are unlikely to respond until they are ready developmentally. Children will respond to instruction and repetitive practice only after they reach the relevant level of motor development. No scientific evidence supports the notion that it is possible to groom a toddler to become a future champion athlete by intensive instruction and practice at a young age. Such experiences have not been shown to accelerate motor development or lead to better sports performance later on.

Although most children acquire the fundamental motor skills at a basic level naturally through play, instruction and practice are necessary to fully develop fundamental motor skills to their most mature level. Each fundamental skill is composed of a series of stages of development of that skill. The sequence for developing the motor skill of kicking is listed in **Table 2.1**. A child who fails to progress through all the stages may not be as proficient in sports activities as one who has fully developed motor skills. Inefficient throwing is a common example of failure to progress to the fully developed stage of throwing, and it can limit a child's proficiency in a variety of physical activities that require throwing or serving motions.

Poor Motor Development

Some children have difficulty achieving the expected level of motor development, and they are often considered clumsy or uncoordinated. Usually the cause is a temporary delay in motor skill development, the result of slow progression through the stages of motor skill development. These children will ultimately catch up to their peers, and they will experience no long-term disadvantage. Infrequently, poor motor skills may be due to an underlying physical or neurologic abnormality. In some children, poor motor skill development is caused by developmental coordination disorder, a learning disability that affects motor skill development. Children with this disorder often have problems learning both gross and fine

TABLE 2.1
Developmental Sequence of Kicking

Stage	Description
1	With no leg windup, the child pushes the ball with his or her foot from a stationary position. He or she usually steps back afterward to regain balance. Most boys and girls reach this stage at about age 2 years.
2	The child again begins from a stationary position, but in preparing to kick, there is both leg windup to the rear and some opposition of the arms and legs. Balance is recovered by stepping backward or to the side. Most boys reach this stage by age 3½; most girls reach it by age 4.
3	The child takes a step or two to approach the ball. The kicking foot stays close to the ground until the moment of contact. After the kick, the child steps forward or to the side to regain balance. Most boys achieve this stage by age 4½, compared with age 6 for most girls.
4	The child approaches the ball with several rapid steps, leaps before the kick, and usually hops on the support leg afterward. The body generally inclines backward during the windup. Most boys reach this stage by age 7, most girls by age 8.

Copyright 1992 by the New York Times Co. Reprinted with permission.

motor skills. They are most often identified because they have difficulty with fine motor skills, such as handwriting and tying their shoes. Interventions such as appropriate selection of physical activities and physical therapy help these children; however, evidence suggests that children with this disorder do not simply outgrow the problem. Children with poor motor skills will have the best experiences in activities that do not require complex motor skills, such as walking, cycling, and swimming; in individual rather than team sports; in noncompetitive physical activities; and in participating with younger children whose skills may be equivalent.

PREDICTING SPORTS READINESS

At what age is a child ready to begin participation in a specific activity? Although this is a commonly asked question, there is no answer from a neurodevelopmental standpoint. If sports readiness cannot be predicted on the basis of age or other specific parameters, how is a child's readiness to learn certain skills or participate in certain sports activities determined? The best answer is that sports activities should match, or should be modified to match, the developmental capabilities of the individual child. Sports activities that require skills beyond the developmental level of the participants are unlikely to be successful. When given the opportunity, children naturally select and modify activities so that they can participate successfully and have fun. Therefore, modification of equipment and rules should be made to suit the developmental level of the participants. Examples of such modifications might include smaller balls, smaller fields, shorter games and practices, fewer participants playing at the same time, frequent changing of positions, and less emphasis on keeping score. One such adaptation is the game of T-ball, in which children hit a stationary baseball mounted on a stand rather than a pitched ball, which would require the child to possess more advanced visual tracking skills.

Selection of appropriate sports activities for children can be guided by an understanding of the developmental skills and limitations of specific age groups. This information is summarized in **Table 2.2**.

Early Childhood (2 to 5 Years)

Attempts to master the basic fundamental skills are the focus of children's sports activities. Balance is poor because the children are just starting to integrate visual, vestibular, and proprioceptive cues. Children younger than age 6 or 7 years are farsighted. Imprecise eye movements limit their ability to track and judge the speed of moving objects. Fundamental motor skills can be improved through active play and do not require organized sports activities. Toddlers who participate in organized sports programs do not gain any long-term advantage for future sports performance. For instance, toddlers who have practiced throwing a ball are no better at throwing than their peers when they reach school age. Appropriate sports activities emphasize fundamental skills such as running, swimming, tumbling, throwing, and catching. Children at this age have short attention spans and learn best by exploration, experimentation, and mimicking others. Accordingly, instruction should be limited, follow a show-and-tell format, and be followed by play time. Competition should be avoided, and parental involvement should be encouraged for role modeling.

Middle Childhood (6 to 9 Years)

At this age, children begin to master transitional skills, which are fundamental skills that are performed in various combinations and with variations, such as throwing for distance or accuracy. These skills are required for participation in organized sports activities. Rapid improvement in running occurs in this age group. Vision is almost mature, but children in this age group still have difficulty determining the direction in which a moving object is traveling. Sports that can be adapted to be played at a basic level and that emphasize fundamental motor skills with few variables are the most appropriate; such sports include running, swimming, soccer, baseball, tennis, gymnastics, martial arts, and skiing. Sports that require complex visual and motor skills, rapid decision making, or detailed strategies or teamwork (football, basketball, hockey, volleyball) will be difficult unless greatly modified. Rules should be flexible and should promote success, action, and participation.

Late Childhood (10 to 12 Years)

Children at this age have the cognitive ability to understand and remember strategies for sports such as football and basketball. Their vision is fully mature. They are generally ready to participate in most sports activities that require more complex motor and cognitive skills. Coaches can begin to incorporate instruction on tactics and strategy. However, most experts believe that skill development, fun, and participation should take priority over competition.

Some children in this age group may be entering their pubertal growth spurt, during which there may be a temporary decline in coordination and balance may temporarily worsen. A child's resulting inability to perform a skill as effectively as in the previous sports season can be a frustrating experience if it is misinterpreted as a lack of talent or effort.

During the pubertal growth spurt, the physical differences between children, particularly boys of the same age, can be dramatic and often have implications for choice of appropriate sports activities. Boys who begin their pubertal growth spurt ahead of other boys their age will be temporarily taller, heavier, and stronger. However, this should not be equated with superior ability or talent. Success due to advanced physical maturity can lead to unrealistic expectations that these boys will continue to be outstanding athletes. Attempts should be made for these boys to participate and compete with boys at a similar state of maturation. Similarly, boys who mature later may experience a temporary physical disadvantage in sports that should not be misinterpreted as a lack of talent or ability. These boys should be encouraged to participate initially in sports that place less emphasis on physical size, such as racquet sports, soccer, martial arts, wrestling, and certain track events.

THE BEST SPORTS

Although parents often ask what sports or physical activities are best for their child, there is no best physical activity. Any physical activity that the child enjoys and that is safe and developmentally appropriate will be

TABLE 2.2

Developmental Skills for Sports and Sports Recommendations during Childhood

EARLY CHILDHOOD (AGES 2 TO 5 YEARS)

Motor skills	Limited fundamental skills
	Limited balance skills
Learning	Extremely short attention span
	Poor selective attention
	Egocentric learning: Trial and error
	Visual and auditory cues are important
Vision	Not fully mature; before ages 6 to 7 years (farsighted)
	Difficulty tracking and judging velocity of moving objects
Sports recommendations	Emphasize fundamental skills with minimal variation and limited instruction
	Emphasize fun, playfulness, exploration, and experimentation rather than competition
	Activities: Running, swimming, tumbling, throwing, catching

MIDDLE CHILDHOOD (AGES 6 TO 9 YEARS)

Motor skills	Continued improvement in fundamental skills
	Posture and balance become more automatic
	Improved reaction times
	Beginning transitional skills
Learning	Short attention span
	Limited development of memory and rapid decision making
Vision	Improved tracking
	Limited directionality
Sports recommendations	Emphasize fundamental skills and beginning transitional skills
	Flexible rules of sports
	Allow free time in practices
	Short instruction time
	Minimal competition
	Activities: running, swimming, skiing, entry-level soccer, baseball, tennis, gymnastics, martial arts

LATE CHILDHOOD (AGES 10 TO 12 YEARS)

Motor skills	Improved transitional skills
	Ability to master complex motor skills
	Temporary decline in balance control at puberty
Learning	Selective attention
	Able to use memory strategies for sports such as football and basketball
Vision	Adult patterns
Sports recommendations	Emphasis on skill development
	Increasing emphasis on tactics and strategy
	Emphasize factors promoting continued participation
	Activities: entry level for complex skill sports (football, basketball, hockey, volleyball)

Adapted from Nelson MA: Developmental skills and children's sports. *Physican Sportsmed* 1991; 19:67-79, with permission from Vendome Group.

beneficial. The most important goal is to encourage participation and enjoyment in physical activities in general. Physical activities that are sustainable over a lifetime are ideal, such as walking, hiking, cyling, rollerblading, dancing, and swimming.

COED SPORTS PARTICIPATION

Sex-based differences in aerobic capacity and muscle strength become apparent at puberty, as a result of the increase in muscle mass in boys and the increase in body fat in girls. Before puberty, there are no appreciable differences between boys and girls in endurance, strength, height, or body mass, so coeducational participation does not place girls at a physical disadvantage or at increased risk of injury. However, some girls may prefer not to play on coed teams with boys, who tend to be more physically aggressive than girls at young ages. After puberty, most girls are unlikely to compete on an equal basis from a physical standpoint with boys their age and may be at increased risk of injury as a result of discrepancy in strength and size.

CONTACT SPORTS

Should young children (for example, aged 9 years) participate in contact sports such as football? When parents ask this question, their main concern is risk of injury. They can be reassured that young children actually have a lower risk of injury in contact sports such as football than older children because they do not have the size and strength to generate forces great enough to cause serious injury. In addition, the marked physical mismatch that could put a smaller child at increased risk of injury does not occur until puberty. A more relevant concern is whether the physical contact and associated aggressiveness and competition is developmentally appropriate, and whether it enhances the value of the experience at this age. The child's enjoyment and eagerness to participate are some of the best indicators of the appropriateness of the activity.

There may be dramatic physical differences between individuals of the same sex, particularly boys, because children enter puberty across a wide age spectrum. For this reason, adolescents' participation in contact sports should be matched on the basis of size and maturational stage, not necessarily on the basis of chronologic age alone. Skeletally immature athletes should be counseled about the potential risks of injury from competing in contact sports against athletes who are physically more mature.

ORGANIZED COMPETITIVE SPORTS

When considering organized or community sports programs, parents should look for programs that encourage participation for everyone and that emphasize age-appropriate skill development rather than competition and winning. They should ensure that appropriate safety issues are addressed, and that the coaching and structure are appropriate for the child's age. The participating children's levels of enjoyment and fun are the best indicators of a good program.

Motivational factors for children's participation in sports include fun, success, skill development, variety, freedom, participation with family or friends, and enthusiastic leadership. Conversely, failure, embarrassment, competition, boredom, and regimentation discourage participation. In general, children are much more interested in personal involvement and action than in winning and scores. Most children would rather play more on a losing team than less on a winning team. Emphasis on winning should be downplayed, and children should not be placed in a competitive win-lose situation until they understand that their self-worth is not based on the outcome of the activity. Attrition in children's sports occurs largely because of lack of playing time, feelings of failure, and overemphasis on competition. Sports programs for children should be designed with these factors in mind in order to promote long-term involvement.

When given the opportunity, children naturally select and modify activities so that they can participate successfully and have fun. However, the structure of organized sports often impedes the ability of children to play at their own developmental level. It is estimated that by age 15, 75% of children who had been involved in organized sports have dropped out. This suggests that many youth sports programs are organized in ways that do not promote the interests of the children, but rather those of the adults involved. Game structures and adults' expectations for performance should be revised to match the interests and developmental capabilities of the children so that positive sports experiences during childhood provide a basis for lifelong involvement. The key principles governing appropriate sports activities for children are summarized in **Table 2.3.**

SPORTS SPECIALIZATION AND INTENSIVE TRAINING

At what age is it appropriate for a child to specialize in a single sport, train year round, or participate in programs that require daily practices, or many hours of participation per week?

TABLE 2.3

Bill of Rights of Young Athletes

- The right to participate in sports
- The right to participate at a level commensurate with each child's developmental level
- The right to have qualified adult leadership
- The right to participate in safe and healthy environments
- The right to share in the leadership and decision making of their sports participation
- The right to play as a child and not as an adult
- The right to proper preparation for participation in sports
- The right for equal opportunity to strive for success
- The right to be treated with dignity
- The right to have fun in sports

Reprinted from *Guidelines in Children's Sports* (1979) with permission from the National Association for Sport and Physical Education (NASPE), 1990 Association Driver, Reston, VA 20191-1599.

Most parents' main concern about such programs is the risk of injury. Intuitively, it would seem that young children, whose bodies are not fully developed and who are smaller, lighter, and weaker than older children, would be more vulnerable to injuries. However, the opposite is true. Injury rates are lowest for younger children and increase as children get older, particularly during adolescence. Younger children are less prone to injuries from overtraining because they lack the body size, strength, and speed to generate forces great enough to lead to severe injury. In addition, the immature musculoskeletal system of young children is generally more flexible and resilient than that of older children, making serious injuries such as ligament tears, cartilage damage, and broken bones less likely to occur—and less severe when they do occur. Injury risk from overtraining increases dramatically at puberty as a result of musculoskeletal changes associated with the adolescent growth spurt.

From a practical standpoint, intensive training of children has a low yield. Before puberty, the gains in strength and endurance that are the result of training are relatively small and unlikely to confer any significant performance advantages. Children are more likely to improve sports performance by practicing and perfecting the skills of the sport itself, rather than from additional strength and endurance training.

Early specialization in a single sport, intensive training, and year-round training should be undertaken cautiously because they may result in an increased risk of psychological stress and burnout. Specialization in a single sport may preclude development of a variety of motor skills obtained from participation in several different sports. Parents should evaluate the reasons for increased involvement against the potential risks and benefits for their child. An important concern is whether the sport requires too much time at the expense of time available for other experiences that comprise a well-rounded lifestyle, such a school, friends, family, and unstructured time. Readiness for more intensive participation is best determined by the child's skill development, physical and emotional maturity, and self-motivation, not by being in a particular age category. If the coaching is appropriate for the child's age, if the emphasis is on fun and skill development, and, most importantly, if the child enjoys the experience, then it may be fine to participate at a higher level.

SUMMARY POINTS

- Children should participate in physical activities that are fun, developmentally appropriate, and sustainable over a lifetime.

- Children should participate in activities that promote physical fitness and the acquisition of sports skills.

- To encourage long-term participation, sports programs for children should emphasize personal involvement, variety, success, and fun rather than competition, regimentation, and winning.

- Modification of equipment and rules should be made to suit the developmental level of the participants.

- Safety should be a priority with regard to appropriate setting, equipment, protective gear, program design, and rules of play.

- Before puberty, there are no appreciable differences between boys and girls in endurance, strength, height, or body mass, and boys and girls can compete equally together.

- For optimal physical matching of adolescents in contact sports, chronologic age, body size, and maturational stage should all be considered.

- Early specialization in a single sport, intensive training, and year-round training should be undertaken cautiously to avoid overuse injury, psychological stress, and burnout.

- Children should not be placed in a competitive win-lose situation until they understand that their self-worth is not based on the outcome of the activity.

- Levels of enjoyment and fun experienced by participating children are the best indicators of a good sports program.

SUGGESTED READING

American Academy of Pediatrics, Committee on Sports Medicine and Fitness. Intensive training and sports specialization in young athletes. *Pediatrics.* 2000;106:154-157.

American Academy of Pediatrics, Committee on Sports Medicine and Fitness. Organized sports for children and preadolescents. *Pediatrics.* 2001;107:1459-1462.

American Academy of Pediatrics, Committee on Sports Medicine and Fitness. Overuse injuries, overtraining, and burnout in child and adolescent athletes. *Pediatrics.* 2007; 119:1242–1245.

Bale P. The functional performance of children in relation to growth, maturation, and exercise. *Sports Med.* 1992;13:151-159.

Branta C, Haubenstricker J, Seefeldt V. Age changes in motor skills during childhood and adolescence. *Exerc Sport Sci Rev.* 1984;12:467-520.

Gould D. Understanding attrition in children's sport. In: Gould D, Weiss MR, eds. *Advances in Pediatric Sport Sciences.* Champaign, IL: Human Kinetics; 1987;2:61-86.

Harris SS. Developmental and maturational issues. In: Puffer JC, ed. *Twenty Common Problems in Sports Medicine.* New York: McGraw-Hill; 2000:337-352.

Nelson MA. Developmental skills and children's sports. *Phys Sportsmed.* 1991;19:67-79.

Seefeldt V, Haubenstricker J. Patterns, phases, or stages: an analytical model for the study of developmental movement. In: Kelso JAS, Clark JE, eds. *The Development of Movement Control and Coordination.* Chichester, NY: John Wiley; 1982:309-318.

Willoughby C, Polatajko HJ. Motor problems in children with developmental coordination disorder: review of the literature. *Am J Occup Ther.* 1995;49:787-794.

CHAPTER 3

Growth and Maturation

Jorge E. Gómez, MS, MD

Questions about sports preparedness, training capabilities, and skill development are all directly related to age-specific changes in the neuromotor, cardiovascular, and cognitive-integrative systems. To best answer these questions, the physician must understand the normal development of these systems as they relate to sports participation.

INFANCY (BIRTH TO 2 YEARS)

Many parents are concerned about whether real or perceived aberrancies in neuromotor or musculoskeletal development during their child's first year of life will have bearing on later sports competencies.

An infant's natural curiosity and drive to attain self-sufficiency provide the impetus for trying increasingly complex patterns of movement. Attainment of gross and fine motor milestones in infancy follows a predictable pattern. The mean age at which infants begin to walk independently is about 13 months (range, 9–17 months). Late walking is probably not related to neuromotor retardation, but it may be the result of an inherited dependent behavioral style or lack of parental emphasis on gross motor skills. Conversely, genetics may explain why African American, Mexican, East Indian, and Middle Eastern infants achieve gross motor milestones earlier than white North American infants. Cultural customs of infant swaddling or carrying, which limit movement, do not seem to affect the age at which the child learns to walk.

Encouragement and training of motor skills at this age in an attempt to produce early development—for example, the use of infant walkers—appears to have no effect on the age of walking, or may even delay it. Walking at an early age has not been shown to predict earlier achievement of complex sports-related skills. Similarly, the arm and leg movements demonstrated by infants who are placed in water are purely reflexive and do not predict swimming aptitude.

EARLY CHILDHOOD (2 TO 5 YEARS)

Physical Changes

The preschool years are most notable for a dramatic change in body composition and an improvement in gait and specific motor skills. Both fat mass and fat-free mass gradually increase with body size between ages 2 and 6 years. The percentage of fat, however, declines between the ages of 3 and 6 years, more so for boys than for girls, coinciding with decreased caloric intake and increased energy expenditure.

Between ages 2 and 3 years, the child's normal bow legs will slowly evolve into a nearly straight quadriceps angle on the way to a maximum average valgus angle of 12° by approximately age 3 years (**Figure 3.1**). Persistence or worsening of the bow legs beyond age 2 warrants investigation for pathologic causes, such as epiphyseal dysplasia (eg, Blount disease) (**Figure 3.2**).

Development of Walking Skills and Handedness

Increases in limb and stride length between ages 2 and 4 years parallel the refinement in walking skill. As walking proficiency develops, the base of support is narrowed, and arm movements become more synchronous with the stride. By age 4, most children achieve an adult walking pattern. The arms can now be used for increasingly complex tasks. Handedness is usually established by about age 2 years, but it is often not firmly established until ages 3 or 4. Handedness is largely predetermined, and right- or left-handedness does not affect success.

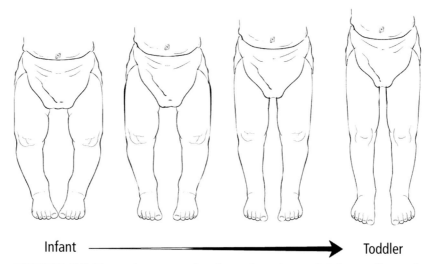

Infant ──────────────────────────────▶ Toddler

FIGURE 3.1 Normal progression from bow legs of infancy through slow evolution to a physiologic valgus angle of about 12° at age 3 (toddlers).

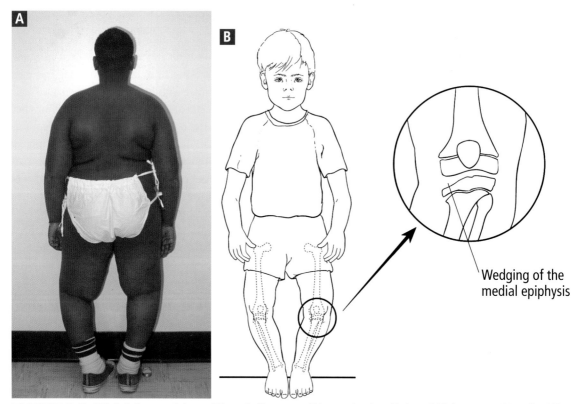

Wedging of the medial epiphysis

FIGURE 3.2 (A) Adolescent-type Blount disease with marked unilateral tibia vara. (B) Infantile-type Blount disease, which is often bilateral. Radiographs may show wedging of the medial epiphysis and a beaking of the proximal metaphysis.

Gender Differences

Gross motor development during the preschool years is fairly uniform in boys and girls, but there are some differences in development of sport-specific skills. The age at which 60% of boys achieve a mature running pattern is about 4 years, 2 months, whereas for girls it is about 5 years. Most boys achieve a mature throwing pattern by age 6 years, whereas girls this age still tend to throw with the feet fixed and with little trunk rotation. Jumping and catching develop at the same rate in boys and girls. Girls tend to be proficient in skipping and hopping earlier than boys, and by age 6 years, kicking and striking are more advanced in boys.

Skill Development

New skills are learned by application of fundamental movements to new situations. The freedom to try new things, move, and explore is essential for motor development. Observation of toddler play reveals the fundamental conflict of dependence versus independence when the child is exploring. The child moves away from the parent, tries something new, returns to the parent for approval and reassurance, and repeats the cycle. For this cycle to lead to successful motor learning, the parent must be willing to both reassure the child and give up control. Excessive parental guidance and monitoring squelch the child's sense of self-discovery, making learning or mastering new skills boring and unrewarding. Criticism or ridicule over mistakes in the performance of motor skills deters future willing participation in these skills.

Growing Pains

The leg aches referred to as growing pains are most common during this period. The cause of this condition is unknown. Although children diagnosed with growing pains should fulfill the criteria in **Table 3.1**, growing pains remain a diagnosis of exclusion. Children often find massage comforting, and parents often administer acetaminophen or ibuprofen, which may or may not help. Passive stretching of the quadriceps, hamstrings, and calves at bedtime may benefit some children. Health care providers should reassure parents about the benign and self-limited nature of this condition.

MIDDLE TO LATE CHILDHOOD (6 TO 12 YEARS)

Physical Changes

Growth is fairly steady during the elementary school years. Toward the end of this period, it is common for girls to become temporarily taller and heavier than boys of the same age because of the earlier onset of puberty. Percentage of fat mass actually declines or remains steady, with girls always having a slightly higher percentage. Flexibility may increase. The incidence of generalized joint hypermobility, defined as the ability to extend the hands and thumbs parallel to the forearm, hyperextension of the knees and elbows, and the ability to touch the palms to the floor, is highest in school-age children (5%–7%). Children with hypermobility often complain of musculoskeletal pain and may be at increased risk of glenohumeral and patellar subluxation or dislocation, but the risk of most other injuries is not increased.

Strength and Speed

Grip, arm, shoulder, and quadriceps strength begins to diverge in boys and girls between ages 6 to 12 years, but these differences are small compared with those seen in adolescence. Performance on tasks that depend on explosive power, such as the vertical jump, long jump, and throw for distance, also diverges slowly, with boys always having a slight edge. Running speed is nearly equal between boys and girls between ages 9 and 11 years, and girls tend to have better balance than boys of the same age. Although children at this age tend to have playmates of the same sex, boys and girls are able to compete together on an equal level.

Motor Skills

Most children achieve mature patterns of fundamental motor skills during elementary school. Most girls achieve a mature throwing technique by age 8 years; 60% of children achieve mature kicking and striking patterns at about age 7 for boys and age 8 for girls. Mature hopping and catching patterns are achieved between ages 7 and 8 years for most boys and girls.

TABLE 3.1
Diagnostic Criteria for Growing Pains

- Pain does not occur with activity.
- Pain usually occurs at night.
- Pain is localized to the thighs, knees, or calves.
- Pain is usually relieved with massage and over-the-counter analgesics.
- Child is active during the day.
- Review of systems indicates that the pains are completely benign.
- Physical examination reveals nothing abnormal.

Aerobic and Anaerobic Capacities

Capacities for aerobic and anaerobic exercise slowly increase during middle childhood but are limited compared with adolescent capacities. This limitation probably has little impact on play and sports activities because most play during early and middle childhood is at submaximal cardiorespiratory function. Analysis of movement patterns during free play of young children indicates that they are active in short bursts, with 95% of the high-intensity bursts lasting less than 15 seconds. Most of their activities, however, are in the low- to moderate-intensity range. Children at this age are physiologically more suited for activities that are intermittent in nature. They usually prefer activities of low to moderate intensity, with occasional bursts of high-intensity activity.

It was once thought that children were "metabolic nonspecialists," the idea being that a child who was more anaerobically gifted (say, a sprinter) could more easily become a highly developed aerobic athlete (a distance runner) with training than could an adult. However, on the basis of limited data, this does not appear to be the case. Although children's fitness test scores for aerobic and anaerobic tasks tend to correlate strongly with each other, top performance in strength, endurance, and short-burst activities tends to track into adulthood, with no greater capacity to cross over during childhood than later, reflecting the fact that the ratios of fast-twitch to slow-twitch fibers do not change from childhood to adulthood.

Skill Development

Mastering new skills becomes more significant during middle childhood, when success and mastery become closely linked with the child's sense of self-worth. The drive to achieve self-efficacy and to acquire social acceptance explains why children at this age are able to immerse themselves in academic, artistic, and athletic activities with great energy and for prolonged periods. Sports and dance may provide opportunities for mastery of neuromotor skills and for social recognition and interaction, which build self-efficacy.

The child of elementary school age generally has an internal locus of control for performing feats of physical exertion; children at this age rarely push themselves physically beyond the limits of comfort. Maximal effort usually occurs as a result of intense urging by authority figures. This is in contrast with adolescents, who often push themselves physically beyond the limits of comfort to fulfill personal goals, without prodding from adults.

There appear to be critical periods between ages 10 to 12 years and early adolescence during which acquisition of some specific skills is easiest and after which acquisition of those skills to the same degree is either extremely difficult or impossible. Such skills include hitting a baseball or tennis ball and shooting a basketball. However, the precise ages at which this window occurs and the time frame of such a window has not been studied. Therefore, active time for the school-age child should emphasize learning and refining sport-specific skills.

Developmental Coordination Disorder

During the early elementary school years, children with developmental coordination disorder may exhibit failure or delay in developing normal skills such as skipping, jumping, or ball handling (**Table 3.2**). The diagnosis is difficult to make and should include a differential diagnosis that includes neurological problems, mental retardation, autism, and attention-deficit/hyperactivity disorder. Early recognition followed by appropriate therapy may enable these children to engage in age-appropriate sporting activities.

EARLY ADOLESCENCE (13 TO 15 YEARS)

Physical Changes

The increases in muscle mass, muscle strength, and cardiopulmonary endurance that occur during puberty are greater than those that occur at any other age. Both fat mass and fat-free mass continue to increase in both boys and girls during early and midadolescence. With the onset of puberty, girls tend to accumulate fat mass faster than boys. By the end of high school,

---

TABLE 3.2

Diagnostic Criteria for Developmental Coordination Disorder

- Performance in daily activities that require motor coordination is substantially below that expected given the person's chronologic age and measured intelligence, as evidenced by motor delay, clumsiness, poor performance in sports, or poor handwriting.
- The disturbance significantly interferes with academic or athletic achievement or activities of daily living.
- The disturbance is not due to another medical condition (eg, cerebral palsy, hemiplegia, muscular dystrophy).
- If mental retardation is present, the motor difficulties exceed those usually associated with it.

most girls have nearly twice the percentage of body fat as boys.

Muscle strength accelerates dramatically in boys during puberty. Girls continue to increase their muscle strength during this time, but the increase is more gradual. These differences in muscle strength gains are reflected in differences in performance of tasks requiring muscle power, defined as the product of strength and velocity of contraction. During puberty, boys have a sharp increase in the performance of vertical or horizontal jumping, throwing, and sprinting, whereas girls show gradual improvement or reach a plateau in their performance of these skills.

Increased tightness of the hamstrings and ankle dorsiflexors occurs during puberty and is greatest during the height spurt that occurs around age 12 in girls and age 14 in boys. Dancers and gymnasts may be most sensitive to the loss of flexibility associated with the height spurt. Hamstring tightness may contribute to increased stress at the patellofemoral joint, leading to patellofemoral pain, which becomes increasingly common during this age.

Maturational Differences

Differences in physical performance early in adolescence are more strongly influenced by the age at onset of puberty than by chronologic age. Boys who mature early tend to be taller; to have greater muscle mass and fat mass; and to have better arm, grip, and explosive strength (jumping and sprinting) than boys who mature later. Girls who mature early tend to be taller and to have greater fat mass and fat-free mass than average- or late-maturing girls but have only a modest advantage in strength. Girls who mature later perform better on tests of upper extremity strength than average-maturing girls, perhaps because of a lower ratio of fat to fat-free mass, and they generally perform better on tasks requiring balance.

Aerobic and Anaerobic Capacities

The strongest predictor of changes in aerobic capacity (maximal oxygen uptake, or $\dot{V}o_2$max) during early adolescence is stage of maturity. Increases in $\dot{V}o_2$max result from the development of pulmonary ventilation, cardiac output, muscular oxygen extraction, and oxidative metabolism, which are strongly related to physical maturity. The increase in $\dot{V}o_2$max during adolescence, in comparison with the lack of change in $\dot{V}o_2$max per kilogram of body weight, indicates that the increase in aerobic power is directly related to dimensional changes in the oxygen delivery and muscular systems. Levels of physical activity and fat correlate much less strongly with increasing aerobic power during puberty than do visceral and muscular growth. The capacity for

anaerobic (intense, short burst) exercise increases more gradually than does aerobic capacity.

Maturational Status

Questions often arise about whether early- versus late-maturing boys and girls are better suited to certain sports. Data from cross-sectional studies of pubertal athletes have generally shown that early-maturing boys tend to excel in sports that require speed and strength. Elite-level male track-and-field performers aged 10 to 15 are more mature for their age than average. Elite female track-and-field athletes have average skeletal maturity for their age, but throwers (eg, shot, discus) were more mature than average. In contrast, elite female gymnasts have later onset of menarche and narrower hips and shoulders than average girls. For most athletes, it is unlikely that the choice of sport or the intensity of training causes premature or delayed onset of puberty in either male or female athletes.

Mismatching children by maturity status during early adolescence results in an unfair competitive advantage to those who are more mature; however, there is little evidence that such mismatching increases the risk of injury to those who are less mature. The incidence of musculoskeletal injury is lower during early adolescence than during middle or late adolescence.

Pubertal Changes in Leg Alignment in Girls

During puberty, the knee in girls develops an increased quadriceps angle (Q-angle) (**Figure 3.3**). This is measured as the angle between two lines: one from the anterior superior iliac spine to the center of the patella, and the other from the center of the patella to the tibial tuberosity. The increased Q-angle during puberty results primarily from the increased valgus angle of the knee. The increased Q-angle during puberty predisposes to patellofemoral pain syndrome and lateral patellar subluxation and dislocation. There is some evidence that the increased valgus angle of the knee, and the accentuation of this valgus angle during landing from a jump, may increase the risk of anterior cruciate ligament injuries in adolescent female athletes. In addition, this malalignment of the legs predisposes girls to a variety of overuse conditions of the legs.

LATE ADOLESCENCE (16 TO 20 YEARS)

Physical Changes

Boys' strength, speed, and size continue to increase during late adolescence, although the rate of increase is not nearly as great as during puberty. Girls do not have significant

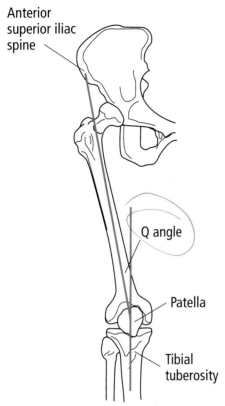

FIGURE 3.3 Q-angle of the knee.

increases in fat-free mass during late adolescence but continue to accumulate fat mass, which often has an adverse effect on performance. In general, both muscular strength and aerobic capacity continue to increase into adulthood, but the rate of increase is much more gradual than during puberty.

Maturational Status

Differences in boys' stature associated with differences in the age of onset of puberty will vanish by late adolescence. Children with familial late maturation or constitutional growth delay can be reassured that they will catch up to their peers by high school. However, some functional differences will persist. Even in late adolescence, early-maturing boys will continue to be heavier and continue to outperform average- or late-maturing boys on tests of arm strength.

Role of Continued Sports Participation

Whether an adolescent remains active into young adulthood may depend on whether athletics helps him or her deal with the developmental tasks of adolescence,

including emancipating from the family, forming a sexual identity, identifying with a peer group, developing the capacity for intimacy, and preparing for adult education and employment. Most older adolescents are not motivated to be physically active by a desire to compete on the playing field. Rather, older adolescents should be encouraged to view athletics as a means for relieving stress, maintaining vigor, and providing social interactions.

SUMMARY POINTS

- Attainment of motor milestones in childhood occurs in a largely predetermined, predictable pattern.

- Choice of sport or intensity of training is unlikely to cause either premature or delayed onset of puberty for most athletes.

- Increases in strength, muscle mass, and cardiopulmonary endurance are greatest during puberty.

- Mismatching competitors of different physical maturity levels does not appear to increase the risk of injury to the less mature athlete. However, mismatching athletes in this way does put the less mature player at a competitive disadvantage.

- Normal growth and maturation influence the timing of acquisition of an athlete's skills and influence the risk of various injuries at different ages.

SUGGESTED READING

Bailey RC, Olson J, Pepper SL, Porszasz J, Barstow TJ, Cooper DM. The level and tempo of children's physical activities: an observational study. *Med Sci Sports Exerc.* 1995;27:1033-1041.

Dixon SD, Stein MT, eds. *Encounters With Children: Pediatric Behavior and Development.* 2nd ed. St Louis, MO: Mosby Year Book; 1992.

Malina RM, Bouchard C, eds. *Growth, Maturation, and Physical Activity.* Champaign, IL: Human Kinetics; 1991.

Morrissy RT, ed. *Lovell and Winter's Pediatric Orthopaedics.* 3rd ed. Philadelphia, PA: JB Lippincott; 1990.

Noyes FR, Barber-Westin SD, Fleckenstein C, Walsh C, West J. The drop-jump screening test: difference in lower limb control by gender and effect of neuromuscular training in female athletes. *Am J Sports Med.* 2005;33: 197-207.

Polatajko HJ, Cantin N. Developmental coordination disorder (dyspraxia): an overview of the state of the art. *Semin Pediatr Neurol.* 2005;12:250-258.

Rowland TW, ed. *Developmental Exercise Physiology.* Champaign, IL: Human Kinetics; 1996.

Rowland TW. On being a metabolic non-specialist. *Pediatr Exercise Sci.* 2002;14:315-320.

CHAPTER 4

Promoting Physical Activity

Barbara J. Long, MD, MPH

Physicians and other primary care providers who work with children and adolescents have traditionally been responsible for providing a broad range of anticipatory guidance in areas such as child growth and development, accident and injury prevention, dietary counseling, and parenting issues. Because there is sufficient evidence that the processes of cardiovascular disease begin in childhood, prevention has become another important counseling area for physicians. Even though lipid screening, nutrition counseling, obesity treatment, and regular exercise are all important, it is not clear to what degree or how effectively physicians address these areas. This chapter covers issues surrounding the promotion of regular physical activity and presents an outline for a behaviorally oriented approach intended to help physicians effectively promote physical activity among youths.

DEFINING PHYSICAL ACTIVITY

Physical activity is any body movement produced by skeletal musculature that results in energy expenditure. Physical fitness is the ability to perform physical activity. Exercise is planned, structured, and repetitive body movement done to improve or maintain physical fitness. Physical fitness is a physiologic trait; physical activity is a behavior. Physical activity can occur during exercise, during the routine activities of daily living (walking, climbing stairs, performing occupational work), and during the free play of children and youths. Physicians should counsel children and their parents to promote or increase physical activity. The goal is to involve all children in a variety of activities that will enhance their current physical and psychological well-being and to promote active lifestyle choices that will continue into adulthood.

EPIDEMIOLOGY OF PHYSICAL ACTIVITY

Two large US population-based studies, the National Children and Youth Fitness Study (NCYFS) and the Youth Risk Behavior Survey (YRBS), have helped delineate patterns of physical activity among youths. In the mid-1980s, the NCYFS measured the physical fitness and physical activity habits of a national sample of children aged 10 to 18 years. Results showed that students between grades 7 and 12 reported spending an average of 1.8 hours per day on physical activity outside of physical education (PE) classes. The YRBS, sponsored by the Centers for Disease Control and Prevention (CDC), was first administered in 1990 and was repeated in 1991 and every 2 years thereafter. The most recent survey was done in 2007.

The 2007 YRBS defined the recommended physical activity level as "any physical activity that made you breath hard some of the time for a total of at least 60 minutes per day on 5 or more days of the 7 days preceding the survey." Results from the 2007 YRBS (**Table 4.1**) showed that only 34.7% of youth reported meeting this level of recommended physical activity. More boys (43.7%) than girls (25.6%) reported this level of physical activity. Looking at these figures by age and sex helps delineate the trends in physical activity; 44.4% of ninth-grade boys and 31.5% of ninth-grade girls reported meeting this recommendation. The percentages dropped by the twelfth grade to 38.7% of boys and 20.6% of girls. By race and sex, the highest rate of exercise was reported by white boys (46.1%), black boys (41.3%), and Hispanic boys (38.6%), followed by rates reported by white girls (27.9%), Hispanic girls (21.9%), and black girls (21%).

Involvement in daily physical activity at school also decreases during adolescence. Forty percent of girls and 39.7% of

TABLE 4.1

Percentage of Young People Meeting Current Recommendations for Physical Activity*

Demographic Group	2007 YRBS	
	%	95% CI
Overall	34.7	32.5-37.0
Sex		
Male	43.7	41.1-46.4
Female	25.6	22.8-28.6
Race/ethnicity		
White, non-Hispanic		
Male	46.1	42.6-49.6
Female	27.9	23.7-32.6
Total	37.0	33.9-40.3
Black, non-Hispanic		
Male	41.3	38.9-43.7
Female	21.0	18.1-24.2
Total	31.0	29.3-32.9
Hispanic		
Male	38.6	35.5-41.9
Female	21.9	18.7-25.4
Total	30.2	27.6-33.0
Grade in school—boys		
9	44.4	41.2-47.7
10	45.1	41.8-48.3
11	45.2	41.0-49.4
12	38.7	34.7-42.8
Grade in school—girls		
9	31.5	27.6-35.8
10	24.4	20.4-28.9
11	24.6	21.2-28.3
12	20.6	17.2-24.4

From Youth Risk Behavior Survey 2007, Centers for Disease Control and Prevention. * Defined as "Any physical activity that made you breathe hard some of the time for a total of at least 60 minutes per day on 5 or more days of the 7 days preceding the survey." YRBS indicates Youth Risk Behavior Survey; 95% CI, 95% confidence interval.

boys reported that they had PE classes daily during the ninth grade. By the twelfth grade this had decreased to 20.2% of girls and 27.5% of boys. The 2007 YRBS also showed that 24.9% of youth did not participate in 60 or more minutes of physical activity on any day in the 7 days before the survey. This percentage was higher in girls (31.8%) than in boys (18%).

The number of girls participating in organized team sports has increased more than 900% since the passage of Title IX in 1972, compared with a 19% increase in the number of boys participating in organized sports over the same time period. The 2007 YRBS reported that 50.4% of girls reported participating in one or more sports teams during the past 12 months. Even though more girls are involved in sports, the YRBS data showed that their participation in team sports decreased from grades 9 to 12 (54.7% to 41.9%). In the 2007 YRBS the percentage of boys participating in organized sports was 62.1%. Their participation also decreased from grades 9 to 12 (63.4% to 56.2%), although less so than in girls.

These surveys reveal several important trends. Although children are active, especially when compared with adults, physical activity decreases significantly during adolescence. This decline is consistent across participation in PE classes, involvement in vigorous or moderate activity, and participation in team sports. Boys are more active than girls across all ages, and the decline in activity across adolescence is more marked for girls than for boys, particularly minority girls. Because this decline continues into adulthood, promotion of physical activity should begin during childhood and adolescence.

PHYSICIAN BEHAVIOR

Because of the many short- and long-term benefits of physical activity, its promotion should be a priority in every physician setting. However, it is often hard to fit this type of counseling into the list of tasks that need to be addressed during a well-child visit, especially when time and money are not allocated for health promotion counseling.

The counseling behaviors of physicians in terms of the frequency and quality of physical activity counseling are related to their training, perceived effectiveness at changing patient behavior, practice settings, and personal physical activity practices. There is a gap between physicians' recognition of the importance of promoting regular activity and the perception of their effectiveness at changing patient behavior. In studies of physician counseling behaviors with adults, frequently cited barriers to counseling included lack of time, lack of training, lack of standardized recommendations and counseling techniques, lack of reimbursement, and lack of effectiveness at changing patient behavior. These barriers need to be addressed to facilitate adequate counseling within the clinical setting about physical activity.

The following sections review current physical activity guidelines for youths and strategies that can be used to address some of these known barriers to counseling.

BASIC RECOMMENDATIONS FOR PROMOTING ACTIVITY

Guidelines have been developed to establish parameters for promoting physical activity among youth. They provide information that could be used to address public health needs and to help clinicians recommend physical activity to their patients. These guidelines define the quantity and quality of activity needed to optimize physical fitness and to identify the health-related benefits of physical activity. They incorporate expert opinion and the findings published in the current scientific literature, but they also acknowledge the gaps in research. Although the recommendations vary, all of them emphasize daily physical activity. Participating in regular physical activity is probably more important than intensity for obtaining health-related benefits.

The Dietary Guidelines for Americans are published every 5 years. These guidelines, which were built on previous recommendations and were published in 2000 and updated in 2005, recommended that "Children and adolescents engage in at least 60 minutes of physical activity on most, preferably, all days of the week." This amount was thought to achieve the health-related benefits of physical activity and would help prevent excessive weight gain.

On the basis of the scientific literature, the Council for Physical Education for Children, within the National Association for Sport and Physical Education, wrote a position statement directed at physical activity guidelines for younger children.

In 2004 the National Association of Sports and Physical Education (NASPE) updated its guidelines for appropriate physical activity for children aged 5 to 12. NASPE made the following recommendations: (1) Children should accumulate at least 60 minutes, and up to several hours, of age-appropriate physical activity on most or all days of the week. This daily accumulation should include moderate and vigorous physical activity, with most time spent on intermittent, rather than sustained, activity. (2) Children should participate in several bouts of physical activity lasting 15 minutes or more each day. (3) Children should participate each day in a variety of age-appropriate physical activities designed to help them achieve optimal health, wellness, fitness, and performance benefits. (4) Extended periods of inactivity (periods of 2 or more hours) are discouraged for children, especially during the day.

The CDC convened an expert panel in 2004 to review the current state of the scientific literature and develop an evidence-based recommendation. It concluded that "school age youth should participate every day in 60 minutes or more of moderate to vigorous physical activity that is developmentally appropriate, enjoyable, and involves a variety of activities."

Moderate activity is defined as an activity that increases the heart rate to between 50% and 70% of the estimated maximum heart rate (with maximum heart rate estimated as 220 minus the age in years). At this activity level, the intensity of the activity should permit the individual to hold a conversation. Examples include brisk walking (3.5 mph), slow bicycling ($<$10 mph), light weight lifting, hiking, or dancing. Vigorous activity increases the heart rate to more than 70% of the maximum, and it is more difficult to maintain a conversation during this type of activity. Examples include fast walking (4.5 mph), running or jogging (5 mph), bicycling ($>$10 mph), swimming, basketball, and most competitive sports.

Regular activity performed at a moderate level of intensity will provide most health-related benefits of physical activity. Additional benefits and fitness levels can be obtained by more vigorous levels of activity. Although obtaining or enhancing physical fitness is a desirable goal, the more important goal is establishing regular physical activity patterns that maintain fitness levels and prevent the decline of activity levels through the adolescent years.

Recommendations for youth should focus on promoting a variety of activities that are fun and can be easily incorporated into their lifestyle. These activities may include team sports, individual sports, and recreational or lifetime activities, such as walking, bicycling, and swimming. The best forms of physical activity are regular, enjoyable, and sustainable. Parents and youth coaches should avoid the use of exercise as punishment for bad behavior. This implies that exercise is not fun—the opposite of what should be promoted.

ASSESSMENT OF CURRENT ACTIVITY

The patient's level of physical activity should be assessed at every well-child visit. This can be part of a standard health assessment form completed by the patient or parent in the waiting room, part of the nursing assessment, or part of the physician interview. Additional assessment can be made by the physician or office staff if the initial assessment identifies a child or adolescent who is sedentary or only intermittently active. As part of identifying the problem, it is important to determine the child's readiness to make a behavior change and to identify potential barriers to change. Inactive youth can be asked whether they are interested in becoming more active. Those who are active can be asked how likely it is they will continue their activity over the next 3 to 6 months. A counseling approach that is based on current activity and readiness to change or maintain behavior can then be used. Creating solutions is a joint effort between the physician and child that should optimally include the parents.

INTERVENTIONS

Most physicians are good at identifying problems. It is harder to provide useful solutions or effective health promotion interventions within the confines of a busy clinical setting. Some restraints, such as time and reimbursement, cannot be changed until practice styles and reimbursement patterns are redefined. Efforts therefore need to be focused on brief, effective interventions that easily can be incorporated into current practice patterns.

Promoting physical activity starts with providing educational literature in the waiting room that emphasizes healthy lifestyles and physical activity. Posters or pictures showing different types of activities, both vigorous and moderate, being done by a variety of children and adolescents with and without adults send a healthy message to patients and their families.

Readiness and Behavior Modification

Successful models in adult physical activity counseling have incorporated concepts from stages of change theory, social cognitive theory, and behavior modification techniques. These include identifying the patient's readiness to make a behavioral change, setting goals, creating contracts, addressing barriers, and enlisting social support. These concepts can easily be incorporated into brief clinical counseling interventions and can be adapted to a variety of health behaviors.

Youngsters who are already meeting the recommended levels of activity should receive reinforcement about their healthy lifestyle and encouragement about continuing their activity. For inactive children or adolescents who are not ready to change, identifying potential benefits and current barriers to activity can be an important first step. Often physical activity can be recommended for a medical reason, such as an increase in weight disproportionate to an increase in height, high blood pressure for age, or a family history of cardiovascular disease or diabetes. Because young people are much more focused on the present than on potential long-term benefits of physical activity, emphasizing immediate and short-term benefits can be a more effective motivation than the prevention of chronic diseases in the distant future (**Table 4.2**). For this group, identifying salient benefits and briefly addressing the

---

TABLE 4.2

Immediate and Short-term Benefits of Physical Activity

- Having fun
- Spending time with friends
- Improving body image
- Maintaining healthy weight
- Increasing energy levels
- Increasing endurance for sports or hobbies
- Improved self-image
- Feeling stronger
- Getting muscles or definition
- Just feeling better about oneself

---

barriers can be the first step toward getting the individual or family to think about becoming more physically active (**Table 4.3**). This targeted approach is more satisfying for patients and physicians, is a much better use of valuable counseling time, and allows physicians to spend the most time with patients who are ready to make positive changes.

Physical Activity Prescription

A physical activity prescription is needed only for patients who are ready to make a change. For inactive or intermittently active youngsters who are interested in increasing their activity level, counseling should include an actual activity plan or physical activity prescription. Presenting recommendations as a prescription is a useful concept. Writing a patient a prescription uses a medical model that patients are familiar with. It takes advantage of the authority of the physician and reinforces to patients the notion that physical activity is as important to their health as any medication that might be prescribed. Allowing the patient, and parents when appropriate, to participate in setting the goal of the physical activity will help with compliance. For many children, parents play an important role in any behavioral change, so counseling needs to target both the child and the parent. Adapting simple concepts of behavior change into counseling will help make the limited time available for counseling more effective.

Because this group of patients is ready to change, any counseling or direction provided is much more likely to translate into a behavior change. Focus should be placed on the goal of increasing moderate to vigorous physical

TABLE 4.3

Suggested Solutions to Common Barriers to Physical Activity

Barrier	Suggested Solution
I don't have time.	• Build activity into your day; walk or ride your bike for transportation. • Get off the bus a stop early. • Take the stairs whenever possible. • Plan fun, active activities with friends. • Sign up for physical education at your school. • Walk around the mall twice before you start shopping.
I don't like sports.	• Choose an activity that you enjoy. It does not have to be a sport. • Walking, dancing, or swimming are great activities. • Consider active hobbies or volunteer work.
My neighborhood isn't safe.	• Use a workout video or DVD within your home. • Dance at home to your favorite music. • Find a Y, Boys & Girls Club, or community recreation center in your neighborhood. • Sign up for school activities such as physical education or after-school programs.
I'm not good at any sports.	• You don't have to play a sport to be active. • Walking, dancing, swimming–anything that gets you moving counts. • Find a friend, sibling, or family member to be an activity buddy, and schedule a fun activity 2 or 3 times a week.
I'm overweight or out of shape.	• Start slowly, with 10 or 15 minutes of activity until the activity is comfortable. • Build short activity breaks into your day. • Count up your daily sedentary activities (computer, video games, TV time) and decrease by 30 minutes. • Consider after-school programs or community programs that involve activity or learning a new skill–get a friend to go with you.

activity to 60 minutes per day. This can be accomplished by accumulating several bouts of 10 to 15 minutes of activity. Gradually increasing the total time or number of days per week improves the individual's ability to achieve and maintain a positive health behavior change. It is important

to have the child be as clear as possible regarding the plan, including type of activity and intensity, location, when he or she is going to be active, and for how long. To make the plan detailed, the child will need to anticipate barriers and create solutions. The most common reported barriers to physical activity include lack of time, lack of access to facilities, unsafe neighborhoods, transportation needs, cost, and dislike of exercise. Asking about barriers and helping patients create solutions are key components of counseling. The more detailed the plan, the more likely the child will meet the goal.

Recommendations for At-Risk or Overweight Youth

The obesity epidemic among youth in the United States is a major health concern that affects their current and future health. Regular physical activity must be part of any program to help maintain appropriate weight. Overweight youth face all the barriers to activities that normal-weight youth face, such as lack of time, unsafe neighborhoods, and lack of facilities. They also report being self-conscious regarding their bodies, experiencing teasing from peers, experiencing discomfort as a result of poor physical conditioning, and having lower self-efficacy for participation in activities and sports.

Although the recommended level of activity is 60 minutes of moderate to vigorous activities per day, obese children may need 60 to 90 minutes of daily activity to assist in weight maintenance or weight loss. Given the low level of physical activity frequently reported in this population, this duration of activity appears overwhelming, so it is important to start slowly with achievable goals to reinforce positive changes, no matter how small. As with any patient receiving physical activity recommendations, physicians should begin by identifying the current amounts of daily activity and sedentary activity. Many youth do not identify nonathletic activities, such as walking, as physical activity. Helping them broaden their view of what comprises activity will help them identify more options to increase their activity levels. The scientific literature supports the value of decreasing sedentary activities as an important component of weight control. Particularly important is reducing the amount of time spent sitting in front of a TV or computer screen. The American Academy of Pediatrics recommends limiting television, video games, and computer time (not related to schoolwork) to less than 2 hours per day.

In all cases, it is important to assess the patient's readiness to make a change. Addressing any health issues related to their high body mass index, such as poor fitness, high blood pressure, orthopedic issues, problems with their feet, or the risk of diabetes, should be addressed to encourage patients to increase their physical activity levels. However, as seen in their normal-weight peers, the immediate benefits of physical activity, such as having fun, having more energy, and spending time with friends, are often stronger motivators. If patients are interested in making a change, then an activity prescription should be written. They should plan to start or add 10 to 15 minutes of activities to their daily routine. This will allow them to feel successful and to avoid injury or discomfort, thus improving the chances they will maintain the activity. Each week, they should increase daily activity by about 10% until they have reached the goal of 60 to 90 minutes of moderate-intensity activity per day. Recommending small bouts of activity throughout the day—taking the stairs, taking walks with friends, dancing—will help the patient build a more active lifestyle. Active participation in PE classes and after-school or community-based activity programs should be discussed. The plan for activity should be as specific as possible regarding the activity's type, intensity, location, time, and duration. Identifying and addressing barriers to the plan is a key component.

Physical activity should be gradually increased over time. Encouraging a variety of activities that are fun, identifying an activity buddy (such as a family member or peer) to provide support, and establishing realistic goals for physical activity and weight loss are also important. For at-risk or overweight children, weight maintenance may be the primary goal. If weight loss is indicated, the goal should be slow and steady weight loss (1–2 pounds per month). Patients should be asked about physical activity at subsequent visits, and any positive changes (large or small) should be reinforced. If possible, a follow-up visit should be scheduled to monitor progress, reinforce positive changes, address barriers, and adjust plans and goals.

Creating a Social Climate for Physical Activity

Physical activity needs to be fun and accessible to the participant if it is to be continued. It is important to help children choose activities that are fun, developmentally appropriate, and realistic given their individual, family, and community resources. One method that has been frequently used in exercise prescriptions for adults, but that can also be used for children, incorporates the mnemonic FITT: frequency, intensity, time (duration), and type of activity (**Table 4.4**). This can be used to help create a physical

TABLE 4.4

FITT Mnemonic

Frequency	The goal should be to include some type of physical activity daily. It is important to educate patients that activities of daily living (ie, walking or bicycling for transportation) count as physical activity.
Intensity	The goal should be for the daily activity to be of at least moderate intensity, with ideally several bouts of more vigorous activity over the week. Vigorous activity is defined as activity that makes you breathe hard and sweat. Intensity is less important than establishing and maintaining regular activity.
Time (duration)	The goal should be the accumulation of 60 minutes of activity daily. Acknowledge that accumulation of activity in 10- to 15-minute bouts provides nearly all the health benefits of longer bouts of sustained activity. This can be a great way to encourage physical activity in individuals who are less inclined to participate in more organized team sports or to engage in longer bouts of sustained activity. This concept may also lead to the incorporation of lifestyle activities that may be more easily maintained over time.
Type	The activities can include a variety of team sports, individual sports, recreational activities, family activities, and lifestyle activities such as walking or bicycling for transportation, household chores, and taking the stairs. Several bouts a week of weight-bearing activities that promote muscle strength, flexibility, and bone health are desirable. Involvement in a variety of activities may help by decreasing burnout and overuse syndromes, increasing enjoyment in the activity, and promoting maintenance of the activities. Injuries and lack of enjoyment are frequently cited as reasons adolescents quit participating in activities.

activity prescription, and it can be used as a simple way to record recommendations.

Suggestions for increasing physical activity can include walking or bicycling for transportation and planning physically active rather than sedentary activities with friends. Many adolescents, especially girls, may not be active because they think organized sports are the only type of exercise that counts. Therefore, it is important to help adolescents identify the physical activity they may already be getting, such as walking, and to reinforce the benefits of other lifetime activities, such as bicycling, dancing, skating, and swimming.

Identifying ways to incorporate increased physical activity into the activities of daily living can also be useful. Examples include taking the stairs whenever possible, getting off the bus a stop earlier, taking walks with friends rather than talking on the telephone, and walking at least one lap of the mall before shopping.

Social support has been identified as an important component in making a successful behavior change. Adolescents may want to consider finding an activity buddy. Parents of younger children should plan time together with their children where they are active. This increases their children's activity level and models desirable behavior.

SAFETY CONCERNS

Examples of safety concerns that should be addressed with patients include using appropriate protective gear, using developmentally appropriate and correctly sized equipment and field size, and having access to proper hydration. Larger community-based issues include advocating for proper education and training for adults working with youth sports programs. Physicians should provide literature or information to patients and families about basic first aid for activity-related injuries. If needed, patients should be encouraged to seek medical care and rehabilitation to decrease the risk of chronic problems; and patients should be counseled to modify or discontinue activities if they are injured.

Concern about neighborhood safety is a barrier for many youth and their families. Activities that can be done indoors, such as exercise videos or DVDs and dancing to popular music, may be recommended. Identifying activities that take place in a safe, controlled space under the supervision of adults, such as after-school or community recreation programs, are also good alternatives. Recommending participation in daily PE classes throughout elementary and secondary school is another safe alternative.

SEDENTARY BEHAVIOR

Decreasing the amount of time spent in sedentary behaviors, such as watching television, talking on the telephone, and playing computer or video games, especially in the late afternoon and early evening, to less than 2 hours a day will result in more accumulated daily activity. Riding a stationary bicycle or stretching while watching TV are easy ways to increase activity during an otherwise sedentary time. Although the link between physical activity and watching TV is not clear, increased watching has been linked to obesity.

Primary care providers should talk with all their patients about the time spent in sedentary behaviors. The AAP has recommended limiting screen time to less than 2 hours per day.

The pediatrician should be addressing amount of time spent in sedentary behaviors with all patients. The use of a similar approach to that used to counsel for increased physical activity—identifying current behavior, identifying the benefits of more exercise, addressing barriers to change, and evaluating self-efficacy to make a change—may be used to help patients decrease the amount of time spent in sedentary behaviors.

REINFORCEMENT

When physicians ask about physical activity at each office visit, it sends an important message to the patient about the priority placed on physical activity as an important health behavior. For inactive patients, repeating the reasons they should consider increasing activity is important. For patients who received an activity prescription, positive changes should be reinforced, and addressing barriers, making adjustments, and emphasizing the benefits they are receiving, no matter how small, are vital to their success.

The behavior of the child or adolescent who is appropriately active should be reinforced. Often it is helpful to identify the health benefits of regular activity, such as maintenance of appropriate weight, increased energy, improved sense of well-being, and heightened self-esteem. It can also be useful to assess how confident a patient is that he or she will remain active and to provide solutions for any identified potential barriers to maintaining that activity.

Physicians and other health care providers need to be good role models for their patients and their families. This includes a personal plan for incorporating physical activity within their own busy schedules. Studies with internists show that physicians who exercise regularly are more likely to provide more frequent and more aggressive physical activity counseling to their patients.

COMMUNITY AND SCHOOLS

Physicians can play an important role in promoting physical activity by being good role models for an active lifestyle and being advocates for physical activity in other arenas. Children and adolescents spend most of their time attending school. Physicians need to advocate for more health education and physical education that includes aerobic lifestyle activities (ie, walking, jogging,

---

TABLE 4.5

Keys to Promoting Physical Fitness and Activity

In the Clinic

- Ensure that the clinical setting stresses physical activity by including posters, videos, pictures, magazines, and other patient education materials that promote physical activity and healthy lifestyle choices.

- Be a good role model. Physicians who incorporate 30 minutes of moderate activity into their daily routines on most days of the week will be better counselors and healthier individuals.

- Assess and record the level of physical activity at all well-child visits.

- If a patient is inactive and not interested in changing, give the patient some reasons to reconsider, and address any identified barriers to activity.

- If a patient is inactive and ready to change, help the patient create an activity plan that is fun, developmentally appropriate, and realistic.

- As part of any activity plan, identify FITT: frequency, intensity, time (duration), type.

- Identify a social support, or activity buddy, for the patient. This could be a friend or a family member.

- Record recommendations in the medical chart, and follow up with patients at subsequent visits.

- Advocate for physical activity counseling to be part of managed care service requirements and thus reimbursable.

In the Community

- Be an advocate in community schools for more physical education and health education classes, including classes that encourage lifetime activities as well as competitive sports.

- Be an advocate in the community for safe and convenient venues for activity, including parks, recreation centers, bicycle lanes, after-hours access to school facilities, and playgrounds for after-school activities.

- Become familiar with resources in the community, including the Y, community recreation departments, community sports programs, and other youth programs.

---

dancing) as well as teaches sport-specific skills. In addition, physicians can become more involved with teachers and coaching staffs. This communication improves the care of the young athlete and increases the effectiveness of the adults working with these children. Changes in school policy can reach more children than promoting physical activity in individual patients in the office. Physicians are also important advocates for the availability of safe and accessible places for physical activity to occur within the community, such as open spaces, parks, recreation centers, community centers, and school playgrounds after hours.

Guidelines exist for establishing appropriate health education and physical education curricula, and physicians can be valuable advocates for promoting these guidelines and encouraging daily physical education within local schools. CDC guidelines promote physical activity within schools and communities, and the American Academy of Pediatrics has developed a list of recommendations that physicians can use in the office setting to assess physical activity and fitness. **Table 4.5** incorporates many of those recommendations, but it focuses on ways physicians in the clinical setting and in the community can promote regular physical activity.

SUMMARY POINTS

- Physical activity decreases significantly during adolescence for both sexes, but particularly for girls. Because this decline continues into adulthood, physical activity promotion should begin during childhood and adolescence.

- Although published recommendations vary somewhat, all recommendations emphasize daily physical activity. Participating in regular physical activity is probably more important for obtaining health-related benefits than the intensity of the activity.

- Although obtaining or enhancing physical fitness is a desirable goal, the more important goal is establishing regular enjoyable physical activity patterns that maintain fitness levels and prevent the decline of activity levels through the adolescent years.

- Physicians and other health care providers are an important part of a national effort to increase physical activity among the population.

- Levels of physical activity should be assessed in the office, and inactive youth should be encouraged to increase their activity. A written physical activity prescription helps patients who demonstrate a willingness to change their behavior.

- Physicians should assess levels of sedentary behaviors and counsel patients to decrease them, including reducing time in front of TV and computer screens to 2 hours a day or less.

- Involvement with schools and communities to create policies that promote physical activity is an effective way to promote physical activity in large numbers of children.

- By promoting lifetime activities as well as organized sports and athletics, physicians can positively affect the current health and well-being of youth, which in turn will help prevent chronic diseases in adulthood.

SUGGESTED READING

2008 Physical Activity Guidelines for Americans. http://www.health.gov/PAGuidelines.

American Academy of Pediatrics, Committee on Public Education. Children, adolescents and television. *Pediatrics.* 2001;107:423-427.

American Academy of Pediatrics, Committee on Sports Medicine and Fitness and Committee on School Health. Organized sports for children and preadolescents. *Pediatrics.* 2001;107:1459-1462.

American Academy of Pediatrics, Council on Sports Medicine and Fitness, Council on School Health. Active healthy living: prevention of childhood obesity through increased physical activity. *Pediatrics.* 2006;117:1834-1842.

Biddle S, Sallis J, Cavill N, eds. *Young and Active? Young People and Health-Enhancing Physical Activity: Evidence and Implications.* London, England: Health Education Authority; 1998.

Centers for Disease Control and Prevention. Guidelines for school and community programs to promote lifelong physical activity among young people. *MMWR Morb Mortal Wkly Rep.* 1997;46:1-36.

Centers for Disease Control and Prevention. Increasing physical activity: a report on recommendations of the Task Force on Community Preventive Services. *MMWR Morb Mortal Wkly Rep.* 2001;50:1-16.

Childhood Obesity—Advancing Effective Prevention and Treatment: An Overview for Health Professionals. Washington, DC: National Institute for Health Care Management; 2003.

Division of Nutrition, Physical Activity and Obesity, Centers for Disease Control and Prevention Web site. http://www.cdc.gov/nccdphp/dnpa/index.htm. Accessed May 21, 2008.

Healthy Youth! Physical Activity Publications. http://www.cdc.gov/HealthyYouth/physicalactivity/publications.htm. Accessed May 21, 2008.

Katz DL, O'Connell M, Yeh MC, et al, Task Force on Community Preventive Services. Public health strategies for preventing and controlling overweight and obesity in school and worksite settings: a report on recommendations of the Task Force on Community Preventive Services 11. *MMWR Morb Mortal Wkly Rep.* 2005;54(RR-10):1-12.

Koplan JP, Liverman CT, Kraak VI. *Preventing Childhood Obesity: Health in the Balance.* Washington, DC: National Academies Press; 2005.

National Association for Sport and Physical Education. *Physical Activity for Children: A Statement of Guidelines.* 2nd ed. Reston, VA: National Association for Sport and Physical Education; 2004.

National Centers for Chronic Disease Prevention and Health Promotion. *Physical Activity and Health: A Report of the Surgeon General.* Atlanta, GA: US Department of Health and Human Services, Centers for Disease Control and Prevention; 1996.

Patrick K, Spear B, Holt K, Sofka D, eds. *Bright Futures in Practice: Physical Activity.* Arlington, VA: National Center for Education in Maternal and Child Health; 2001. http://www.brightfutures.org/physicalactivity/about.htm. Accessed May 21, 2008.

President's Council on Physical Fitness and Sports Web site. http://www.fitness.gov/. Accessed May 21, 2008.

Promoting Better Health for Young People through Physical Activity and Sport. A Report to the President from the Secretary of Health and Human Services and the Secretary of Education. 2000. http://www.cdc.gov/healthyyouth/physicalactivity/promoting_health/. Accessed May 21, 2008.

Sallis JF, Patrick K. Physical activity guidelines for adolescents: consensus statement. *Pediatr Exerc Sci.* 1994;6:434-447.

Strong WB, Malina RM, Blimkie CJ, et al. Evidence based physical activity for school-age youth. *J Pediatr.* 2005;146:732-737.

VERB—a media campaign promoting physical activity in 9-13 year olds (tweens). http://www.cdc.gov/youthcampaign/. Accessed May 21, 2008.

CHAPTER 5

The Preparticipation Physical Evaluation

Eric W. Small, MD

More than 6 million high school students participate in sports each year. With this many participants, the preparticipation physical evaluation (PPE) is one of the most commonly performed examinations. Over the past decade, the PPE has evolved to allow physicians to provide consistent, high-quality examinations nationwide. In the early 1990s, the American Academy of Family Physicians, the American Academy of Pediatrics, the American Medical Society for Sports Medicine, the American Orthopaedic Society for Sports Medicine, and the American Osteopathic Academy of Sports Medicine formed the Preparticipation Examination Task Force to standardize the conduct and content of these examinations. In 1992 the task force published recommendations for the PPE on the basis of the consensus of the current literature. These guidelines were updated in 1997, 2002, and 2004 and serve as the basis for the current PPE.

GOALS OF THE PREPARTICIPATION PHYSICAL EVALUATION

The purpose of the preparticipation physical evaluation (PPE) is not to disqualify athletes; less than 2% are actually disqualified on the basis of the evaluation's results. Rather, the primary goals of the PPE are to detect conditions that might predispose the athlete to injury, to detect conditions that might be life-threatening or disabling, and to meet legal or insurance requirements. The secondary goals are to determine general health, to counsel athletes on health-related issues, and to assess fitness level.

Identifying athletes who may need further diagnostic testing, counseling, or rehabilitation is the primary goal of

the PPE, but there are many other expectations. Sometimes, parents expect the PPE to be a comprehensive evaluation of the athlete's health, including areas that may be considered unrelated to sports participation, such as teenage sexuality, substance abuse, immunizations, and others. Parents frequently think of the PPE as the only medical evaluation their child or adolescent needs, and they expect it to be comprehensive. In contrast, many physicians view the PPE as a cursory examination that is intended only to detect conditions that might limit or impair athletic endeavors. Common questions parents have about the PPE, and their answers, are provided in **Table 5.1**.

Because parents and physicians view the evaluation differently, parents must be advised about the intent of the PPE, and the PPE's scope and purpose must be made clear to them. The most recent PPE guidelines suggest creating a medical home for all athletes.

CONDUCTING THE PPE

Methods

The PPE is typically conducted in 1 of 3 ways: the locker room method, the station method, or the office-based method.

In the locker room method, athletes traditionally line up single file, and the physician examines each athlete individually. One benefit of this method is that it requires few personnel and can be done with little preparation. However, it affords little privacy for the athlete, it is usually noisy so that the physician has a hard time auscultating the heart and lungs, and it is often too brief.

The station method divides the examination into several components with physicians, nurses, athletic

TABLE 5.1

Common Questions Parents Have about the Preparticipation Physical Evaluation (PPE)

My son had a physical examination for participation in football last year. Does he still need to see his physician this year?

Although the PPE is comprehensive, it was never designed to take the place of a regular physician visit. The setting or time allocation for the PPE is often not conducive to discussions of health issues that are of primary importance during the adolescent years, such as drug and alcohol use, smoking, sexual activity education, safety issues, and diagnosis of depression.

When should my child have a PPE relative to the beginning of an athletic season?

The best time for the PPE is about 4 to 6 weeks before the beginning of the athletic season. This allows enough time for thorough evaluations, consultations, and rehabilitation of any identified musculoskeletal injuries.

Do I need to attend the PPE with my child?

Although you may not be asked to attend the PPE with your child, it is important that you review the accuracy and completeness of the medical history and family history that are given. Your child may not know or remember some of the history. Most of the important information obtained in the PPE is obtained from the history.

How often will my son or daughter need a PPE?

The frequency of required evaluations varies by state. Most commonly, a physical evaluation is required every year. To determine the requirements of your state, check with the school district or the state high school athletic association.

Will my child need to undergo any laboratory or radiographic studies at the PPE?

Routine laboratory studies and radiographs are not generally performed. On the basis of information obtained during the history and physical examination, however, your physician may think that further studies are indicated.

trainers, and coaches each assigned to a single task. This method is ideally suited for screening large numbers of athletes. Two benefits of this method are its relative efficiency and its good ability to identify abnormalities. However, this method affords less rapport with athletes, and like the locker room method, there is a lack of privacy. Athletes have little opportunity to ask questions of the physicians regarding their own health or other medical or personal issues.

The office-based method is an individual physical examination and has the advantage of an established physician-patient relationship in which the medical history is known and continuity of care is fostered. Disadvantages include a lack of consistency among physicians, potential unfamiliarity of the physician with the sport and its disqualifying conditions, and its lack of cost-effectiveness.

Timing

Ideally, the PPE is performed early enough before the sport's season begins to ensure that athletes who have medical problems can be thoroughly evaluated and treated, but not so early that intervening injuries are likely to occur. The best time for the evaluation to take place is 4 to 6 weeks before the first scheduled practice.

Although the current guidelines of the American Academy of Pediatrics suggest that the PPE should be performed every year, other sources suggest that the PPE be conducted before the beginning of each new level of competition (ie, middle school or junior high, high school, and college), with annual updates of the history and targeted physical examinations of areas of concern. However, most state high school athletic associations require annual evaluations. A recent survey of all 50 states and the District of Columbia found that 65% of states require annual examination of all athletes competing in high school sports.

EVALUATION

History

As with any health evaluation, the history identifies most potential problems for young athletes. Most experts agree that despite the best screening of athletes to prevent sudden death, only a few who die would have been detected through history and physical examination. The key to identifying these problems is the questionnaire that systematically screens for conditions that frequently cause problems in athletes or that could lead to sudden death during athletic activity. **Table 5.2** lists some of the most important questions to ask during the examination. The PPE forms provided by state high school athletic associations often do not incorporate all of the screening questions recommended by the Preparticipation Examination Task Force. (The form that should be used is provided in **Figure 5.1**).

TABLE 5.2

Medical History Questions

Question	Reason
1. Injury or illness since last checkup?	Targets potential physical examination concerns
2. Chronic illnesses, hospitalizations, or surgeries?	Identifies potential counseling or rehabilitation issues
3. Any medications or supplements of any type?	Identifies drugs that may inhibit or interfere with sports participation
4. Allergies to medications, insects, food?	Alerts physicians and trainers for potential allergic reactions
5. Dizziness or chest pain with exercise or after exercise; history of sudden death in a close relative <50 years old?	Identifies potential causes of sudden death due to cardiovascular problems
6. Fainting or passing out during or after exercise?	Targets cardiovascular concerns
7. History of hypertension or murmur?	Targets cardiovascular concerns
8. Family history of Marfan syndrome	Targets cardiovascular concerns
9. Ever been restricted from sports by physician?	Identifies potential disqualifying problems
10. Any skin problems?	Identifies potential transmittable disease during contact
11. Concussion, knocked out, unconsciousness, or memory loss, seizure, or severe/frequent headache?	Targets neurologic concerns
12. Stinger, burner, pinched nerve, numbness/tingling in extremities?	Targets neurologic concerns
13. Problems while exercising in the heat?	Targets heat illness concerns
14. Asthma, allergies, wheezing, difficulty breathing, chest pain?	Identifies potential for exercise-induced asthma
15. Special equipment or devices not usually used in your sport?	Identifies potential concerns for physician follow-up
16. Glasses, contacts, or vision or eye problems?	Identifies ophthalmologic concerns
17. Strain, sprain, fracture, joint pain, or swelling?	Identifies potential musculoskeletal problems
18. Concerns about weight: Do you lose weight regularly for your sport?	Identifies potential disordered eating
19. Feel stressed out?	Clue to ask follow-up questions regarding drug use, eating problems, sexuality, home/school problems
20. Recent immunizations (tetanus, measles, hepatitis B, chickenpox)	Health maintenance issues
21. Girls only: menstrual history	Identifies oligomenorrhea and amenorrhea and potential risk for poor nutrition, stress fractures
22. Do you wear protective braces, splints?	Identifies injuries that have not been fully rehabilitated

Adapted with permission from the American Academy of Family Physicians, American Academy of Pediatrics, American Medical Society for Sports Medicine, American Orthopaedic Society for Sports Medicine, Osteopathic Academy of Sports Medicine. The PPE physical examination. In: *Preparticipation Physical Examination*. 2nd ed. Minneapolis, MN: McGraw-Hill; 1997:17-27.

Athletes typically complete their history forms without input from their parents. One study showed that only 40% of PPE forms matched when filled out independently by parent and child. The athlete and the parents should therefore complete the form together to obtain a thorough and accurate history.

Physical Examination

Two key components of the physical examination (cardiovascular and musculoskeletal) identify most athletes who warrant further evaluation or disqualification. The medical evaluation form recommended by the Preparticipation Examination Task Force is shown in **Figure 5.2**.

Cardiovascular Examination The cardiovascular examination should include evaluation of peripheral pulses, murmurs,

and blood pressure. **Table 5.3** summarizes important aspects of the cardiovascular examination screening. Coarctation of the aorta may present with decreased intensity of femoral pulses, but it may also present more subtly with brachial-femoral pulse delay. All diastolic murmurs and grade 3/6 systolic murmurs warrant further evaluation. Hypertrophic cardiomyopathy may produce a systolic murmur that cannot be distinguished from an innocent murmur. The murmur of hypertrophic cardiomyopathy increases in intensity with a Valsalva maneuver (decreased ventricular filling, increased obstruction) and decreases with squatting (increased ventricular filling, decreased obstruction). It will also increase in intensity when the athlete moves from a squatting to standing position.

Blood pressures obtained during the PPE are often high. Sometimes this is the result of using a blood pressure cuff that is too small, particularly in large adolescents. However,

Preparticipation Physical Evaluation

HISTORY FORM

DATE OF EXAM_____

Name_____ Sex_____ Age_____ Date of birth_____
Grade_____ School_____ Sport(s)_____
Address_____ Phone_____
Personal physician_____
In case of emergency, contact:
Name_____ Relationship_____ Phone (H)_____ (W)_____

Explain "Yes" answers below.
Circle questions you don't know the answers to.

	Yes	No
1. Has a doctor ever denied or restricted your participation in sports for any reason?	☐	☐
2. Do you have an ongoing medical condition (like diabetes or asthma)?	☐	☐
3. Are you currently taking any prescription or nonprescription (over-the-counter) medicines or pills?	☐	☐
4. Do you have allergies to medicines, pollens, foods, or stinging insects?	☐	☐
5. Have you ever passed out or nearly passed out DURING exercise?	☐	☐
6. Have you ever passed out or nearly passed out AFTER exercise?	☐	☐
7. Have you ever had discomfort, pain, or pressure in your chest during exercise?	☐	☐
8. Does your heart race or skip beats during exercise?	☐	☐
9. Has a doctor ever told you that you have (check all that apply):		

☐ High blood pressure   ☐ A heart murmur
☐ High cholesterol   ☐ A heart infection

	Yes	No
10. Has a doctor ever ordered a test for your heart? (for example: ECG, echocardiogram)	☐	☐
11. Has anyone in your family died for no apparent reason?	☐	☐
12. Does anyone in your family have a heart problem?	☐	☐
13. Has any family member or relative died of heart problems or of sudden death before age 50?	☐	☐
14. Does anyone in your family have Marfan syndrome?	☐	☐
15. Have you ever spent the night in a hospital?	☐	☐
16. Have you ever had surgery?	☐	☐
17. Have you ever had an injury, like a sprain, muscle or ligament tear, or tendinitis, that caused you to miss a practice or game? If yes, circle affected area below:	☐	☐
18. Have you had any broken or fractured bones or dislocated joints? If yes, circle below:	☐	☐
19. Have you had a bone or joint injury that required x-rays, MRI, CT, surgery, injections, rehabilitation, physical therapy, a brace, a cast, or crutches? If yes, circle below:	☐	☐

Head	Neck	Shoulder	Upper arm	Elbow	Forearm	Hand/ fingers	Chest
Upper back	Lower back	Hip	Thigh	Knee	Calf/ shin	Ankle	Foot/ toes

	Yes	No
20. Have you ever had a stress fracture?	☐	☐
21. Have you been told that you have or have you had an x-ray for atlantoaxial (neck) instability?	☐	☐
22. Do you regularly use a brace or assistive device?	☐	☐
23. Has a doctor ever told you that you have asthma or allergies?	☐	☐

	Yes	No
24. Do you cough, wheeze, or have difficulty breathing during or after exercise?	☐	☐
25. Is there anyone in your family who has asthma?	☐	☐
26. Have you ever used an inhaler or taken asthma medicine?	☐	☐
27. Were you born without or are you missing a kidney, an eye, a testicle, or any other organ?	☐	☐
28. Have you had infectious mononucleosis (mono) within the last month?	☐	☐
29. Do you have any rashes, pressure sores, or other skin problems?	☐	☐
30. Have you had a herpes skin infection?	☐	☐
31. Have you ever had a head injury or concussion?	☐	☐
32. Have you been hit in the head and been confused or lost your memory?	☐	☐
33. Have you ever had a seizure?	☐	☐
34. Do you have headaches with exercise?	☐	☐
35. Have you ever had numbness, tingling, or weakness in your arms or legs after being hit or falling?	☐	☐
36. Have you ever been unable to move your arms or legs after being hit or falling?	☐	☐
37. When exercising in the heat, do you have severe muscle cramps or become ill?	☐	☐
38. Has a doctor told you that you or someone in your family has sickle cell trait or sickle cell disease?	☐	☐
39. Have you had any problems with your eyes or vision?	☐	☐
40. Do you wear glasses or contact lenses?	☐	☐
41. Do you wear protective eyewear, such as goggles or a face shield?	☐	☐
42. Are you happy with your weight?	☐	☐
43. Are you trying to gain or lose weight?	☐	☐
44. Has anyone recommended you change your weight or eating habits?	☐	☐
45. Do you limit or carefully control what you eat?	☐	☐
46. Do you have any concerns that you would like to discuss with a doctor?	☐	☐

FEMALES ONLY

	Yes	No
47. Have you ever had a menstrual period?	☐	☐

48. How old were you when you had your first menstrual period?_____
49. How many periods have you had in the last 12 months?_____

Explain "Yes" answers here:_____
_____
_____
_____
_____
_____

I hereby state that, to the best of my knowledge, my answers to the above questions are complete and correct.
Signature of athlete_____ Signature of parent/guardian_____ Date_____

© 2004 American Academy of Family Physicians, American Academy of Pediatrics, American College of Sports Medicine, American Medical Society for Sports Medicine, American Orthopaedic Society for Sports Medicine, and American Osteopathic Academy of Sports Medicine.

FIGURE 5.1 Medical history form. Adapted with permission from the American Academy of Family Physicians, American Academy of Pediatrics, American Medical Society for Sports Medicine, American Orthopaedic Society for Sports Medicine, Osteopathic Academy of Sports Medicine. The PPE physical examination. In: *Preparticipation Physical Examination*. 3rd ed. Minneapolis, MN: McGraw-Hill; 2005:93.

Preparticipation Physical Evaluation

PHYSICAL EXAMINATION FORM

Name_____Date of birth_____

Height_____Weight_____% Body fat (optional)_____Pulse_____BP____/____ (____/____ , ____/____)

Vision R 20/____ L 20/____   Corrected: Y   N   Pupils: Equal ____ Unequal ____

Follow-Up Questions on More Sensitive Issues:	Yes	No
1. Do you feel stressed out or under a lot of pressure?	☐	☐
2. Do you ever feel so sad or hopeless that you stop doing some of your usual activities for more than a few days?	☐	☐
3. Do you feel safe?	☐	☐
4. Have you ever tried cigarette smoking, even 1 or 2 puffs? Do you currently smoke?	☐	☐
5. During the past 30 days, did you use chewing tobacco, snuff, or dip?	☐	☐
6. During the past 30 days, have you had a least 1 drink of alcohol?	☐	☐
7. Have you ever taken steroid pills or shots without a doctor's prescription?	☐	☐
8. Have you ever taken any supplements to help you gain or lose weight or improve your performance?	☐	☐
9. Questions from the Youth Risk Behavior Survey (http://www.cdc.gov/HealthyYouth/yrbs/index.htm) on guns, seatbelts, unprotected sex, domestic violence, drugs, etc.	☐	☐

NOTES: _____

_____

_____

	NORMAL	ABNORMAL FINDINGS	INITIALS*
MEDICAL			
Appearance			
Eyes/ears/nose/throat			
Hearing			
Lymph nodes			
Heart			
Murmurs			
Pulses			
Lungs			
Abdomen			
Genitourinary (males only)†			
Skin			
MUSCULOSKELETAL			
Neck			
Back			
Shoulder/arm			
Elbow/forearm			
Wrist/hand/fingers			
Hip/thigh			
Knee			
Leg/ankle			
Foot/toes			

*Multiple-examiner set-up only.
†Having a third party present is recommended for the genitourinary examination.

Notes: _____

_____

Name of physician (print/type)_____ Date_____

Address_____ Phone_____

Signature of physician_____ , MD or DO

© 2004 American Academy of Family Physicians, American Academy of Pediatrics, American College of Sports Medicine, American Medical Society for Sports Medicine, American Orthopaedic Society for Sports Medicine, and American Osteopathic Academy of Sports Medicine.

FIGURE 5.2 Physical examination form. Adapted with permission from the American Academy of Family Physicians, American Academy of Pediatrics, American Medical Society for Sports Medicine, American Orthopaedic Society for Sports Medicine, Osteopathic Academy of Sports Medicine. The PPE physical examination. In: *Preparticipation Physical Examination.* 3rd ed. Minneapolis, MN: McGraw-Hill; 2005:94.

TABLE 5.3

Cardiovascular Screening in Athletes

Condition	Cardiovascular Examination	Abnormality
Hypertension	Blood pressure	Varies with age—general guideline is >135/85 mm Hg in adolescents
Coarctation of aorta	Femoral pulses	Decreased intensity of femoral pulse; brachial-femoral pulse delay
Hypertrophic cardiomyopathy	Auscultation with provocative maneuvers (standing, supine, Valsalva maneuver)	Systolic ejection murmur that intensifies with standing or Valsalva maneuver; murmur may be absent
Marfan syndrome	Auscultation	Aortic (decrescendo diastolic murmur) or mitral insufficiency (holosystolic murmur); murmur may be absent; individuals with Marfanoid body habitus may require evaluation for silent aortic root dilation

Adapted with permission from Maron BJ, Thompson PO, Puffer JC. Cardiovascular preparticipation screening of competitive athletes: a statement from the Sudden Death Committee [clinical cardiology] and Congenital Cardiac Defects Committee [cardiovascular disease in the young], American Heart Association. *Circulation*. 1996;94:850-856.

sometimes the athlete's blood pressure is truly high when an age-based table of norms is consulted. Hypertension is rarely severe enough to disqualify an athlete from participation, but it needs to be identified and followed by the athlete's regular physician. Weight training activities should be restricted in patients who have severe hypertension. Recent cardiovascular research shows that screening for sudden cardiac death that includes a standardized history, physical examination, and electrocardiogram in a homogenous population may help prevent sudden death due to cardiomyopathy.

Sudden cardiac death in young athletes is rare, but a history of syncope, chest pain with exercise, or a family history of sudden death under age 50 should be evaluated. Many individuals with Marfan syndrome will have significant aortic root dilation without the characteristic murmur of aortic insufficiency. Athletes with suggestive Marfanoid body habitus should be evaluated for silent aortic root dilations, which could increase the risk of sudden death during athletic participation.

Musculoskeletal Examination The musculoskeletal examination is particularly important because it typically accounts for 50% of the abnormal physical findings identified on the PPE. The examination should focus on previously injured or symptomatic areas. Ninety-two percent of orthopedic injuries are detected by history alone.

Some authorities suggest a sport-specific approach to the physical examination. This method emphasizes the areas that are most commonly affected or injured in each specific sport. For example, a swimmer's examination would focus on the shoulders and ears (otitis externa), whereas a football

player's examination would include evaluation of neurologic conditions and musculoskeletal injuries.

Table 5.4 lists special considerations for the examination of injured or symptomatic joints.

Laboratory Studies

Laboratory studies have not been shown to be cost-effective or warranted in young asymptomatic athletes. Routine urinalysis and hematocrit for all athletes have been largely abandoned because these tests do not identify athletes who require disqualification, and they have a high rate of false-positive results. Similarly, electrocardiogram, echocardiogram, and stress testing are not suggested as screening tests in asymptomatic individuals because of the high rate of false-positive findings and their high cost.

TABLE 5.4

Special Considerations for the Examination of Injured or Symptomatic Joints

Inspect for visual deformity, muscle mass, asymmetry, and swelling.

- Palpate for localized areas of tenderness, warmth, and effusion.
- Assess range of motion (eg, an athlete with hip pain should be tested for loss of internal rotation and abduction, which can be seen in slipped capital femoral epiphysis and Legg-Calvé-Perthes disease).
- Test neurovascular status by evaluating muscle strength, sensation, reflexes, and pulses of the involved limb (eg, an athlete with a history of burners or stingers should undergo complete neurovascular testing of the neck and upper extremities).
- Test joint stability (eg, an athlete with knee pain should undergo tests for valgus and varus stress, Lachman test, and posterior drawer test), as discussed in Chapter 40.

SPORTS CLASSIFICATION

Sports are classified on the basis of the likelihood of collision injury and the strenuousness of the exercise. These classifications are used to guide physicians on the risk of injury and the degree of cardiopulmonary fitness required to successfully engage in the sport. The American Academy of Pediatrics has established classification guidelines by contact and intensity (**Table 5.5** and **Figure 5.3**).

CLEARANCE TO PLAY

Few athletes are disqualified from activity on the basis of conditions identified during the PPE. **Table 5.6**, which is designed to be understood by both medical and nonmedical personnel, lists the most current recommendations regarding medical conditions and contraindications to participation. It is important to work with athletes to find safe, enjoyable sports that they can participate in. If possible, and depending on the condition that is detected, sports participation should not be eliminated altogether. For athletes with specific cardiac conditions, refer to Chapter 19. **Figure 5.4** provides a sample clearance to return to play form.

Occasionally, an athlete or parent will disagree with a physician's recommendation for restricting participation in a particular sport. The parent and the athlete can decide to let the athlete play "against the medical advice" of the physician. In these cases, it is important to fully explain the reasons for the recommendation and to consider having the athlete and parent sign a document acknowledging that this discussion occurred and that they were informed of the risks. Athletes who request a second opinion should be encouraged to do so. Ultimately, the team physician is responsible for ensuring that athletes are able to participate safely and without undue risk of injury.

SPECIAL CONSIDERATIONS

Nutritional Supplements

Sports supplements have become a billion-dollar industry. Athletes as young as 11 years are taking performance-enhancing supplements. Sports supplements contain impurities, and when taken inappropriately, they may result in adverse side effects. Side effects can include muscle cramps, dehydration, abdominal bloating, tachycardia, arrhythmia, and even death. Supplement use should be discouraged. If a young athlete is taking supplements, he or

TABLE 5.5

Classification of Sports According to Contact

Contact	Limited Contact	Noncontact
Basketball	Adventure racing[a]	Badminton
Boxing[b]	Baseball	Bodybuilding[c]
Cheerleading	Bicycling	Bowling
Diving	Canoeing or kayaking (white water)	Canoeing or kayaking (flat water)
Extreme sports[d]	Fencing	Crew or rowing
Field hockey	Field events	Curling
Football, tackle	High jump	Dance
Gymnastics	Pole vault	Field events
Ice hockey[e]	Floor hockey	Discus
Lacrosse	Football, flag or touch	Javelin
Martial arts[f]	Handball	Shot put
Rodeo	Horseback riding	Golf
Rugby	Martial arts[f]	Orienteering[g]
Skiing, downhill	Racquetball	Power lifting[c]
Ski jumping	Skating	Race walking
Snowboarding	Ice	Riflery
Soccer	Inline	Rope jumping
Team handball	Roller	Running
Ultimate Frisbee	Skiing	Sailing
Water polo	Cross-country	Scuba diving
Wrestling	Water	Swimming
	Skateboarding	Table tennis
	Softball	Tennis
	Squash	Track
	Volleyball	
	Weight lifting	
	Windsurfing or surfing	

[a]Adventure racing has been added since the previous statement was published and is defined as a combination of two or more disciplines, including orientation and navigation, cross-country running, mountain biking, paddling, and climbing and rope skills.
[b]The American Academy of Pediatrics opposes participation in boxing for children, adolescents, and young adults.[2]
[c]The American Academy of Pediatrics recommends limiting bodybuilding and power lifting until the adolescent achieves sexual maturity rating 5 (Tanner stage V).
[d]Extreme sports has been added since the previous statement was published.
[e]The American Academy of Pediatrics recommends limiting the amount of body checking allowed for hockey players 15 years and younger, to reduce injuries.
[f]Martial arts can be subclassified as judo, jujitsu, karate, kung fu, and tae kwon do; some forms are contact sports and others are limited-contact sports.
[g]Orienteering is a race (contest) in which competitors use a map and a compass to find their way through unfamiliar territory.

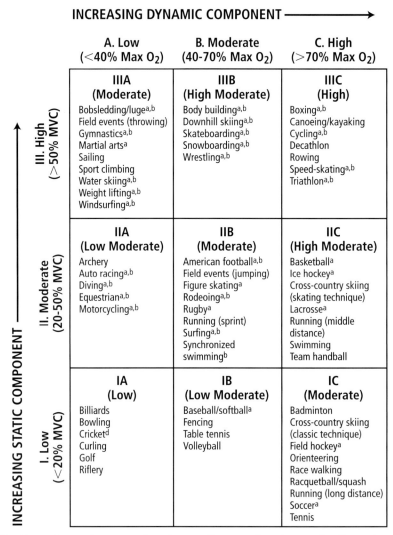

INCREASING DYNAMIC COMPONENT ———→

	A. Low (<40% Max O$_2$)	**B. Moderate** (40-70% Max O$_2$)	**C. High** (>70% Max O$_2$)
III. High (>50% MVC)	**IIIA** **(Moderate)** Bobsledding/luge[a,b] Field events (throwing) Gymnastics[a,b] Martial arts[a] Sailing Sport climbing Water skiing[a,b] Weight lifting[a,b] Windsurfing[a,b]	**IIIB** **(High Moderate)** Body building[a,b] Downhill skiing[a,b] Skateboarding[a,b] Snowboarding[a,b] Wrestling[a,b]	**IIIC** **(High)** Boxing[a,b] Canoeing/kayaking Cycling[a,b] Decathlon Rowing Speed-skating[a,b] Triathlon[a,b]
II. Moderate (20-50% MVC)	**IIA** **(Low Moderate)** Archery Auto racing[a,b] Diving[a,b] Equestrian[a,b] Motorcycling[a,b]	**IIB** **(Moderate)** American football[a,b] Field events (jumping) Figure skating[a] Rodeoing[a,b] Rugby[a] Running (sprint) Surfing[a,b] Synchronized swimming[b]	**IIC** **(High Moderate)** Basketball[a] Ice hockey[a] Cross-country skiing (skating technique) Lacrosse[a] Running (middle distance) Swimming Team handball
I. Low (<20% MVC)	**IA** **(Low)** Billiards Bowling Cricket[d] Curling Golf Riflery	**IB** **(Low Moderate)** Baseball/softball[a] Fencing Table tennis Volleyball	**IC** **(Moderate)** Badminton Cross-country skiing (classic technique) Field hockey[a] Orienteering Race walking Racquetball/squash Running (long distance) Soccer[a] Tennis

INCREASING STATIC COMPONENT ———↑

FIGURE 5.3 Classification of sports according to cardiovascular demands (based on combined static and dynamic components).* This classification is based on peak static and dynamic components achieved during competition. It should be noted, however, that the higher values may be reached during training. The increasing dynamic component is defined in terms of the estimated percentage of maximal oxygen uptake (Max O$_2$) achieved and results in increasing cardiac output. The increasing static component is related to the estimated percentage of maximal voluntary contraction (MVC) reached and results in increasing blood pressure load. Activities with the lowest total cardiovascular demands (cardiac output and blood pressure) are shown in Box IA, and those with the highest demands are shown in box IIIC. Boxes IIA and IB depict activities with low/moderate total cardiovascular demands; boxes IIIA, IIB, and IC depict high/moderate total cardiovascular demands. These categories progress diagonally across the graph from lower left to upper right.

[a] Danger of bodily collision

[b] Increased risk if syncope occurs.

[c] Participation is not recommended by the American Academy of Pediatrics.

[d] The American Academy of Pediatrics classifies cricket in the IB box (low static component and moderate dynamic component). (American Academy of Pediatrics. General physical activities defined by level of intensity. Available at: www.aap.org/sections/seniormembers/docs/Fit-actvsIntensity.pdf. Accessed October 2, 2007.)

* American College of Cardiology Foundation. 36th Bethesda Conference: eligibility recommendations for competitive athletes with cardiovascular abnormalities. *J Am Coll Cardiol*. 2005;45 (8):1313-1375.

Reproduced with permission from Mitchell JH, Haskell W, Snell P, Van Camp SP. 36th Bethesda Conference. Task force 8: classification of sports. *J Am Coll Cardiol*. 2005;45(8):1364-1367.

TABLE 5.6

Medical Conditions and Sports Participation

Condition	May Participate
Atlantoaxial instability (instability of the joint between cervical vertebrae 1 and 2)	Qualified yes
Explanation: Athlete (particularly if he or she has Down syndrome or juvenile rheumatoid arthritis with cervical involvement) needs evaluation to assess the risk of spinal cord injury during sports participation, especially when using a trampoline.[1-4]	
Bleeding disorder	Qualified yes
Explanation: Athlete needs evaluation.[5,6]	
Cardiovascular Disease	
Carditis (inflammation of the heart)	No
Explanation: Carditis may result in sudden death with exertion.	
Hypertension (high blood pressure)	Qualified yes
Explanation: Those with hypertension >5 mm Hg above the 99th percentile for age, gender, and height should avoid heavy weight lifting and power lifting, bodybuilding, and high-static component sports. Those with sustained hypertension (>95th percentile for age, gender, and height) need evaluation.[7-9] The National High Blood Pressure Education Program Working Group report defined prehypertension and stage 1 and stage 2 hypertension in children and adolescents younger than 18 years of age.[7]	
Congenital heart disease (structural heart defects present at birth)	Qualified yes
Explanation: Consultation with a cardiologist is recommended. Those who have mild forms may participate fully in most cases; those who have moderate or severe forms or who have undergone surgery need evaluation. The 36th Bethesda Conference[9] defined mild, moderate, and severe disease for common cardiac lesions.	
Dysrhythmia (irregular heart rhythm)	Qualified yes
Long-QT syndrome	
Malignant ventricular arrhythmias	
Symptomatic Wolff-Parkinson-White syndrome	
Advanced heart block	
Family history of sudden death or previous sudden cardiac event	
Implantation of a cardioverter-defibrillator	
Explanation: Consultation with a cardiologist is advised. Those with symptoms (chest pain, syncope, near-syncope, dizziness, shortness of breath, or other symptoms of possible dysrhythmia) or evidence of mitral regurgitation on physical examination need evaluation. All others may participate fully.[10-12]	
Heart murmur	Qualified yes
Explanation: If the murmur is innocent (does not indicate heart disease), full participation is permitted. Otherwise, athlete needs evaluation (see structural heart disease, especially hypertrophic cardiomyopathy and mitral valve prolapse).	
Structural/acquired heart disease	
Hypertrophic cardiomyopathy	Qualified no
Coronary artery anomalies	Qualified no
Arrhythmogenic right ventricular cardiomyopathy	Qualified no
Acute rheumatic fever with carditis	Qualified no
Ehlers-Danlos syndrome, vascular form	Qualified no
Marfan syndrome	Qualified yes
Mitral valve prolapse	Qualified yes
Anthracycline use	Qualified yes
Explanation: Consultation with a cardiologist is recommended. The 36th Bethesda Conference provided detailed recommendations.[9,10,12-15] Most of these conditions carry a significant risk of sudden cardiac death associated with intense physical exercise. Hypertrophic cardiomyopathy requires thorough and repeated evaluations, because disease may change manifestations during later adolescence.[9,10,14] Marfan syndrome with an aortic aneurysm also can cause sudden death during intense physical exercise.[15] Athlete who has ever received chemotherapy with anthracyclines may be at increased risk of cardiac problems because of the cardiotoxic effects of the medications, and resistance training in this population should be approached with caution; strength training that avoids isometric contractions may be permitted.[16,17] Athlete needs evaluation.	
Vasculitis/vascular disease	Qualified yes
Kawasaki disease (coronary artery vasculitis)	
Pulmonary hypertension	
Explanation: Consultation with a cardiologist is recommended. Athlete needs individual evaluation to assess risk on the basis of disease activity, pathologic changes, and medical regimen.[18]	

TABLE 5.6

Medical Conditions and Sports Participation—cont'd

Condition	May Participate
Cerebral palsy	Qualified yes
Explanation: Athlete needs evaluation to assess functional capacity to perform sports-specific activity.	
Diabetes mellitus	Yes
Explanation: All sports can be played with proper attention and appropriate adjustments to diet (particularly carbohydrate intake), blood glucose concentrations, hydration, and insulin therapy. Blood glucose concentrations should be monitored before exercise, every 30 min during continuous exercise, 15 min after completion of exercise, and at bedtime.	
Diarrhea, infectious	Qualified no
Explanation: Unless symptoms are mild and athlete is fully hydrated, no participation is permitted, because diarrhea may increase risk of dehydration and heat illness (see fever).	
Eating disorders	Qualified yes
Explanation: Athlete with an eating disorder needs medical and psychiatric assessment before participation.	
Eyes	Qualified yes
Functionally 1-eyed athlete	
Loss of an eye	
Detached retina or family history of retinal detachment at young age	
High myopia	
Connective tissue disorder, such as Marfan or Stickler syndrome	
Previous intraocular eye surgery or serious eye injury	
Explanation: A functionally 1-eyed athlete is defined as having best-corrected visual acuity worse than 20/40 in the poorer-seeing eye. Such an athlete would suffer significant disability if the better eye were seriously injured, as would an athlete with loss of an eye. Specifically, boxing and full-contact martial arts are not recommended for functionally 1-eyed athletes, because eye protection is impractical and/or not permitted. Some athletes who previously underwent intraocular eye surgery or had a serious eye injury may have increased risk of injury because of weakened eye tissue. Availability of eye guards approved by the American Society for Testing and Materials and other protective equipment may allow participation in most sports, but this must be judged on an individual basis.[19,20]	
Conjunctivitis, infectious	Qualified no
Explanation: Athlete with active infectious conjunctivitis should be excluded from swimming.	
Fever	No
Explanation: Elevated core temperature may be indicative of a pathologic medical condition (infection or disease) that is often manifest by increased resting metabolism and heart rate. Accordingly, during athlete's usual exercise regimen, the presence of fever can result in greater heat storage, decreased heat tolerance, increased risk of heat illness, increased cardiopulmonary effort, reduced maximal exercise capacity, and increased risk of hypotension because of altered vascular tone and dehydration. On rare occasions, fever may accompany myocarditis or other conditions that may make usual exercise dangerous.	
Gastrointestinal	Qualified yes
Malabsorption syndromes (celiac disease or cystic fibrosis)	
Explanation: Athlete needs individual assessment for general malnutrition or specific deficits resulting in coagulation or other defects; with appropriate treatment, these deficits can be treated adequately to permit normal activities.	
Short-bowel syndrome or other disorders requiring specialized nutritional support, including parenteral or enteral nutrition	
Explanation: Athlete needs individual assessment for collision, contact, or limited-contact sports. Presence of central or peripheral, indwelling, venous catheter may require special considerations for activities and emergency preparedness for unexpected trauma to the device(s).	
Heat illness, history of	Qualified yes
Explanation: Because of the likelihood of recurrence, athlete needs individual assessment to determine the presence of predisposing conditions and behaviors and to develop a prevention strategy that includes sufficient acclimatization (to the environment and to exercise intensity and duration), conditioning, hydration, and salt intake, as well as other effective measures to improve heat tolerance and to reduce heat injury risk (such as protective equipment and uniform configurations).[21,22]	
Hepatitis, infectious (primarily hepatitis C)	Yes
Explanation: All athletes should receive hepatitis B vaccination before participation. Because of the apparent minimal risk to others, all sports may be played as athlete's state of health allows. For all athletes, skin lesions should be covered properly, and athletic personnel should use universal precautions when handling blood or body fluids with visible blood.[23]	

Continued

TABLE 5.6

Medical Conditions and Sports Participation—cont'd

Condition	May Participate
HIV infection	Yes
Explanation: Because of the apparent minimal risk to others, all sports may be played as athlete's state of health allows (especially if viral load is undetectable or very low). For all athletes, skin lesions should be covered properly, and athletic personnel should use universal precautions when handling blood or body fluids with visible blood.[23] However, certain sports (such as wrestling and boxing) may create a situation that favors viral transmission (likely bleeding plus skin breaks). If viral load is detectable, then athletes should be advised to avoid such high-contact sports.	
Kidney, absence of one	Qualified yes
Explanation: Athlete needs individual assessment for contact, collision, and limited-contact sports. Protective equipment may reduce risk of injury to the remaining kidney sufficiently to allow participation in most sports, providing such equipment remains in place during activity.[19]	
Liver, enlarged	Qualified yes
Explanation: If the liver is acutely enlarged, then participation should be avoided because of risk of rupture. If the liver is chronically enlarged, then individual assessment is needed before collision, contact, or limited-contact sports are played. Patients with chronic liver disease may have changes in liver function that affect stamina, mental status, coagulation, or nutritional status.	
Malignant neoplasm	Qualified yes
Explanation: Athlete needs individual assessment.[24]	
Musculoskeletal disorders	Qualified yes
Explanation: Athlete needs individual assessment.	
Neurologic Disorders	
History of serious head or spine trauma or abnormality, including craniotomy, epidural bleeding, subdural hematoma, intracerebral hemorrhage, second-impact syndrome, vascular malformation, and neck fracture.[1,2,25-27]	Qualified yes
Explanation: Athlete needs individual assessment for collision, contact, or limited-contact sports.	
History of simple concussion (mild traumatic brain injury), multiple simple concussions, and/or complex concussion	Qualified yes
Explanation: Athlete needs individual assessment. Research supports a conservative approach to concussion management, including no athletic participation while symptomatic or when deficits in judgment or cognition are detected, followed by graduated return to full activity.[25-29]	
Myopathies	Qualified yes
Explanation: Athlete needs individual assessment.	
Recurrent headaches	Yes
Explanation: Athlete needs individual assessment.[30]	
Recurrent plexopathy (burner or stinger) and cervical cord neuropraxia with persistent defects	Qualified yes
Explanation: Athlete needs individual assessment for collision, contact, or limited-contact sports; regaining normal strength is important benchmark for return to play.[31,32]	
Seizure disorder, well controlled	Yes
Explanation: Risk of seizure during participation is minimal.[33]	
Seizure disorder, poorly controlled	Qualified yes
Explanation: Athlete needs individual assessment for collision, contact, or limited-contact sports. The following noncontact sports should be avoided: archery, riflery, swimming, weight lifting, power lifting, strength training, and sports involving heights. In these sports, occurrence of a seizure during activity may pose a risk to self or others.[33]	
Obesity	Yes
Explanation: Because of the increased risk of heat illness and cardiovascular strain, obese athlete particularly needs careful acclimatization (to the environment and to exercise intensity and duration), sufficient hydration, and potential activity and recovery modifications during competition and training.[34]	
Organ transplant recipient (and those taking immunosuppressive medications)	Qualified yes
Explanation: Athlete needs individual assessment for contact, collision, and limited-contact sports. In addition to potential risk of infections, some medications (eg, prednisone) may increase tendency for bruising.	
Ovary, absence of one	Yes
Explanation: Risk of severe injury to remaining ovary is minimal.	
Pregnancy/postpartum	Qualified yes
Explanation: Athlete needs individual assessment. As pregnancy progresses, modifications to usual exercise routines will become necessary. Activities with high risk of falling or abdominal trauma should be avoided. Scuba diving and activities posing risk of altitude sickness should also be avoided during pregnancy. After the birth, physiological and morphologic changes of pregnancy take 4 to 6 weeks to return to baseline.[35,36]	

TABLE 5.6

Medical Conditions and Sports Participation—cont'd

Condition	May Participate
Respiratory Conditions	
Pulmonary compromise, including cystic fibrosis	Qualified yes
Explanation: Athlete needs individual assessment but, generally, all sports may be played if oxygenation remains satisfactory during graded exercise test. Athletes with cystic fibrosis need acclimatization and good hydration to reduce risk of heat illness.	
Asthma	Yes
Explanation: With proper medication and education, only athletes with severe asthma need to modify their participation. For those using inhalers, recommend having a written action plan and using a peak flowmeter daily.[37-40] Athletes with asthma may encounter risks when scuba diving.	
Acute upper respiratory infection	Qualified yes
Explanation: Upper respiratory obstruction may affect pulmonary function. Athlete needs individual assessment for all except mild disease (see fever).	
Rheumatologic diseases	Qualified yes
Juvenile rheumatoid arthritis	
Explanation: Athletes with systemic or polyarticular juvenile rheumatoid arthritis and history of cervical spine involvement need radiographs of vertebrae C1 and C2 to assess risk of spinal cord injury. Athletes with systemic or HLA-B27–associated arthritis require cardiovascular assessment for possible cardiac complications during exercise. For those with micrognathia (open bite and exposed teeth), mouth guards are helpful. If uveitis is present, risk of eye damage from trauma is increased; ophthalmologic assessment is recommended. If visually impaired, guidelines for functionally 1-eyed athletes should be followed.[41]	
Juvenile dermatomyositis, idiopathic myositis	
Systemic lupus erythematosus	
Raynaud phenomenon	
Explanation: Athlete with juvenile dermatomyositis or systemic lupus erythematosus with cardiac involvement requires cardiology assessment before participation. Athletes receiving systemic corticosteroid therapy are at higher risk of osteoporotic fractures and avascular necrosis, which should be assessed before clearance; those receiving immunosuppressive medications are at higher risk of serious infection. Sports activities should be avoided when myositis is active. Rhabdomyolysis during intensive exercise may cause renal injury in athletes with idiopathic myositis and other myopathies. Because of photosensitivity with juvenile dermatomyositis and systemic lupus erythematosus, sun protection is necessary during outdoor activities. With Raynaud phenomenon, exposure to the cold presents risk to hands and feet.[42-45]	
Sickle cell disease	Qualified yes
Explanation: Athlete needs individual assessment. In general, if illness status permits, all sports may be played; however, any sport or activity that entails overexertion, overheating, dehydration, or chilling should be avoided. Participation at high altitude, especially when not acclimatized, also poses risk of sickle cell crisis.	
Sickle cell trait	Yes
Explanation: Athletes with sickle cell trait generally do not have increased risk of sudden death or other medical problems during athletic participation under normal environmental conditions. However, when high exertional activity is performed under extreme conditions of heat and humidity or increased altitude, such catastrophic complications have occurred rarely.[5,46-49] Athletes with sickle cell trait, like all athletes, should be progressively acclimatized to the environment and to the intensity and duration of activities and should be sufficiently hydrated to reduce the risk of exertional heat illness and/or rhabdomyolysis.[22] According to National Institutes of Health management guidelines, sickle cell trait is not a contraindication to participation in competitive athletics, and there is no requirement for screening before participation.[50] More research is needed to assess fully potential risks and benefits of screening athletes for sickle cell trait.	
Skin infections, including herpes simplex, molluscum contagiosum, verrucae (warts), staphylococcal and streptococcal infections (furuncles [boils], carbuncles, impetigo, methicillin-resistant Staphylococcus aureus [cellulitis and/or abscesses]), scabies, and tinea	Qualified yes
Explanation: During contagious periods, participation in gymnastics or cheerleading with mats, martial arts, wrestling, or other collision, contact, or limited-contact sports is not allowed.[51-54]	
Spleen, enlarged	Qualified yes
Explanation: If the spleen is acutely enlarged, then participation should be avoided because of risk of rupture. If the spleen is chronically enlarged, then individual assessment is needed before collision, contact, or limited-contact sports are played.	
Testicle, undescended or absence of one	Yes
Explanation: Certain sports may require a protective cup.[19]	

This table is designed for use by medical and nonmedical personnel. "Needs evaluation" means that a physician with appropriate knowledge and experience should assess the safety of a given sport for an athlete with the listed medical condition. Unless otherwise noted, this need for special consideration is because of variability in the severity of the disease, the risk of injury for specific sports listed in Table 5.5, or both.

1 American Academy of Pediatrics, Committee on Injury and Poison Prevention, Committee on Sports Medicine and Fitness. Trampolines at home, school, and recreational centers. *Pediatrics*. 1999;103(5):1053-1056.

2 Maranich AM, Hamele M, Fairchok MP. Atlanto-axial subluxation: a newly reported trampolining injury. *Clin Pediatr* (Phila). 2006;45 (5):468-470.

3 American Academy of Pediatrics, Committee on Sports Medicine and Fitness. Atlanto-axial instability in Down syndrome: subject review. *Pediatrics*. 1995;96 (1):151-154.

4 American Academy of Family Physicians, American Academy of Pediatrics, American College of Sports Medicine, American Medical Society for Sports Medicine, American Orthopaedic Society for Sports Medicine, American Osteopathic Academy of Sports Medicine. *Preparticipation Physical Evaluation*. 3rd ed. New York, NY: McGraw-Hill; 2004.

5 Mercer KW, Densmore JJ. Hematologic disorders in the athlete. *Clin Sports Med*. 2005;24 (3):599-621.

6 National Hemophilia Foundation. *Playing It Safe: Bleeding Disorders, Sports and Exercise*. New York, NY: National Hemophilia Foundation; 2005.

7 National High Blood Pressure Education Program Working Group on High Blood Pressure in Children and Adolescents. The fourth report on the diagnosis, evaluation, and treatment of high blood pressure in children and adolescents. *Pediatrics*. 2004;114 (2 suppl):555-576.

8 American Academy of Pediatrics, Committee on Sports Medicine and Fitness. Athletic participation by children and adolescents who have systemic hypertension. *Pediatrics*. 1997;99 (4):637-638.

9 American College of Cardiology Foundation. 36th Bethesda Conference: eligibility recommendations for competitive athletes with cardiovascular abnormalities. *J Am Coll Cardiol*. 2005;45 (8):1313-1375.

10 Maron BJ, Thompson PD, Ackerman MJ, et al. Recommendations and considerations related to preparticipation screening for cardiovascular abnormalities in competitive athletes: 2007 update: a scientific statement from the American Heart Association Council on Nutrition, Physical Activity and Metabolism: endorsed by the American College of Cardiology Foundation. *Circulation*. 2007;115 (12):1643-1655.

11 American Academy of Pediatrics, Committee on Sports Medicine and Fitness. Cardiac dysrhythmias and sports. *Pediatrics*. 1995;95 (5):786-788.

12 Freed LA, Levy D, Levine RA, et al. Prevalence and clinical outcome of mitral-valve prolapse. *N Engl J Med*. 1999;341 (1):1-7.

13 Maron BJ. Sudden death in young athletes. *N Engl J Med*. 2003;349 (11):1064-1075.

14 Maron BJ. Hypertrophic cardiomyopathy: a systematic review. *JAMA*. 2002;287 (10):1308-1320.

15 Pyeritz RE. The Marfan syndrome. *Annu Rev Med*. 2000;51 :481-510.

16 American Academy of Pediatrics, Council on Sports Medicine and Fitness. Strength training by children and adolescents. *Pediatrics*. 2008;121 (4):835-840.

17 Steinherz L, Steinherz P, Tan C, et al. Cardiac toxicity 4 to 20 years after completing anthracycline therapy. *JAMA*. 1991;266 (12):1672-1677.

18 Newburger JW, Takahashi M, Gerber MA, et al. Diagnosis, treatment, and long-term management of Kawasaki disease: a statement for health professionals from the Committee on Rheumatic Fever, Endocarditis, and Kawasaki Disease, Council on Cardiovascular Disease in the Young, American Heart Association. *Pediatrics*. 2004;114 (6):1708-1733.

19 Gomez JE. Paired organ loss. In: Delee JC, Drez D Jr, Miller MD, eds. *Delee and Drez's Orthopaedic Sports Medicine: Principles and Practice*. 2nd ed. Philadelphia, PA: Saunders; 2003:264-271.

20 American Academy of Pediatrics, Committee on Sports Medicine and Fitness. Protective eyewear for young athletes. *Pediatrics*. 2004;113 (3):619-622.

21 American Academy of Pediatrics, Committee on Sports Medicine and Fitness. Climatic heat stress and the exercising child and adolescent. *Pediatrics*. 2000;106 (1):158-159.

22 Bergeron MF, McKeag DB, Casa DJ, et al. Youth football: heat stress and injury risk. *Med Sci Sports Exerc*. 2005;37 (8):1421-1430.

23 American Academy of Pediatrics, Committee on Sports Medicine and Fitness. Human immunodeficiency virus and other blood-borne viral pathogens in the athletic setting. *Pediatrics*. 1999;104 (6):1400-1403.

24 Dickerman JD. The late effects of childhood cancer therapy. *Pediatrics*. 2007;119 (3):554-568.

25 Wojtys EM, Hovda D, Landry G, et al. Current concepts: concussion in sports. *Am J Sports Med*. 1999;27 (5):676-687.

26 McCrory P, Johnston K, Meeuwisse W, et al. Summary and agreement statement of the 2nd International Conference on Concussion in Sport, Prague 2004. *Clin J Sport Med*. 2005;15 (2):48-55.

27 Aubry M, Cantu R, Dvorak J, et al. Summary and agreement statement of the 1st International Symposium on Concussion in Sport, Vienna 2001. *Clin J Sport Med*. 2002;12 (1):6-11.

28 Herring SA, Bergfeld JA, Boland A, et al. Concussion (mild traumatic brain injury) and the team physician: a consensus statement. *Med Sci Sports Exerc*. 2006;38 (2):395-399.

29 Guskiewicz KM, Bruce SL, Cantu RC, et al. National Athletic Trainers' Association position statement: management of sport-related concussion. *J Athl Train*. 2004;39 (3):280-297.

30 Lewis DW, Ashwal S, Dahl G, et al. Practice parameter: evaluation of children and adolescents with recurrent headaches: report of the Quality Standards Subcommittee of the American Academy of Neurology and the Practice Committee of the Child Neurology Society. *Neurology*. 2002;59 (4):490-498.

31 Castro FP Jr. Stingers, cervical cord neuropraxia, and stenosis. Clin Sports Med. 2003;22 (3):483-492.

32 Weinberg J, Rokito S, Silber JS. Etiology, treatment, and prevention of athletic "stingers." *Clin Sports Med*. 2003;22 (3):493-500, viii.

33 Hirtz D, Berg A, Bettis D, et al. Practice parameter: treatment of the child with a first unprovoked seizure: report of the Quality Standards Subcommittee of the American Academy of Neurology and the Practice Committee of the Child Neurology Society. *Neurology*. 2003;60 (2):166-175.

34 American Academy of Pediatrics, Council on Sports Medicine and Fitness and Council on School Health. Active healthy living: prevention of childhood obesity through increased physical activity. *Pediatrics*. 2006;117 (5):1834-1842.

35 American College of Obstetricians and Gynecologists, Committee on Obstetric Practice. ACOG committee opinion: exercise during pregnancy and the postpartum period. *Obstet Gynecol*. 2002;99 (1):171-173.

36 Morales M, Dumps P, Extermann P. Pregnancy and scuba diving: what precautions? [in French]. *J Gynecol Obstet Biol Reprod* (Paris). 1999;28 (2):118-123.

37 National Heart, Lung, and Blood Institute. National Asthma Education and Prevention Program Expert Panel Report 3: *Guidelines for the Diagnosis and Management of Asthma: Full Report*. Bethesda, MD: National Institutes of Health; 2007. Available at: www.nhlbi.nih.gov/guidelines/asthma/asthupdt.htm. Accessed October 2, 2007.

38 American College of Allergy, Asthma, and Immunology. *Asthma Disease Management Resource Manual*. Arlington Heights, IL: American College of Allergy, Asthma, and Immunology. Available at: www.acaai.org/Member/Practice_Resources/manual.htm. Accessed November 17, 2006.

39 Storms WW. Review of exercise-induced asthma. *Med Sci Sports Exerc*. 2003;35 (9):1464-1470.

40 Holzer K, Brukner P. Screening of athletes for exercise-induced bronchospasm. *Clin J Sport Med*. 2004;14 (3):134-138.

41 Giannini MJ, Protas EJ. Exercise response in children with and without juvenile rheumatoid arthritis: a case-comparison study. *Phys Ther*. 1992;72 (5):365-372.

42 Tench C, Bentley D, Vleck V, McCurdie I, White P, D'Cruz D. Aerobic fitness, fatigue, and physical disability in systemic lupus erythematosus. *J Rheumatol*. 2002;29 (3):474-481.

43 Carvalho MR, Sato EI, Tebexreni AS, Heidecher RT, Schenckman S, Neto TL. Effects of supervised cardiovascular training program on exercise tolerance, aerobic capacity, and quality of life in patients with systemic lupus erythematosis. *Arthritis Rheum*. 2005;53 (6):838-844.

44 Hicks JE, Drinkard B, Summers RM, Rider LG. Decreased aerobic capacity in children with juvenile dermatomyositis. *Arthritis Rheum*. 2002;47 (2):118-123.

45 Clarkson PM, Kearns AK, Rouzier P, Rubin R, Thompson PD. Serum creatine kinase levels and renal function measures in exertional muscle damage. *Med Sci Sports Exerc*. 2006;38 (4):623-627.

46 Pretzlaff RK. Death of an adolescent athlete with sickle cell trait caused by exertional heat stroke. *Pediatr Crit Care Med*. 2002;3 (3):308-310.

47 Kark J. Sickle Cell Trait. Washington, DC: Howard University School of Medicine; 2000. Available at: http://sickle.bwh.harvard.edu/sickle_trait.html. Accessed November 17, 2006.

48 Kerle KK, Nishimura KD. Exertional collapse and sudden death associated with sickle cell trait. *Am Fam Physician*. 1996;54 (1):237-240.

49 Bergeron MF, Cannon JG, Hall EL, Kutlar A. Erythrocyte sickling during exercise and thermal stress. *Clin J Sport Med*. 2004;14 (6):354-356.

50 National Heart, Lung, and Blood Institute. The Management of Sickle Cell Disease. 4th ed. Bethesda, MD: National Institutes of Health; 2002:15-18. NIH publication 02-2117.

51 Mast EE, Goodman RA. Prevention of infectious disease transmission in sports. *Sports Med*. 1997;24 (1):1-7.

52 Sevier TL. Infectious disease in athletes. *Med Clin North Am*. 1994;78 (2):389-412.

53 Centers for Disease Control and Prevention. Methicillin-resistant Staphylococcus aureus infections among competitive sports participants: Colorado, Indiana, Pennsylvania, and Los Angeles County, 2000-2003. *MMWR Morb Mortal Wkly Rep*. 2003;52 (33):793-795. Available at: www.cdc.gov/mmwr/preview/mmwrhtml/mm5233a4.htm. Accessed November 17, 2006.

54 Centers for Disease Control and Prevention. Community-associated MRSA information for clinicians. Available at: www.cdc.gov/ncidod/dhqp/ar_mrsa_ca_clinicians.html. Accessed November 17, 2006.

Source: American Academy of Pediatrics, Council on Sports Medicine and Fitness. Medical conditions affecting sports participation. *Pediatrics*. 2008, 121:841-848.

Clearance to Return to Play

Name _____ Date _____

Diagnosis _____

May return to: ☐ Full participation in _____ on _____
(sport or activity)   (date)

☐ Limited participation (with the following restrictions):
_____

☐ Not cleared to participate until _____

Special Instructions:

General conditioning exercises that can be continued during recovery:
_____

Rehabilitation exercises:_____

Recommendation for taping, pads, and/or protective equipment:
_____

Medications (or other treatments) that may need to be taken during school or available at practice/games:
_____

Suggested number of practices to complete before returning to games or competition: _____

Medical follow-up with: _____ Date: _____

Physician name _____ Phone _____

Address _____

Signature _____

FIGURE 5.4 Sample clearance for return to play form.

she should be told about their possible ill effects. The PPE is an ideal time to briefly question athletes about supplement use.

Obesity

Childhood obesity has reached epidemic proportions. As many as 30% of children are obese, and many of these youngsters are seeking to participate in sports. Obesity is not a contraindication to sports participation unless there is a comorbid finding such as severe hypertension. Obese children are at increased risk of heat injury and should be counseled accordingly. Sports participation with emphasis on activities that improve fitness should be encouraged for the obese child.

Concussion

History of previous concussions should be addressed during the PPE. Consensus about concussion has been updated from the former 3 grades of severity to 2: simple and complicated. Complicated concussion includes amnesia, loss of consciousness, seizure, or prolonged symptoms. Neuropsychological testing is suggested with repeat concussion or complicated concussion. Patients must meet 3 criteria to return to play: asymptomatic at rest, asymptomatic with exercise, and no neurocognitive deficits (memory loss, concentration problems, fatigue, fogginess, confusion) (see Chapter 20, "Head Injuries").

The Medical Home

The single most underserved population in health care today is adolescents. Often, their only contact with the medical system is the PPE. However, it is important to refer all young athletes to a primary care provider for routine care and for follow-up of any ongoing medical conditions.

Electronic Version of the PPE

It is the goal to have an electronic version of the PPE available in the future for several reasons. First, there would be a standardized history and physical, so better data collection can be achieved. Second, athletes who graduate or move from one community to the next would be able to have a portable record. Finally, it could be used as a data base for clinical research regarding prediction of injury.

SUMMARY POINTS

- A PPE is performed to prevent injury and assess medical conditions; it is not performed primarily to disqualify an athlete.

- A PPE should ideally be performed by one physician, even if there is a mass screening.

- Sudden cardiac death in young athletes is a rare event, but a history of syncope or chest pain with exercise, or a family history of sudden death under age 50, should be evaluated.

- The musculoskeletal history and physical examination are the best ways to pick up on orthopedic problems.

- Concussion, heat injury, and use of nutritional supplements are topics that need to be discussed and emphasized during the PPE.

SUGGESTED READING

American Academy of Family Physicians, American Academy of Pediatrics, American College of Sports Medicine, American Medical Society for Sports Medicine, American Orthopaedic Society for Sports Medicine, American Osteopathic Academy of Sports Medicine. *The Preparticipation Physical Evaluation.* 3rd ed. Minneapolis, MN: McGraw-Hill; 2005.

American Academy of Pediatrics, Council on Sports Medicine and Fitness. Medical conditions affecting sports participation. *Pediatrics.* 2008;121:841-848.

American College of Cardiology Foundation. 36th Bethesda Conference: Eligibility recommendations for competitive athletes with cardiovascular abnormalities. *J Am Coll Cardiol.* 2005;45(8):1313–1375.

Corrado D, Basso C, Pavei A, Michieli P, Schiavon M, Thiene G. Trends in sudden cardiovascular death in young competitive athletes after implementation of a preparticipation screening program. *JAMA.* 2006;296:1593-1601.

Fahrenbach MC, Thompson PD. The preparticipation sports examination: cardiovascular considerations for screening. *Cardiol Clin.* 1992;10:319-328.

Glover DW, Maron BJ. Profile of preparticipation cardiovascular screening for high school athletes. *JAMA.* 1998;279:1817-1819.

Grafe MW, Paul GR, Foster TE. The preparticipation sports examination for high school and college athletes. *Clin Sports Med.* 1997;16:569-591.

Maron BJ, Thompson PD, Ackerman MJ, et al. Recommendations and considerations related to preparticipation screening for cardiovascular abnormalities in competitive athletes: 2007 update: A scientific statement from the American Heart Associations Council on Nutrition, Physical Activity, and Metabolism:

Endorsed by the American College of Cardiology Foundation. *Circulation.* 2007;115(12):1643-1655.

McCrory P, Johnston K, Meeuwisse WH, et al. Summary and agreement statement of the 2nd International Conference on Concussion in Sport, Prague 2004. *Br J Sports Med.* 2005;39:196-204.

Mitten MJ, Maron BJ, Zipes DP. Task Force 12: legal aspects of the 36th Bethesda Conference recommendations. *J Am Coll Cardiol.* 2005;45:1373-1375.

Smith DM, Kovan JR, Rich BSE, Tanner SM, eds. *Preparticipation Physical Evaluation.* 2nd ed. Minneapolis, MN: McGraw-Hill; 1997.

Wingfield K, Matheson GO, Meeuwisse WH. Preparticipation evaluation: an evidence-based review. *Clin J Sport Med.* 2004;14:109-122.

SECTION 2

Training Issues

CHAPTER 6

Aerobic and Anaerobic Trainability

Thomas W. Rowland, MD

The athlete who engages in a program of repeated bouts of exercise supposes that this physical training will result in favorable anatomic and physiologic adaptations, which in turn will lead to improvement in sports performance. Indeed, this is the essence of athletic training: improvements in function as body tissues and organ systems respond to the stresses of repeated exercise. These alterations are highly sport specific: the distance runner needs to place endurance loads on the cardiovascular system, for example, while the power lifter must emphasize maximum force production to improve skeletal muscle strength.

The characteristics and training regimens necessary to evoke these improvements have been well described in adults. There is some evidence, however, that certain aspects of physiologic responses to physical training may be different in youth, particularly before the age of puberty. Recognizing such variations in training responses may be important because these differences could dictate appropriate training regimens for children.

Indeed, there are a number of interesting and pertinent questions surrounding athletic training in children. How much of a child athlete's improvements as he or she grows are related to training and how much to genetic-based capabilities? Can (or how can) these abilities be detected in the young child destined for sports stardom? Children normally improve in motor performance (ie, endurance run times, muscle grip strength) as they grow even without any training at all. So what is the purpose of athletic training in children—to enhance ultimate performance ability? Or simply to accelerate the rate of improvement over time to an already genetically determined ceiling? The answers to these questions, which clearly have implications for applying appropriate training models in youth, are currently unclear.

This chapter focuses on what is known about the physiologic responses to exercise training in children in 2 realms: activities that use aerobic metabolic pathways for energy utilization (endurance running, swimming) and those that rely on anaerobic metabolism (short-burst activities such as sprints). Information is reviewed that considers whether these responses differ from those in adults and how they may affect field performance.

AEROBIC TRAINABILITY

Endurance exercise is not typical of the daily activities of children. Still, considerable research has focused on aerobic fitness in this age group as a result of the increasing involvement by prepubertal athletes in intensive endurance training regimens and as a result of the possible health implications of cardiovascular fitness in this age group.

Physiologic Fitness

The greatest amount of oxygen that one's body can use to support endurance exercise is termed maximal oxygen uptake, or $\dot{V}o_2max$. $\dot{V}o_2max$ is determined by measuring expired gases during a treadmill or cycle exercise test, and it is the single best physiologic indicator of aerobic fitness. It represents the combined peak function of the many components of the oxygen delivery chain (lungs, heart, blood volume, muscle enzyme capacity) and is closely associated with performance in endurance activities in both adults and children.

$\dot{V}o_2max$ normally improves as children age as a consequence of growth of the contributors to oxygen delivery, most particularly the heart, lungs, and skeletal muscle mass. The 6-year-old boy with an absolute $\dot{V}o_2max$ of 1.2 L min^{-1} will have a value of 2.7 L min^{-1} at age 12. Values for girls are generally about 200 mL min^{-1} lower at any given age before puberty. When expressed relative to body mass, $\dot{V}o_2$max on treadmill testing remains stable in boys throughout the childhood years (about 50 mL kg^{-1} min^{-1}), but it decreases progressively in girls from an average of 48 mL kg^{-1} min^{-1} at age 8 years to 42 mL kg^{-1} min^{-1}. These sex differences are largely an expression of variations in body composition (ie, greater lean body mass and lower body fat in boys).

Training Effects

When a previously sedentary adult is placed in a moderately intense endurance exercise program 3 times a week for 2 or 3 months, the functional capacity of these components improves, and $\dot{V}o_2$max typically increases by 15% to 30%. This aerobic fitness effect is expected to result in improvements in endurance events. Typically, the degree of training-induced increase in $\dot{V}o_2$max is inversely related to the pretraining level—that is, those with poorer aerobic fitness to start with will improve more.

But this physiologic response to endurance training seems to be blunted in prepubertal boys and girls. Among the many training studies that have been performed in young children (using a program originally designed for adults), some have failed to demonstrate a change in $\dot{V}o_2$max (**Table 6.1**). Overall, the average improvement in physiologic aerobic fitness has averaged about 5%.

The existence of a ceiling for aerobic trainability in children is supported by findings that values of $\dot{V}o_2$max in trained child endurance athletes are typically less than those observed in adult athletes (**Figure 6.1**). In addition, the difference between $\dot{V}o_2$max in child athletes and nonathletes is smaller than that between trained and untrained adults.

Effects of Growth

As a result of physiologic changes during growth, $\dot{V}o_{2max}$ and many of its determinants normally improve as a child ages, even if he or she avoids physical activity altogether

TABLE 6.1

Recent Studies Examining Changes in $\dot{V}o_2$max in Response to Endurance Training in Prepubertal Children

Study	Subjects, n	Sex	Duration, wk	$\dot{V}o_{2max}$ Change, %
McManus AM, Cheung CH, Leung MP, Yung TC, MacFarlane DJ. Improving aerobic power in primary school boys: a comparison of continuous and interval training. Int J Sports Med. 2005;26:781-786.	10	M	8	7.5
George KP, Gates PE, Tolfrey K. The impact of aerobic training upon left ventricular morphology and function in pre-pubescent children. Ergonomics. 2005;48:1378-1389.	25	F	12	NS*
Obert P, Mandigout S, Nottin S, Vinet A, N'Guyen L-D, Lecoq A-M. Cardiovascular response to endurance training in children: effect of gender. Eur J Clin Invest. 2003;33:199-208.	19	M, F	13	15, 8
McManus AM, Armstrong N, Williams CA. Effects of training on the anaerobic power and anaerobic performance of prepubertal girls. Acta Paediatr. 1997;86:456-459.	12	F	8	7.8
Welsman JR, Armstrong N, Withers S. Responses of young girls to two modes of aerobic training. Br J Sports Med. 1997;31:139-142.	17	F	8	NS*
Tolfrey K, Campbell IG, Batterham AM. Aerobic trainability of prepubertal boys and girls. Pediatr. Exerc. Science. 1998;10:248-263.	12, 14	M, F	12	NS,* 7.9
Rowland TW, Martel L, Vanderburgh P, Manos T, Charkoudian N. The influence of short-term aerobic training on blood lipids in healthy 10-12 year old children. Int J Sports Med. 1996;17:487-492.	31	M, F	13	5.4
Ignicio AA, Mahon AD. The effects of a physical fitness program on low-fit children. Res Q Exerc Sport. 1995;66:85-90.	18	M, F	10	NS*
Yoshizawa S, Honda H, Nakamura N, Itoh K, Watanabe N. Effects of an 18-month endurance run training program on maximal aerobic power in 4- to 6-year old girls. Pediatr Exer Science. 1997;9:33-43.	8	F	72	18.9
Mobert J, Koch G, Humplik O, Oyen E-M. Cardiovascular adjustment to supine and seated postures: effects of physical training. In: Children and exercise XII. S. Oseid and K-H Carlsen (eds). Champaign, IL: Human Kinetics. 1989, p. 165-182.	12	M	28	12.2

* NS indicates no significant change.

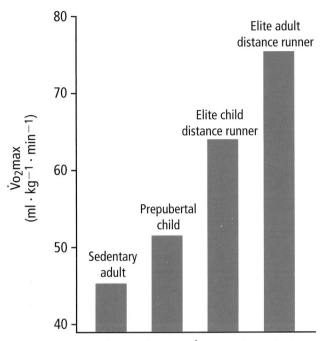

FIGURE 6.1 Typical values of $\dot{V}O_2$max in untrained children and adults (males) compared with endurance-trained athletes. From T.W. Rowland, 1990, Exercise and Children's Health, page 57, figure 4.6. © 1990 by Thomas W. Rowland. Reprinted with permission from Human Kinetics (Champaign, IL).

TABLE 6.2

Comparison of Expected Responses to a Period of Endurance Training and Those Occurring with Normal Growth and Development during Childhood

Response	Normal Growth	Aerobic Training
Maximal oxygen uptake $\dot{V}O_2$max	+	+
Maximal cardiac output	+	+
Maximal minute ventilation	+	+
Maximal arterial venous oxygen difference	0	0
Maximal heart rate	0	0
Submaximal energy economy	+	0/+
Lower resting, submaximal heart rate	+	+
Blood volume	+	+

+ indicates increases; 0 indicates no change.

(**Table 6.2**). Changes in aerobic fitness observed in response to a period of endurance training, then, must be distinguished from those that are normally expected with growth and development.

Effects of Habitual Activity

The explanation and implications of this dampened $\dot{V}O_2$max response to endurance training in prepubertal children remain problematic. Some have considered that the high daily physical activity of children, compared with adults, provides a training stimulus, and therefore less improvement will be observed when a child begins a formal training program. This is unlikely, however, because the short-burst characteristics of daily activity are not expected to trigger aerobic physiologic responses. In addition, little association exists between level of habitual physical activity and $\dot{V}O_2$max in children.

Duration of Training

It may be that the duration of training needs to be longer in children. This is suggested by the observation that the three longest training studies in prepubertal children (15, 18, and 72 weeks) triggered the highest responses in $\dot{V}O_2$max change (+10.3%, +12.2%, and +18.9%, respectively). Why such a maturity-related difference should exist, however, is unknown.

Biological Limitations

It is possible that biological differences account for children's dampened $\dot{V}O_2$max response to aerobic training, although this is hard to assess because the basic mechanisms underlying the aerobic fitness effect are not well understood. Sexual maturation may influence aerobic trainability. Interest has therefore focused on the potential effects of endocrine changes at the time of puberty. For instance, both estrogen and testosterone, which increase at sexual maturation, influence plasma volume. Autonomic differences between children and adults might modulate heart rate responses to training. Possible maturational differences in vascular conductance, muscle capillarization, and skeletal muscle pump function also need to considered. In addition, animal studies indicate that the magnitude of improvements in skeletal muscle aerobic enzyme activity with physical training are directly related to body size, although no research has yet directly examined these possibilities in a human model.

Genetic Influences

In adults, genetic influences clearly contribute to the magnitude of $\dot{V}O_2$max response to training. Whether these inherent controls operate during childhood is unknown. A considerable variation in $\dot{V}O_2$max response to training is observed in children, as it is in adults. In one study, 12 weeks of endurance training in prepubertal children resulted in changes $\dot{V}O_2$max in that varied from −3% to +21%.

Association between Endurance Training, $\dot{V}o_2$max, and Endurance Performance

It is not clear whether the dampened responses of $\dot{V}o_2$max with endurance training in children before puberty mean that children have an inferior ability to improve in endurance performance. Although $\dot{V}o_2$max plays a key role in determining such performance, other factors, such as exercise economy, substrate utilization, and aerobic enzyme capacity, are also important. During the normal course of childhood, endurance performance improves dramatically (ie, 1-mile run times in boys shorten by half between ages 5 and 15 years), as does running economy (energy needed to run a particular speed), with no improvements in size-adjusted $\dot{V}o_2$max (**Figure 6.2**). Studies addressing performance changes with training are confounded by a large variety of factors, such as normal improvements with growth, adaptation of running skills (ie, pacing and strategy), motivation, and environmental factors. The key question of whether children can substantially improve endurance running, bicycling, or swimming performance with training beyond the normal improvements that come with growth remains unanswered.

Implications for Endurance Training Programs

Important implications exist for the design of endurance training programs for prepubertal athletes. If aerobic trainability—both physiologic changes and improved performance—is limited in this age group, it would make better sense for training regimens in child athletes to focus on skill and strategy rather than training volume. This is particularly important considering the possible physical and psychological risks of high-volume intensive training in youth. Clarification of the issue of aerobic trainability in prepubertal athletes awaits future research information.

ANAEROBIC TRAINABILITY

Physiologic Fitness

Performance on short-burst activities lasting from a few seconds to 1 to 2 minutes, which rely predominantly on glycolytic metabolic energy pathways, are expressions of anaerobic fitness. Unlike aerobic fitness, there is no primary physiologic indicator of anaerobic capacity, and anaerobic fitness has been defined by biochemical markers (eg, lactate production), short all-out exercise tests (eg, Wingate 30-second test), and field performance (eg, sprints) (**Table 6.3**). Interestingly, although short-burst exercise is typical of their daily activity patterns, children demonstrate low levels of anaerobic fitness by all these markers, although such fitness improves as they grow.

Effects of Training

A period of high-intensity training in adults has been reported to increase anaerobic enzyme activity, fast-twitch muscle size, lactate production, and performance in short-burst activities. Whether prepubertal children can similarly improve anaerobic fitness with training depends on what is being considered. Biochemically, a period of highly intense training in youth typically causes no changes in exercise-induced blood lactate levels, although the activity of glycolytic enzymes may improve. Small (3%-8%) enhancements in power production during the Wingate cycling test have been reported in children after training. Plyometric (jumping) performance of children has been shown to improve with training, as has high-intensity treadmill running. But no changes have been observed in swim or field sprint times after training.

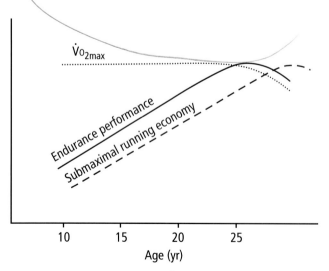

FIGURE 6.2 Changes in $\dot{V}o_2$max (maximal oxygen uptake), endurance performance, and running economy with age. From T.W. Rowland, 1990, Exercise and Children's Health, page 56, figure 4.5. © 1990 by Thomas W. Rowland. Reprinted with permission from Human Kinetics (Champaign, IL).

TABLE 6.3

Markers of Anaerobic Fitness

- Anaerobic enzyme activity
- Lactate production
- Fast-twitch muscle fiber population
- Short-burst all-out cycle tests (Wingate test)
- Sprint performance

Sex effects on anaerobic trainability in children have not been studied. All of these investigations are hampered by the lack of a clearly defined standard for frequency, duration, and intensity in anaerobic training regimens.

important for people who coach young athletes because differences in aerobic and anaerobic trainability in children might influence training regimens specifically designed for this age group.

SUMMARY POINTS

- Maximal oxygen uptake $\dot{V}o_2$max and its many determinants normally improve as a child ages, regardless of level of physical activity.

- The effects of endurance training on aerobic fitness must be distinguished from improvements that are expected on the basis of growth alone.

- Physiologic responses to a period of aerobic and anaerobic training may differ in immature athletes compared with their adult counterparts, but the nature and extent of these maturity-related variations are unclear.

- Physiologic aerobic adaptations to endurance exercise training, as manifested by changes in $\dot{V}o_2$max, are typically less in prepubertal children than in young adults.

- It is unclear whether anaerobic (short-burst activity) fitness in children can be improved with training compared with adults.

- The implications of physiologic differences in response to training with respect to performance outcomes remain to be determined. This issue is particularly

SUGGESTED READING

Katch VL. Physical conditioning of children. *J Adolesc Health Care.* 1983;3:241-246.

Obert P, Mandigout S, Nottin S, Vinet A, N'Guyen LD, Lecoq AM. Cardiovascular response to endurance training in children. Effect of gender. *Eur J Clin Invest.* 2003;33:199-208.

Payne VG, Morrow JR. The effect of physical training on prepubescent $\dot{V}o_2$max: a meta-analysis. *Res Q Exerc Sport.* 1993;64:305-313.

Rowland TW. Aerobic response to endurance training in prepubescent children: a critical analysis. *Med Sci Sports Exerc.* 1985;17:493-497.

Tolfrey K, Campbell IG, Batterham AM. Aerobic trainability of prepubertal boys and girls. *Pediatr Exerc Sci.* 1998;10:248-263.

Van Praagh E. Development of anaerobic function during childhood and adolescence. *Pediatr Exerc Sci.* 2000;12:150-173.

CHAPTER 7

Strength Training

Teri M. McCambridge, MD

Although strength training was formerly discouraged in preadolescents because of concerns about injury to the developing skeleton, this activity is now considered safe and appropriate for adolescents and preadolescents. Before embarking on a strength training program, the athlete's expectations need to be in line with the results: children will experience an improvement in strength but not an increase in bulk. Medical providers need to be comfortable discussing the risks, benefits, and essential components of a strength training program in preadolescents and adolescents. Physicians should also counsel athletes and their parents on reputable organizations that provide strength training certification so that they can ensure that the coaches are qualified to teach proper technique and can design age-appropriate exercise progressions.

In the early 1980s, strength training was discouraged in the preadolescent by the leading sports medicine authorities within the American Academy of Pediatrics (AAP) because of theoretical risks to the developing skeleton, such as loss of flexibility, risks of growth plate arrest, and stunted linear growth, and because there was insufficient evidence for significant strength gains. However, studies conducted in the early 1990s demonstrated strength gains of 30% to 50% in the preadolescent. These gains are above and beyond the gains associated with normal growth and development and are seen in both boys and girls. **Table 7.1** lists the common myths associated with youth strength training.

DEFINITIONS

Strength training (also known as resistance training) is a specialized form of conditioning used to increase the ability to exert or resist a force. The resistance can be supplied by

TABLE 7.1
Common Myths Associated with Strength Training in Youth

Myth	Reality
It is dangerous to the immature skeleton.	In a properly designed program with proper supervision, there have been no reports of epiphyseal injuries. Research has demonstrated it is safer than contact sports such as soccer, football, and basketball.
Participation will decrease flexibility.	Research has refuted this claim and has demonstrated that incorporation of a stretching program into the weight program has resulted in improved flexibility.
No significant strength changes will be achieved until adolescence.	Studies have reproducibly demonstrated strength gains in the preadolescent of 30% to 50% above normal growth and development with a program of proper duration, intensity, frequency, and progression.

one's own weight, elastic bands or tubing, free weights, or weight machines. There are benefits and drawbacks for each type of resistance. For example, free weights are cheap and permit intensity modifications with small weight increments, but their use requires qualified spotters and the ability to balance, which is hard for younger children. In contrast, weight machines do not require spotters or good balance, but they are sized for adults, and weights typically increase in large 5- or 10-pound increments.

The AAP's Council on Sports Medicine and Fitness supports strength training in children and adolescents as an adjunct to youth fitness programs, conditioning for sports programs, health promotion, and injury prevention. However, the AAP does not condone youth participation in Olympic weight lifting, power lifting, or bodybuilding until full skeletal and developmental maturity have been reached (Tanner stage 5). (See **Table 7.2** for definitions of these activities.) These events are competitive, and they require ballistic maneuvers through extremes of joint motion and 1-repetition maximums. These events may affect the immature skeleton, especially the spine, if lifting is performed improperly. Children who participate may also be tempted to use anabolic steroids in an attempt to achieve proper muscle definition and size.

SAFETY

Concerns regarding the safety of weight training for children arose after data from the Consumer Product Safety Commission National Electronic Injury Surveillance System (NEISS) reported about 20,500 injuries related to weight lifting equipment from 1978 to 1998. Children younger than 6 years old had 6 times the injury risk of the other age groups when they used home weight equipment.

However, the applicability of these findings to strength training safety is questionable because the data from the NEISS do not distinguish between strength training and competitive forms of weight lifting, bodybuilding, and power lifting, or between supervised and unsupervised injuries. Nor did the NEISS assess whether the weight

equipment was used properly. Well-supervised and well-designed strength training programs have a lower injury rate compared with contact sports such as football.

BENEFITS

Reasons for beginning a strength training program are many. Obvious goals include strength enhancement, improved body composition, and improved physique. Preadolescent athletes must have realistic expectations of strength training: they will experience an improvement in strength but not an increase in bulk. The increase in strength achieved in the preadolescent occurs through neuromuscular adaptations rather than changes in muscle size (muscular hypertrophy), as documented by computed tomographic scans. These neuromuscular adaptations include increased motor unit activation and coordination, increased recruitment and firing, and intrinsic muscle adaptations.

Strength training has many benefits, including improved self-esteem, improved cardiovascular fitness, increased bone density, improved blood lipid profiles, and increased lean body mass. Pediatric primary care providers should consider recommending strength training as an activity appropriate for overweight or obese patients because it is low impact.

Improving sports performance is an additional goal of strength training. Improvement has been demonstrated in specific measurable motor skills such as the long jump, the vertical jump, the 30-m dash, and agility runs. However, a direct correlation between strength training and better performance in sports has not been proved.

Preventing injury is another goal of strength training. Prehabilitation is a strength training program that addresses common areas subjected to overuse in specific sports (eg, development of a scapular stabilization program before the swimming season begins, to prevent shoulder pain). Adolescents who undergo prehabilitation may have fewer injuries, but such training in the preadolescent has not been studied. Strength training has not been shown to prevent catastrophic injuries, but recent research suggests that strength training combined with specific plyometric exercises may reduce the risk of anterior cruciate ligament tears in the knees of adolescent female athletes.

RISKS

The biggest risk with strength training, as with any sport, is injury. The most common reported injuries in well-supervised, well-designed strength training programs are muscle strains, which comprise about 60% to 75% of all

TABLE 7.2	
Definition of Terms	
Term	**Definition**
Strength training	The use of resistance methods to increase one's ability to exert or resist force
Core strengthening	A focused strength training program for the muscles, stabilizing the trunk of the body (abdominals, lower back, stomach)
Olympic weight lifting	A competitive sport that involves maximum lifting ability (snatch, clean and jerk)
Power lifting	A competitive sport that involves maximum lifting ability (dead lift, squat, bench press)
Bodybuilding	A competition judging muscle size, symmetry, and definition

injuries. The lower back is the most frequently injured area. Injuries reported in unsupervised strength training programs on home equipment or in athletes who use improper form or ballistic movements have included ruptured intervertebral disks, spondylolysis (stress fracture of the spine), spondylolisthesis (slippage of the spinal vertebral bodies), fractures (iliac spine avulsions, radius, ulna, clavicle, and metatarsal), dislocations, osteolysis of the distal clavicle (stress reaction with distal resorption of the clavicle), cartilage tears in the knee, tendon ruptures, and, rarely, death. Despite concerns that strength training can result in stunted growth, no studies have demonstrated an effect on height.

Inappropriate use of anabolic steroids and androgen precursor supplements, which are taken to increase muscle strength or to enhance physique, may also be a risk of strength training, but it is more commonly a problem in competitive weight lifting, power lifting, and bodybuilding. Primary care providers must be able to recognize the side effects of steroid use (**Table 7.3**) and provide resources to educate students and parents on the risks of their use. The AAP does not recommend the use of supplements (ergogenic aids) in children because of unidentified risks to the immature skeleton and a lack of substantial research in this patient population.

CONTRAINDICATIONS

Although weight training is a relatively safe activity, a few medical conditions preclude participation because of acute change in cardiac output with relatively little change in systemic vascular resistance, which leads to transient hypertension. Hypertension is the most common disorder that a primary care provider may encounter that may be a contraindication to participation. The AAP recommends that children with persistent hypertension (140 mm Hg systolic or 90 mm Hg diastolic blood pressure) undergo a comprehensive medical examination before they participate. Moderate hypertension in the absence of end-organ disease is not a contraindication to participation, although strength training in youth with poorly controlled hypertension may worsen their condition.

When a strength training program is initiated, individuals with a history of childhood cancers treated with anthracyclines (adriamycin, daunomycin, idarubicin, and possibly mitoxantrone) may have an asymptomatic subclinical cardiomyopathy until clinical decompensation occurs. Youths treated with these chemotherapeutic agents must be cleared by their cardiologist or oncologist before participation.

Athletes with Marfan syndrome and a dilated aortic root should also refrain from participating. Children with

---

TABLE 7.3

Common Side Effects Associated with Anabolic Steroid Use

* Rapid strength or weight gain
* Edema
* Severe cystic acne
* Striae
* Premature physeal closure
* Mood swings
* Aggression
* Hypertension
* Hypercholesterolemia
* Myocardial ischemia
* Liver dysfunction
* Hepatomas
* Tendon ruptures
* Death

Boys only
* Gynecomastia
* Testicular atrophy
* Priapism
* Impotence

Girls only
* Male pattern boldness
* Hirsutism
* Breast atrophy
* Voice deepening
* Clitoromegaly
* Amenorrhea

---

complex heart disease (cardiomyopathy or pulmonary hypertension) should have a consultation with a pediatric cardiologist before beginning a strength training program. Finally, individuals with a poorly controlled seizure disorder should refrain from training with free weights, but they may participate in strength training with properly fitted weight machines.

GUIDELINES FOR PROGRAM DEVELOPMENT

The American College of Sports Medicine, the AAP, the American Orthopaedic Society for Sports Medicine, and the National Strength and Conditioning Association suggest that with proper program design and adult supervision, strength training in children and adolescents is safe and worthwhile.

The proper age to enroll a child in a strength training program depends on the individual child. Such a decision is based on maturity, attainment of appropriate developmental milestones, and the most likely type of sports participation. General guidelines for readiness include a desire to participate, the discipline needed to perform resistance training several times a week, and the capacity to listen and follow directions. Most individuals will have these characteristics and will have proper balance and postural control at about age 7 or 8. The AAP continues to discourage participation in power lifting, bodybuilding, competitive weight lifting, or 1-repetition maximums until Tanner stage 5 has been achieved.

Before beginning a strength training program, the athlete should undergo a complete physical examination, the goal of which is to identify any contraindications to participation, to provide anticipatory guidance, and to detect any unrehabilitated injuries.

The design and progression of the strength training program is critical to its effectiveness. The program should last at least 8 weeks, with each session 20 to 30 minutes in length. The American College of Sports Medicine recommends a minimum frequency of 2 times a week; 3 times a week is generally thought to be the most efficacious. The program design must include the initial weight intensity (amount of weight to be lifted), the type of resistance (free weights, body weight, machines, Thera-Bands, weighted balls), the volume desired (sets and repetitions), exercise selection and order, and the amount of rest between sets. Exercises need to be appropriately selected to include the core musculature and all major muscle groups.

The initial program should include 6 to 8 exercises. The exercises should incorporate both single and multijoint exercises through the full range of motion of the joint. Proper technique and form should be emphasized throughout the program, rather than the amount of weight or the number of repetitions. Varying any component affects effectiveness and results; for example, shortening the rest periods between sets increases the aerobic component of the program. Increases in weight intensity should be in increments of 5% to 10% and may be difficult for young children to achieve with standard-size weight machines, which are fitted to adults. The program should begin with a 10-minute warm-up and end with a cooldown.

The program itself should be altered over time to prevent boredom and to optimize performance. Progression can be

achieved by increasing the weight, number of sets, exercises, or training sessions. Injuries can be prevented in strength training by following the suggestions in **Table 7.4**.

DETRAINING

Detraining is defined as the temporary or permanent withdrawal of the training stimulus that resulted in strength changes. In preadolescent athletes, strength gains achieved through strength training are not permanent and will not be maintained, even if the child participates in sports such as football, basketball, and soccer. A complete loss of strength gains will occur 8 weeks after the resistance training program is completed. To maintain strength gains, strength training should be performed twice a week; once a week is not enough.

RECOMMENDED CERTIFICATIONS

Adults who provide strength and conditioning instruction to children have varied backgrounds and expertise. Strength training consultants may work at a local gym, a school, a personal training studio, or a youth fitness center. Primary care providers should recommend that, at a minimum, their patients use trainers who have credentials through an organization certified by the National Commission for Certifying Agencies (NCCA). This certifying board ensures minimum standards for licensure,

---

TABLE 7.4

Prevention of Strength Training Injuries

- Use proper technique (straight back and slightly flexed extremities).
- Ensure proper adult supervision (maximum youth-adult ratio, 10:1).
- Ensure that a spotter is present for heavy lifts or free weights.
- Ensure a proper 10-minute warm-up and stretching before beginning.
- Perform movements in slow, controlled motions.
- Avoid hyperventilation and Valsalva maneuvers during lifting.
- Avoid ballistic weight lifting before the skeleton has matured (Tanner stage 5).
- Wear shoes with good traction, and avoid loose, baggy clothing.
- Stop lifting if there is pain.
- Do not exercise the same muscle group more than 3 times a week.
- Include core stabilization in the weight training program.
- Do not use anabolic steroids or hormone precursors.

which include continuing education credits and proctored examinations. However, the certifying standards are extremely variable, even within those organizations that have NCCA certification. The best-qualified strength training coaches will have a certification that requires competence in CPR, a bachelor's degree, and practicum hours in addition to the minimum standards just described. Certifications through the National Strength and Conditioning Association, the American Council on Exercise, and the American College of Sports Medicine all meet these standards. The Web site for the National Organization for Competency Assurance (http://www.noca.org/ncca/accredorg.htm) has more information about the certification process.

SUMMARY POINTS

- Preadolescents undertaking a strength training program should have realistic expectations of improved strength without a significant change in body habitus per se.

- Children and adolescents should be allowed to participate in well-supervised and well-designed strength training programs.

- Children and adolescents should not be allowed to participate in Olympic weight lifting, power lifting, or bodybuilding until skeletal maturity.

- Contraindications to participation include poorly controlled hypertension, hypertension with end-organ damage, previous treatment with anthracyclines, aortic root dilatation in patients with Marfan's syndrome, and a poorly controlled seizure disorder.

- Children with complex heart disease (cardiomyopathy or pulmonary hypertension) should have a consultation with a pediatric cardiologist before beginning a strength training program.

- Athletes participating in strength training should receive anticipatory guidance on supplements and anabolic steroids, and the use of such substances should be discouraged.

SUGGESTED READING

American Academy of Pediatrics. Strength training by children and adolescents. *Pediatrics.* 2008;21: 835-840.

American Academy of Pediatrics Committee on Sports Medicine and Fitness. Adolescents and anabolic steroids: a subject review. *Pediatrics.* 1997;99:904-908.

American Academy of Pediatrics Council on Sports Medicine and Fitness. Use of performance-enhancing substances. *Pediatrics.* 2005;115:1103-1106.

Benjamin HJ, Glow KM. Strength training for children and adolescents. *Phys Sports Med.* 2003;31(9):19-26.

Faigenbaum AD. Pediatric and adolescent sports injuries: strength training for children and adolescents. *Clin Sports Med.* 2000;19:593-619.

Faigenbaum AD, Kraemer WJ, Cahill B, et al. Youth resistance training: position statement paper and literature review. *J Strength Cond.* 1996;18:62-75.

Guy JA, Micheli LJ. Strength training for children and adolescents. *J Am Acad Orthop Surg.* 2001;9:29-36.

Risser W. Weight training injuries in children and adolescents. *Am Fam Phys.* 1991;44:2104-2110.

CHAPTER 8

Thermoregulation

Ron Feinstein, MD

Environmental conditions can not only have a detrimental effect on athletic performance, but they may also pose a significant health risk to athletes. Temperature and humidity can affect the athlete's training and performance as well as the body's ability to maintain heat balance and organ function. Although some athletes are at greater risk than others under stressful environmental conditions, even an athlete in excellent physical condition who is optimally trained will be affected by the environment, and all athletes need to take precautions in environments of extreme humidity, heat, or cold.

Almost all environmentally related illnesses are preventable. Although regimens in the past sometimes used extremes in training, ostensibly to toughen up athletes (eg, failing to provide water during practices; training during the hottest part of the day; requiring athletes to wear complete uniforms at all practices even in hot conditions; and continuing wind sprints until a large number of the athletes vomited, developed muscle cramps, or collapsed), the science of sports medicine has shown most of these training methods to be dangerous. However, because athletes are often asked to perform in high-risk conditions, parents, coaches (both in schools and communities), and health care professionals should be aware of the signs, symptoms, and treatment of these environmentally related illnesses. Adults working with young athletes should be knowledgeable about the environmental conditions that predispose athletes to morbidity and possible mortality and how to avoid them.

TEMPERATURE

The body's metabolism produces heat. Heat balance is maintained through the processes of conduction, convection, radiation, and evaporation. In conduction, heat equilibrium is established when objects are in contact. This process is particularly important in water. Convection, the transfer of heat by circulation of a liquid or gas, is the mechanism by which hot air warms and frigid air cools. Radiation is the transfer of heat in the form of infrared heat rays, such as from an athlete's body to the surrounding air. Evaporation is a liquid's phase change to a gas. It is the most important cooling mechanism in hot conditions. Dripping sweat affords no benefit; only sweat that evaporates will provide cooling.

Body temperature is determined by the balance between heat generation and heat dissipation. Almost all energy released by the body's metabolism of nutrients is eventually converted into body heat. Typically, radiation accounts for up to 60% of heat loss when ambient temperature is lower than skin surface temperature. When ambient temperature is equal to or higher than skin surface temperature, evaporation is the sole mechanism available to the body to dissipate heat. If the humidity is 75% or greater, the surrounding air is so saturated with water that sweat can no longer evaporate, leaving the body with no effective means of maintaining heat balance.

All athletes need to become acclimated to extreme environmental conditions. This involves progressively exposing the athlete to extremes over 1 or 2 weeks. When exposed to hot environments, sweat glands adapt so that the amount of salt lost is only a small fraction of that lost before acclimatization. This process results from increased aldosterone secretion by the adrenal cortex.

When children and adults perform under mild or moderate environmental conditions, thermoregulation tends to be similar in both groups. In extreme environmental conditions—either very hot or very cold—children are at a disadvantage compared with adults when performing physical activity. The unique features of thermoregulation in children are listed in **Table 8.1**.

EXERTIONAL HEAT-RELATED ILLNESS

Along with head and neck trauma and heart conditions, exertional heatstroke is one of the most common causes of death in young athletes. Exertional heat-related illnesses (EHRIs) are also frequent reasons for emergency department visits and on-site treatments by team physicians, athletic trainers, and coaches. EHRI occurs when thermoregulatory mechanisms are impaired or when the heat generated by the ambient temperature or exercise exceeds the amount of heat that can be dissipated.

Exercising muscles produce 10 to 20 times the heat generated by resting muscles. Radiant heat (from direct sunlight) or reflected heat (from surfaces such as artificial turf or sand) contributes to increasing the body's core temperature. During exercise, in most environmental conditions, radiation of heat and evaporation of sweat are the primary methods of dissipating excess body heat. When it is very hot, radiation, convection, and conduction lose their effectiveness and cannot adequately dissipate heat, and when it is humid, evaporation of sweat becomes less effective as a means of cooling.

TABLE 8.1

Unique Features of Thermoregulation in Preadolescents and Early Adolescents[a]

• Lower sweating rate (absolute and per sweat gland) that potentially decreases the capacity to dissipate heat through evaporation of sweat

• More energy used, and consequently more heat generated, in order to move, as a result of relative mechanical inefficiency compared with adults

• Greater body surface area to mass ratio than adults, which can result in excessive heat gain from the environment on a hot day and heat loss to the environment on a cold day

• Lower cardiac output, which reduces capacity for heat transport from the body's core to the skin during strenuous exercise

• Acclimatize to exercising in heat more slowly than adults; the degree of acclimatization achieved in 6 days by young men requires 12 days for 8- to 10-year-old boys

[a] A child in early adolescence either has not begun or is just beginning to develop secondary sexual characteristics.

Heat Cramps

Heat cramps are painful muscle contractions associated with intense exercise and possible muscle fatigue. Cramping is probably the result of dehydration and electrolyte disturbances. Such cramps are usually brief, and they most often affect the legs, arms, and abdomen. A mass may be palpable in the muscle. Body temperature remains in the normal range. Cramps may occur during or after exercise, sometimes when the youth is relaxing or showering. Cramps usually occur in clusters and will usually continue until the athlete is adequately rehydrated and muscle fatigue has resolved. This condition may be a sign of impending heat exhaustion if it is associated with intense exercise under environmental stress.

Supportive treatment of heat cramps involves stopping the exercise, massaging and stretching the involved muscle, and rehydrating by drinking cold water or an appropriate carbohydrate-electrolyte drink.

Heat Exhaustion

Heat exhaustion occurs in athletes who sweat profusely and experience mild to moderate volume depletion. Core body temperature generally ranges from 38°C to 40°C (100.4°F-104°F). Symptoms include nausea, vomiting, headache, dizziness or syncope, weakness, and mild changes in mental status such as confusion or inattention. Heat exhaustion may progress to heatstroke if it is not recognized and treated.

To treat heat exhaustion, the athlete should stop exercising and be moved to a cool, shaded environment. On-site cooling (eg, ice bags, fans, ice bath) should be initiated. Unnecessary clothing and equipment should be removed. Rehydration should begin with cold water or an appropriate carbohydrate-electrolyte drink. If intravenous rehydration is begun, emergency medical services should be contacted. If the athlete's rectal temperature exceeds 40°C (104°F), immediate arrangements should be made to transport the youth to the hospital for intravenous hydration and close monitoring.

Heatstroke

Heatstroke is a life-threatening, acute medical emergency with a mortality rate of about 10% despite good medical management. Heatstroke is defined clinically as a core body temperature above 40°C (104°F) and is accompanied by hot, dry skin and central nervous system abnormalities such as delirium, confusion, seizures, or coma. Susceptibility to heatstroke varies greatly from individual to individual. The most serious complications of heatstroke are associated with multiorgan dysfunction, including rhabdomyolysis;

acute renal failure; myocardial injury; and hepatic, intestinal, and pancreatic ischemia and infarction. Complications may also be hemorrhagic, especially disseminated intravascular coagulation and extreme thrombocytopenia. **Table 8.2** lists the conditions that contribute to an increased risk of EHRI.

Time and cooling are crucial in the treatment of heatstroke. In the field, the diagnosis should be established. If the youth has collapsed or is unconscious, cardiac arrhythmia needs to be excluded as a cause. While the youth is awaiting transport to an emergency medical facility, cooling should be initiated with ice bags or ice water baths. In the hospital, rapid cooling should be continued. When core temperature has fallen to 38.3°C (101°F), the youth should be monitored for hypothermia that may result from the cooling. Seizures need to be controlled. The airway should be protected, and oxygen may need to be provided. Organ perfusion should be restored by volume expansion or perhaps treatment with vasopressors. The youth should be monitored for signs of myoglobin-induced renal failure, life-threatening cardiac arrhythmias, and recovery of organ function.

MEASURING ENVIRONMENTAL HEAT STRESS

The gold standard measurement of heat stress is the wet bulb globe temperature (WBGT). It is a measurement of ambient air temperature (T), radiation (G), and humidity (WB). The heat stress index is calculated by the following equation:

$$WBGT = (0.7 \times WB\ temp) + (0.2 \times G\ temp) + (0.1 \times temp)$$

The most practical approach to measuring WBGT is with a sling psychrometer. This inexpensive, compact instrument allows for immediate on-the-field determination. Several different sets of standards can be used to determine whether it is safe to hold practice or competition (**Table 8.3** and **Table 8.4**).

PREVENTION OF EHRI

To prevent EHRI, exercise should be scheduled during the coolest times of day, usually before 10:00 AM and after 6:00 PM. However, in some regions, environmental conditions, particularly heat and humidity, may always be at high-risk levels. Activities should be canceled when environmental conditions are extreme; the local Department of Public Health may be able to advise when conditions are unsuitable for exercise.

If young athletes are just beginning a strenuous exercise program or have traveled to a warmer climate, the intensity and duration of exercise should be limited at first, then gradually increased over 10 to 14 days to help them acclimate to the heat. When such a period is not available, the length of time of participation should be shortened.

TABLE 8.3

Wet Bulb Globe Temperature Guide to Activity

Under 60°F	Safe, but always observe athletes
61°F to 65°F	Observe players carefully
66°F to 70°F	Caution
71°F to 75°F	Shorter practice sessions; more frequent water and rest breaks
Above 75°F	Danger level and extreme caution

Reproduced with permission from Fox, EL, Mathews, DK, eds. *The Physiological Basis of Physical Education and Athletics.* 3rd ed. 1981. Reproduced with permission of The McGraw-Hill Companies.

TABLE 8.2

Conditions Contributing to Increased Risk of Exertional Heat-Related Illness

- Dehydration (febrile state, diabetes, gastrointestinal infection)
- Suboptimal sweating (spina bifida, sweating insufficiency syndrome)
- Excessive sweating (selected cyanotic congenital heart defects)
- Diminished thirst (cystic fibrosis)
- Acute febrile illness
- Chronic illnesses (sickle cell disease, inflammatory bowel disease)
- Inadequate fluid intake (mental retardation, young children)
- Abnormal hypothalamic thermoregulatory function (anorexia nervosa, undernutrition, previous exertional heat-related illness)
- Obesity
- Legal and illegal drug use; see Table 8.5

TABLE 8.4

Weather Guide for Activities Lasting 30 Minutes or More

Air Temperature (°F)	Relative Humidity (%)	
	Danger Zone	Critical Zone
70	80	100
75	70	100
80	50	80
85	40	68
90	20	40
100	10	30

Reproduced with permission from Fox, EL, Mathews, DK, eds. *The Physiological Basis of Physical Education and Athletics.* 3rd ed. 1981. Reproduced with permission of The McGraw-Hill Companies.

Young athletes should be well hydrated before beginning prolonged activity. During the activity, coaches and trainers should ensure that the athletes periodically drink cold water or an appropriate carbohydrate-electrolyte drink. They should drink 5 to 8 ounces every 20 minutes, even if they do not feel thirsty. Special guidelines for fluid replacement during marathon running address the unique problems that develop during this activity, particularly hyponatremia. Weighing youth before and after an activity that lasts longer than 30 minutes can verify hydration status if the individual is weighed while wearing little or no clothing.

Clothing should be light-colored, lightweight, and limited to one layer of absorbent material to facilitate evaporation of sweat. Young athletes should replace sweat-saturated garments with dry garments. They should never wear rubberized sweat suits to lose weight.

Children should be encouraged to eat a balanced diet and not to skip meals. A basic healthy nutrition plan can usually provide necessary salts, minerals, and vitamins. Salt tablets may be dangerous and should not be taken to replace salt lost through exercise or sweating. **Table 8.5** lists drugs associated with heat intolerance.

COLD-RELATED ILLNESS

The increased popularity and participation in activities in cold climates, such as skiing, backpacking, and mountain climbing, have led to a dramatic increase in the number of youth at risk for developing a cold-related illness. The 2 most common cold-related illnesses are hypothermia and frostbite.

Thermoregulation in cold weather differs from that in warm weather in 3 principal ways. First, shivering generates additional muscular heat, requiring additional energy expenditure. Second, substantial respiratory heat loss occurs in cold weather. Third, adding or removing additional clothing efficiently helps thermoregulation.

Even in extremely cold conditions, properly clothed young athletes can exercise enough to raise their core temperature. Overheating becomes a problem if too much clothing is worn for the climatic conditions and the level of exertion. If the athlete is forced to markedly reduce his or her level of exercise or remove clothing, excessive cooling can occur. Cold-weather athletes must be allowed to add and remove layers of clothing as conditions change during competition.

Fluid losses can be substantial if exercise is prolonged in cold weather, especially if relative humidity is low. Acclimatization to cold conditions is limited. Studies in adults have shown some acclimatization effect, but it is not known whether youth can similarly adapt.

Hypothermia

Hypothermia, or a core body temperature of <36°C (97°F), can occur in any setting in which the environmental temperature is below the core body temperature. It can have a rapid onset from immersion in cold water or severe cold exposure, or a slow onset from prolonged exposure. Death occurs in approximately 30% of affected individuals. Patients with a pulse at the initial examination have better survival rates; the longer the duration of hypothermia, the greater the rate of morbidity and mortality.

Hypothermia can be classified into 3 categories of severity: mild (32°C-35°C, 89.6°F-95°F), which results in tachycardia, tachypnea, shivering, and dysarthria; moderate (28°C-32°C, 82.5°F-89.6°F), which results in

---

TABLE 8.5

Drugs Associated with Heat Intolerance

- Phenothiazines (haloperidol, perphenazine, thioridazine, chlorpromazine)
- Anticholinergic agents (benztropine, atropine, belladonna extracts)
- Beta-blockers, diuretics, laxatives, antihistamines, methyldopa, MAO inhibitors, tricyclic antidepressants, vasoconstrictors
- Amphetamines
- Lithium plus fluoxetine (Prozac)
- Miscellaneous agents (cannabinoids, phencyclidine , phentermine, Ecstasy, alcohol, cocaine, LSD, opiates [withdrawal])

Adapted with permission from Epstein Y: Heat intolerance: Predisposing factor or residual injury? *Med Sci Sports Exerc* 1990; 22:29-35.

TABLE 8.6

Predisposing Factors for Developing Hypothermia

- Environmental temperature <18°C (<64°F), especially in wet conditions and during prolonged endurance events
- Extremes of age
- Cold water immersion (heat loss is 32 times greater than in the air)
- Athletes with decreased metabolic rates (hypothyroidism)
- Large body surface to mass ratio
- Athletes with depleted glycogen stores resulting from prolonged physical exertion or shivering
- Derangement of normal central metabolic control (head injury)
- Drugs (alcohol, phenothiazines, barbiturates, caffeine)

TABLE 8.7

Treatment of Hypothermia

Initial Treatment

- Ensure that personnel prioritize their own safety and protection.
- In the field, prevent further core temperature cooling and cardiac arrhythmia.
  - Handle youth gently.
  - Remove wet clothes.
  - Cover the child with insulating material.

Definitive Treatment

- Monitor core temperature with a rectal thermometer.
- Replace volume losses
- Handle youth gently because the hypothermic heart is more susceptible to arrhythmia caused by excessive movement.
- Order laboratory evaluations that monitor multiorgan involvement, especially cardiac, renal, respiratory, and central nervous system involvement.
- Do not provide topical or systemic agents.
- Rewarm the child in a controlled manner.

Rewarming

- For mild hypothermia, provide a warm, dry environment after removing wet clothing, then cover the child in blankets (passive external rewarming); raise core temperature 0.5°C to 2°C (1°F-3.5°F) per hour.
- For moderate hypothermia, provide heating blankets, radiant heat from a light source, or a heated air system (active external rewarming); raise core temperature 0.8°C (1.5°F) per hour.
- For severe hypothermia, provide active internal rewarming (eg, cardiopulmonary bypass, warmed intravenous fluids, heated humidified oxygen, peritoneal lavage, gastrointestinal irrigation).

an altered level of consciousness and an absence of shivering; and severe (<28°C, 82.4°F), which results in arrhythmia or coma. **Table 8.6** lists the predisposing factors for developing hypothermia. **Table 8.7** lists the treatment for hypothermia.

Localized Cold Injury

The body responds to cold exposure by shunting blood away from peripheral organs, thus protecting the core temperature. Such changes can potentially expose peripheral tissues to extremely cold temperatures. Freezing of human tissue, including intracellular contents, occurs at −0.6°C (31°F) and results in direct cellular toxicity and progressive microvascular thrombosis.

Evidence suggests that although direct cold injury is usually reversible, permanent tissue damage actually occurs during

rewarming. Partial thawing and refreezing results in severe thrombosis and vessel damage, often resulting in severe injury.

Frostnip Frostnip is a precursor to frostbite. It usually affects the nose, ears, face, and fingers. It is associated with reversible numbness, tingling, and blanching. No tissue death occurs, and the affected areas usually respond to rewarming.

Frostbite Frostbite is defined as the crystallization of fluids in the skin or subcutaneous tissue after exposure to temperatures below freezing. Risk factors for frostbite include previous frostbite (2-fold increase); altered mental status, including alcohol intoxication; outdoor sports; and outdoor occupational activities. **Table 8.8** outlines treatment for frostbite.

TABLE 8.8

Treatment for Frostbite

Initial Treatment

- Remove the individual from the cold environment.
- Remove wet clothing.
- Warm the involved extremity against an unaffected body part.
- Protect exposed skin under dry clothes.
- Avoid vigorous rubbing and massaging because they can make the injury worse.
- Rewarming should be attempted in the field only if it can be ensured that refreezing will not occur on the way to definitive care.

Definitive Treatment

- Rapidly rewarm the affected area with circulating water at 40°C to 42°C (104°F-108°F) for 15 to 30 minutes.
- Continue rewarming until capillary refill returns and the tissue is supple.
- Do not use dry or excessive heat because it may worsen the condition.
- Do not disrupt any blisters.
- Provide analgesia during the rewarming process.
- Consider the use of tissue plasminogen activator to reduce vascular thrombosis.
- Consider the possibility of the individual also having hypothermia, and treat accordingly.

Postthaw Treatment

- Handle the injured tissue gently, and cover with dry, sterile dressing.
- Splint and elevate hands and feet to prevent edema.
- Separate digits with sterile gauze.
- Monitor compartment pressure.
- Provide daily whirlpool with physical therapy.

Prognosis

Early intervention is critical for those suffering from the effects of extreme cold. A delay of more than 24 hours greatly increases the need for surgical intervention. An initial physical examination has limited value, although a poor prognosis is usually associated with nonblanching cyanosis, hemorrhagic blisters, and impaired sensation. Long-term sequelae are common and include cold hypersensitivity, decreased sensation, and impaired ability to work.

CONCLUSION

Exposure to environmental stress continues to be a major source of morbidity and mortality among young athletes. Careful attention to the temperature and humidity should be of the utmost importance to the athlete, parent, coach, and physician, and working together, they can prevent almost all environmentally related illnesses.

SUMMARY POINTS

- Environmental conditions can adversely affect even the athlete who is in excellent physical condition and optimally trained.

- When children and adults perform physical activity in extreme environmental conditions, children are more susceptible to environmentally related illnesses than adults.

- Heatstroke is an acute medical emergency.

- The key to successful treatment of EHRI is early recognition.

- Contingencies should be developed to cancel, postpone, or modify events in the face of adverse environmental conditions.

- Both temperature and humidity must be measured to accurately assess environmental heat stress.

- Athletes who have experienced one episode of EHRI are at a higher-than-average risk for another episode.

- Hypothermia can have a rapid onset due to immersion in cold water or severe cold exposure, or a slow onset due to prolonged exposure.

- Cold-weather athletes should be allowed to add and remove layers of clothing as conditions change during competition.

- Prolonged exercise in cold weather can result in substantial fluid losses, especially if relative humidity is low.

- Rewarming frostbitten extremities should be attempted in the field only if it can be ensured that refreezing will not occur on the way to definitive care.

SUGGESTED READING

American Academy of Pediatrics, Committee on Sports Medicine and Fitness. Climatic heat stress and the exercising child and adolescent. *Pediatrics.* 2000;106:158-159.

American College of Sports Medicine. Youth football: heat stress and injury risk. *Med Sci Sports Exerc.* 2005;37(5):1421-1430.

Bouchama A, Knochel JP. Heat stroke. *N Engl J Med.* 2002;346:1978-1988.

Guyton AC, Hall JE. *Human Physiology and Mechanisms of Disease.* 6th ed. Philadelphia, PA: WB Saunders; 1997.

Knoechel JP. Dog days and siriasis. *JAMA.* 1975;233: 513-515.

National Athletic Trainers' Association Web site. Inter-Association Task Force on Exertional Heat Illness. http://www.nata.org/consumer/heatillness/index.htm. Accessed May 27, 2008.

Ulrich AS, Rathlev NK. Hypothermia and localized cold injuries. *Emerg Med Clin North Am.* 2004;22:281-298.

CHAPTER 9

Sports Nutrition

Michele LaBotz, MD

Good nutrition plays an important role in growth and overall development as well in the development of peak athletic performance. Although many young athletes (and even some parents) seek nutritional shortcuts for enhanced athletic performance, the best results are obtained by consistently applying basic, sound nutrition principles. This chapter provides the practitioner with practical information on how to advise young athletes about their sports-related nutrition concerns.

DIETARY REQUIREMENTS

Fluid

Fluids and adequate hydration play a vital role in maintaining optimal athletic performance. Diminished athletic performance, particularly endurance, may occur at approximately 1% dehydration. However, thirst is activated only when dehydration reaches about 3% of total body weight. Therefore, thirst is not a good marker for hydration status, and athletes should drink water before, during, and after the activity, without waiting for thirst to prompt them.

Sweat losses and fluid requirements vary greatly and depend on activity, heat acclimatization, fitness, and a variety of intrinsic factors. General guidelines for fluid intake are provided in **Table 9.1**. These are particularly important when activity lasts for more than an hour.

Children are better able to maintain appropriate hydration status if they are given adult guidance on the importance of drinking fluids during exercise and are provided with palatable fluids. Water is appropriate for activities lasting less than 60 to 90 minutes, but children

tend to drink less water than other fluids that contain flavor, color, sodium, and carbohydrate (CHO). Strategies for optimizing fluid intake in young athletes are listed in **Table 9.2**.

The risk for exertional hyponatremia may be a concern in some athletic populations. Although certain individuals may be at increased risk, exertional hyponatremia most often affects endurance and ultraendurance athletes who are involved in events that last for more than 4 hours. Most young athletes, who are involved in shorter and more intermittent training sessions, and who are not excessively restricting dietary sodium, are at very low risk.

Carbohydrates

CHOs serve several related functions that are of particular interest to the young athlete. They are the primary fuel source for most athletic activity, and they spare muscle tissue from catabolism. When inadequate amounts of CHOs are ingested, athletic performance and overall activity levels may suffer. General guidelines recommend that adult and adolescent athletes consume 6 to 10 g of CHOs per kilogram of body weight per day. **Table 9.3** and **Table 9.4** provide helpful information for those who counsel athletes on CHO intake.

The significance of CHOs in pretraining meals and the roles they play in bolstering blood glucose and muscle glycogen are often intuitive for young athletes and their parents. But athletes are often less familiar with the importance of CHOs during and after exercise. Although it is well known that CHO intake during exercise is beneficial for activities lasting longer than 60 minutes, recent evidence shows it may be beneficial during shorter bouts as well. If

TABLE 9.1

General Recommendations for Fluids in Athletes[a]

Timing	Fluid Volumes
1-2 hours before exercise	• Body weight <40 kg: 3-6 oz
	• Body weight >40 kg: 6-12 oz
During exercise	• Body weight <40 kg: 4 oz every 20 minutes
	• Body weight 40-60 kg: 5-7 oz every 20 minutes
	• Body weight >60 kg: 8 oz every 20 minutes
After exercise	• Replace losses: 500-650 mL/0.5 kg body weight lost (~16-20 oz per pound lost)

[a] The above recommendations can be individualized by having the athlete record body weight in dry clothes before and after workouts. Each pound of body weight lost indicates that the athlete fell behind by about 16 oz of fluid, and this volume should be replaced before the next workout. Athletes can also be advised to maintain a clear or very pale urine color.

TABLE 9.2

Strategies for Enhancing Fluid Intake in Young Athletes

• Provide opportunities for young athletes to drink at least every 15-20 minutes.

• Do not use fluid restriction for discipline.

• To enhance greater voluntary fluid intake, provide fluid that contains color and flavor and that also contains 10-20 mmol/L Na.

• Provide fluids containing 6%-8% carbohydrates to enhance gastric emptying.[a]

[a] This is the concentration of carbohydrates found in most sports drinks, but it can also be obtained by diluting fruit juice with an equal volume of water.

TABLE 9.3

Common High-Carbohydrate Foods

Food	Amount	Grams of Carbohydrate
Beans		
Navy beans	1/2 cup	24
Kidney beans	1/2 cup	20
Garbanzo beans (chickpeas)	1/2 cup	22
Pinto beans	1/2 cup	22
Breads, Cereals, Grains		
Rice	1 cup cooked	50
Spaghetti	1 cup cooked	34
Flour tortilla	1	15
Waffle	2	17
Bagel	2 oz	31
Breadsticks	4 sticks	30
Whole wheat bread	2 slices	24
Fig bar	1	10
Cheerios	1/2 cup	8
Oatmeal	1/2 cup	13
Shredded wheat	1 biscuit	18
English muffin	1	30
Graham crackers	2 squares	11
Oatmeal raisin cookie	1	9
Popcorn	1 cup	6
Pretzels	1 oz	21
Fruits		
Apple	1 medium	21
Dried apricot	1/2 cup	40
Banana	1 medium	27
Cantaloupe	1/2 cup	7
Cranberry juice	1/2 cup	19
Orange	1 medium	16
Orange juice	1/2 cup	12
Peach	1 medium	10
Pear	1 medium	30
Raisins	1/2 cup	57
Vegetables		
Baked potato	Large	50
Corn	1/2 cup	21
Carrot	1 medium	8
Dairy		
Yogurt (fruit)	1 cup	42
Yogurt (frozen, low fat)	1 cup	34

hydration is maintained with recommended fluid volumes of a 6% to 8% CHO beverage (ie, sports drink), no additional CHOs are needed. Gastric tolerance of these food and fluid recommendations is a problem for many athletes, particularly athletes who participate in sports involving running (**Figure 9.1**).

The importance of the postexercise meal in replenishing muscle glycogen and providing fuel for the next day's workout is often underappreciated. This is particularly important for athletes who train on consecutive days.

Ideally, recommended amounts of CHOs should be ingested as soon as possible after a workout, while the muscles still have the optimum capacity for taking up glucose. Within an hour after exercise, muscle tissue becomes more resistant to insulin, and its ability to replenish glycogen diminishes. This diminishes fuel availability for the next day's training session.

TABLE 9.4

Carbohydrate Recommendations before, during, and after Exercise

Timing	Carbohydrate Amount	Example for 40-kg Athlete
3-4 hours before exercise	4 g CHO/kg body weight	• 160 g CHO desired • 160 g CHO × 4 kcal/g CHO = 640 CHO calories • This is approximately the amount of CHO found in 2 c pasta (68 g CHO) + 1 c pasta sauce (34 g CHO) + 1 dinner roll (15 g CHO) + apple (21 g CHO) + 8 oz 1% milk (12 g CHO)
1-2 hours before exercise	0.5-1 g CHO/kg body weight	• 20-40 g CHO desired • 20-40 g CHO × 4 kcal/g CHO = 80-160 CHO calories • 1 medium banana (29 g CHO)
During exercise	0.7 g/kg body weight/h every 15-20 minutes	• 28 g CHO desired • 28 g CHO × 4 kcal/g CHO = 112 CHO calories • About 16 oz of most sports drinks (28-30 g CHO)
After exercise	1-1.5 g CHO as soon as possible after exercise and again 2 hours later	• 40-60 g CHO desired • 40-60 g CHO × 4 kcal/g CHO = 160-240 CHO calories • One 3½ inch bagel (38 g CHO) + 2 tbsp peanut butter (6 g CHO)

CHO indicates carbohydrate.

Protein

Data in adults demonstrate that protein requirements in athletes are greater than the requirements for a sedentary population (**Table 9.5**). These additional requirements are due to protein accretion, which results from increased muscle mass; protein turnover, which results from the tissue breakdown that occurs with training; and use of certain amino acids as a fuel source. Despite their bodies' requirements, athletes often consume too much or too little protein. Athletes who are primarily interested in gains in strength and power may consume diets that contain far more protein than the current recommendations, whereas athletes who are primarily concerned with endurance performance or who are trying to lose weight may ingest far less.

Athletes can usually meet the protein requirements easily by eating a balanced, omnivorous diet. Vegetarian diets may require additional planning to ensure that appropriate amounts of all essential amino acids are included, and serious athletes who are vegetarians (especially vegans, who ingest no animal products) may benefit from consultation with a registered dietitian.

As much as possible, young athletes should be encouraged to obtain their protein from dietary sources (**Table 9.6**) rather than protein supplements. However, some athletes have a hard time getting the recommended protein amounts in their daily diets, and such athletes should enhance their diet with protein. One easy way to supplement protein is by enriching food with nonfat dry milk, which contains 11 g of protein per ¼ cup and can be added to a variety of foods, such as milk, soup, pasta sauce, and cereal. Instant breakfast packets prepared with milk can be used as protein shakes; these typically contain about 12 g of protein per serving.

Despite the variety of dietary protein sources, commercial protein supplements are popular among adolescent athletes. Although they may be helpful for some athletes to meet their protein requirements, the American Academy of Pediatrics (AAP) recommends that primary care providers take a strong stand against supplement use in their young athletes. **Table 9.7** lists some talking points about protein supplementation.

Many young athletes have concerns not only about the amount of protein ingested but also about the timing of protein intake. Protein ingestion should be spread throughout the day to allow the body free access to necessary amino acids as it undergoes repair during the time between workouts. Protein ingested shortly before workouts may lead to gastric upset and is often broken down as fuel for the exercising muscles. However, some evidence suggests that small amounts of protein added to adequate pre- and postexercise CHOs may have a muscle-sparing effect. The clinical and performance significance of this is yet to be determined.

WEIGHT CONTROL

Dissatisfaction with body weight is ubiquitous among adolescents in American culture. Although athletes generally have a better body image compared with their sedentary peers, many adolescent athletes actively seek changes in body weight in hopes of improving athletic performance. In some sports, such as wrestling, gymnastics, and endurance running, athletes and coaches associate optimal performance with a relatively low body mass. In other sports, particularly contact and collision sports such as football, increased body mass is often encouraged. **Table 9.8** lists measures in common use to assess body size or composition.

ENHANCING GASTRIC TOLERANCE IN ATHLETES

Intense physical activity

↓

Delay in gastric motility

↓

Food and fluid:

Not absorbed, and therefore desired benefits not provided

May cause nausea/gastric upset

Emphasize to athletes and parents:

- The significance of maintaining hydration and fuel source during activity (particularly in events lasting more than 60 minutes).

- The ability to enhance gastric tolerance with practice, but trial and error is often part of the process.

- Commercially available sports drinks, bars, or gels may be helpful for some athletes, but are not necessary.

The following techniques may be attempted to enhance gastric emptying/comfort:

1. Minimize fat and protein in pretraining meals and snacks.

    a. Carbohydrates (CHOs) empty faster than either protein or fat.

2. Fluids containing 4%–8% CHOs empty faster than either water or higher CHO fluids.

    a. 6%–8% CHOs can be found in most sports drinks or by diluting many fruit juices with an equal volume of water.

    b. Recommended fluid volumes of 6%–8% CHO beverages provide as much CHO as the stomach can empty. Therefore, additional food during exercise does not provide significant performance benefit.

3. Tepid fluids empty faster than ice-cold beverages.

    a. Some athletes tolerate CHOs containing sucrose or glucose better than fructose, the primary sweetener used in many sports drinks and energy bars.

4. Empty stomachs have lower motility than those containing some volume (~600 mL).

    a. Maintain regular meal schedule earlier in the day (ie, breakfast and lunch for late afternoon practice).

FIGURE 9.1 Strategies for enhancing gastric comfort during exercise.

TABLE 9.5

Protein Requirements in Select Populations

Population	Protein RDA (g protein/kg body weight/d)
Child aged 4-13 years	0.95
Adolescent aged 14-18 years	0.85
Adult	0.80
Endurance-trained athlete	1.2-1.4
Weight-trained athlete	1.2-1.7
Novice athlete (just beginning training program)	1.0-1.5

RDA indicates recommended daily allowance.

TABLE 9.6

Protein Content in Common Foods

Food	Amount	Grams of Protein
Meat, Fish, Poultry		
Lean beef	1 oz	8
Chicken	1 oz	8
Turkey breast	1 oz	8
Fish	1 oz	7
Eggs	1	6
Beans, Nuts		
Kidney beans	1/2 cup	9
Navy beans	1/2 cup	7
Garbanzo beans (chickpeas)	1/2 cup	6
Tofu	2 oz	5
Peanut butter	1 tbsp	4
Dairy		
Low-fat cottage cheese	1/2 cup	13
Milk, whole, skim	1 cup	8
Yogurt	1 cup	8
Cheddar cheese	1 oz	7
Ice cream	1/2 cup	4
Frozen yogurt	1/2 cup	4
American cheese	1 oz	3
Breads, Cereals Grains		
Macaroni and cheese	1/2 cup	6
Spaghetti	1 cup cooked	8
Bagel	2 oz	6
Raisin bran	1 oz (2/3 cup)	3
Rice	1 cup cooked	3
Bread	1 slice	2
Vegetables		
Baked potato	1 large	4
Peas, green	1/2 cup	4
Corn	1/2 cup	2
Lettuce	1/4 head	1
Carrot	1 large	1
Fruits		
Banana	1 medium	1
Orange	1 medium	1
Apple	1 medium	1

For athletes and parents struggling with weight-related issues, it may help to emphasize that the optimal weight for a given athlete depends on a variety of individual factors. These include developmental stage, body composition, sport and position choice, and a variety of intrinsic factors. Use of universal target body composition measures for optimal sport performance is not supported by medical evidence and is fundamentally different from measures used to certify minimal weight classification in wrestling and other sports. Most sports-governing bodies (eg, National Federation of State High School Associations [NFHS], National Collegiate Athletic Association [NCAA]) recommend against routine body composition assessment, particularly in girls, except when required for weight certification. Measures of athletic performance, such as speed, jump height, and agility, are better indicators of optimal weight than body composition measures. If body composition measures are used, the AAP recommends that they be performed no more than twice a year.

Changes in body weight should occur at a maximal rate of 1.5% body mass per week (usually 1-2 lb per week).

Weight Loss

Young athletes use a variety of weight loss strategies, some of which result in rapid loss of fluid weight, while others use more gradual methods to produce reductions in fat mass. Of these 2 strategies, the latter is obviously better. However, athletes sometimes use the process of rapid weight loss, often described as cutting weight, when they need to achieve a certain weight within a short period of time, as in wrestling and other weight-classified sports. This loss of fluid weight places athletes at increased risk for adverse activity-related consequences due to dehydration and heat illness. Techniques used to cut weight include excessive exercise, possibly in a heated environment or using other measures to enhance sweat production (eg, rubberized suits, saunas); spitting; using diuretics or laxatives; and vomiting. These practices have come under close scrutiny by the NFHS, the NCAA, and USA Wrestling. The prevalence of weight loss issues in wrestling prompted the NFHS to nationally mandate a process for weight certification in wrestling. Although these rules are refined on an annual basis, Table 9.9 and Table 9.10 outline the fundamentals.

TABLE 9.7

Talking Points for Patients and Family Considering Use of Protein Supplements

- Protein from supplements is not better than that found in foods containing all essential amino acids (complete proteins—eg, meat, dairy, soy).
- Protein in amounts above daily requirements does not enhance gains in muscle mass or performance but is either used for energy or turned into fat.
- Protein from supplements is more expensive than dietary protein.
- Protein type (soy vs whey) does not appear to be important in determining increases in muscle mass or athletic performance.
- Dietary protein supplements are not regulated and are occasionally found to contain potentially harmful impurities.

Weight Gain

For athletes who are interested in gaining weight, it is important to emphasize the differences between gains in lean body mass compared with gains in fat mass. These are outlined in **Table 9.11**.

Most athletes who are seeking to gain weight desire the outcomes associated with increases in lean mass rather than increases in fat mass. However, the methods used by many athletes to gain weight (especially when rapid weight gain is the goal) often produce greater gains in fat than in lean muscle. Reviewing the principles outlined in **Table 9.12** on how to optimize lean mass accumulation can be helpful for these athletes and their parents.

TABLE 9.8

Measures in Common Use to Assess Body Size or Composition

Measure	Advantages	Disadvantages
Weight	• Easy to use • Typically followed longitudinally in pediatric practices	• Does not reflect body composition
Body mass index percentile	• Easy to use • Reasonable representation of obesity or obesity risk in population of average build	• Overestimates body fat in muscular athletes • Inaccurate in athletes with eating disorders
Skinfold measures	• Used in some sports for weight certification • Provides readily available measure of body composition • Equipment and training are cheap and readily accessible	• Equations not universal (depends on sex, race/ethnicity, development) and are validated only for specific populations • Operator dependent • Need to perform in conjunction with hydration assessment
Hydrostatic weighing	• Greater accuracy for determination of body composition	• Expensive and inconvenient
Bioelectrical impedance scale	• Convenient • Cheap equipment • Used in some sports for weight certification	• Often inaccurate and dependent on fluid status • Proprietary formulas (located within the scales) are often not validated in children
Dual energy x-ray absorptiometry (DEXA)	• Most accurate in determining body composition and specific components including fat mass, lean muscle mass, and bone mineral density	• Calculation formulas not validated in children • Expensive • Radiation exposure (minimal)

TABLE 9.9

Weight Certification Procedures in High School Wrestling

Allowed minimum weights for wrestlers are established during the preseason.

- Hydration status is assessed via urine specific gravity determination.
  - Specific gravity <1.025 is required to proceed with body composition assessment.
- Body composition and lean body mass are calculated.
  - Bioelectrical impedance or skinfold measurements are the most commonly used methods.
  - Measurements are often performed by trained health professionals (usually certified athletic trainers, physical therapists, or physicians).

This calculated lean body mass is then used to determine the minimum allowed wrestling weights for athletes (**Table 9.10**).

- The minimum allowed weight must be equal to or greater than 12% body fat in girls and 7% body fat in boys.
- The weight obtained by a "monitored weekly weight loss plan" is not to exceed 1.5% of total body weight per week (also known as a "descent plan").

If a wrestler is naturally below the minimum fat percentiles, the athlete's physician may be asked to certify that the athlete is able to participate in the sport, but this certification will not affect the wrestler's weight classification.

TABLE 9.10

Calculations for Minimum Wrestling Weight

$$FM = TBM \times (\% \text{ Body Fat}/100)$$
$$LBM = TBM - FM$$

For boys:

$$\text{Minimum Wrestling Weight} = LBM/0.93$$

For girls:

$$\text{Minimum Wrestling Weight} = LBM/0.88$$

Where:

$$FM = \text{Fat Mass}$$
$$TBM = \text{Total Body Mass}$$
$$LBM = \text{Lean Body Mass}$$

For athletes who are having a hard time gaining weight, the following tips can be helpful: do not skip breakfast; increase the frequency of meals and snacks; aim to eat every 2 to 3 hours or about 5 to 9 times a day; increase the caloric density of foods; enrich milk with flavorings or instant breakfast; add high-density foods such as dried fruits and nuts to cereal and sandwiches; use milk or evaporated milk

TABLE 9.11

Comparison of Effects of Increases in Lean Mass Versus Fat Mass

Gains in Lean Body Mass (Muscle)	Gains in Fat Mass
• Often associated with gains in strength and power. • May negatively affect endurance performance. • Tissue is metabolically active and therefore contributes to resting metabolic rate.	• Does not contribute directly to strength and power development. • Often decreases strength-weight ratio. • May negatively affect athletic performance measures such as jump height, agility, endurance performance. • Fat tissue is not metabolically active, and excessive increases in body fat during adolescence have been associated with early development of cardiovascular risk.

instead of water for reconstituting condensed soups and making hot cereal; and choose dense cereals and grain products (ie, granola instead of puffed rice and thick-sliced full-grain bread instead of white bread).

MICRONUTRIENTS

Minerals

Although the sports medicine literature is rife with references to the poor iron and calcium status of young athletes, particularly girls, inadequate intake of these minerals is actually ubiquitous in the young American population; it is a universal issue, not one limited to girls and athletes. Less than half of US adolescent girls get more than 55% of the recommended daily allowance (RDA) of iron. Less than half of boys and girls older than 6 years get their RDA of calcium.

When addressing nutrition concerns in young athletes, the physician should be able to assess the athletes' iron and calcium intake, advise them about appropriate amounts, and suggest foods and serving sizes. In addition, iron and calcium are often poorly absorbed, and a review of factors that affect dietary absorption may also help athletes adjust their diets appropriately.

Athletes with poor caloric intake may also be at increased risk for inadequate intake of other minerals, such as zinc and magnesium.

TABLE 9.12

Principles of Maximizing Gains in Lean Mass in Young Athletes

Gains of approximately 1.5% body weight/week (about 1-2 lb/wk) are reasonable initial goals for adolescent athletes who wish to minimize fat gains. This requires:

1. Resistance training of sufficient intensity to stimulate muscle growth
   a. Muscle hypertrophy is best achieved with multiple sets of 8-15 repetitions.
   b. Strength/power is best achieved with multiple sets of 4-6 repetitions.
2. Sufficient rest between sessions to allow for tissue repair and recovery
   a. Allow at least 48 hours between hard workouts for a given body part.
3. Adequate calories and carbohydrates (especially before training) to protect muscle tissue from catabolism
   a. For athletes who are currently maintaining their body weight, intake can be increased by 300-400 calories/d over any increased expenditures.
      i. Two servings of most instant breakfast or liquid meal replacement food products (eg, Carnation Instant Breakfast or Ensure) provide enough protein and calories for lean muscle growth.
   b. Weight-gain supplements often provide 500-2000 calories per serving, and when taken as directed, they often result in excess gains of fat mass.
4. Adequate protein to support tissue growth (usually 1.5-1.8 g protein/kg body weight/d)
5. Rate of lean mass gain is highly individualized and depends on a variety of factors. Some people gain weight quickly while others gain more slowly, and athletes often find this frustrating. Some of the factors that contribute to these differences include:
   a. Endogenous anabolic hormone production, which is affected by
      i. Developmental stage
      ii. Sex
      iii. Genetic factors
   b. Training history
      i. Novice athletes often experience rapid gains at the initiation of training, which then slows with increased training experience.

TABLE 9.13

Dietary Iron Recommendations[a]

Age and Sex	Iron Intake
>9-13 Years Old	
Boys	8 mg/d
Girls	8 mg/d
14-18 Years Old	
Boys	11 mg/d
Girls	15 mg/d

[a] Amounts provided are the current US recommended daily allowances for iron. Vegetarians may need almost twice these amounts as a result of the poor bioavailability of plant-based nonheme iron.

and possibly select laboratory testing, such as a complete blood count, with or without additional iron studies. Although the prevalence of iron-deficiency anemia appears to be the same in athletes and nonathletes, the detection rates of iron deficiency anemia may be higher in the athletic population because early symptoms are often related to exertion. Current controversy exists about the role nonanemic iron deficiency (ie, low ferritin with normal hemoglobin) may play in reducing athletic performance.

In athletes with a known or suspected iron deficiency, it is important to perform a dietary screening, with particular attention paid to iron content in the diet (**Table 9.14** and **Table 9.15**). In addition, iron is often poorly absorbed, and athletes and parents often benefit from counseling on how to increase the absorption of dietary iron (**Table 9.16**).

Calcium

Calcuim is an important nutrient for growing athletes. Athletes should be screened for adequate calcium in their diet (**Tables 9.17 and 9.18**) and counseled regarding dietary factors that affect calcium absorption and excretion (**Table 19.19**)

TABLE 9.14

Screening for Dietary Iron

Screening question:
   How many servings of iron-rich food do you get per day on most days?
Recommended intake:
   Many iron-rich foods contain about 3 mg iron/serving.
Therefore:

In 9- to 13-year-olds:	at least 2 servings/d
In 14- to 18-year-olds:	
Boys	at least 3 servings/d
Girls	at least 4 servings/d

Iron

Although some endurance athletes lose blood and iron through the gastrointestinal and genitourinary tracts, this is not an issue for most child and adolescent athletes. Iron requirements in the young recreational or competitive athlete do not appear to be higher than those of the general population (**Table 9.13**).

Iron status frequently comes up when a young athlete is evaluated for fatigue or decreased performance. These athletes and their parents will often seek care, concerned about the presence of anemia or other iron-deficient state. In these athletes, the initial evaluation often includes a history (with dietary assessment); a physical examination;

TABLE 9.15

Iron Content of Some Common Foods[a]

Food	Serving Size	Iron Content (mg)
Beef, lean	3 oz	3
Turkey	3½ oz	2
Chicken	3½ oz	1
Lentils, cooked	½ cup	3
Beans/legumes	1 cup	3-5
Tofu, firm	½ cup	3
Spinach, cooked	½ cup	3
Molasses, blackstrap	1 tbsp	3
Tomato puree	½ cup	2 mg

[a] For many young athletes, fortified cereals are important sources of iron and may contain anywhere from 3-18 mg iron/serving.

TABLE 9.16

Issues Affecting Absorption of Dietary Iron

1. Heme iron from meat protein is about 15%-35% absorbed.
2. Nonheme iron from vegetable sources is 2%-20% absorbed.
3. Nonheme iron absorption may be enhanced by simultaneous ingestion of
   a. Vitamin C
   b. Meat proteins
4. Nonheme iron absorption is decreased by many things, including
   a. Calcium
   b. Phytates in legumes and whole grains
   c. Some soy proteins
   d. Tannins (in tea)

TABLE 9.17

Screening for Dietary Calcium

Screening question:
   How many servings of calcium-rich foods do you get on most days?
Recommended intake:
   Many calcium-rich foods contain about 300 mg calcium/serving.
Therefore:
   Four or more servings on most days of the week should supply adequate calcium amounts.
In 9- to 18-year-olds: 1300 mg/d to meet USDA recommended daily allowance

TABLE 9.18

Sample Servings of Calcium-Rich Foods[a]

Food	Serving Size
Milk, any type	8 oz
Cheese	
Parmesan/Romano	1 oz
Cheddar/Swiss	1½ oz
Yogurt, low fat	6 oz
Orange juice, calcium fortified	8 oz
Soy milk, calcium fortified	8 oz (but may vary widely)
Tofu, prepared with calcium	¾ cup
Sardines, canned with bones	4 oz
Collard greens, cooked	1 cup

[a] Approximately 300 mg calcium per serving. A number of cereal and bread products are calcium fortified and may contain up to 300 mg or more of calcium per serving.

TABLE 9.19

Issues Affecting Absorption and Excretion of Dietary Calcium

- Age affects calcium absorption: up to 60% absorbed in young children, decreasing to 15%-20% in adulthood.
- Efficiency of calcium absorption decreases with increased calcium content of a given meal.
- Calcium found in many vegetable sources is poorly absorbed as a result of the presence of phytates and oxalates, which bind calcium.
- High-protein and high-sodium diets increase calcium excretion.
- Increasing potassium may decrease calcium excretion.
- Some uncertainty exists regarding the effect of phosphorus on net calcium accretion; in many adolescents, high-phosphorus soft drinks displace consumption of milk and other high-calcium fluids.
- Fiber (especially wheat bran) may decrease calcium absorption. However, most young Americans do not consume enough fiber for this to affect calcium absorption.

Although the interactions among activity, calcium intake, and bone density are unclear, adequate calcium intake and weight-bearing activity appear to be synergistic in enhancing bone density. Even when calcium intake is suboptimal, many young athletes are found to have increased bone density relative to their sedentary peers. This is likely an important protective mechanism, given the increased risk for both acute trauma and chronic stress injury to bone in athletes.

Although calcium supplementation is common (and should be suggested to young athletes who do not get enough calcium in their diet), doubts have been cast on the efficacy of calcium supplementation in bringing about

The low intake of calcium in most US children has raised concern regarding the ability of this population to attain peak bone mass during their adolescent years. Peak calcium accretion occurs at about 12.5 years of age in girls and at about 14 years of age in boys.

long-term improvements in bone density as compared with the known benefits of a diet that consistently provides adequate levels of calcium intake.

Vitamins

A comprehensive discussion of vitamins is beyond the scope of this text. However, some vitamins have been directly implicated in issues of specific concern to young athletes, and these are reviewed in **Table 9.20**.

TABLE 9.20

Vitamins of Particular Relevance to Young Athletes

Vitamin	Description
B	• Involved in many energy-generating reactions in the body.
	• Supplementation has not been shown to enhance athletic performance.
	• Exercise may result in increased turnover and utilization of B vitamins in athletes.
	• In adults, the American College of Sports Medicine recommends up to twice the RDA; unclear whether this applies to children and adolescents.
	• Vegetarians may need supplements for vitamin B_{12} needs.
	• If eating balanced diet and not calorie restricting, RDA for B vitamins is generally achieved by meeting caloric needs.
A, C, E	• Recognized as antioxidants that may reduce damage to muscle and other tissues during exercise (although athletes already have enhanced antioxidant mechanisms).
	• Current evidence does not support increased antioxidant requirements in athletes, and supplementation does not appear to improve athletic performance.
D	• Important in bone formation and maintenance.
	• Regulates phosphorus and calcium levels.
	• Most important source for most young athletes in outdoor sports is sunlight.
	• Adequate intake provided with 10-15 minutes' sun exposure on face, arms, hands, or back twice a week.
	• Vitamin D synthesis decreased by sunscreen, cloud cover, increasing latitude, and pollution.
	• Dietary sources important for those who live in northern states (especially during winter) and others who do not get adequate sun exposure.
	• May be obtained by fortified milk and cereal.
	• May be obtained by eating some kinds of fish (mackerel, sardines, tuna canned in oil).

SUMMARY POINTS

● Fluid recommendations should be individualized as much as possible. The easiest way to do this is to have athletes weigh themselves before and after workouts and replace each pound lost with about 16 oz of fluid.

● Replenishment of CHO stores as soon as possible after exercise is the key to providing fuel for the next day's workout.

● Young athletes need more protein than their sedentary peers. This protein is ideally obtained from dietary sources and is spread throughout the day.

● Changes in weight should be no greater than 1.5% body weight per week (1-2 lb per week). Weight loss faster than this is mostly fluid loss. Weight gain faster than this results in increased fat mass.

● Inadequate iron and calcium intake is a problem among American children and adolescents and should be addressed in athletes and nonathletes alike.

SUGGESTED READING

American Academy of Pediatrics Committee on Sports Medicine and Fitness. Promotion of healthy weight-control practices in young athletes. *Pediatrics.* 2005;116:1557-1564.

American Dietetic Association, Dietitians of Canada, American College of Sports Medicine. Nutrition and athletic performance. *J Am Diet Assoc.* 2000;100: 1543-1556.

Kleinman RE, ed. Sports nutrition. In: American Academy of Pediatrics Committee on Nutrition. *Pediatric Nutrition Handbook.* 6th ed. Elk Grove Village, IL: American Academy of Pediatrics; 2008.

Lukaski HC. Vitamin and mineral status: effects on physical performance. *Nutrition.* 2004;20:632-644.

Petrie HJ, Stover EA, Horswill CA. Nutritional concerns for the child and adolescent competitor. *Nutrition.* 2004;20:620-631.

CHAPTER 10

Performance-Enhancing Substances

Bernard A. Griesemer, MD

Young athletes today are participating in increasingly competitive sports in elementary school, middle school, and high school. The perceptions that performance-enhancing substances are of value at these levels of sports participation, or that use of these substances will provide a competitive advantage in progressing to elite levels of competition, are becoming increasingly common topics of discussion among child athletes, their parents, and their coaches.

Performance-enhancing substances are considered to have a positive ergogenic (meaning "to make work") effect if it can be proved scientifically that they increase power, endurance, or mental focus. They also may be ergogenic in sports if they decrease a perception of fatigue, decrease pain, release inhibition, decrease the catabolic effect of exercise on skeletal muscle, decrease fine motor tremulousness, or slow an athlete's heart rate. A product that is ergogenic in one competitive scenario may result in performance deterioration in other sports or may even have varying positive and negative effects in a single competitive scenario, depending on the duration of the activity. In many instances, the ergogenic effect of a compound may not be the substance's original intended use, but rather a secondary result.

Individuals and corporations who derive significant income from marketing substances with purported ergogenic benefits seldom include information that details the limits of these products on the incremental ergogenic gain that a young athlete can realize when the effect of these products is compared with appropriate fluid and calorie intake, strength training and conditioning, and skill development. At elite levels of Olympic, collegiate, and professional sports, even the small incremental gain possible with most ergogenic aids may provide a competitive advantage. At the middle school and high school levels of competition, the incremental gain from ergogenic aids is far less likely to be a significant factor in winning margins of competition. Controlled studies that specifically delineate the ergogenic effects and the detrimental effects of many of these products in child athletes are extremely limited.

Many products that have ergogenic properties are not monitored or controlled by federal agencies that have oversight responsibilities in the pharmaceutical industry. The Dietary Supplement Health and Education Act of 1994 removed many of these products from significant government oversight. Consequently, when a physician is asked by an athlete, coach, or parent about the content and safety of these so-called nutraceuticals, it is difficult to approve the use of these compounds, much less encourage or endorse their use. Physicians who care for child athletes thus need to be familiar with substances that are used to enhance athletic performance so that they can effectively counsel their patients regarding the effects of these substances.

Athletes, coaches, and medical support staff should contact their sport's governing body to determine the status (prohibited or allowed) of substances used to enhance performance. The United States Anti-Doping Agency provides information about many drugs that are used to enhance sports performance, with particular relevance for young athletes who are participating in sports sanctioned by sport federations that comprise the United States Olympic Committee.

ERGOGENIC COMPOUNDS

Anabolic Steroids

The use of anabolic-androgenic steroids for sports performance enhancement has been reported in the medical literature for decades. These compounds are anabolic (increase protein synthesis in skeletal muscle and decrease catabolism of skeletal muscle in exercise scenarios) and androgenic (shift muscle and fat into a masculine pattern). However, the exact ergogenic potential of these products in children has not been determined. In general, they increase muscle size and strength when—and only when—they are combined with adequate calories and strength training. Anabolic-androgenic steroids do not significantly enhance aerobic capabilities and thus may be of little performance-enhancing value to young athletes who are participating in the most common sports (basketball, soccer) that have a component of endurance. Ergogenic benefits are mostly observed in athletic activities in which brief, explosive power provides a competitive advantage.

Usage trends are difficult to determine as a result of the wide variation in the use of these compounds among various sports, player position in team sports, and the level of competition. Rates of use by high school athletes vary widely, from 1.1% to 8.0% overall. Middle school use of these compounds has been reported as 2.7%. The overall rates of use in children have not appreciably increased or decreased over time.

Many factors influence use patterns and rates, including age and makeup of the study population; association with a peer group that uses steroids; knowledge of the beneficial effect of these substances; denial of the detrimental effects; association with other risk-taking behaviors; and dissatisfaction with current size and overall body image. Young athletes generally obtain information about the onset of action, duration of action, potential side effects, and options for administration from peers, coaches, strength training specialists, or muscle magazines rather than from medical authorities. Adolescents and young adults usually obtain information from the supplement industry and from the Internet; neither source provides accurate information about safety and efficacy.

Use of anabolic-androgenic steroids cuts across all socioeconomic strata; further, not only athletes use them. Increasingly, adolescents and young adults are using anabolic-androgenic steroids for cosmetic reasons, seeking to enhance their physiques.

Methods of Administration Anabolic-androgenic steroids can be taken orally or injected. The principal differences between the 2 forms include onset of action, duration of action, and the length of time during which detection is possible. Injectable forms are considered to be more potent and longer lasting but also of higher risk. Infection can develop at the site of injection, and needle sharing among athletes carries the risk of HIV and hepatitis B virus transmission.

Oral anabolic-androgenic steroids, including the 17α steroid derivatives and androstenediol, androstenedione, and dehydroepiandrosterone, are converted by the liver to testosterone after ingestion. Most injectable forms do not require hepatic conversion to an active form.

Adverse Effects Adverse effects from anabolic-androgenic steroid use have been reported in virtually every organ system of the body (**Table 10.1**). Some adverse effects are reversible; others are not.

One serious and irreversible adverse effect unique to the skeletally immature individual is physeal closure. A single cycle of anabolic-androgenic steroids may result in permanent epiphyseal closure and arrest of linear growth. Tendon strains and subsequent ruptures have also been associated with anabolic-androgenic steroid use. These have been attributed to muscle strength gains that exceed the strength of the related tendon.

Effects on the cardiovascular system include predictable but reversible increases in blood pressure, increases in total cholesterol, and a reduction in high-density lipoprotein levels. A higher risk of arteriosclerotic heart disease and possible cardiomyopathy are also concerns. An increased risk also exists of thromboplastic events in the coronary arteries due to increased production of thrombin and plasmin caused by anabolic-androgenic steroid use.

Negative effects on the hepatobiliary system include transient increases in liver enzymes and bilirubin. Peliosis hepatis (blood-filled cysts in the liver) has been associated with traumatic rupture and may result in fatal hemorrhage. Liver tumors, such as benign hepatoma or potentially fatal hepatic carcinoma, have also been reported, although their true incidence in young people is unknown.

Dermatologic problems, including acne and male-pattern baldness, are not life-threatening, but they may be the most obvious clinical signs.

In girls, the androgenic effect of anabolic-androgenic steroids results in masculinization, including irreversible hypertrophy of the clitoris, irreversible thickening of the vocal cords, and hirsutism. In boys, the genitourinary system is adversely affected in many ways. Testicular

TABLE 10.1

Body Systems Affected by Anabolic Steroid Use

Body System	Effect
Dermatologic	• Increased acne • Male-pattern baldness (in girls) • Hirsutism (in girls)
Cardiovascular	• High blood pressure • Increased cholesterol • Decreased high-density lipoprotein • Possible cardiomyopathy • Increased risk of thromboembolism
Musculoskeletal	• Epiphyseal closure in skeletally immature athletes • Tendon strain/rupture
Genitourinary	• Hypertrophy of clitoris (in girls) • Testicular atrophy (in boys) • Oligospermia (in boys)
Hepatobiliary	• Increased liver enzymes • Increased bilirubin • Peliosis hepatis • Liver tumors
Psychological	• Aggression • Emotional instability • Altered libido • Depression
Infectious disease (injectable drugs)	• Soft tissue abscess • HIV • Hepatitis B, C

atrophy, oligospermia, abnormal sperm morphology, prostatic hypertrophy, and prostatic cancer have all been reported in adults. In younger people, additional study is required to determine the effects of these drugs on the genitourinary system, the degree to which they adversely affect fertility, and the degree to which the effects are reversible.

Psychological effects are a common, but not always predictable, consequence of anabolic-androgenic steroid use. Aggression (known as 'roid rage), emotional instability, altered libido, and even steroid-induced psychosis have been reported. Depression may occur as part of a withdrawal syndrome. The risk of drug dependency is higher in individuals who start taking anabolic-androgenic steroids before age 16. Additional research is needed to learn whether athletes who abuse these substances at earlier ages and pubertal stages are at increased risk, compared with the adult population, for adverse effects on organ systems other than the musculoskeletal system. Because of the ethical and medicolegal issues inherently involved with giving these products to otherwise healthy young athletes in controlled scientific studies, the extent of these risks will most likely always have to be extrapolated from the use of these compounds in pathological states.

Physicians who care for young athletes are more likely to encounter individuals who are using, or who have questions about, anabolic-androgenic precursors that were widely available in the retail market in the past 2 decades. Androstenediol, androstenedione, and dehydroepiandrosterone (DHEA) received heavy media attention because many high-profile professional athletes openly acknowledged using these compounds. These products are directly metabolized to testosterone. Although these compounds are less effective than pharmaceutical-grade anabolic-androgenic drugs, young athletes need to be aware that if they are taking enough of the precursors to achieve an anabolic-androgenic effect, they are taking enough of the product to be at risk for the same adverse effects of anabolic-androgenic drugs. The original 1994 Dietary Supplement Health and Education Act removed these compounds from control of the US Food and Drug Administration. However, recent legislation (the Anabolic Steroid Act of 2004) placed these compounds under the Controlled Substances Act as class III drugs.

β2 Agonists

Another drug that has anabolic effects but that is not in the steroid family is clenbuterol, a β2 agonist approved for treatment of asthma in some countries. This medication can have anabolic effects in that it promotes protein synthesis and increases lean body mass. With oral and inhaled routes of administration, clenbuterol also has abuse potential for its stimulant effects. Physicians also need to be aware of certain restrictions placed on the use of other inhaled β2 agonists in elite competition. If young athletes are competing at the Olympic level and require the use of β2 agonists for control of reactive airway disease, athletes must request a therapeutic use exemption from their sport's appropriate governing body before competition.

STIMULANTS

Caffeine

Because many consumer products contain caffeine, stimulants are perhaps the most widely available ergogenic substances. Caffeine, a xanthine derivative in the same family of alkaloids as theophylline, is found in coffee, tea, chocolate, soft drinks, and prescription and over-the-counter drugs. The ergogenic effect of caffeine is derived from multiple actions, including central nervous system stimulation, delayed onset of fatigue, and increased metabolism of free fatty acids for energy while sparing glycogen stores. The average amount of caffeine in a cup of coffee (approximately 100 mg) has a small ergogenic effect for endurance activities. Some highly caffeinated soft drinks contain as much as 71.5 mg of caffeine per 12-oz serving. Over-the-counter drugs specifically intended to be used as stimulants contain as much as 200 mg of caffeine per tablet.

Ingesting any combination of beverages or medications that contain a total of approximately 800 mg of caffeine can result in a positive drug test in events that are subject to testing for performance-enhancing substances. However, caffeine levels do not have to be illegally high to have adverse effects. Caffeine acts as a diuretic, which can result in dehydration. This can lead to diminished muscular strength and endurance, as well as greater risk of a heat-related injury.

Energy drinks may contain an array of stimulants, including taurine, glucuronolactone, and caffeine. Data from Europe concerning risk of dehydration and catastrophic events in athletes prompted a warning at the 36th Bethesda Conference from the task force that reviewed drugs and performance-enhancing substances. Whether younger athletes are also at increased risk for catastrophic events from these products (relative to the adult athlete) is unknown.

Nicotine

Nicotine is another widely available stimulant used by many young people. Smokeless tobacco is often an attractive alternative to cigarettes to young athletes who underestimate its dangers. The health risks outweigh any benefit from the stimulant effect.

Ephedrine

Ephedrine, a chemical found in the plant genus *Ephedra*, was formerly contained in many nonprescription drugs, foods, and nutritional supplements. Because ephedrine is a major ingredient in the illegal production of methamphetamine, legislation has significantly restricted its availability. Ephedrine has ergogenic properties similar to amphetamines. Young athletes are likely to consume products containing ephedrine and pseudoephedrine in herbal teas, medications (eg, ma huang, ginseng, *Ginkgo biloba*), nonprescription cold medications, and nonprescription medications used specifically to attempt to reduce fatigue and to enhance mental alertness.

Amphetamines

Amphetamines are the most potent ergogenic drugs in the stimulant category. Illicit production of methamphetamine in home-based laboratories has increased its availability to all age groups. Amphetamines increase cardiac output and metabolism of free fatty acids. Central nervous system stimulation from amphetamines can increase aggression, increase mental alertness, and decrease perception of fatigue. Heat-related injury may occur from high metabolic activity and alterations in cooling. These compounds cause tachyarrhythmias that may potentially lead to catastrophic events during practice and competition. Athletes in a withdrawal phase of amphetamine abuse may experience depression and a marked reduction in athletic performance.

One area of medical and ethical controversy is the use of amphetamine derivatives and other related medications (eg, methylphenidate) in athletes with attention-deficit/hyperactivity disorder (ADHD). In athletic competition where complicated play strategy and team member assignments require concentration, athletes with ADHD would presumably perform better with medical treatment. Increasing the dose of methylphenidate for athletes with ADHD during competition has not been proved to be necessary to maintain attention. Likewise, increasing the dosage immediately before or during competition has not been proved to be safe in terms of cardiac- or heat-related complications of athletic competition. Therefore, young athletes who regularly receive methylphenidate to treat ADHD should be allowed to continue their usual dose of medication on days of athletic competition. Young athletes who are competing at the Olympic level should be aware that methylphenidate and other medications used for treating ADHD are banned substances.

NONSTEROID, NONSTIMULANT ERGOGENIC DRUGS

β-Blockers

β-blockers are compounds that slow the heart rate and lower blood pressure. β-blockers have little ergogenic potential except in sports such as shooting, archery, and combination sports (eg, biathlon) in which fine motor control and decreased tremulousness are critical components of competition. Physicians who care for athletes in these sports should be aware that β-blockers are prohibited substances in these sports.

Human Growth Hormone

Human growth hormone is a polypeptide hormone produced endogenously by the anterior lobe of the pituitary gland. With the increasing use of recombinant DNA technology, human growth hormone has become more widely available to athletes. Both the natural compound and the synthetic drug accelerate linear growth in the skeletally immature individual and increase body weight and muscle mass, regardless of skeletal maturity status. Researchers are investigating the degree to which rDNA HGH increases muscle strength and $\dot{V}o_2$max.

Athletes may use a wide variety of substances that may promote—or are dubiously purported to promote—production and secretion of endogenous growth hormone. L-Dopa, propranolol, arginine, clonidine, 5-hydroxytryptophan, insulin, caffeine, and a wide variety of dietary supplements have been used by athletes of all ages in attempts to achieve increases in endogenous growth hormone. The extent to which use of these products results in incremental gains in endogenous growth hormone production to levels that enhance performance is unclear, especially in the younger athlete.

Detection of polypeptide hormones by conventional urine drug screening is complicated by the fact that little of the parenterally administered product is excreted in the urine, and the synthetic product is difficult to distinguish from the naturally occurring compound.

Although increased linear growth and muscle size may enhance performance in selected sports, an insulin-like effect on glucose metabolism may hurt performance. Other significant side effects of exogenous human growth hormone supplementation include increased serum cholesterol and triglycerides, cardiac enlargement, hypogonadism, and acromegaly.

Blood Doping

Use of exogenous erythropoietin (EPO) or blood transfusions to enhance performance in endurance sports has been observed for decades. Both techniques are referred to as blood doping. Increasing the hematocrit and hemoglobin concentration improves the availability of oxygen to the exercising muscle and consequently improves aerobic capacity and muscle endurance. Physicians who care for young athletes are less likely to encounter blood doping techniques that involve medications (eg, RSR-13, a methylpropionic allosteric modifier of hemoglobin) that

are used to shift the O_2 dissociation curve in an attempt to derive performance enhancement in endurance sports by increasing the amount of oxygen available to skeletal muscle.

EPO is a glycoprotein produced endogenously by the kidneys. The synthetic compound is a product of recombinant DNA technology and is difficult to distinguish from the naturally occurring substance. Production of red blood cells increases in direct proportion to the dose of EPO used and can result in a hematocrit exceeding 60%. Autologous blood transfusions rarely increase the hematocrit to above 55%.

Blood components for transfusions are obtained from donors or are collected from the athlete approximately 6 weeks in advance and are then reinfused before competition. Blood doping detection techniques include analysis of red blood cell types (for homologous transfusions) and cell age (for autologous transfusions). Detection of EPO, although expensive, is becoming increasingly sensitive and accurate.

In athletes, dehydration during competition increases hematocrit. A hematocrit above 55% increases the risk for hyperviscosity syndrome and subsequent stroke, heart failure, and even death. Young athletes who use blood doping as an ergogenic aid are at increased risk for hyperviscosity syndrome because of their higher sweating rates and the consequent risk of dehydration with exercise.

Blood doping transfusions carry the added risk of HIV or hepatitis B infection. Physicians who care for young endurance athletes should be aware of the potential abuse of EPO and blood transfusions and should counsel their patients regarding the dangers of this practice.

Diuretics

Diuretics may be used in sports to reduce body weight, reduce fluid retention from anabolic-androgenic steroid use, or serve as a masking agent for drug testing. In sports with weight categories, such as wrestling, football, and crew, young athletes may use diuretics as part of a strategy to reach the lowest possible weight. Diuretics may also be abused in sports such as bodybuilding, gymnastics, and ballet, in which lower weight or a leaner appearance is rewarded. These products may also be used to control fluid retention or hypertension in individuals who use anabolic-androgenic steroids. Diuretics may be used as a masking agent in an attempt to circumvent detection of other substances in doping control, so agents such as furosemide are banned in competitions subject to doping control programs.

Physicians are more likely to encounter young athletes who are misusing diuretics when the medical staff is participating in minimum weight certification for sports in which competition parameters are defined by weight.

Dietary Supplements

Dietary supplements are oral compounds that do not require a prescription. The classification of a product as a dietary supplement often is determined more on the basis of legal or political considerations than on the biochemistry of the compound in question. They are loosely regulated under the Dietary Supplement Health and Education Act of 1994. Research studies have documented the high error rates in content and labeling of these products.

It is difficult, if not impossible, for physicians to determine whether an individual product is safe or free of substances that are banned by sports-governing bodies. It is also difficult to determine whether these compounds have any ergogenic effects in young athletes. For example, protein supplementation to a balanced diet has not been shown to significantly enhance performance. Likewise, vitamin and mineral products (including chromium) have not been shown to significantly contribute to athletic performance, especially in younger athletes. To be significantly ergogenic from the perspective of youth sports, these products should have a demonstrated incremental ergogenic effect over gains that can be achieved by adequate baseline nutrition, training, and skill development, yet such effects are difficult to confirm, even in the adult athlete, for most vitamin, mineral, and protein supplements. Reproducible, scientifically controlled studies of the ergogenic gains from these products in children and adolescents are virtually nonexistent.

Creatine, a nucleic acid in the guanidino family, has been touted as a performance-enhancing substance for the past 2 decades; it was first described in the medical literature in 1835. Its ergogenic effects have been found to be inconsistent, with only about 70% of test subjects showing 5% to 7% improvement in brief exercise activity. Athletes in endurance sports (cycling, swimming, middle- and long-distance running) are more likely to see performance degradation. The exact causes of the performance degradation are being investigated and may include factors such as increased weight. Creatine and other products that have a high osmotic load may also place younger athletes at a higher risk of dehydration and subsequent heat-related illness.

Because of the high rate of product contamination, adulteration, and mislabeling, further studies and closer quality control may be needed to determine the extent to which any of these compounds truly enhances performance in any athlete, child or adult.

DRUG TESTING

Drug testing for ergogenic substances is expensive and complex. However, young athletes who compete in events sanctioned by national sports federations may be selected for drug testing according to standards set by the governing body for each sport.

Some categories of drugs are restricted only in specific sports, such as β-blockers in shooting sports. Other drugs, such as amphetamines and anabolic steroids, are banned in all sports. Because many prescription and nonprescription drugs have effects that may enhance performance, young athletes who are subject to drug testing should contact their sports-governing body or doping control unit to determine whether medications they may be considering contain banned substances.

In recent years, school systems and youth organizations have instituted voluntary drug testing for young athletes in an effort to curb abuse and provide athletes with an additional weapon to combat peer pressure to use drugs. These programs typically focus on psychoactive substances. They are less likely to screen for drugs used exclusively for ergogenic purposes, such as anabolic steroids.

The text appendix includes a policy statement from the American Academy of Pediatrics that specifically addresses steroid use. Ergogenic products that are truly effective in enhancing sports performance (eg, anabolic-androgenic steroids, methamphetamine) are uniformly banned in youth sports at all levels of play. State high school activity associations and their parent organization, the National Federation of High Schools, also have published position papers condemning the use of prohibited ergogenic drugs.

Categories of ergogenic drugs and supplements are listed in **Table 10.2** and **Table 10.3.**

CONCLUSION

The use of performance-enhancing substances and other doping techniques is unethical, unhealthy, and potentially life-threatening. Physicians need to be aware of the potential for abuse of these substances by both athletes and nonathletes. Many substances have ergogenic effects and may be banned for competitors at national and international events. Physicians should be aware of drug control policies for their athletes and avoid prescribing or recommending a medication that may disqualify the athlete from an event. Counseling and sound medical advice are critical for athletes who are using or contemplating the use of performance-enhancing substances.

TABLE 10.2

Common Performance-Enhancing Substances

Category	Compounds	Ergogenic Effect

Anabolic-androgenic steroids	• Oral
	  • 17α methyl testosterone (eg, Android)
	  • 17α ethyl testosterone (eg, Maxi Bolin)
	  • 1-Methyl testosterone (eg, Primobolan)
	  • Androstenediol (eg, Andro food supplements)
	  • Androstenedione
	  • Dihydroepiandrosterone (eg, DHEA food supplements)
	• Injectable
	  • 19-Nortestosterone ester derivatives (eg, Durabolin)
	  • Testosterone ester derivatives (eg, Oreton)
	  • Testosterone cypionate derivatives (eg, Virilon)
	  • Boldenone (eg, Equipoise)
		• Increased muscle mass
		• Increased muscle strength
		• Redistribution of fat in a characteristically male pattern for cosmetic reasons
		• Increased aggressiveness, allowing for more intense training and competitive effort

Stimulants	• Amphetamines (eg, Adderall) • Caffeine (eg, NoDoz, Vivarin, Excedrin, Midol) • Methylphenidate (eg, Ritalin) • Pemoline (eg, Cylert) • Ephedrine derivatives (eg, pseudoephedrine) • β2 agonists (eg, albuterol, clenbuterol)	• Decreased perception of fatigue • Increased metabolism of free fatty acids • Increased aggressiveness, allowing for more intense training and competitive effort • Increased cardiac output • Increased skeletal muscle contractility • Heightened awareness • Weight reduction in weight-categorized competition
β-Blockers	• Propanolol	• Decreased fine motor tremulousness • Decreased heart rate

Polypeptide and glycoprotein hormones	• Human growth hormone (HGH)
	• Adenocorticotropic hormone (ACTH)
	• Human chorionic gonadotrophin (hCG)
		• Increased muscle mass
		• HGH
		  • Increased O_2 capacity
		  • Increased linear growth in skeletally immature individuals
		  • Increased cardiac output
		  • Increased red blood cell mass
		  • Increased circulatory volume
		  • Decreased body fat

Blood doping	• Erythropoietin (EPO) • Autologous blood transfusions • Homologous blood transfusions • Hemoglobin-O_2 affinity modifiers • Plasma expanders	• Increased aerobic capacity • Increased endurance
Diuretics	• Furosemide • Hydrochlorothiazide • Mannitol • Spironolactone • Acetazolamide	• Decreased weight in weight-categorized competition • Increased muscle definition for cosmetic reasons • Doping control masking agent

TABLE 10.3

Vitamins, Minerals, and Other Performance-Enhancing Supplements

Category	Compounds	Ergogenic Effect
Vitamins	• Vitamin C–ascorbic acid • Vitamin E–α tocopherol • B vitamins–thiamine, riboflavin, niacin, pyridoxine	• Antioxidant • Improved immune system[a] • Improved metabolism[a]
Minerals	• Chromium • Iron	• Increased lean muscle mass[a] • Increased red cell mass in iron-deficient state only
Amino acids	• Arginine, ornithine, and lysine • Aspartates • Valine, leucine, isoleucine • Glutamine • L-Carnitine • β-Hydroxyl-β-methylbutyrate (HMB)	• Increase in lean muscle by stimulating endogenous growth hormone[b] • Reduced fatigue[b] • Reduced levels of tryptophan leading to reduced central fatigue[b] • Improved immune system, reduced infection risk • Decreased blood lactate[b] • Increased maximum O_2 uptake[b] • Decreased muscle catabolism from exercise • Increased muscle strength
Protein supplements	• Whey protein	• Increased weight • No clear advantage over adequate baseline diet
Nucleic acid supplements	• Creatine (methyl guanidine acidic acid) • Guanadino compounds	• Increased myofibril synthesis • Increased power in brief explosive competition • Increased weight
Other	• Sodium bicarbonate • Coenzyme Q-10 (ubiquinone)	• Sodium supplementation to reduce risk of hyponatremia • Increased exercise tolerance • Antioxidant[a]

[a] No ergogenic effect in young athletes substantiated by research.
[b] Not substantiated by research.

Providing medical information should not be construed as tacit approval for the use of performance-enhancing substances. Conversely, the use of scare tactics that emphasize the negative side effects of illicit ergogenic substances is ineffective as a deterrent to their use in young athletes.

Changes in the pattern of use by young athletes are more likely to be achieved by providing positive counseling regarding alternatives to illegal and dangerous techniques. Healthy alternatives include programs in strength training and conditioning, programs in sports nutrition, and camps or coaching in which emphasis is placed on acquiring sports skill and training.

SUMMARY POINTS

● Athletes must get the basics down (proper nutrition and fluid intake, skills development, proper strength and conditioning), or the tricks (performance-enhancing substances) don't work.

● If the athlete has the basics down, the tricks are of little incremental value in performance enhancement in a young athlete.

● The relative lack of product content quality control in the dietary supplement industry has resulted in major concerns regarding the safety of the use of these products in young athletes.

- If the athlete ingests a performance-enhancing substance in sufficient quantities to get an effect, he or she is taking enough to result in adverse effects.

- Use of illicit performance-enhancing substances is cheating.

SUGGESTED READING

American Academy of Pediatrics Committee on Sports Medicine and Fitness. Adolescents and anabolic steroids: a subject review. *Pediatrics.* 1997;99:904-908.

American Academy of Pediatrics Committee on Sports Medicine and Fitness. Use of Performance-Enhancing Substances. *Pediatrics.* 2005;115:1103-1106.

Faigenbaum A, Zaichkowsky L, Gardner D, Micheli L. Anabolic steroid use by male and female middle school students. *Pediatrics.* 1998;101:e6-e10.

Green G, Catlin DH, Starcevic B. Analysis of over-the-counter dietary supplements. *Clin J Sports Med.* 2001;11:254-259.

Johnson MD. Anabolic steroid use in adolescent athletes. *Pediatr Clin North Am.* 1990;37:1111-1123.

Pasquale M. Stimulants and adaptogens: part 1. *Drugs Sports.* 1992;1:26.

United States Anti-Doping Agency Web site. http://www.usantidoping.org/. Accessed May 28, 2008.

CHAPTER 11

Psychological Issues

Daniel Gould, PhD

Russell Medbery, MS, PhD

Opinions vary as to whether organized sports for children are beneficial or harmful. The potential beneficial effects include character development, confidence, leadership, teamwork, and achievement orientations; however, these attributes do not simply appear as a result of participating in sports. Similarly, participation in organized sports does not necessarily foster an environment of excessive stress, lower self-esteem, or apathy. Research has shown that the psychological benefits are more likely to occur when competent adult supervision is supplied by coaches and parents who understand children and who know how to structure programs that result in a positive learning experience. When these adults fail to understand the unique psychological makeup of the young athlete or treat children like elite adult athletes, negative effects are likely to occur.

Physicians caring for young athletes can provide qualified youth sport leadership in the psychological domain by helping parents understand the psychology of young athletes; helping to create developmentally appropriate policies, regulations, and coaching; and recognizing and managing psychological issues of concern, referring young athletes to pediatric mental health experts when appropriate. Many excellent references address the diagnosis and management of specific clinical disorders, including depression, substance abuse, and anorexia or bulimia. This chapter focuses on psychological issues related to children's participation in sports that can be recognized and managed by primary care physicians.

For conditions that require more specialized care, educational or clinical sport psychology experts should be consulted. Clinical sport psychologists are licensed to diagnose and treat individuals with emotional disorders (eg, severe depression, suicidal tendencies). In addition to extensive training in psychology, they receive additional training in sport and exercise psychology and the sport sciences.

Educational sport psychology consultants, however, are not trained to treat individuals with emotional disorders, nor are they licensed psychologists. Rather, they have specialized training in sport and exercise science and the psychology of human movement. These specialists may have graduate training in psychology and counseling. They are mental coaches who, through group and individual sessions, educate athletes about psychological skills and their development, including anxiety management, confidence and self-esteem development, and improved communication.

Although there will be times when a young athlete should be referred to a sport psychology specialist, in most instances the physician should be able to serve as an educational resource for parents and coaches of young athletes. This chapter, which is based on the latest pediatric sport psychology research and the professional opinions of leading developmental sport psychologists, focuses on 10 common issues that physicians are most frequently asked about children's sports.

COMPONENTS OF A YOUTH SPORTS PROGRAM

Parents should learn as much as they can about the philosophy of the overall sports program, particularly that of the coach. Signs of a desirable coach include considerable positive interaction with the athletes; strong emphasis on teaching sports skills and sportsmanship; and a consistent philosophy that puts the young athlete's physical, social, and psychological development before winning. Discipline has its place, but it should be used infrequently and never in a demeaning way. Ineffective or undesirable coaches provide little effective teaching and commonly use negative feedback and punishment, often conveyed in a demeaning manner. They also espouse a philosophy that places winning before the child's development.

One of the best ways for parents to learn about a coach is to ask specific questions about the coach's philosophy of coaching. What are the coach's objectives in working with young athletes? How does he or she achieve these objectives in practices and games? How much does each child play and how is playing time determined? Do children get individual attention? What role does the coach expect parents to assume? If possible, parents should be encouraged to attend several practice sessions to observe the type of interaction that occurs between the coach and the athletes. If this is not possible, parents should meet with the parents of other team members to inquire about the program and coach. **Table 11.1** outlines questions parents should ask when assessing coaches.

THE ROLE OF PARENTS IN A CHILD'S SPORT EXPERIENCE

Parents should be involved in their child's youth sport experience. Research shows that physically active parents are more likely to have physically active children and that parental support is critical for children's initial and

TABLE 11.1
What Parents Should Look for in a Youth Sport Coach
• Does the league offer coaching education?
• Has the coach had any coaching education?
• If yes, what coaching education?
• If no, what experiences qualify him or her to coach?
• Does the coach clearly outline his or her objectives for working with youth in sport?
• Do the coach's objectives match your child's?
• Do children get individual attention?
• Are you comfortable with the coach teaching your child?
• How are the coaching objectives achieved in practices and games?
• How much does each child play, and how is playing time determined?
• What role does the coach expect from the parents?
If you have 2 or more no's, you should consider finding another team, league, or sport.

continued involvement in organized sports. However, research has shown that too little or too much involvement can have negative psychological effects. For example, overinvolvement can lead to increased stress and burnout, which is physical or emotional withdrawal from a previously enjoyable activity as a result of long-term stress. Recent research also reveals that as many as 3 out of 10 parents are overinvolved in their children's sports and do things like criticize their child, interfere with practices, or pressure their child to win. Underinvolvement can negatively affect the child's sports participation and motivation, and underinvolved parents also have no way of knowing what is happening in their child's program.

Table 11.2 lists potential parent roles and responsibilities developed by the American Sport Education Program as part of its sport parent program. Using these guidelines, parents can achieve an appropriate balance between too little and too much involvement. The guidelines can also be used to learn how to respond to the child's sports experience.

PARENT AS COACH

Parents are appropriate and often necessary in the role of coach to their children in entry-level sports. In fact, 60% of the estimated 2.5 million volunteer youth sport coaches in the United States coach their own children. Because most parents have no formal training as coaches, participation in a youth sport coaching certification program and a first aid program are recommended prerequisites.

As children become more intensely involved in sports, the issue of parent as coach becomes more problematic. Although many outstanding athletes were coached by a parent, coaching one's own child can lead to increased stress and burnout. Children may confuse coaching feedback and criticism with a lack of unconditional parental love. Parent coaches also face the dilemma of remaining impartial, trying not to show favoritism toward their own child but also not overcompensating by being extra hard on their own child.

Given these concerns, parents should be encouraged to coach their children in sports at entry levels of play. However, as children move to higher levels of play, it is often easier to provide unconditional support if the child plays for another coach.

EMOTIONS AND THE CHILD ATHLETE

Emotions are an integral component of sport. From joy and excitement to sadness and frustration, athletes experience a wide range of emotions as they participate

TABLE 11.2

Parent Responsibilities and Code of Conduct for Children in Sports

Responsibilities

- Encourage your children to play sports, but do not exert undue pressure. Allow your child to choose to play, and to quit, if he or she wants.
- Understand what your child wants from sports and provide a supportive atmosphere for achieving his or her goals.
- Set limits on your child's participation in sports. You need to determine when your child is physically and emotionally ready to play and to ensure that the conditions for playing are safe.
- Ensure that the coach is qualified to guide your child through the sports experience.
- Keep winning in perspective, and help your child do the same.
- Help your child set realistic performance goals.
- Help your child understand the valuable lessons sports can teach.
- Help your child meet the responsibilities to the team and the coach.
- Discipline your child appropriately when necessary.
- Allow coaches to do the coaching—do not meddle or coach from the stands.
- Supply the coach with information about any injuries or other medical conditions your child may have.
- Ensure that your child takes any necessary medications to games and practices.

Code of Conduct

- Remain in the spectator area during games.
- Do not advise the coach on how to coach.
- Do not make derogatory comments to coaches, officials, or parents of either team.
- Do not try to coach your child during the contest.
- Do not drink alcohol at contests or come to a contest after drinking too much.
- Cheer for your child's team.
- Show interest, enthusiasm, and support for your child.
- Be in control of your emotions.
- Help when asked by coaches or officials.
- Thank coaches, officials, and other volunteers who conduct the event.

From American Sport Education Program. *Sport Parent*. Champaign, IL: Human Kinetics; 1994:29. Reprinted with permission from Human Kinetics.

in a sport. There are 2 aspects to emotions that affect participation in sports for children: the experience of these emotions and the effect these emotions have on sport participation and performance. The experience of emotion has 3 components: (1) an appraisal of an event, (2) an arousal factor, and (3) an emotional behavior. For example, a child might see a coach yell at a player to try harder. The child views this yelling as scolding and experiences an increase in arousal, causing tension. The child, fearful of the coach, then tries to avoid making mistakes around the coach. Another child could see the same event, but she interprets the yelling as positive encouragement. She also feels an increase in energy, but it is a positive feeling of determination. Because of the many different aspects of emotional experiences that a child may feel in sports, it is important to listen to what children have to say about experiences that occur during their participation.

Emotions also play a role in the performance of athletes. Adult and adolescent athletes experience a range of emotions as they compete. Although there is no single constellation or pattern of emotions that works well for performance, each athlete has an individualized constellation and zone of optimal emotional functioning that help enhance performance. Parents and coaches must help older children understand how emotions can affect performance and enjoyment in sport.

STRESS AND SPORTS

Pediatric sport psychology research clearly shows that most children who participate in sports do not experience excessive stress. Therefore, children should not be discouraged from participating in sports because of competitive stress concerns. However, this research has also shown that excessive stress can be a problem for certain children in specific situations. If only 10% of children experience excessive stress, this could still translate to millions of children nationwide. To increase awareness and to help reduce stress from sports, sport psychologists have identified personal and situational factors associated with heightened stress in young athletes (**Table 11.3**). Physicians who are familiar with this profile are better able to identify children who are experiencing unhealthy levels of stress and are at risk.

To help children with stress or who are at high risk of experiencing stress, parents and coaches need to be educated about what situations create stress for young athletes and what strategies are effective for reducing stress. A positive sports environment, without negative feedback or criticism, can bolster confidence and enjoyment while reducing stress. Stress can also be alleviated by reducing social evaluation (eg, "How did you play?" not "Did you win?") and the importance placed on winning (eg, no more fiery pregame pep talks). Finally, sport psychologists can adapt adult anxiety reduction techniques, such as progressive muscle relaxation, breath control, and mental training strategies, for use with children. General directions like "Just relax!" or "You can do it!" are not enough to help children manage stress.

CHILDREN AND BURNOUT

Burnout is a growing concern in competitive sports for children. It is thought to occur when early specialization in a sport and long, intense hours of training cause children to lose interest in the sport. Children as young as 4 years begin participating in sports such as gymnastics, swimming, or tennis and may be competing at an international level by their early teens. When careers end early or performance declines prematurely, burnout is suspected.

Recent studies have contributed to the general understanding of burnout as a special case of sport withdrawal in which a young athlete discontinues or curtails sport involvement that was once considered pleasurable. Although children withdraw from sports for reasons other than burnout, burnout should be suspected when other reasons for withdrawal are not apparent.

Adolescents who experience burnout typically have a 1-dimensional view of themselves as athletes rather than

TABLE 11.3

Characteristics of Children at Risk for Stress During Competitive Situations

Personal Characteristics

- High trait anxiety disposition (a personality disposition that predisposes a child to see competition and social evaluation as psychologically threatening)
- Low self-esteem
- Perfectionistic personality
- Low performance expectancies relative to his or her team
- Low self-performance expectancies
- Frequent worries about failure
- Frequent worries about adult expectations and social evaluation by others
- Less perceived fun
- Less satisfaction with his or her performance, regardless of winning or losing
- Perceived importance to parents that he or she participate in sport
- Outcome goal focus (places a great deal of focus on winning and losing, as opposed to self-improvement)

Situational Characteristics

- Defeat or victory—children experience more stress after losing than winning
- Event importance—the more importance placed on a contest, the higher the state of anxiety experienced by the participants
- Sport type—other things being equal, individual sports are more stressful than team sports

From Weinberg RS, Gould D. *Foundations of Sport and Exercise Psychology.* 4th ed. Champaign, IL: Human Kinetics; 2007:522-523. Reprinted with permission from Human Kinetics.

students, family members, musicians, or school activity leaders. In addition, these young athletes often have a limited sense of control of their own destinies, both in and out of sports. Their parents and/or coaches make the important decisions regarding their lives, with little or no input from them. Some burned-out young athletes also feel trapped; they stay involved in the sport only because they think that they cannot discontinue it. Prominent factors associated with burnout are listed in **Table 11.4**. Unlike the transient stress experienced by most athletes before a contest, the child with burnout has stress that constantly builds.

ENCOURAGING CHILDREN TO PARTICIPATE IN SPORTS

American children are increasingly sedentary, and as a result, they have greatly increased their health risks. In addition, children who do not participate in sports cannot derive the social and psychological benefits that come from well-run programs. Therefore, parents should encourage their children to become involved in sports.

One of the best ways to encourage children to become involved in sports and physical activities is for parents to engage in those activities with them. Parents are encouraged to engage in physical play with very young children (girls as well as boys), play ball with them, swim, dance, bike, run, and hike. Sharing in an active lifestyle sends a message to children that physical activity is fun and rewarding.

Although parental involvement typically increases a child's activity level, some children may still prefer more sedentary activities, such as watching television or playing video games. Potential conflict may be the result. Studies have shown that children who are pushed into activities that they do not want to do or that they dislike are not likely to develop the intrinsic motivation needed to sustain a lifetime of involvement. At the same time, if children are not exposed to sports, they will never fully appreciate what they are missing. Parents must then walk a fine line between encouraging and exposing children to sports without pushing them into activities they have no interest in. One possible solution is to ask children to select from one of several activities, with the understanding that if they do not enjoy the activity after 2 or 3 weeks, they do not have to continue. Moreover, the coach should be informed of the child's reluctance to participate so that he or she can be sure to provide a positive, encouraging environment. More often than not, children want to continue with an activity after a low-pressure trial period. However, if they still have no interest in the program after trying it for the designated time, they should be allowed to stop participating. This may be followed with an opportunity to try a different sport while assuring them that they can always go back to the first sport again if they wish.

Although patience and persistence may pay off, parents may reach a point when they realize that despite active encouragement to participate, competitive sports may not be right for their child. Nonetheless, children should still be encouraged to engage in some regular physical activity. Free play, recreational sports, and individual exercise programs provide healthy options for children who are not interested in or ready for competitive sports.

QUITTING SPORTS

Children cite many reasons for participating in sports, including fun, improving skills, friendship, fitness, challenge, and feeling worthy or successful. A strong sense of self and competence are particularly important for children to remain interested in participating. Children usually quit when they do not feel worthy relative to the activity ("I don't play well"), when one or more of their important motives for participating are not met ("My friends quit"), or when they become interested in other activities ("Scouts and soccer meet at the same time, and I like Scouts more"). Finally, studies have shown that children often quit one sport only to continue on in another, a phenomenon that has been labeled *sports transferring*.

TABLE 11.4

Factors Associated with Burnout in Young Athletes

- Very high self- and external expectations
- Win-at-all-costs attitude
- Parental pressure
- Long practices with little variety
- Inconsistent coaching practices
- Overuse injuries
- Excessive time demands
- High travel demands
- Love from others determined by winning and losing
- Perfectionism

From Weinberg RS, Gould D. *Foundations of Sport and Exercise Psychology.* 4th ed. Champaign, IL: Human Kinetics; 2007:522-523. Reprinted with permission from Human Kinetics.

Children may discontinue a sport for many good reasons, but if they quit because they have a bad experience or if they have a low sense of self-worth, the basis for these feelings should be addressed. If the basis for these feelings cannot be reversed, the child may be best served by sitting out for the season. After the decision to discontinue is made, a search should be undertaken for more positive options.

Children's physical self-worth is also highly related to their physical competence, so it is critical that novice athletes receive good instruction in fundamental skills. Children must not only be active but must develop a skill base that will equip them for lifelong involvement in physical activity.

DEVELOPING SELF-ESTEEM IN SPORTS

One of the greatest potential benefits of youth sports participation is the development of self-esteem and self-worth. Parents and coaches play a role in ensuring that this occurs, while the physician plays an important role in identifying children with low self-esteem.

Symptoms of low self-esteem include low levels of self-confidence, often expressed with phrases such as "I can't," "I'm no good," and "I stink." These children may also have difficulty making friends, are often afraid to take risks or engage in activities in which their performance is critically evaluated, and are generally anxious about participating in sports. Young athletes with low self-esteem may exhibit little effort because they feel that, despite their best efforts, they will fail. If a more positive experience is not found, referral to a sport psychology specialist should be considered.

Coaches and parents are particularly important in helping build self-esteem in these children. Coaches use the following strategies on a regular basis to enhance self-esteem in young athletes: ensuring success by breaking down skills into smaller parts so that they can be more easily learned and mastered; modifying activities so that children can be more successful (eg, lower baskets in basketball); providing plenty of rewarding statements; ensuring that praise is sincere; maintaining realistic expectations; rewarding effort as much as outcome; creating an environment that reduces fear of trying new skills; and being enthusiastic.

WHEN A CHILD FAILS IN SPORTS

A difficult situation for parents is knowing what to say when their child fails in sports. Every child reacts differently to failure; some may appear unaffected, whereas others have trouble coping.

Parents must show unconditional love and emotional support when their child fails or feels as if he or she has failed a sport. Involved parents need to be aware of the possibility of getting so caught up in their child's athletic success that they subtly—or not so subtly—convey their disappointment in the child when the child loses or fails. Generally, parents should refrain from giving corrective advice because the child often misinterprets this advice as criticism. Although some parents wait to give advice until after the child has had time to deal with the mistake or loss, a better solution may be to let the coach provide the advice; after all, that is the coach's job.

Parents who feel compelled to give advice should follow the so-called 3-fold psychological sandwich approach to error correction. First, mention what the child did correctly ("Good try—you stayed right in there on that pitch") because this will help reduce the child's frustration in making the error. Second, provide information to correct the error made ("Watch the ball all the way"). End with an encouraging remark ("Stick with it—it's tough, but you'll get it"). Parents should also wait until the child is emotionally calm before conveying any advice.

LEARNING THE RIGHT VALUES THROUGH SPORTS

Most parents want their children to develop character and good moral values such as honesty, integrity, and compassion through their sports participation. Although a child has the potential to develop such attributes and values, these values must be taught and modeled; they do not simply appear with participation in sports.

Parents should first identify the values they would most like to instill in their child, then assess the values of the organization and the coaches who are working with their children. Studies have shown that young athletes model the values of the people they spend time with and admire. At the organizational level, parents should become familiar with league rules and talk with other parents to find out how athletes, coaches, and parents are treated. At the team level, parents should learn what values the coach emphasizes; whether his or her actions are consistent with those values; and whether the players, parents, and coaches are treated with respect. On the field, parents should learn whether rules are reinforced and whether all players are treated in a fair, consistent manner. They should also observe the types of values the coaches and other parents display in front of the athletes and determine whether winning is given more importance than effort, improvement, and enjoyment.

Finally, parents should play a role in reinforcing desirable values, identifying undesirable behaviors, and serving as appropriate role models.

SUMMARY POINTS

- Participation in organized sports has many potential benefits for psychological development in young athletes. However, benefits will be derived only if competent, qualified adult leadership is provided throughout the youth sports experience.

- The physician plays an important role in educating parents and coaches in the best strategies for ensuring that the best possible psychological development is provided to young athletes.

- Parents should know the reasons why their child participates in sports and should be aware that these reasons may change over time.

- Parents should talk with and listen to their child about his or her feelings about participation in sports. This can help avert burnout.

- The child is not a professional athlete. Parents need to find ways to focus on successes, which can be used to help the child build the confidence needed to work on areas of challenge.

- Corrective advice from a parent is often misinterpreted by the child as criticism.

- The Sport Parent Responsibilities and Code of Conduct can help parents practice supportive behaviors for their child (**Table 11.2**).

- Sports are an opportunity to teach character development, such as commitment and integrity, not a path for financial return.

- Most children who participate in sports do not experience excessive stress.

- Children should never be forced to participate in sports. Children should be offered a variety of activities and permitted to select one or more to try. Often children will agree to join activities with their friends.

- Parents should teach by example by being active.

- Organized sports are not for everyone. Children can still be physically active by participating in other nonsports activities and free play.

SUGGESTED READING

American Academy of Pediatrics Committee on Sports Medicine and Fitness. Intensive training and sports specialization in young athletes. *Pediatrics.* 2000;106: 154-157.

American Academy of Pediatrics Council on Sports Medicine and Fitness. Overuse injuries, overtraining, and burnout in child and adolescent athletes. *Pediatrics.* 2007;119:1242-1245.

American Sport Education Program. *Sport Parent.* Champaign, IL: Human Kinetics; 1994.

Association for Applied Sport Psychology Web site. http://www.aaasponline.org/. Accessed May 30, 2008.

Gould D. Intensive sport participation and the prepubescent athlete. In: Cahill BR, Pearl AJ, eds. *Intensive Participation in Children's Sports.* Champaign, IL: Human Kinetics; 1993:19-38.

Gould D, Lauer L, Rolo C, Jannes C, Pennisi NS. Understanding the role parents play in tennis success: a national survey of junior tennis coaches. *Br J Sports Med.* 2006;40:632-636.

Hanin Y. *Emotions in Sport.* Champaign, IL: Human Kinetics; 2000.

Petlichkoff LM. The drop-out dilemma in youth sports. In: Bar-Or O, ed. *The Child and Adolescent Athlete.* Cambridge, MA: Blackwell Science; 1996:418-430.

Smoll FL, Smith RE. *Children and Youth in Sport: A Biopsychological Perspective.* Madison, WI: Brown & Benchmark Publishers; 1996.

Sport Psychology Division of the US Olympic Committee Web site. http://www.usoc.org/teamusanet/TeamUSAnet_46377.cfm. Accessed May 30, 2008.

Weinberg RS, Gould D. *Foundations of Sport and Exercise Psychology.* 4th ed. Champaign, IL: Human Kinetics; 2007:522-523.

Weiss M. Psychological effects of intensive sport participation on children and youth: self-esteem and motivation. In: Cahill BR, Pearl AJ, eds. *Intensive Participation in Children's Sports.* Champaign, IL: Human Kinetics; 1993:39-70.

SECTION 3

Basic Management Concepts

CHAPTER 12

Risks of Injury During Sports Participation

Stephen G. Rice, MD, PhD, MPH

Virtually all physical activities and sports carry some risk of injury or even catastrophic outcome. If prevention of all injuries were the only goal, then the only appropriate solution would be to eliminate sports and recreational activities. Injuries are an inevitable outcome of challenging competition; striving to push the body to its limit entails the risk of exceeding that limit. Loss of control, or facing forces greater than the body or a specific body part can withstand, often results in traumatic injury. Similarly, excessive training may result in an overuse injury rather than the desired conditioning or performance outcome.

More and more young athletes are engaging in intense continuous training or participating in several sports during a single season. Both of these behaviors increase the risk of overuse injuries. In addition, summer sports camps have grown in popularity, but they pose the risk of resulting in acute and overuse injuries if the athlete has not undertaken appropriate sport-specific physical conditioning in the weeks before attending camp.

Physicians seek to provide guidance to parents who ask, "Is this activity safe for my child?" or "Is this activity appropriate for my child?" It is the physician's responsibility to help define reasonableness and the appropriateness of particular activites, depending on the child's physiologic, emotional, and cognitive abilities. Data from epidemiologic studies can be used to help identify the risks of injury in various sports activities. If, after receiving appropriate information regarding the benefits and risks, a parent believes that the benefits clearly outweigh the risks, the activity is worthwhile; if the risks exceed the benefits, then the activity is too dangerous to justify participation. This kind of analysis varies among families, depending on their values and their comfort with risk in sporting activities.

Initial steps toward preventing and managing injuries include the recognition and acceptance by athletes, coaches, and parents that some risk is always present during physical activity. Managing or controlling risk associated with sports activity requires identifying and quantifying such risks, then using methods to minimize them. Risk is assessed, predicted, or measured through careful injury surveillance studies that note the frequency of injury in a given sport, as well as factors leading to or associated with such injury.

When similar definitions and methodologies are used, meaningful comparisons of risk within sports and among sports become feasible. Through analysis of injury data, trends and patterns of related variables may emerge that can lead to the development of specific strategies and interventions designed to reduce the frequency of future injuries. This chapter presents the relative frequency of injuries, including catastrophic injuries, in various sports activities.

DEFINITIONS

An athletic injury is a medical condition, resulting from athletic activity, that causes a limitation or restriction on participation in that activity or for which medical treatment was received. The 2 most common ways to develop a definition of injury in the context of sports activity are an accurate, specific diagnosis and an accounting of time lost from participation. Days of time lost are counted until the athlete returns to full, unrestricted participation. In some studies, any injury that resulted in limitation or restriction on participation was included; in other studies, only injuries that have limitations or restrictions beyond the day of injury merit inclusion.

To establish injury rates, information regarding the total number of participants or the total number of athletic exposures is also required. An athletic exposure—a unit of risk—is defined as one athlete participating in one practice or contest in which he or she is exposed to the possibility of an athletic injury (an opportunity to become injured through participation).

Data about the number of injuries give numerator information; data about the population at risk give denominator information. Injury rate data are usually expressed in terms of injuries per unit of participation or risk, such as injuries per 100 athletes per season or injuries per 1000 athletic exposures. The quality of the denominator often determines the accuracy and power of the data, making injury rate per 1000 athletic exposures a more accurate method of reporting than injuries per 100 athletes per season.

RESULTS OF INJURY SURVEILLANCE STUDIES

Reliable data about the risks of participation are generally lacking in recreational youth sports, including organized, competitive, and team sports. Still, the consensus is that injury rates are low in all organized sports at the youth level because prepubertal athletes do not often generate sufficient force during collisions or falls to cause tissue damage. Injury rates rise dramatically when participants reach puberty because athletes get bigger, stronger, faster, and more aggressive with age. Because the kinetic energy of a collision is related to both mass and velocity, adolescent athletes generate and receive far more force than prepubertal children.

Among children younger than age 10 years, fractures and catastrophic injuries occur more frequently from individual recreational activities than from organized sports. Such injuries often occur from falls or collisions while riding bicycles or horses, from using skateboards or in-line skates, while on trampolines or sleds, while climbing trees and fences, or while generally roughhousing. Many of these injuries occur while the child is learning the activity (during the first week), before full acquisition of the skills has been achieved.

More than 7 million boys and girls participate in interscholastic high school sports every year. Large high school

injury surveillance and epidemiologic studies have resulted in relatively consistent patterns of data. The National Athletic Trainers' Association (NATA) gathered injury data for the period between 1995 and 1997 on 10 sports from more than 200 high schools nationwide that employ certified athletic trainers. The North Carolina High School Athlete Injury Study, funded by the National Institutes of Health, examined 12 sports from 100 high schools between 1996 and 2000. A high school sports-related injury surveillance study, sponsored by a Centers for Disease Control and Prevention (CDC) grant using NATA-certified athletic trainers, was conducted during the 2005-2006 school year using a nationally representative sample of 100 high schools; it studied 9 sports. The Athletic Health Care System (AHCS) studied injuries in all 18 sports among 20 high schools in the Seattle area over 14 years, from 1979 to 1993, using specifically trained coaches and their student athletic trainers as reporters. The AHCS database contains data about nearly 60 000 athletes who have participated in more than 2.5 million days of athletic activity.

Both the original NATA and AHCS studies reveal, for example, that 35% of football players experience at least one time-loss injury per season—the highest among the sports surveyed. About 50% to 80% of reportable injuries in all sports are minor, causing the athlete to miss fewer than 5 to 7 days of participation; between 4% and 15% of injuries entail a time loss of more than 3 weeks. Approximately 55% of injuries in all high school sports (including football) occur in practice, reflecting the greater number of practices compared with games and the participation of all athletes throughout practice compared with a small number on the field at the same time during games. On a minute-by-minute basis, however, game action produces more injuries than practice. In the North Carolina High School Injury Study, preseason injuries are reported at a higher rate than in-season injuries; further, girls had higher rates of injuries than boys during preseason but not during the regular season.

The composite rank order of injury rates among the sports included in all of these four surveillance studies is, in descending order, football, wrestling, girls' soccer, boys' soccer, boys' basketball, girls' basketball, volleyball, girls' softball, and baseball (**Table 12.1**). Fall sports had the highest rates of injury, and spring sports had the lowest. Older students (juniors and seniors) had higher rates of injury than younger students (freshmen and sophomores). Wrestling, football, and gymnastics are high on the list of injury frequency and severity in every injury study. The AHCS study was the only study to include cross-country running, swimming, tennis, and golf. Girls' cross-country had the highest reported rate of injury among all high school sports (injuries per 1000 athletic exposures), with boys' cross-country in fifth place. Girls' soccer (fourth place) and boys' soccer (seventh place) were also in this top tier.

The mass of accumulated data makes it difficult to definitively determine whether girls experience more injuries than boys in soccer, basketball, and track, but there is consensus that the rates of knee surgery for high school girls, particularly for anterior cruciate ligament (ACL) injuries, markedly exceed that of boys, especially in soccer and basketball. ACL injuries in soccer, for both boys and girls, occur significantly more frequently than in basketball. Attention has been focused on understanding and preventing ACL injuries. Detailed biomechanical studies of jumping

and landing in high school athletes have yet to lead to firm evidence-based solutions. Avoiding stiff-legged landings has been recognized as an important safety technique; using plyometric training to teach proper landings is gaining in popularity. Strength in both the quadriceps muscles and hamstring muscles is essential, including an appropriate strength ratio. Core stability, lower extremity motor control, and prioprioception are also critical parameters in reducing stress on the ACL.

Different sports stress different body parts, which results in a variable distribution of injuries among different sports. For example, the NATA data show that 75% of injuries in girls' soccer occur in the lower extremity, compared with 60% to 65% for girls' basketball, volleyball, and field hockey. The AHCS data show that in cross-country running, 94% of injuries involve the lower extremities,

TABLE 12.1

Ranking of All Sports Injury Data, Fall 1979-Spring 1992[a]

Rank[b]	Sport	Season	Total Athletes	Injury Rate/100 Athletes/ Season	Injury Rate/1000 Athletic Exposures	Significant Injury Rate/1000 Athletic Exposures[c]	Major Injury Rate/1000 Athletic Exposures[d]	Different Athletes Injured, %[e]
1	Girls' cross-country	Fall	1299	61.4	17.3	3.3	0.9	33.1
2	Football	Fall	8560	58.8	12.7	3.1	0.9	36.7
3	Wrestling	Winter	3624	49.7	11.8	2.6	1.0	32.1
4	Girls' soccer	Fall	3186	43.7	11.6	2.9	0.7	31.6
5	Boys' cross-country	Fall	2481	38.7	10.5	2.3	0.5	24.6
6	Girls' gymnastics	Winter	1082	38.9	10.0	2.3	0.7	26.2
7	Boys' soccer	Spring	3848	36.4	9.5	2.1	0.4	25.2
8	Girls' basketball	Winter	3634	34.5	7.1	1.7	0.5	24.2
9	Girls' track	Spring	3543	24.8	6.2	1.6	0.3	18.0
10	Boys' basketball	Winter	3874	29.2	5.5	1.3	0.3	22.9
11	Volleyball	Fall	3444	19.9	5.4	1.1	0.3	16.1
12	Softball	Spring	2957	18.3	4.8	1.2	0.3	14.8
13	Boys' track	Spring	4425	17.3	4.4	1.1	0.3	13.6
14	Baseball	Spring	3397	17.1	4.2	1.0	0.3	14.4
15	Fast pitch	Spring	134	11.9	2.4	1.2	0.6	11.9
16	Coed swimming	Winter	4004	8.3	2.2	0.5	0.0	6.4
17	Coed tennis	Fall/Spring	4096	7.0	1.9	0.4	0.1	5.8
18	Coed golf	Fall/Spring	2170	1.4	0.8	0.0	0.0	1.3
	Combined totals		59758	30.6	7.6	1.8	0.5	21.1

[a] Injury implies time loss with no participation and/or limited participation. With a typical high school schedule of participating 5 days per week, this means essentially a 1-week injury for a significant injury and a 3-week injury for a major injury.
[b] Ranking based on injury rate/1000 athletic exposures.
[c] Significant injuries are defined as 5 or more consecutive games and/or practices in which the athlete could not fully participate.
[d] Major injuries are defined as 15 or more consecutive games and/or practices in which the athlete could not fully participate.
[e] Percent of different athletes injured counts the number of different individuals who have been injured during a season.
Data from National Athletic Trainers Associaion, North Carolina High School Athlete Injury Study, Athletic Health Care System, and Centers for Disease Control and Prevention (see Comstock entry in the Suggested Readings).

compared with 80% to 85% for soccer and 70% to 74% for basketball. Swimmers, tennis players, and baseball pitchers tend to experience more upper extremity injuries, whereas gymnasts tend to have an equal distribution between upper and lower extremity injuries. Most injuries in cross-country running are caused by overuse, while most injuries in wrestling are caused by acute trauma.

The most commonly injured body parts vary with age and sports activity. The youngest athletes often experience upper extremity injuries from falling on an outstretched arm, especially fractures to the wrist, forearm, and clavicle. Among older children and adolescents, the lower extremity is more likely to be injured.

The AHCS data on body part distribution of 8479 injuries among all 18 high school sports over an 8-year period indicate that 55% of injuries are to the lower leg (knee and below); 12.6% to the upper leg (thigh, groin, hamstring, and hip); 13% to the back, neck, and head; and 19.4% to the upper extremity (**Table 12.2**). More specifically in the lower extremity, 22.8% of injuries were ankle injuries; 16.7% were knee injuries; 9.8%, shin/calf; and 5.7%, foot. The length of time loss from (or severity of) knee injuries exceeds that of ankle injuries, with 13% of athletes with knee injuries missing more than 3 weeks versus 7% of athletes with ankle injuries. Sprains and strains account for more than half of the injuries in every sport in the NATA, CDC, and North Carolina studies. In the NATA study, the knee is the only body part to have more than 10% of reported injuries in all 10 sports studied. Fractures are the cause of less than 10% of injuries in high school sports.

CATASTROPHIC INJURY STUDIES

The National Center for Catastrophic Sports Injury Research at the University of North Carolina at Chapel Hill tracks and reports annually on catastrophic injuries and sports-related deaths among high school and college athletes. Catastrophic injury is defined as any severe spinal, spinal cord, or cerebral injury. Three categories of outcomes are identified: fatal; nonfatal with permanent disability; and serious, with no permanent functional disability, such as a fractured cervical vertebra with complete recovery. Each year, approximately 175 cases of paraplegia and 75 cases of quadriplegia are related to a sports injury.

Types of Catastrophic Injuries

Catastrophic injuries are divided into 2 categories: direct and indirect cause. Direct injuries are those resulting directly from participation in the skills of the sport, such as tackling in football or making a save in hockey. Trauma is the cause of these injuries. Indirect injuries are caused by a systemic failure as the result of exertion while participating in a sport or activity or by a complication that results from a nonfatal injury. These injuries are nontraumatic. Sudden cardiac death and dehydration/hyperthermia death are examples of indirect catastrophic injury.

Catastrophic injury data among high school athletes from the fall of 1982 through the spring of 2004 are reported in **Table 12.3** and **Table 12.4**. Among boys, gymnasts had the highest rates for direct traumatic fatalities and permanent injuries; ice hockey was second in both categories. Football was fourth in direct fatalities and third

TABLE 12.2

Injuries by Body Part

Body Part	No.	Overall, %	Game, %	Practice, %	1 Day	2-4 Days	5-15 Days	>15 Days
						Length of Injury, %		
Ankle	1937	22.8	30.8	69.2	31.5	37.4	24.3	6.8
Knee	1415	16.7	26.6	73.4	31.7	31.8	23.8	12.7
Hand, wrist, elbow	1126	13.3	29.5	70.5	43.9	27.7	19.7	8.7
Shin, calf	829	9.8	20.3	79.7	33.5	36.3	21.1	9.0
Thigh, groin	623	7.3	15.6	84.4	32.6	43.2	22.0	2.2
Head, neck, collarbone	618	7.3	42.4	57.6	51.3	31.9	12.9	3.9
Shoulder	517	6.1	31.8	68.2	33.7	35.2	22.4	8.7
Foot	485	5.7	17.8	82.2	36.1	36.2	21.9	5.8
Back	484	5.7	25.3	74.7	32.0	38.4	20.5	9.1
Hip	234	2.8	24.2	75.8	37.6	37.2	18.8	6.4
Hamstring	211	2.5	22.4	77.6	27.5	40.3	25.1	7.1
Totals	8479	100	27.2	72.8	35.4	35.0	21.7	7.9

Data from Athletic Health Care System.

TABLE 12.3

Boys' High School Direct and Indirect Injuries, "Fall 1982 to Spring 2005"

Sport	Season	Direct, %			Indirect, %		
		Fatal	Nonfatal	Serious	Fatal	Nonfatal	Serious
Cross-country	Fall	0.00	0.03	0.00	0.38	0.00	0.00
Football	Fall	0.31	0.75	0.76	0.48	0.00	0.01
Soccer	Fall/Spring	0.10	0.03	0.10	0.38	0.00	0.00
Water polo	Fall	0.00	0.00	0.00	1.79	0.00	0.00
Basketball	Winter	0.02	0.03	0.07	0.73	0.00	0.01
Gymnastics	Winter	1.09	2.19	1.09	0.00	0.00	0.00
Ice hockey	Winter	0.33	1.14	1.14	0.65	0.00	0.00
Swimming	Winter	0.00	0.26	0.16	0.05	0.00	0.00
Wrestling	Winter	0.04	0.59	0.33	0.31	0.00	0.02
Baseball	Spring	0.11	0.17	0.20	0.15	0.00	0.00
Lacrosse	Spring	0.31	0.63	0.31	0.63	0.00	0.00
Tennis	Fall/Spring	0.00	0.00	0.00	0.09	0.00	0.00
Track	Spring	0.17	0.13	0.15	0.22	0.00	0.00

Source: Mueller FO, Cantu RC. *Twenty-third Annual Report, Fall 1982-Spring 2005*. Chapel Hill, NC: National Center for Catastrophic Sports Injury Research; 2006. Injury rates are per 100 000 participants. Direct indicates injuries resulting directly from trauma related to participation in the skills of the sport; indirect injuries are caused by a systemic failure resulting from exertion while participating in a sport or activity, or by a complication that resulted from a nonfatal injury; fatal, athlete died; nonfatal, athlete left with permanent disability; and serious, athlete experienced severe injury but recovered, to be left with no permanent functional disability.

TABLE 12.4

Girls' High School Direct and Indirect Injuries, "Fall 1982 to Spring 2005"

Sport	Season	Direct, %			Indirect, %		
		Fatal	Nonfatal	Serious	Fatal	Nonfatal	Serious
Cross-country	Fall	0.00	0.00	0.00	0.14	0.00	0.00
Football	Fall	0.00	0.00	0.00	0.00	0.00	0.00
Soccer	Fall	0.00	0.02	0.00	0.14	0.00	0.00
Volleyball	Fall/Winter	0.00	0.02	0.00	0.02	0.00	0.00
Field hockey	Fall	0.00	0.24	0.00	0.00	0.00	0.00
Water polo	Fall	0.00	0.00	0.00	0.78	0.00	0.00
Basketball	Winter	0.00	0.01	0.03	0.10	0.00	0.01
Gymnastics	Winter	0.00	1.03	0.51	0.00	0.00	0.00
Ice hockey	Winter	0.00	0.00	4.15	0.00	0.00	0.00
Swimming	Winter	0.00	0.16	0.04	0.24	0.00	0.04
Wrestling	Winter	0.00	0.00	0.00	0.00	0.00	0.00
Softball	Spring	0.01	0.03	0.00	0.00	0.00	0.00
Lacrosse	Spring	0.00	0.00	0.24	0.00	0.00	0.00
Tennis	Spring	0.00	0.00	0.00	0.00	0.00	0.00
Track	Spring	0.01	0.01	0.04	0.05	0.00	0.00
Baseball	Spring	0.00	0.00	0.00	0.00	0.00	0.00

Source: Mueller FO, Cantu RC. *Twenty-third Annual Report, Fall 1982-Spring 2005*. Chapel Hill, NC: National Center for Catastrophic Sports Injury Research; 2006. Injury rates are per 100 000 participants. Direct indicates injuries resulting directly from trauma related to participation in the skills of the sport; indirect injuries are caused by a systemic failure resulting from exertion while participating in a sport or activity, or by a complication that resulted from a nonfatal injury; fatal, athlete died; nonfatal, athlete left with permanent disability; and serious, athlete experienced severe injury but recovered, to be left with no permanent functional disability.

in both permanent and serious injuries. Wrestling was eighth in fatalities and fifth in both permanent and serious injuries. For girls' sports, the only sports with direct fatalites were softball and track. Girls' gymnastics had the highest rate of nonfatal permanent injuries, while girls' ice hockey had a high rate of serious injuries. Cheerleading was not included among the sports studied, but evidence indicates that cheerleading accounts for half of the direct catastophic injuries in high school girls.

Indirect Fatalities

Indirect (nontraumatic) fatalities in high school boys are shown in **Table 12.3**. The sports with the highest estimated death rates per 100 000 athletes per year were water polo, basketball, ice hockey, lacrosse, football, cross-country, soccer, and wrestling. Among girls, indirect fatalities were reported in water polo, swimming, cross-country, soccer, track, basketball, and volleyball. The estimated indirect fatality rate for boys is more than 5 times greater than that for girls (**Table 12.3** and **Table 12.4**).

The cause of indirect sports fatalities among young athletes was cardiovascular in 70% to more than 90% of cases, noncardiovascular in 6% to 22%, and undetermined in 4%. Among cardiovascular deaths, hypertrophic cardiomyopathy (HCM) or probable HCM was the leading cause, followed by commotio cordis, coronary artery anomalies, myocarditis, ruptured aortic aneurysm (Marfan syndrome), arrhythmogenic right ventricular cardiomyopathy, aortic stenosis, and cardiomyopathies.

Among noncardiovascular conditions that caused death, hyperthermia, rhabdomyolysis, status asthmaticus, and electrocution were leading causes. Deaths have also resulted from exercise-induced anaphylaxis, aspiration/gastrointestinal bleeding, and Arnold-Chiari type II malformation.

Direct Fatalities and Injuries

Direct traumatic fatalities in high school football have been dramatically reduced since 1976, when spearing (or using the head as the first point of contact) was banned. The death rate decreased by more than 50% immediately and continued to decline steadily during the 1980s through 1994. Since 1994, there have been an average of 4.5 direct fatalities in football annually. Among high school athletes, 90% of the direct deaths between 1960 and 2004 involved the head, neck, and brain stem. Injuries to the heart, kidney, and abdominal organs accounted for the remaining 10% of direct football deaths. The direct fatality rate per 100 000 participants in football over 22 years was 0.31.

Catastrophic cervical spine injuries in football (in which there is incomplete recovery) continue to occur, averaging 10 injuries per year over the 22-year time studied. The direct permanent catastrophic injury rate per 100 000 athletes per year in football is 0.74.

Overall, fall high school sports account for 72% of direct catastrophic injuries and 54% of indirect fatalities. Football is responsible for 99.6% of direct fatalities and injuries and 74% of indirect fatalities during the fall season. Spring sports have the lowest rates of both direct and indirect catastrophic injuries. During winter sports, 78% of the indirect fatalities occur among male basketball athletes, mostly attributable to cardiac etiologies.

HEAD INJURIES

Head injuries have attracted ever-increasing attention, not only with the recognition of the catastrophic second-impact syndrome and the cumulative effects of multiple episodes of closed head trauma but also with better understanding of the pathophysiology and clinical course of concussion. At the professional sports level, especially in the collision sports of football and hockey, the effects of repetitive concussive events have been evident among athletes who have been forced into retirement. Mounting evidence indicates that the young developing brain is more vulnerable to damage from concussion than the adult brains of professional athletes.

The frequencies of these closed head traumatic brain injuries vary widely among various studies. When athletes are questioned directly about previous head injury, the rate is about 20 head injuries per 100 athletes per season in football. When head injuries are tabulated as one part of an injury surveillance reporting system, however, the reported rates are about half or less of those obtained through direct interviews.

Through the use of various diagnostic imaging techniques and neuropsychological testing, the tools available to the physician to assess and manage both mild brain trauma and more severe forms of head injury continue to improve each year. Since 2000, there have been 2 international consensus conferences on concussion and position statements from several major sports medicine organizations and coalitions. Additional information about head injuries is presented in Chapter 20.

CHEERLEADING INJURIES

A cheeerleader has evolved from a service-oriented leader of cheer on the sidelines to a highly skilled competing athlete who performs stunts requiring gymnastic abilities.

About half of the states have a state high school championship for competitive cheer; in 2003-2004, more than 89 000 girls (and 2251 boys) participated, making it the ninth most popular sport for girls. Catastrophic injuries among high school girls, however, continue to be a concern. Of the 73 catastrophic direct high school injuries among girls in the years between 1982 and 2005, more than half occurred in cheerleading. Falling from a pyramid, failing in attempts to complete flips, and flyers not being caught by teammates as they fall are the leading causes of catastrophic injury. Initiating safety guidelines, creating qualification standards for coaches, and requiring preparticipation physical examinations for cheerleaders are several recommendations that have been offered to reduce this injury rate.

RECREATIONAL ACTIVITIES STUDIES

Injury data from organized and unorganized activities are obtained through the Consumer Product Safety Commission (CPSC) and its National Electronic Injury Surveillance System (NEISS). Emergency departments in all regions of the country and of varying population densities participate. These facilities record injuries, which are then tabulated and projected to generate national totals. Significant injury is associated each year with bicycling (falling, collision with a stationary object, hit by a moving vehicle), skateboarding, in-line skating, jumping on a trampoline, snowboarding, skiing, and sledding—all activities done at high speed or with high energy transfer.

In 2005, basketball injuries (512 213) accounted for the greatest number of treatments in hospital emergency rooms in the United States, followed by bicycles (485 669), football (418 260), soccer (174 686), baseball (155 898), skateboards (112 544), trampolines (108 029), softball (106 884), swimming/diving (82 354), horseback riding (73 576), weight lifting (65 716), volleyball (52 091), golf (47 360), roller skating (35 003), wrestling (33 734), gymnastics (27 821), in-line skating (26 935), tennis (19 487), and track and field (17 306). However, there is no method of measuring the number of participants doing each activity, so injury rates cannot be calculated.

Several examples of the clinical applications of epidemiologic research to recreational injuries can be found in bicycling, skateboarding, and all-terrain vehicles (ATVs). The benefit of wearing bicycle helmets to prevent or minimize head injuries is the most obvious case. Skateboarders and in-line skaters who wear protective devices on the head, elbows, wrists, and knees greatly

reduce their risk of injury. The most common skating injuries occur to the wrist and forearm; therefore, the most important piece of equipment, other than a helmet, is wrist guards. When a high number of serious injuries from ATV accidents was discovered, interventions were undertaken. These included modifying the ATVs, recommending a minimum age for drivers, and requiring educational courses for all drivers.

The advent of extreme sports has taken recreational activity and elevated it to a competitive level. By their very nature, these activities are as risky as they are exciting to perform or watch. Extreme sports are individual in nature and lack formal coaching or organization. No evidence-based studies of their injury risk have yet appeared. Skateboarding is the most popular of the sports, with many communities creating special parks for skateboarders. Snowboarding, now an Olympic sport, is challenging downhill skiing in poplarity in many areas among young winter sport participants. There are more wrist and upper extremity injuries among children in snowboarding than skiing but fewer knee sprains, thumb injuries, lacerations, and boot-top injuries. About half of ankle injuries among snowboarders are fractures; 3% of all injuries involve a fracture of the lateral process of the talus, dubbed snowboarder's fracture.

CLINICAL APPLICATIONS AND EXAMPLES

Athletic equipment and/or rule changes are often used to promote safety and prevent injury. Batting helmets in baseball, shin guards in soccer, headgear in wrestling to protect ears, and football and hockey helmets and pads are examples of commonly used safety equipment. When injury surveillance identifies previously unrecognized injuries, questions arise as to whether new equipment or modifications of existing equipment or rule changes could prevent or reduce the severity of such injuries.

On the basis of evidence from injury surveillance studies and the catastrophic injury registry, the elimination of racing starts in shallow pools has reduced catastrophic swimming injuries; educational campaigns to decrease heat-related injury in football and other sports have been initiated; weight-control measures in wrestling that use certification by body fat percentage calculations, proper hydration (urine specific gravity), and graduated weight loss regimens are used in more and more states; and recommendations of eye protection for sports involving sticks (such as field hockey) have been promulgated. Several other examples under consideration include requiring chest protectors for young baseball players to prevent commotio cordis, a fatal cardiac arrhythmia produced by blunt trauma to the chest by a batted or thrown ball; banning aluminum baseball bats from Little League through high school; and altering the ice hockey helmet to provide protection to the carotid arteries to prevent skate blade lacerations, protect the ears, and prevent ruptured eardrums. Only by knowing the mechanism and frequency of such injuries and the efficacy and costs of the new equipment can it be reasonably determined whether such changes are needed and appropriate.

SUMMARY POINTS

- The increasing participation of younger athletes in physical activities and sports at a high level of intensity on a year-round basis or in multiple competitive sports during a single season has led to a rise in the frequency of both acute and overuse injuries. Appropriate prevention, early recognition, and proper management of these injuries can minimize any pain and discomfort the athlete endures while ensuring complete rehabilitation.

- Children younger than 10 years of age are at higher risk of injury from recreational activities than from organized sports.

- Young children usually experience upper extremity injuries, whereas older children and adolescents usually experience lower extremity injuries.

- Between 50% and 60% of all injuries occur during practice. On a minute-by-minute basis, games yield higher rates of injury than practice.

- High school boys have the highest rate of injury per athletic exposure in football. Among girls, the highest injury rate occurs in cross-country running.

- The highest rates of direct catastrophic injuries (traumatic fatalities and permanent injuries) among boys' and girls' sports occur in gymnastics.

- Half of all direct traumatic fatalities and permanent injuries among high school girls have occurred in cheerleading as this sport has evolved toward more difficult stunts and interscholastic competition.

- Concussion (mild traumatic brain injury) associated with sports participation continues to be a major concern because brain healing and full recovery require sufficient brain rest. Symptomatic athletes should never be returned to participation; some mental functions are not fully restored to normal levels even when the patient no longer demonstrates symptoms.

- When participating in organized sports, children should be well coached and supervised, play on a safe playing surface, and be well fitted in appropriately conditioned protective equipment.

- Injury surveillance studies generate data that may help physicians advise parents on the risks of sports participation, but more important, such research leads to improvements in rules and protective equipment to prevent injuries.

- Skateboarding and snowboarding have increased dramatically in participation levels and have become competitive sports. Helmets and wrist guards are essential for minimizing head injuries and wrist trauma. Specially designed skateboard parks and snowboarding areas on the slopes may also help control injuries.

SUGGESTED READING

Athletic Health Care System. Contact: Stephen G. Rice, M.D., Department of Pediatrics, Jersey Shore University Medical Center, Neptune, NJ.

Caine DJ, Caine CG, Lindner KJ, eds. *Epidemiology of Sports Injuries.* Champaign, IL: Human Kinetics; 1996.

Caine DJ, Maffulli N, eds. *Epidemiology of Pediatric Sports Injuries: Individual Sports* (vol 48); *Team Sports* (vol 49). Basel, Switzerland: Karger; 2005. *Medicine and Sport Science*; vols 48-49.

Comstock RD, Knox C, Gilchrist J. Sports-related injuries among high school athletes—United States, 2005-2006 school year. *MMWR Morb Mortal Wkly Rep.* 2006;55(38):1037-1040.

Mueller FO, Cantu RC. *Twenty-third Annual Report, Fall 1982-Spring 2005.* Chapel Hill, NC: National Center for Catastrophic Sports Injury Research; 2006.

Mueller FO, Cantu RC, Can Camp SP, eds. *Catastrophic Injuries in High School and College Sports.* Vol. 8. Champaign, IL: Human Kinetics; 1996.

Mueller FO, Weaver NL, Yang J, et al. *Final Report—The North Carolina High School Athlete Injury Study.* Bethesda, MD: National Institute of Arthritis and Musculoskeletal and Skin Diseases; 2002.

National Center for Catastrophic Sports Injury Research, University of North Carolina, Chapel Hill, NC. http://www.unc.edu/depts/nccsi.

National Collegiate Athletic Association (NCAA) Injury Surveillance System. Available at http://www.ncaa.org/wps/ncaa?ContentID=355.

National Collegiate Athletic Association Injury Surveillance System: (Descriptive Epidemiology of Collegiate Sports Injuries). *J Athl Train. 2007;*42(2):170-319.

NEISS Data Highlight: National Electronic Injury/Illness Surveillance System (NEISS). Bethesda, MD: Bureau of Epidemiology, US Consumer Product Safety Commission; 2006.

Powell JW. Epidemiological research for injury prevention programs in sports. In: Mueller FO, Ryan AJ, eds. *Prevention of Athletic Injuries: The Role of the Sports Medicine Team.* Philadelphia, PA: FA Davis; 1991:11-25.

Rauh MJ, Koepsell TD, Rivara FP, Margherita AJ, Rice SG. Epidemiology of musculoskeletal injuries among high school cross-country runners. *Am J Epidemiol.* 2006;163:151-159.

Rauh MJ, Margherita AJ, Rice SG, Koepsell TD, Rivara FP. High school cross-country running injuries: a longitudinal study. *Clin J Sport Med.* 2000;10:110-116.

Rice SG. Development of an injury surveillance system: results from a longitudinal study of high school athletes. In: Ashare AB, ed. *Safety in Ice Hockey;* vol 3. West Conshohocken, PA: American Society for Testing and Materials; 2000;STP 1341:3-18.

Young CC. Extreme sports: injuries and medical coverage. *Curr Sports Med Rep.* 2002;1:306-311.

CHAPTER 13

General Principles of Injury Prevention

Joel Brenner, MD

Steven J. Anderson, MD

Sally S. Harris, MD, MPH

An approach to injury management that includes prevention distinguishes sports medicine from other disciplines that focus primarily on treating injuries after they occur. In sports, the potential for getting hurt while doing something for fun is a constant reminder of why injury prevention is so critical to ensuring that sports and physical activity are safe and healthy.

Prevention of illness, accidents, and injury is an integral part of pediatrics. However, when it comes to sports injuries, primary care providers and others who care for young people may feel that effective and proven prevention strategies are not readily available. For patients just beginning in sports or for experienced athletes who have already experienced several sports injuries, comprehensive care should include advice on how to reduce risk. General recommendations to "stretch" or "wear a brace" may, unfortunately, fall short of achieving safety goals. Similarly, the preparticipation evaluation (PPE) continues to be mandated and routinely performed, even though there is ongoing debate as to its efficacy in reducing injuries.

One of the limitations of a unidimensional prevention strategy is that injuries are multifactoral in nature. The same injury may have different causes; the same causes can produce different injuries. For an injury prevention program to be effective, it must address as many of the contributing causes of the injury as possible. Solutions may require looking beyond simplistic safety measures or what can be dealt with during a standard office visit. Prevention strategies that address only one component of risk will likely affect only a small subset of injuries. A multifaceted approach is usually necessary to prevent multifaceted problems.

INJURY PREVENTION MODELS

Examples of injury prevention strategies from other venues demonstrate the requirements and benefits of a multifaceted approach. Motor vehicle accidents remain a common cause of serious injuries and fatalities. However, injuries have been reduced in recent years as a result of safer cars, safer roads, and safer drivers. Driving can be compared to a sport, the car can be compared to the equipment that is used to play the sport, and the roads can be compared to the playing fields. With seat belts, air bags, impact zones, and good tires, the car can better avoid or withstand collisions. To make the driving environment safer, roads are contoured and designed for safety; they have warning signs, reflectors, guardrails, and lighting, and they undergo regular maintenance. Driver safety is enhanced by mandatory licensing requirements, vision tests, and adherence to safety rules that address speeding, right of way, and driving while impaired.

The parallels between motor vehicle safety and sports safety are obvious. Helmets, pads, and mouth guards are standard protective equipment for athletes. Shoes, like tires, are a factor in both performance and safety. Fields, playing surfaces, and terrain can be a factor in sports injury, as can variations in ambient temperature, humidity, sun exposure, and other weather conditions. The PPE may be the equivalent of a driver's licensing test.

In an entirely different arena, cancer prevention strategies raise additional parallels to sports safety. Many forms of cancer have been linked to unhealthy behaviors (eg, smoking), unhealthy diets, unhealthy environments, and even a sedentary lifestyle. Prevention focuses on education, reducing dangerous behaviors, reducing exposure to unhealthy environments, and making unhealthy environments safer. In addition, many cancer prevention programs focus on early detection with mammograms, Pap smears, colonoscopies, and analysis of prostate-specific antigen. Recognizing cancer in its early stages can improve treatment outcomes and reduce complications associated with progression to more advanced stages.

In sports settings, there are also risk factors related to the individual lifestyle, behaviors, nutritional status, fitness, and overall health. In sports, as in oncology, there is a premium on recognition and treatment of conditions in the early stages to prevent the progression to something more serious or long-term. Examining injury prevention strategies in other areas provides useful models for planning a broad-based, multifaceted approach to preventing sports injuries.

PRIMARY VERSUS SECONDARY PREVENTION

Reducing overall injuries can be done through both primary and secondary prevention. Primary prevention refers to preventing a first injury. In cancer, primary prevention might take the form of a no-smoking program. In sports, primary prevention might be a program to retrain jumping and pivoting techniques in attempt to prevent anterior cruciate ligament (ACL) tears.

Secondary prevention refers to preventing a recurrent injury or preventing a more serious injury from developing from an earlier, more treatable precursor condition. In cancer, mammograms are a tool for secondary prevention in that they can detect both recurrences and early disease. In sports settings, secondary prevention might be recognizing and treating shin splints to prevent a tibial stress fracture from developing. Secondary prevention may also include recognizing, treating, and fully rehabilitating a mild hamstring strain to prevent either the development of a complete hamstring rupture or low back problems. Over an athlete's career, a high proportion of the injuries are recurrent or secondary to a previous problem. Secondary

prevention refers to preventing a prior injury from recurring or preventing a mild injury from becoming more serious.

RISK FACTOR ANALYSIS

Any prevention program requires identification of risk factors for the injury or condition that is targeted for prevention. The risk factors for a sports injury can be divided into extrinsic and intrinsic categories (**Table 13.1**). Extrinsic risk factors include risks related to the nature and demands of the sport, the equipment used for the sport, the equipment used for protection from injury, and the sports environment. Intrinsic risk factors relate more to the individual participant and include variables such as age, gender, maturation, health, general fitness, psychologic makeup, and anatomic factors (eg, flexibility, strength, joint stability, alignment, and foot type).

Most injuries are due to a combination of extrinsic and intrinsic risk factors. When an injury occurs, the degree to which contributing factors can be identified and corrected will positively correlate with a lower chance of reinjury (secondary prevention). The observation of recurring patterns of risk factors that lead to particular injuries form the basis for primary prevention. Uninjured athletes who possess risk factors similar to injured athletes are logical targets for primary injury prevention programs.

EXTRINSIC RISK FACTORS

Extrinsic risk factors for sports injury can be divided into subcategories related to the sport, the equipment, and sports environment. Further analysis of these important components of injury risk will help in understanding the cause of injuries and will provide a foundation for prevention efforts.

Sport-Related Risks

Within a given sport, there are risks related to the nature and demands of the sport, coaching and training regimens associated with the sport, and rules and supervision related to the sport. Contact and collision sports tend to have higher overall rates of injury than noncontact sports, more injuries in games as opposed to practice, and a higher proportion of acute injuries. Endurance sports tend to have more overuse injuries and a higher proportion of injuries that occur from training rather than competition. Understanding these patterns can be helpful in allocating medical resources, providing advice on preparation and training for the sport, and counseling patients about overall risk and risk of specific injuries.

TABLE 13.1

Risk Factors for Sports Injuries

Domain	Examples
EXTRINSIC FACTORS	
Sport	• Nature of the sport (ie, contact vs. non-contact; aerobic vs. anaerobic; individual vs. team); physical demands of training • Coaching, training techniques • Rules, supervision
Equipment	• Equipment to play sport (eg, bats, balls, racquets, goals, shoes, cleats) • Protective equipment (eg, helmets, face masks, pads, gloves, goggles, mouth guards) • Injury protection equipment (eg, ankle tape, knee brace, cowboy collar, orthotics)
Environment	• Fields, surfaces, terrain • Facility use pattern • Accessibility • Weather conditions (eg, temperature, humidity, wind, lightning)
INTRINSIC FACTORS	
Age	
Gender	
Maturation	
Health/fitness	• Presence of acute or chronic illness • Body composition • Dietary habits and nutritional status • Cardiovascular endurance
Physical characteristics and function	• Flexibility • Joint stability • Muscle strength, endurance • Proprioception • Alignment (eg, genu varus/valgus; internal/external tibial torsion femoral anteversion; Q angle; pes planus, pes cavus)
Prior injury	
Psychological makeup	

Although avoiding high-risk activities may not technically qualify as prevention, information about the relative risk of different activities may allow a patient or family to choose an activity that carries a lower likelihood of becoming injured (see Chapter 12, "Risks of Injury During Sports Participation"). In some cases, the nature and demands of a sport have an unacceptably high risk relative to their particular situation. For example, a patient with a previous concussion may find the risks of football or wrestling to be unacceptably high but could safely compete on the cross-country and swimming teams. A girl with osteopenia and stress fractures may face far greater risks on the gymnastics or cross-country team than on the softball or water polo team. The choice of which sports to play is one way to control injury risk.

The knowledge and experience of the coach can also be a factor in injury risk. Coaches with more than 20 years of experience have nearly 50% fewer injuries on their teams compared to coaches with less than 5 years of experience. This is presumably the result of the experience they have acquired in organizing safe practices, teaching proper techniques, properly fitting and maintaining equipment, and dealing with injuries. Most youth sports coaches don't have more than 20 years of experience. However, coach education programs, first aid training, clinics with more experienced coaches, and involvement of trained medical personnel can help compensate for lack of experience.

Rules are part of all sports, and many rules are designed specifically to make the sport safer. Rules can address unsafe practices such as spearing in football, body checking in youth hockey, or headfirst sliding in Little League baseball. There are also rules governing the size of the fields, length of contests, number of pitches thrown, minimum or maximum number of practices, age and size of competitors, and requirements governing return to play after injury. Rules and their enforcement may vary by sport and level of competition, as well as regionally and nationally. Identifying the applicable safety rules can be a valuable component of overall risk assessment and may reveal opportunities to promote safety.

Equipment

Equipment includes items used to play the sport (eg, bats, balls, goals, racquets, bases, skis, shoes, and cleats); items designed to protect against injury (eg, helmets, face masks, pads, mouth guards, cups, and gloves); and items designed to prevent or protect against further injury (eg, ankle braces, knee braces, neck collars, wrist taping, and shoulder harnesses). Protective equipment is designed to enhance safety without compromising performance. Sports equipment has also been modified with safety goals in mind. In baseball, softer baseballs may reduce the impact from a thrown or hit ball. Breakaway bases can reduce ankle or leg injuries from sliding. Football helmets have more effective shells and padding. Soccer goals have better anchors to prevent them from falling on players.

Safety equipment is appealing because the injury prevention benefits are largely passive: changing behavior is not necessary to realize a safety benefit. However, equipment that is poorly designed, improperly fit, inadequately maintained, or improperly used may fail to yield safety dividends—and in fact may lead to an increased risk of injury.

Environment

Environmental risks include fields, playing surfaces, mixed-use facilities, terrain, temperature, humidity, and weather conditions. Fields that have ruts, sprinkler heads, surface irregularities, fixed obstacles, or movable obstacles can contribute to injuries. A carelessly placed first aid kit, piece of equipment, ball bag, bench, or bicycle can be a hazard if it is too close to the field of play. Surfaces that are too hard, too slippery, too sticky, or too unsanitary may also cause injury. For example, a wrestling mat is a playing surface that can also serve as a source for transmission of serious infections, including methicillin-resistant *Staphylococcus aureus*.

Mixed use of facilities can also be an injury risk factor. A swimming facility that simultaneously has swimmers, divers, water polo players, and aqua joggers vying for pool space can lead to dangerous crossovers. A sports field that has soccer players, runners, and javelin throwers in close proximity can also lead to injuries. Shared practice fields and multiuse facilities are common in youth sports, but related injuries should be preventable with appropriate scheduling and supervision.

Weather conditions can be a factor in injury in both subtle and obvious ways. The glare from a setting sun can leave a baseball outfielder vulnerable to being struck by a ball. Windy conditions for a platform diver can have negative effects on balance, timing, and trajectory. A dark and rainy cross-country course can lead to missteps, falls, and injury.

More serious weather-related injuries result from heat and humidity. Heat-related injury and dehydration are relatively common causes of serious injury and even death. Young people are at greater risk for heat injury than adults. By maintaining adequate hydration and scheduling practices and competition at cooler times of the day, heat injury should be entirely preventable. In extreme weather conditions with heat, humidity, cold, or lightning, guidelines should be in place to postpone activities until a safer time. The absence of such guidelines is an easily corrected extrinsic risk factor for sport injury.

INTRINSIC RISK FACTORS

Intrinsic risks relate to the individual and include factors such as general health, fitness, and psychologic makeup, as well as specific anatomic and biomechanical factors. Intrinsic risk factors have been the focus of most medically based efforts to identify at-risk individuals. Despite extensive research, there are few scientifically established links between intrinsic risk factors and specific injuries or overall injury rate. The role of flexibility in injury has been the most extensively studied. Even though tight muscles are seen in association with many injuries, there is scant evidence to suggest that stretching will prevent injuries. Most of the other intrinsic risk factors appear to contribute to injury in selected individuals in selected sports. As discussed below, none of the intrinsic factors in isolation is a particularly strong determinant of overall injury risk.

Age

Being young does not appear to make an individual more vulnerable to a sports injury. When growth plates (epiphyses, apophyses) are open, a young, skeletally immature athlete may be more likely, when injured, to have the injury affect a growth center. However, the skeletal immaturity of young athletes does not increase the likelihood that they will be injured.

Younger children are more vulnerable to heat injury and less tolerant of endurance sports in the heat. Children may respond differently to strength and endurance training, but this does not increase their risk of injury from strength or endurance training. Because children grow and develop at different rates, disparities in size and strength may contribute to injury in contact and collision sports such as football. When athletes are matched according to size, this risk can be mitigated.

Gender

Gender remains as a controversial risk factor for injuries. Concerns that girls and women might be more vulnerable to injury undoubtedly contributed to delays in the advancement of women's sports. Fortunately, these concerns have diminished as girls and women have gained more experience in sports, received better coaching and training, and have proved that they are capable and fit. Data now show that for comparable sports, girls and boys have similar overall injury rates. Selected injuries may be more common in girls, including patellofemoral stress syndrome and ACL tears. Injuries related to the female athlete triad are a gender-specific risk. Despite some lingering biases regarding girls' vulnerability to injury, there is no basis for restricting sports participation on the basis of gender (see Chapter 16, "Female Athletes").

Health and Fitness

It is not entirely clear whether poor health is a direct risk factor for injury or whether poor health is associated with other factors (such as weak muscles, tight muscles, or poor aerobic fitness) that indirectly contribute to injury risk. Previously sedentary, unfit individuals who suddenly increase their activity level are more likely to develop muscle soreness, strains, tendonitis, apophysitis, shin splints, and other musculoskeletal maladies. Heat-related injury is also more likely in overweight participants and in participants who increase activity without time for acclimatization. If health and fitness are compromised as a result of injury, illness, or poor nutrition, there may also be additional risk for injury associated with the underlying cause.

The effects of health and fitness on injury risk and performance will depend on the demands of the sport or activity. Poor health and fitness is not a contraindication to exercise or sports participation. In fact, increased physical activity may be a valuable component of improving fitness. However, to minimize the risk of injury in this population, particular care must be directed toward identifying and correcting the underlying cause of the unfit state. In addition, it is critical to outline a training and conditioning program that corrects deficits to a level sufficient to meet the demands of the sport or the exercise regimen that the individual plans to undertake.

Musculoskeletal Function and Variation

Injuries have been linked with many different forms of musculoskeletal dysfunction; musculoskeletal structure varies widely. Some of the common musculoskeletal findings linked with injury include tight muscles, hypermobile joints, weak muscles, strength imbalances, scapular dyskinesis, proprioceptive deficits, and core weakness, as well as alignment issues such as hyperpronation, genu valgus, external tibial torsion, femoral anteversion, and leg-length discrepancy. In assessing an individual's risk, these factors warrant consideration as potential risks for their particular situation. However, the connection between any of these musculoskeletal risk factors and a specific injury or overall injury risk is not sufficiently established to warrant restriction of participation.

There is no scientific evidence to support recommendations to stretch as a way to prevent injuries. Similarly, there is no scientific support for restricting loose-jointed individuals from sports, requiring prophylactic orthotics for flat-footed individuals, or placing a lift in the shoe of an asymptomatic patient with a leg-length discrepancy. Again, there may be specific circumstances where recommendations to stretch, restrict activity, wear orthotics, or place a lift may be entirely appropriate and necessary. However, there is simply insufficient evidence to support making these recommendations to members of the general population in hopes of preventing sports injuries.

Contexts for understanding the contribution of intrinsic risk factors to injury can be clarified with clinical examples. Many studies have shown an increased risk of subacromial impingement in athletes who have an unstable scapula or imbalance between the internal and external rotators of the shoulder. Patellofemoral pain appears to be more common in athletes with weak hip abductors. Shin splints are more common in athletes with hyperpronation. However, impingement can also be due to postural abnormalities and abnormal techniques for swimming or throwing. Patellofemoral pain can be due to other causes, including patellar hypermobility, genu valgus, or a tight lateral retinaculum. Shin splints can also occur in patients with a supinated foot. Because the same diagnosis may have different causes and the same biomechanical abnormality may lead to different diagnoses, it remains difficult to link any single risk factor to a specific injury or level of risk for injury. It logically follows that prophylactic correction of any of these risk factors in attempt to reduce overall injury rate is not scientifically supported. Specific corrections or modifications may be warranted on a case-by-case basis.

The lack of scientific proof establishing a role for these intrinsic risk factors in injury should not be construed as evidence that there is no effect. Because injuries are multifactoral, and because it is nearly impossible to carry out a prospective study where all injury risk factors are controlled, a scientifically rigorous study that addresses the actual contribution each of these factors has to injury may not be forthcoming. Therefore, individual circumstances may warrant a level of attention to specific risk factors that is not warranted for the general population.

Prior Injury

Athletes who are injured typically have risk factors that led to their injury, and they may acquire additional risk factors as a result of the injury or injury treatment. The effects of the injury, as well as time off for recovery, can result in loss of flexibility, strength, joint stability, proprioception, and overall fitness. The combination of all these factors makes a history of prior injury an all-encompassing risk factor for subsequent injury. The single question that has the greatest power in predicting future injury is, "Have you previously been hurt?"

Psychological Makeup

Psychological factors have been included on many lists of intrinsic risk factors for injury. Risk takers or sensation seekers may gravitate toward sports with a higher rate of injury, or they may take greater chances in sports. Overly aggressive play can be a risk factor not only for the aggressive participant, but also for the other competitors. Conversely, athletes who are tentative or timid may find themselves vulnerable in situations where more bravado is called for. Stress and anxiety can be caused by competitive sports or may be preexisting and exacerbated by sports participation.

Athletes' desire to please their coach may interfere with their ability to recognize injury or protect themselves from overload and burnout. The maturity and ability necessary to set limits may not be developed in younger athletes. Similarly, the highly driven, "no pain, no gain" approach to sports may interfere with timely recognition and treatment of injuries. Burnout and eating disorders also have psychologic precursors as well as psychologic effects.

Although an athlete's psychologic makeup and maturity may be among the most difficult risk factors to change or modify, recognition of an athlete's psychologic tendencies and vulnerabilities can nonetheless help primary care providers and coaches better prepare for the associated risks.

RISK FACTOR MODIFICATION

While risk factors for injury are numerous and difficult to perfectly predict, many may be mitigated. Risk factors related to the choice of sport, training schedule, or use of protective equipment can all be readily controlled. Preseason conditioning, dealing with prior injuries, and maintaining a healthy diet are also risk factors that can be modified. Rules of the sport, playing surfaces, and experience of the coach may be more difficult to control, particularly for the individual athlete. Physical characteristics such as hyperpronation, genu valgus, or leg-length discrepancy cannot be changed, but their effects, if any, may be mitigated by interventions such as orthotics, exercises, or a lift. In cases where a risk factor is deemed significant but cannot be modified or mitigated, it may be necessary to find a sport or activity where that risk factor is less critical.

OPPORTUNITIES TO IMPLEMENT INJURY PREVENTION STRATEGIES

The lack of simple, quick-fix methods for injury prevention may discourage practitioners from pursuing any injury-prevention effort. Fortunately, there are a number of readily available and user-friendly injury prevention strategies that make the task of safety promotion less daunting. Available settings for implementing injury prevention strategies include providing the PPE, office evaluations for injuries or illness, serving as a team doctor, working as a medical advisor to a sports organization or league, or serving as a sports safety advocate in the community.

Preparticipation Evaluation

The PPE is the most institutionally engrained and frequently used tool for safeguarding athletes from injury. The PPE has traditionally focused more on intrinsic rather than extrinsic risk factors. The overall efficacy of the PPE in injury prevention may be limited by the general nature of the examination, the short amount of time available for the examination, and the relatively small percentage of all athletes who are actually required to have the examination. Even with these limitations, there is no reason why the PPE can't be expanded in content and distribution to make it a more useful tool for injury prevention.

After completing the basic PPE, the examination can be customized to better address the risks that are relevant to the patient being examined. The questions listed in

Table 13.2 can help the examiner better understand the risks and demands of the given sport, the most common injuries associated with the sport or sports being played, and the extrinsic risk factors that are most directly related to the sport. These questions can focus the examination on more sport-specific injury risk factors and identify areas where sport-specific safety recommendations may be applicable. Inquiries about the coach's experience, safety procedures, and medical preparedness can also reveal important risk factors and prevention opportunities that will not be apparent by performing just the basic PPE. Questions that can help expand the role of the PPE in determining injury risk are listed in **Table 13.2**.

The PPE is also an ideal time to discuss risks related to particular sports and to counsel the athletes individually about whether the risks and demands of a given sport are appropriate for their age, maturity, health, and physical makeup. The PPE can help match athletes with sports where they have a better chance to be successful, and where they can participate without disproportionate risks of injury. The PPE is also a good time to point out circumstances when the nature and demands of a sport are not a good match for the individual. Chapter 46 provides valuable assistance in customizing the PPE to address the common injuries in each sport; it also identifies sport-specific injury prevention recommendations.

In general, endurance sports or sports that are repetitive in nature have more opportunities for injury prevention. Running, swimming, and cycling are common endurance sports, and they involve multiple repetitions of controlled movements. If the movements or stresses that lead to injury are known and predictable, it is easier to exert control over these forces through modifying training or technique, or by correcting underlying biomechanical abnormalities. When the forces or mechanisms of injury are variable and unpredictable, the prospects for controlling injuries may rely on restricting exposure or augmenting the ability to withstand injury-producing forces with protective equipment or physical conditioning.

Office Appointments

There is no time when athletes or parents are more motivated to reduce injuries than when they are dealing with the reality of being hurt. When evaluating an injury, the extrinsic and intrinsic factors that led to the original injury need to be identified and addressed as part of comprehensive treatment. In addition, any additional risk factors acquired as a result of the injury also need to be addressed to prevent injury progression or recurrence. The time taken out of the sport for injury treatment affords an opportunity to treat deficits from other injuries and work on cross training or general conditioning to help reduce risks associated with returning to play.

Physical Preparedness

During the course of a PPE or office visit, or while in the role of team doctor or medical advisor, there may be an opportunity to give advice on preparation to play a sport. For all sports, the mantra of "get in shape to play," rather than "play to get in shape," is applicable. Physical preparation should start well before the first day of practice. It should include general conditioning, time to treat injuries or correct residual effects from prior injuries, and time to carry out specific exercises that may help reduce injuries specific to the given sport. Endurance sports require at least 6 weeks to establish a minimum level of aerobic fitness. Strength-dependent sports require a similar amount of time to build baseline strength. Ideally, athletes would already have a level of strength

---

TABLE 13.2

Expanding the Role of the Preparticipation Evaluation in Identifying Risk Factors for Sports Injury

- What sports are being played?
- How long are the seasons? Do sports overlap?
- What are the demands of each sport?
- What are the recommendations for preseason training?
- Which injuries are most common to each sport?
- What are the known extrinsic and intrinsic risk factors for these injuries?
- Are specific safety measures (eg, exercises, technique modifications, equipment) available to reduce these risks?
- What is the coach's level of experience? Is any extra training or opportunity available for coach's training in injury prevention?
- Who is in charge of making sure that the playing fields and equipment are safe and adequately maintained?
- What is the procedure for dealing with injuries and for follow-up after injury?
- Is emergency contact and health information available during all practices and competitions?
- Is a certified athletic trainer or other qualified medical professional available?
- Are specific rules in place to safeguard the athletes? If the rules set limits on exposure, what is the effect of playing on multiple teams or concurrently playing multiple sports?

and fitness sufficient to meet the demands of the first practice—before the first practice occurs.

Playing a different sport during the preseason may partially fulfill the conditioning requirements, but the specific demands of each sport usually dictate the need for additional sport-specific training. For example, running on the cross-country team may help a swimmer with aerobic fitness, but it will not prepare the shoulder girdle for the demands of swimming. Similarly, basketball may help with aerobic fitness and lower-extremity strength, but it will not prepare a pitcher's shoulder for the demands of throwing. Most coaches are delighted to give recommendations to athletes, parents, or medical personnel for preseason conditioning. Further advice on physical preparedness and sport-specific conditioning is provided in Chapter 46 .

Weight Management

Most sports have an optimal weight range for ensuring safety and performance. Many adverse health consequences are associated with weighing too much or weighing too little, or gaining or losing weight too rapidly. Athletes who are unhappy with their weight are likely to take steps to change it. This may or may not take place with medical consultation.

The desire to gain weight is most commonly seen in football players trying to get bigger and stronger for the season. Along with any weight gain program come issues related to growth and maturation, endocrine status, nutrition, supplements, performance-enhancing drugs, and weight lifting or other exercise. Each of these components of a weight gain program carries health risks that can be avoided if the athlete receives sound medical advice.

Weight loss discussions involve the same list of medical issues as weight gain discussions. Weight loss is part of weight-controlled sports such as wrestling or crew. In sports such as gymnastics, diving, and ballet, weight loss may be desired for aesthetic purposes. In endurance sports, weight loss may be attempted to help with performance. Inadequate intake of calories and nutrients while athletes are training or still growing has immediate adverse effects on performance. Long-term states of negative calorie balance have detrimental effects on overall health and are part of the female athlete triad. Bone mass, immunity, and recovery time from injury may all be affected.

The opportunity to discuss weight management may come in the course of performing a PPE, following a school screening test that reveals hypertension, or during an office visit for illness or injury. It may also occur in conjunction with a visit for a weight-related medical problem, or in the rare situation where a patient or family actually schedules an appointment to discuss weight management. All of these scenarios offer opportunities for primary or secondary prevention. With proper medical advice and supervision, virtually all adverse effects related to weight management should be preventable.

Equipment

College and professional athletic teams generally have full-time equipment managers who are responsible for ensuring that equipment is properly fit, properly maintained, and properly used. Despite the numerous equipment-related risks, younger athletes typically do not have the luxury of having a qualified expert to look out for equipment-related risks. Physicians may be uncomfortable in this role, but some directed questions, as listed in **Table 13.3**, can help determine whether there are equipment-related risks.

Sports Environment

Inquiries about safety of the sports environment can take place during patient encounters or while acting as a medical advisor to a team, a school, a sports organization, or a parks and recreation department. The questions in

---

TABLE 13.3

Assessment of Equipment-Related Risks

- What equipment (e.g., bats, balls, racquets, goals, cleats) is used to play the sport? Are there features of this equipment that can factor in injuries?
- What protective equipment is used?
- Does the equipment fit properly? Who is responsible for ensuring proper fit?
- When was the equipment last replaced or refurbished?
- How is the equipment maintained?
- Is there optional equipment that may afford additional protection?
- Is there any current or prior injury that would benefit from protective equipment?
- What type of shoes are appropriate for the sport?
- Are there specific shoe modifications that would help athletes with abnormal foot types or injuries?
- Is an orthotic necessary to provide cushion, support, or control that cannot be achieved with the shoe?

Table 13.4 can help identify whether there are environmental risks that could be corrected or avoided.

Sports Oversight

Another out-of-office opportunity to prevent sports injuries and promote safety can take place in the laboratory, classroom, league office, or boardroom. Decisions to modify rules, limit participation, adopt new safety equipment, educate coaches, and validate the efficacy of prevention programs depend on medical input. Unlike the safety advice given to a particular patient in the office, involvement with safety policy at the sport or community level can reach far greater numbers of individuals.

There are many examples of safety-related discussions where the sporting world has worked collaboratively with medical advisors to arrive at the best possible decision for the health of the athlete. Physician involvement can range from designing a program to prevent ACL tears to consulting on whether a school district should supply automated external defibrillators at all sporting events. Medical guidance is needed when considering eligibility requirements, minimum ages for starting competitive sports, and PPE requirements. Sports such as wrestling need to have medically sound policies on weigh-ins, safe weight loss, curtailing spread of skin infections, blood contamination, and cleaning procedures for wrestling mats. The volleyball

coach may want to know whether the players should all be required to wear prophylactic ankle braces to prevent sprains. A group of soccer parents may want to set limits on the number of games in an attempt to reduce injuries. A school district may need help responding to allegations that lead exposure could occur from playing on artificial turf. The district budget office may want to know whether hiring certified athletic trainers would yield savings in the risk-management office. The league may want to put together a coach education program that includes a medical preparedness plan, first aid, emergency transport, and record-keeping system. Questions like these could potentially arise in any community, and helpful responses can come from a broad range of medical specialties.

Injury Management

The presence or absence of an injury management plan can be considered a risk factor for injury that involves both intrinsic and extrinsic risk factors. For example, a cross-country runner with a bee-sting allergy who gets stung during a race may experience either inconvenience or death, depending on the presence of an injury management plan. If the coach is aware of the problem, has emergency medical contact information readily available, and has epinephrine in the first aid kit, the athlete can be treated and a potentially fatal injury can be averted.

Another example demonstrating the importance of an injury management plan is illustrated by the following scenario involving a high-school football player who experienced a suspected concussion during the prior week's game. The injury did not result in a loss of consciousness, but the athlete was advised to have it "checked out." He returned to practice the day before the next week's game and said that he was "okay" to play. Early in the game, he collapsed and became unconscious after what appeared to be a routine tackle. Despite the advice to have the prior injury looked at, no one was sure if he was actually seen or evaluated. There were no available notes regarding his medical clearance to play. There were no records at the field with information on how to contact his parents or doctor. The athlete was en route to a trauma center while coaches and administrators had already started to nervously question their responsibility for this unfortunate occurrence.

Both these examples clearly show the needs and benefits of an injury management plan. Some simple questions, as listed in **Table 13.5**, can determine whether a reasonable injury management plan is in place or how one might be created.

TABLE 13.4

Assessment of Environment-Related Risks

- Are the fields designed and maintained for the current patterns of use?
- Is the field or playing surface free of obstacles and hazards?
- Are multiple teams or different sports using the fields or facilities at the same time?
- Are the surfaces clean and maintained to standards sufficient to reduce transmission of infectious pathogens?
- Is lighting adequate at all times when the field or playing surface is in use?
- Is fluid (eg, water, sports drinks) available at all times?
- Are there guidelines for modifying practices and games for high-temperature and high-humidity conditions?
- Are there guidelines for lightning?
- Is there access to the field or training/competition site for medical emergencies?

TABLE 13.5

Assessment of Medical Preparedness and Injury Management Procedures

- Is there a requirement for a preparticipation evaluation?

- Is baseline medical information and emergency contact information available at all practices and competition?

- Is a mechanism for communication and accessing medical assistance available at all practice and competition sites?

- Is a procedure in place for handling medical emergencies? Is first aid equipment available? Is equipment available for patient stabilization and transport? Is access available for emergency medical services?

- Are there particular injuries or conditions (such as concussions) that routinely warrant medical evaluation before an athlete can return to play? If so, is the policy describing the conditions and requirements communicated to athletes, parents, coaches, and medical providers?

- Is there a policy or procedure for determining readiness to return to play after injury or illness?

- Is a coach, medical specialist, or other person assigned to handle medical supplies, maintain records and correspondence, and coordinate emergency protocols?

- Is a team doctor available to assist with evaluating injuries and creating prevention programs? Is a doctor available to consult with coaches or team trainers?

- Are athletes and coaches aware of early warning signs of common injuries and criteria for seeking medical attention?

- Are athletes and coaches aware of injury mechanisms for serious injuries and recommended prevention strategies for these injuries?

SUMMARY POINTS

- Successful injury prevention strategies must be based on identification and remediation of the *causes* of injury.

- Most injuries have several contributing causes. Even the best-conceived injury prevention program cannot prevent all injuries. However, the efficacy of prevention strategies increases in relation to the number of contributing causes that can be identified and addressed.

- Injury risk factors can be divided into categories of extrinsic and intrinsic risk. Extrinsic risk relates to the sport, equipment, and sports environment. Intrinsic risk relates to the age, gender, maturation, health, and physical makeup of the individual participant.

- The total burden of injury may be reduced by primary and secondary prevention. In primary prevention, the athlete is prevented from sustaining a first injury.

Secondary prevention addresses "second" injuries, which may include recurrent injuries or mild injuries that become worse over time.

- Environment- and equipment-related injuries constitute a large portion of preventable injuries. To take full advantage of these prevention opportunities, it may be necessary to expand the scope of one's practice beyond the office or clinic setting.

- As a result of the multifactoral nature of injuries, effective prevention strategies need to address the full spectrum of intrinsic and extrinsic risk factors and use both primary and secondary prevention methods. Chapter 46 offers more details on both general and sport-specific prevention methods.

- Physicians can help athletes, teams, sports organizations, and communities carry out a broad and thorough analysis of sports injury risk. From this analysis can come an organized and proactive approach to injury prevention and management.

SUGGESTED READING

Abernethy L, Bleakley C. Strategies to prevent injury in adolescent sport: a systematic review. *Br J Sports Med.* 2007;41:627-638.

American College of Sports Medicine. The prevention of sport injuries of children and adolescents. *Med Sci Sports Exerc.* 1993;25(8 Suppl):1-7.

Cahill BR, Griffith EH. Effect of preseason conditioning on the incidence and severity of high school football knee injuries. *Am J Sports Med.* 1978;6:180-183.

Emery CA. Injury prevention and future research. *Med Sport Sci.* 2005;49:170-191.

Ergen E, Ulkar B. Proprioception and ankle injuries in soccer. *Clin Sports Med.* 2008;27:195-217.

Etty Griffin LY. Neuromuscular training and injury prevention in sports. *Clin Orthop Relat Res.* 2003;(409):53-60.

Fradkin AJ, Gabbe BJ, Cameron PA. Does warming up prevent injury in sport? The evidence from randomised controlled trials. *J Sci Med Sport.* 2006;9:214-220.

Hart L. Effect of stretching on sport injury risk: a review. *Clin J Sport Med.* 2005;15:113.

Kelly AK. Anterior cruciate ligament injury prevention. *Curr Sports Med Rep.* 2008;7:255-262.

Lysens RJ, de Weerdt W, Nieuwboer A. Factors associated with injury proneness. *Sports Med.* 1991;12:281-289.

Lysens RJ, Ostyn MS, Vanden Auweele Y, et al. The accident-prone and overuse-prone profiles of the young athlete. *Am J Sports Med.* 1989;17:612-619.

McGuine TA, Keene JS. The effect of a balance training program on the risk of ankle sprains in high school athletes. *Am J Sports Med.* 2006;34:1103-1111.

Meeuwisse WH. Predictability of sports injuries. What is the epidemiological evidence? *Sports Med.* 1991;12:8-15.

Niemuth PE, Johnson RJ, Myers MJ, Thieman TJ. Hip muscle weakness and overuse in juries in recreational runners. *Clin J Sport Med.* 2005;15:14-21.

Olson OC. The Spokane Study: high school football injuries. *Phys Sportsmed.* 1975;7:75-82.

Parkkari J, Kujala UM, Kannus P. Is it possible to prevent sports injuries? Review of controlled clinical trials and recommendations for future work. *Sports Med.* 2001;31:985-995.

Renstrom P, Ljungqvist A, Arendt E, et al. Non-contact ACL injuries in female athletes: an International Olympic Committee current concepts statement. *Br J Sports Med.* 2008;42:394-412.

Shrier I. Stretching before exercise does not reduce the risk of local muscle injury: a critical review of the clinical and basic science literature. *Clin J Sport Med.* 1999;9:221-227.

Small K, McNaughton L, Matthews M. A systematic review into the efficacy of static stretching as part of a warm-up for the prevention of exercise-related injury. *Res Sports Med.* 2008;16:213-231.

Taimela S, Kujala UM, Osterman K. Intrinsic risk factors and athletic injuries. *Sports Med.* 1990;9:205-215.

Thacker SB, Gilchrist J, Stroup DF, Kimsey CD Jr. The impact of stretching on sports injury risk: a systematic review of the literature. *Med Sci Sports Exerc.* 2004;36:371-378.

van Mechelen W, Hlobil H, Kemper HC. Incidence, severity, aetiology and prevention of sports injuries. A review of concepts. *Sports Med.* 1992;14:82-99.

Veigel JD, Pleacher MD. Injury prevention in youth sports. *Curr Sports Med Rep.* 2008;7:348-352.

Witvrouw E, Lysens R, Bellemans J, Cambier D, Vanderstraeten G. Intrinsic risk factors for the development of anterior knee pain in an athletic population. A two-year prospective study. *Am J Sports Med.* 2000;28:480-489.

CHAPTER 14

Return-to-Play Decisions

Steven J. Anderson, MD

When an athlete has been injured or ill or has an underlying medical condition, physicians are frequently called upon to declare whether it is safe for the athlete to return to participation in sports. Although there are published guidelines that address many playability issues, these guidelines may not always be sufficiently specific or relevant to existing concerns.

For many injuries or illnesses, the risks associated with sports participation are unknown. In such cases, it may be tempting to take a conservative approach and simply prohibit participation. However, to completely restrict participation when the risks are unknown can be every bit as harmful as permitting participation when the risks are unacceptably high.

Liability concerns add to the anxiety that accompanies return-to-play decisions. Physicians are challenged to encourage sports participation while discouraging their patients from taking undue participation-associated risks. Denying participation may be perceived as discriminating against physically disabled individuals, even if the basis for denial is to safeguard the athlete from further injury. Claims have been made that the failure to grant clearance to participate has prevented athletes from advancing their sports career, qualifying for a select team, earning a college scholarship, or even obtaining professional contracts. Yet if athletes become seriously injured or disabled when they were inappropriately cleared to participate, the treating physician may be held accountable. Even if the patient or family pressured the doctor to permit an early return to play, the responsibility for a bad outcome will invariably fall on the physician.

In the interest of making the task of return-to-play decisions less daunting, a list of 10 general questions is offered in an attempt to simplify the process. When faced with a return-to-play decision for any injury or illness, the answers to these questions can serve as a framework for gathering the information that will help physicians make more thoughtful, reasoned, sound, and defensible recommendations. The 10 questions are listed in **Table 14.1**. These questions are crafted to encourage a thorough and thoughtful analysis of the important return-to-play issues and to allow flexibility, discretion, and reasonable interpretation by the treating physician.

The risk of injury is not an all-or-nothing matter. Accordingly, return-to-play decisions that are based on injury risk cannot be absolute. The inexactness of risk assessment and return to play is a source of frustration and anxiety among patients and physicians. Some may expect that a systematic approach to return to play should yield a definitive answer. Unfortunately, even return-to-play decisions that seem the most clear-cut may be challenged, debated, or overturned.

Many return-to-play decisions relate to unique or unprecedented situations. The information available in the published literature cannot speak to every return-to-play decision that may occur. With injury risk that is rarely absolute and published guidelines that may be inapplicable or nonexistent, return-to-play decisions must often be made by using the best available information interpreted in the most objective manner possible. If there is bias introduced into the process, it should favor the health and well-being of the athlete.

TABLE 14.1

Ten Questions That Help Determine Readiness to Return to Play

1. What is the diagnosis?
2. How does the condition affect the ability to perform the sport?
3. What is the risk of the condition getting worse from playing?
4. What is the risk of secondary injury?
5. What has been the effect of treatment?
6. Can the sport or level of participation be modified to be safer?
7. Are there published guidelines that address the return-to-play decision?
8. Is the risk for further injury disproportionately high?
9. Is there informed consent?
10. Does the athlete want to play?

The care provider should carefully document the rationales that underlie return-to-play decisions, including the basis for the decision, supporting evidence, and acknowledgment of unknown factors. A discussion of known and unknown risks should take place. The patients' and families' understanding and acceptance of these risks should be documented.

TEN QUESTIONS THAT HELP DETERMINE READINESS TO RETURN TO PLAY

1. What Is the Diagnosis?

Establishing the correct diagnosis is critical to assessing risk, evaluating the adequacy of response to treatment, and ultimately determining readiness to return to play. A diagnosis should convey information about the cause of the problem, the pathophysiology of the problem, the effect of the condition on physiology and/or function, and the expected evolution or natural history of the problem. For example, a "grade II hamstring strain" meets the criteria for an adequate diagnosis, while "muscle spasm" does not. The diagnosis of "muscle spasm" describes only the symptoms of a problem without specifying the cause, the effect on performance, or the expected recovery. Furthermore, when the cause of an injury or illness is not identified, it is difficult to know how subsequent injury can be avoided if the athlete returns to the activity that caused the original problem. Understanding the cause of injury may also be helpful in recognizing injury patterns on a team and in preventing injuries to other participants with similar training regimens or exposure.

An adequate diagnosis should also indicate the pathophysiology of the problem. The underlying pathophysiology determines the effect that the injury or condition will have on musculoskeletal function and physiology. The underlying pathologic deficits must be identified to plan treatment and to determine when the deficits have been sufficiently restored to allow for normal function before returning to play.

A diagnosis should also indicate a natural history of the injury or illness associated with that diagnosis. The natural history includes the usual time for healing, with and without treatment, as well as the potential for full restoration of function. If a broken bone has the potential to heal completely, complete bony union should be the standard for return to play. If a sprained ankle ligament is likely to be permanently more lax, then normal ligamentous stability is not a realistic standard for return to play. If a herniated lumbar disk diagnosed by magnetic resonance imaging (MRI) is unlikely to appear normal on a follow-up MRI, then other criteria should be used to measure recovery and readiness to return to play.

The success of treatment is measured by how effective it is at helping the patient reach optimal recovery from the condition at hand. If the deficits from an injury or illness are not understood, if the effects on physiology and function are not understood, and if the expected level of recovery is not understood, it is difficult to determine when it is appropriate to clear an athlete to return to play. Therefore, a diagnosis that includes the cause and pathogenesis of injury as well as a natural history for recovery is critical for all return-to-play decisions.

2. How Does the Condition Affect the Ability to Perform the Sport?

Once a diagnosis has been established, the effect of that diagnosis on sports training and competition must be assessed. With an adequate diagnosis, there should be specific physiologic and/or functional deficits associated with that diagnosis. The effect of the condition will vary according to the demands of the sport. A condition that affects the cardiovascular system will have a greater effect on an athlete who participates in endurance sports. A hand injury will affect a baseball or tennis player more than a cross-country runner. A leg or ankle injury will affect an athlete in running or jumping sports more than a swimmer.

To appreciate the effect of various conditions on sport, it is necessary to know the sport, including the typical demands of training, practice, and competition. Sports have been classified as noncontact, contact, and collision; they are also classified by their intensity. These classifications are listed in Table 5.5 and Table 5.6, Chapter 5. If this classification system provides an insufficient understanding of the nature and demands of the sport, it is reasonable to simply ask the athlete to describe a typical week in his or her training regimen, including what is done during practice, what comprises the warm-up, what conditioning is undertaken outside of formal practices, and what the competition schedule is. The history should also include whether the athlete participates on multiple teams or in multiple sports.

When the deficits from an injury or illness are measured against the demands of a particular sport or training regimen, the discrepancy represents a specific target for treatment and a reference point for determining readiness to return to play.

3. What Is the Risk of the Condition Getting Worse from Playing?

Implicit in a proper diagnosis should be an identification of the vulnerabilities or deficits associated with that diagnosis. The list of known vulnerabilities should be compared against the list of demands associated with the patient's sport to determine the risk of the condition getting worse from playing. If a muscle strain makes the muscle tight and weak, any activity that places high demand on the injured muscle is likely to make the injury worse. Similarly, if a high-impact activity like basketball caused a stress fracture to develop, continued high-impact activity to a weakened bone may lead to a complete fracture or a nonunion of a stress fracture. Conversely, a runner who falls and accidentally dislocates his or her shoulder is unlikely to make the condition worse by returning to running because running places low demands on the shoulder. This is in contrast to a wrestler with a dislocated shoulder. Stress on the shoulder is an inherent part of wrestling, and returning to wrestling after a shoulder dislocation carries a definite risk of the condition getting worse.

The restrictions necessary after injury or illness are relative to the risks and demands of the particular activity in question. The process of identifying the necessary restrictions can also reveal activities that can safely be continued during the recovery process.

4. What Is the Risk of Secondary Injury?

An injury or illness can have direct consequences on sports performance, become worse as a result of further activity, or contribute to secondary injury. An assessment of the potential for secondary injury should be part of a return-to-play decision. A skier may be able to ski with a shoulder separation. However, if the skier falls and fails to extend an arm to break the fall, a secondary injury to the head or neck may occur. Runners with a painful hip, knee, or foot may compensate by altering their gait and develop a lower

back injury. A baseball pitcher with a painful or weak shoulder may compensate by placing more stress on the forearm or elbow and develop an injury in that area.

Secondary injuries can also apply to teammates and competitors. A football lineman who cannot maintain an effective block may put the quarterback at risk. A cheerleading team with an injury to a team member may put others at risk during lifts or stunts. A ballet dancer with a painful back or weak shoulder may inadvertently injure a dance partner during a lift.

Another source of secondary injury is when an athlete has a communicable disease. An active herpes lesion in a wrestler presents a clear risk to competitors who routinely come into close contact with the lesion. However, the same lesion on a member of the golf team or cross-country team may not require any restrictions. An HIV-positive patient presents a risk to others if there is direct contact with infected blood, although transmission of HIV through sports contact has not been reported. Patients with mononucleosis could spread the infection to others and may be at risk themselves if they have an enlarged spleen.

Finally, any injury or illness that requires extended time off can result in deconditioning. Resuming a vigorous training program after a disruption of training is associated with a greater overall risk for both acute and overuse injuries. A new or different injury that occurs as a result of resuming activity too quickly could be considered a secondary injury. Assessing the risk for secondary injury requires investigation and consideration of issues that extend well beyond the initial problem.

5. What Has Been the Effect of Treatment?

The functional limitations and the risks of further injury associated with a given diagnosis can likely be reduced with treatment. The degree to which treatment has mitigated or eliminated adverse effects from injury or illness will factor into return-to-play decisions. The series of questions about treatment provided in **Table 14.2** can help assess the effect of treatment on readiness to return to play.

The specific answers to these inquiries are not as important as the process of asking these questions and reasonably assessing the responses. The goal is to ensure that when athletes have a treatable condition, they have carried out a reasonable course of the treatment available for that condition and have recovered to a level sufficient to meet the demands of the sport. If the treatment creates any additional risks, or if it is ineffective at restoring baseline function, the level of clearance for return to play should be commensurate with these limitations.

TABLE 14.2

Questions to Help Assess the Effect of Treatment on Readiness to Return to Play

- Is treatment available for the condition in question?
- Has treatment been carried out?
- Has treatment been completed? If not, how far has treatment progressed?
- How did the patient respond to the treatment?
- What are side effects of treatment, and how do they affect performance and injury risk?
- Has the outcome of treatment been measured objectively?
- Has the patient reached maximal medical improvement?
- Has treatment restored normal function?
- Is there equipment (ie, braces, splints, pads, face protectors) that will protect the injured area and permit an earlier return to play?
- Does the protective equipment have any effect on performance or risk for further injury?
- Is the treatment legal under the guidelines for the patient's sport?
- Does the treatment need to continue after clearance to return to play has been granted?
- Is ongoing treatment or follow-up evaluation necessary for the patient to maintain his or her clearance to participate?

6. Can the Sport or Level of Participation Be Modified To Be Safer?

The rules and basic nature of a sport are unlikely to be changed to accommodate an injury. However, the athlete may be able to temporarily change the training regimen, position played, or level of participation to accommodate the injury. A baseball catcher with knee pain from squatting may be able to return to the lineup sooner if he switches to another position. A baseball pitcher with elbow pain may be able to tolerate the lower throwing demands of first base while recovering from the injury. A dancer with a painful great toe may be able to keep dancing by avoiding pointe work and limiting ballet class or emphasizing other disciplines such as modern or jazz dance. A springboard diver with a lumbar disk injury may have to limit pike dives but may continue with back dives or dives in a tuck position. A swimmer with shoulder impingement may have to limit the amount of butterfly stroke during practice. A football player with an unstable shoulder may be able to play on the offensive line while wearing a shoulder harness but is unlikely to be able to play running back or wide receiver.

The level of participation can also be modified. A soccer player with shin splints who plays on 2 teams may have to temporarily stop playing on one of the teams or substitute low-impact conditioning in practices. A swimmer with tendonitis may have to temporarily stop twice-a-day practices.

All of these examples demonstrate opportunities to allow continued participation without jeopardizing the treatment or recovery from a specific injury. The purpose of suggesting these modifications is not to push injured athletes back into play before they are ready. Rather, permitting a modified level of participation keeps the patient involved with the activity, minimizes the risk of deconditioning, and facilitates the transition back to full activity once the injury has healed. Restrictions that are perceived as overly broad or arbitrary will prompt patients to shop around for doctors and may adversely affect the physician's credibility when it comes to subsequent treatment recommendations.

7. Are There Published Recommendations That Address the Return-to-Play Decision?

There are return-to-play or eligibility questions related to particular injuries, particular individuals, and particular sports that occur frequently enough to have been addressed in the medical literature; in addition, several authoritative bodies have issued policy statements. Return to play after a concussion has received much attention. Policy statements for sports participation for numerous conditions have been published by the American Academy of Pediatrics (Table 5.6, Chapter 5). There are also American Academy of Pediatrics policies for sports participation referenced according to age group, including guidelines for preschool and school-aged athletes and guidelines related to specific sports or training activities, including statements on soccer, hockey, wrestling, triathlons, baseball and softball, boxing, and weight lifting (Appendix A).

When available, existing standards or policies should be considered when formulating a return-to-play decision. If existing statements are too general to address a specific return-to-play decision, then the background information and foundation underlying these recommendations can still be useful and can be incorporated into new guidance for the patient.

8. Is the Risk for Further Injury Disproportionately High?

After establishing the diagnosis, assessing the effect of the condition on performance, determining the risk of the condition becoming worse as a result of participation, evaluating the effect of treatment, and considering the options for modifying participation, a composite risk score should be developed. Recognizing the risk for serious or disabling injury is paramount, but identifying the risk of compromised performance and secondary injury should also factor into the overall risk assessment. Rehabilitation and other therapies can reduce the risk for subsequent injury, but even with optimal treatment, there may still be residual risks associated with returning to play.

The basis for medically restricting return to play after injury or illness is the risk for further injury. When the risks are disproportionately high, restrictions are warranted. However, even when the risk is not high, there still remains some baseline risk associated with sports participation. The highest achievable standard for risk reduction after injury or illness is for the risk to return to baseline—that is, the risks faced by average, healthy, uninjured players who participate in the same sport at the same level of competition as the patient in question. The baseline risk of injury varies from sport to sport (see Chapter 12) and increases with increasing intensity of training and increasing levels of competition.

When the baseline risks of a given sport are openly recognized and confronted, some patients and families may not only be surprised, but they may also deem the risk of further participation to be unacceptable. Patients should be aware of baseline risks and, with medical guidance, should have an opportunity to accept, reject, or try to modify those risks. However, when the risk of further injury is disproportionately high, the decision to return to play requires more than the acceptance of the patient and family. When the risk for further injury is disproportionate, the permission to return to play requires medical clearance. The level of clearance may vary according to magnitude of risk and seriousness of the consequences.

When the risk for serious or long-term injury is disproportionately high, clearance to return to play should be denied. In some situations, the restrictions on participation may be permanent. This may be the case in athletes who have experienced multiple concussions or a spinal cord injury. Over time and with treatment, the level of risk may change and the level of restriction may need to be modified accordingly.

In some cases, there may be a recommendation for further treatment or further modification of participation while waiting for the risk to return to an acceptable, baseline level. Again, the athlete's return-to-play status may change according to his or her response to treatment.

Regardless of the level of justification for restricting participation, there may be disagreement and resistance on the part of the patient or family. The disappointment may be mollified by identifying options for eventually removing the restrictions and by letting the patient know which activities he or she can continue to participate in without restriction. Patients often get a second opinion in hopes of finding a more favorable dispensation. The physician should not actively discourage second opinions because it may decrease the opportunity to communicate important facts and findings from the first opinion.

9. Is There Informed Consent?

The risks of further participation and the effect of an injury on performance must be determined and communicated to the patient and family. In the same sense that a preparticipation examination cannot indemnify an athlete against injury or illness, a return-to-play decision cannot guarantee that the patient will be free from further adversity. The difference between baseline risk and disproportionate risk must be made clear to the patient and family. Patients and families should have an opportunity to determine what level of baseline risk is acceptable. The physician can provide background information that will permit a decision to be made about participation. When the risk is disproportionate, the physician has a more prominent role in making the ultimate decision.

Sample language covering a range of risks and recommendations for participation is provided in **Table 14.3**. There are also examples of injuries or injury scenarios that illustrate an appropriate level of restriction. Documenting the recommendations and their underlying rationales can provide a valuable defense if the return-to-play decision is challenged.

10. Does the Athlete Want to Play?

Perhaps this should be the first question because if the athlete does not want to return to play, the responses to the other 9 questions may be irrelevant. Athletes who enjoy sports participation are usually anxious to resume play after an injury or illness. When athletes are not enthusiastic about returning to play—particularly when they could be medically cleared—alarms should go off. The reasons for not wanting to return to play are varied. It may be that athletes do not feel they are physically or mentally ready to resume the rigors of training and competition. They may think they have fallen too far behind their teammates or competitors. They may fear further injury, or they may simply be tired and frustrated with injuries that have

TABLE 14.3

Communicating Return-to-Play Recommendations

Level of Risk	Sample Language	Examples
Risk is not disproportionate.	"We believe that your injury/condition has sufficiently improved and that you can return to participation with a level of risk for further injury that is similar to the baseline risk for other athletes on your team."	• Sprained finger in cross-country runner • Iliac crest contusion in football player • Rib fracture in cyclist
Risk is not disproportionate, but baseline risk is higher than expected.	"Your injury/condition has sufficiently improved to permit medical clearance to return to play. However, you have had multiple injuries in this sport and you have chosen to play a sport associated with a higher-than-average rate of injury. An option to reduce risk for further injury would be to choose a sport associated with a lower overall injury rate."	• Football player with multiple injuries throughout the season; no single injury prohibits play • Female cross-country runner with amenorrhea and history of multiple stress fractures
Risk is disproportionately high but temporary.	"We believe that your injury/condition has improved to a level that will allow you to return to a modified level of play with the restrictions that we have discussed. With further time for injury treatment and healing, we will reevaluate your status, and we hope to later provide clearance to return to full participation without restrictions."	• Hamstring strain • Ankle sprain • Chondromalacia of patella • Splenomegaly from mononucleosis • Rib fracture in football player
Risk is mildly to moderately high and most likely permanent.	"Your condition has reached maximal medical improvement. There are limitations and risks for injury that are disproportionately high. You may be able to continue to play at a reduced level, play in a different position, or choose a sport that has fewer risks."	• Osteochondritis dissecans in a pitcher's elbow • Herniated lumbar disk • Hip arthritis • Lacerated kidney • Spondylolisthesis
Risk for severe or disabling injury is disproportionately high and permanent.	"You have a condition that has not sufficiently improved to make it safe for you to return to your sport. With ongoing treatment and monitoring, there may be other sports or activities that you should be able to safely participate in."	• Recurrent or severe concussion • Spinal stenosis • Hypertrophic cardiomyopathy • Marfan syndrome

already occurred. They may be feeling pressures or unrealistic expectations from parents, family, friends, fellow athletes, or coaches. They may also be burned out or interested in pursuing other activities.

Regardless of the medical readiness to return to play, if athletes do not feel ready or if they do not express a desire to return, then they should not be cleared to return to play. Athletes who are hesitant to return to play should not be pressured to change their minds. Rather, the underlying reasons for the decision should be explored, and the position should be supported medically.

Medical support for decisions to not return to play may include helping the athlete understand and address the underlying reasons. It is not the duty of the physician to challenge the decision, override it, or take sides with other interested parties. Occasionally, telling athletes that they do not have to return to their sport is a tremendous relief. Lingering and otherwise unexplained symptoms may abate when the pressure to return to play is removed. Paradoxically, supporting a decision to not return to play a given sport can

be the most effective means of getting patients ready to return to participation in the activities they want to do.

SUMMARY POINTS

- Return-to-play decisions require a detailed assessment of risk and thoughtful interpretation of that risk in the context of the athlete's involvement in sports. The risks may be limitations of performance, the risk of the injury becoming worse, or the risk of secondary injury.

- To adequately assess these risks, it is necessary to have an accurate diagnosis, an understanding of the nature and demands of the sport, the effect of the condition on participation, the efficacy of treatment, and the degree to which risks have returned to baseline levels.

- When risks are disproportionately high, modification or restriction of participation may be necessary. The goal of medicine is to minimize risk without placing unnecessary restrictions on participation.

- Patients and families need to understand that all risks cannot be eliminated and that clearance to return to play does not guarantee immunity from further injury.

- Return-to-play decisions that are too lenient or too strict are a disservice to the athletes being cared for and a liability for the physicians responsible for those decisions.

SUGGESTED READING

American Academy of Pediatrics, Committee on Sports Medicine and Fitness. Cardiac dysrhythmias and sports. *Pediatrics.* 1995;95(5):786-788.

American Academy of Pediatrics, Committee on Sports Medicine and Fitness. Climatic heat stress and the exercising child and adolescent. Pediatrics. 2000;106:158-159.

American Academy of Pediatrics, Committee on Sports Medicine and Fitness. Human immunodeficiency virus and other blood-borne viral pathogens in the athletic setting. *Pediatrics.* 1999;104(6):1400-1403.

American Academy of Pediatrics, Committee on Sports Medicine and Fitness. Injuries in youth soccer: a subject review. *Pediatrics.* 2000;105:659-661.

American Academy of Pediatrics, Committee on Sports Medicine and Fitness. Medical conditions affecting sports participation. *Pediatrics.* 2008;121(4):841-848.

American Academy of Pediatrics, Committee on Sports Medicine and Fitness. Participation in boxing by children, adolescents, and young adults. *Pediatrics.* 1997;99(1):134-135.

American Academy of Pediatrics, Committee on Sports Medicine and Fitness. Risk of injury from baseball and softball in children. *Pediatrics.* 2001;107:782-784.

American Academy of Pediatrics, Committee on Sports Medicine and Fitness. Safety in youth ice hockey: the effects of body checking. *Pediatrics.* 2000;105:657-658.

Bolin D, Goforth M. Sideline documentation and its role in return to sport. *Clin J Sport Med.* 2005;15(6):405-409.

Cantu RC. Guidelines for return to contact sports after a cerebral concussion. *Phys Sports Med.* 1986;14:75-83.

Cantu RC. Stingers, transient quadriplegia, and cervical spinal stenosis: return to play criteria. *Med Sci Sports Exerc.* 1997;29(7 suppl):S233-S235.

Garrick, JG. Determinants of return to athletic activity. *Ortho Clin North Amer.* 1983;14:317.

Guskiewicz KM, Bruce SL, Cantu RC, et al. National Athletic Trainers' Association position statement: management of sport-related concussion. *J Athl Train.* 2004;39(3):280-297.

Hartigan EH, Hurd W, Snyder-Mackler L. Return to play: screening strategy directs successful rehab. *Biomechanics.* 2006;6(8):18-28.

Kelly JP, Nichols JS, Filey CM, Lillei, KO, Rubinsten D, Kleinschmidt-Demasters BK. Concussion in sports: guidelines for the prevention of catastrophic outcome. *JAMA.* 1991;266(20):2867-2869.

McCrea M, Kelly JP, Kluge J, Ackley B, Randolf C. Standardized assessment of concussion in football players. *Neurology.*1997;48(3):586-588.

McFarland EG. Return to play. *Clin Sports Med.* 2004;23(3):321-502.

Morganti C. Recommendations for return to sports following cervical spine injuries. *Sports Med.* 2003;33(8):563-573.

Murphy NA, Carbone PS, and The Council on Children with Disabilities. Promoting the participation of children with disabilities in sports, recreation, and physical activities. *Pediatrics.* 2008;121:1057-1061.

Orchard J, Best TM, Verrall GM. Return to play following muscle strains. *Clin J Sport Med.* 2005;15(6):436-441.

Putukian M. Repeat mild traumatic brain injury: how to adjust return to play guidelines. *Curr Sports Med Rep.* 2006;5(1):15-22.

Torg JS, Ramsey-Emrhein JA. Management guidelines for participation in collision activities with congenital, developmental, or post-injury lesions involving the cervical spine. *Clin Sports Med.* 1997;16(3):501-530.

Torg JS, Sennett B, Pavlov H, Leventhal MR, Glasgow SG. Spear tackler's spine. An entity precluding participation in tackle football and collision activities that expose the cervical spine to axial energy inputs. *Am J Sports Med.* 1993;21(5):640-649.

Valovich McLeod TC, Barr WB, McCrea M, Guskiewicz KM. Psychometric and measurement properties of concussion assessment tools in youth sports. *J Athl Train.* 2006;41(4):399-408.

CHAPTER 15

Medical Management on the Sidelines

Larry G. McLain, MD, MBA

In the past, most team physicians, particularly at the high school level, have been orthopedic surgeons. However, because so many sporting events require a medical presence, family physicians and others with an interest in sports medicine have also served as team physicians. These physicians are well qualified because they can handle the medical and psychological issues of the young athlete and the injury issues related to physical and skeletal immaturity. With the proper dedication and commitment, these physicians can be good advocates for young athletes in caring for musculoskeletal injuries, injury prevention, fitness promotion, and school health.

GENERAL ATTRIBUTES

Team physicians must be dedicated; available; committed to self-education about sports medicine issues; willing to develop and work with a sports medicine team (athletic trainers, coaches, administrators, physical therapists, and athletes and their parents); and possess a calm, diplomatic approach to clinical problem solving. However, standards for training and assessing the competence of team physicians are not well defined. Many physicians who are currently team physicians have learned by doing. Physicians in training now have greater elective opportunities in sports medicine and the option of participating in sports medicine fellowship programs. Additional training in sports medicine is available through continuing education programs or team physician courses sponsored by national-level sports medicine organizations.

BENEFITS

Serving as a team physician provides a valuable service to schools, teams, and athletes. It also offers many benefits, such as access to adolescents in a nonoffice setting, an opportunity to build and promote a practice in the community, and the personal satisfaction and enjoyment that comes from working with young athletes.

RISKS

Despite the many positive aspects of being a team physician, concerns about liability and the adequacy of professional training and preparation remain. Physicians making medical diagnoses, recommending treatment, and determining readiness to return to play are expected to adhere to the same standards on the sidelines as they would use in their offices. On the sidelines, many diagnostic tools are obviously lacking, such as the controlled environment of the office and the immediate availability of imaging modalities. In addition, the physician on the sidelines is often pressured to make an immediate decision regarding the athlete's return to play, and often the patient is uncooperative. However, these compromises in the medical setting do not justify compromises in medical decision making. Rather, the challenges of the sideline setting demand a greater reliance on clinical acumen.

Although these daunting legal challenges cannot be eliminated, they can be mitigated by ensuring that the athlete's best interests always come first. An athlete should not be allowed to return to play until a diagnosis is known and the risk of further injury has been identified. In addition, a record of the decisions and recommendations made on the sidelines should be maintained. Open communication with the athlete, parents, coach, and/or athletic trainer can help prevent or resolve any conflicts or misunderstandings that can jeopardize optimal medical care.

So-called Good Samaritan legislation offers some protection for volunteer physicians rendering emergency care. However, these statutes vary between states and cannot be relied on to cover all of the team physician's activities. Team physicians who are paid for their work or who have formal contracts to provide sports medicine services tend not to be covered under Good Samaritan laws. Because malpractice coverage varies by policy and state, team physicians should review their policies before committing to a team.

DUTIES AND RESPONSIBILITIES

Team physicians are responsible for the events they cover medically and may be responsible for determining an athlete's ability to safely participate. These responsibilities should be specified in advance to ensure that athletes, coaches, parents, athletic trainers, and administrative staff all understand and agree.

After clarifying duties and responsibilities, the team physician can begin the planning process. Planning issues involve personnel, equipment, procedures, and documentation. Sideline settings will vary according to what is necessary and what is available. Some of the more common emergency situations are listed in **Table 15.1**. Knowing what to

expect and having an emergency plan in place can greatly decrease the anxiety associated with potentially catastrophic injuries.

SIDELINE ORGANIZATION

All aspects of field supervision must be well organized before the start of competition. Although the incidence of catastrophic injury is low, the potential for serious injury exists, and plans to handle the worst-case scenario must be in place. Led by the team physician, precompetition planning sessions with school administrators, coaches, athletic trainers, and the emergency medical system (EMS) in the area must occur to clarify roles. It is advisable to stage a mock emergency on the practice field to prepare for the possibility of such an event. This could include stabilization, movement, and even cardiopulmonary resuscitation for an athlete with serious head and/or neck injuries. Other clinical situations to be considered include caring for an athlete with asthma, heatstroke, severe traumatic musculoskeletal injury, or cardiac arrhythmia.

The use of aluminum-titanium bats in baseball from T-ball through college has increased the number of serious injuries and deaths in young ballplayers. The increased bat speed leads to greater ball velocity off the bat, with decreased reaction time for the defender. The position of pitcher is at greatest risk, and if hit in the chest, the pitcher may experience a condition called commotio cordis, a disruption of the cardiac electrical system that can cause sudden death. The availability and use of automated external defibrillators in this case should be considered.

TABLE 15.1

Medical, Neurologic, and Orthopedic Emergencies

Medical	Neurologic	Orthopedic
• Sudden cardiac death, cardiac arrest	• Head injuries (concussion)	• Unstable extremity fractures
• Exercise-induced asthma	• Cervical spine injuries	• Difficult joint dislocations (neurovascular compromise)
• Acute episode of asthma		
• Diabetes mellitus (hypoglycemia)		
• Syncope		
• Seizures		
• Heat illness and dehydration		
• Bee sting allergy and other anaphylactic reactions		
• Blunt abdominal trauma		
• Traumatic ocular injuries		

Heatstroke continues to be a major concern for the team physician. New advances in cooling techniques look to be beneficial. The Australian Institute of Sport has created a cooling jacket made of wet-suit material that is designed to be packed with ice. Teams playing in the hottest months could benefit by having these jackets available so players can be cooled before playing, thereby staving off heatstroke, and to treat those who become hyperthermic.

A cluster of outbreaks of methicillin-resistant *Staphylococcus aureus* has occurred in athletes. Some of these infections have led to life-threatening conditions. Team physicians need to be aware of the potential severity of these seemingly innocuous infections. Suspected cases can be treated initially with clindamycin or sulfamethoxazole-trimethoprim, while awaiting cultures. Most of the serious infections require intravenous antibiotics. Linezolid (Zyvox) is a first-line alternative drug that is available in an oral form; however, it is very expensive. This drug could be added to the team physician's bag if traveling to remote destinations.

Team physicians must coordinate a group of competent, well-qualified health care professionals to care for athletes on an emergency basis. Sideline organization also includes coordination with the EMS team to ensure that the proper equipment is on site, that the hospital has been notified and is on alert during the competition, that the EMS response time is acceptable, and that EMS is available on an on-call basis or at the site of the competition. Finally, the team physician must check the availability and function of the equipment that must be present on the sidelines (**Table 15.2**).

THE SIDELINES MEDICAL BAG

In addition to the equipment on the sidelines, the team physician must have a personal medical bag. Experience has shown that the old black bag is both too small and highly susceptible to the elements. The medical bag that is favored by many experienced team physicians is a fishing tackle–type box, which can be found in sporting goods or hardware stores. Advantages of this type of bag are size, its ability to be locked, and the capacity to withstand the elements.

Table 15.3 lists suggested equipment and drugs for the medical bag. Because this list represents the minimum requirements and is not intended to be all inclusive, contents should be adjusted to preference. Contents may also vary depending on the sport, level of competition, and availability of EMS. Most clinical situations on the

TABLE 15.2
Suggested Sidelines Equipment
• Stretcher
• Backboard
• Cervical spine immobilizer (C collar)
• Blankets
• Crutches (adjustable)
• Slings
• Splints (upper and lower extremity)
• Elastic bandages
• Ice, plastic bags
• Compression dressings
• Blood contamination kit
• Knife or clippers for face mask removal
• Bag for disposal of contaminated waste
• Disposable gloves

sidelines do not usually require the team physician to render lifesaving care. The medical bag should thus contain only the essential supplies for dealing with an emergency until help arrives.

BEFORE A COMPETITION

The team physician should arrive at least 30 minutes before the start of competition and perform the duties outlined in **Table 15.4**.

DURING A COMPETITION

Once the competition begins, the team physician should be stationed on the sidelines with an unobstructed view of the playing field and should have easy access to the field. Anticipation of possible injuries is a valuable habit to acquire, and the physician must concentrate only on the action on the field. If the team physician is examining an athlete on the sidelines, someone else should be designated to watch the field.

An important responsibility of the team physician is to determine the extent of any injury or illness occurring during the game and to determine the diagnostic and therapeutic intervention the situation requires. The team physician must also decide whether the injured athlete is able to return to play. The circumstances dictate that the

TABLE 15.3

Suggested Contents for the Sidelines Medical Bag

Equipment
- Stethoscope
- Otoscope/ophthalmoscope
- Penlight
- Tongue blades
- Tape
- Needles[a]
- Syringes[a]
- Thermometer
- Blood pressure cuff
- Reflex hammer
- Finger splints
- Latex-free disposable gloves
- Sterile gloves
- Steri-Strips
- Scalpel[a]
- Forceps[a]
- Suture set[a]
- Nylon suture[a]
- Bandage scissors
- Cotton swabs—1 box
- Betadine
- Eye shield
- Saline irrigation solution
- Automated external defibrillator[a]

Cardiopulmonary Resuscitation Equipment
- Airway/endotracheal tube[a]
- Laryngoscope[a]
- Bulb syringe
- Self-inflating bag-valve-mask resuscitator (Ambu bag)[a]

Medications[a]
- Atropine (1-mg prefilled syringe)
- Epinephrine (1:10 000 solution)
- Lidocaine (100-mg prefilled syringe)

General Medications[a]
- Analgesics: acetaminophen (325-mg tablets), ibuprofen (600-mg tablets), acetaminophen with codeine
- Antibiotics: cephalexin, azithromycin, amoxicillin-clavulanate, sulfamethoxazole-trimethoprim

Skin Preparations
- Soap and water or alcohol-based antiseptic hand wash
- Corticosteroid cream[a]
- Silver sulfadiazine cream[a]
- Insect repellent[a]
- Antifungal cream[a]
- Steri-Strips
- Skin glue[a]

Gastrointestinal Medications[a]
- Antacids
- Loperamide
- Promethazine

Eyes, Ears, Nose, Throat
- Antibiotic eyedrops[a]
- Antibiotic eardrops[a]
- Proparacaine eyedrops[a]
- Ophthalmic irrigating solution and eye cup
- Fluorescein strips and ultraviolet light[a]

Miscellaneous
- Albuterol inhaler
- Diphenhydramine
- Dexamethasone[a]
- EpiPen
- Insulin, regular[a]
- Glucagon[a]
- Diazepam[a]

[a] These medications and equipment are optional, given the sideline setting and the proximity to resources that have or can supply these medications.

physician must have total authority to make this decision. The game setting is often highly charged and emotional, but the team physician should not be unduly influenced by nonmedical issues. Calm, rational, and objective decisions are necessary to safeguard both the athlete and the physician.

TABLE 15.4

Team Physician Duties Before a Competition

- Survey the playing field for any dangerous conditions.
- Check all medical supplies and equipment.
- Check the availability of telephones to ensure that EMS is available.
- Conduct introductions with the visiting coaches because the visiting team may not have its own team physician.
- Conduct introductions with the officials and referees and inform them of where the medical team will be on the sidelines during the game.
- Develop and agree with officials on guidelines about when to stop play to allow the medical team access to the field.
- Clarify that the physician has the ultimate authority regarding return-to-play decisions for injuried athletes.

CONCLUSION

The requirements for a team physician include dedication, availability, and commitment to providing high-quality medical care to young athletes. The responsibility is great, but the benefits of being a team physician are many. Physicians who are considering accepting this responsibility should review their malpractice insurance before accepting.

Efficient, effective management on the sidelines is an essential component of providing proper care to the injured athlete. Developing a well-organized, team approach that includes appropriately trained personnel who are available to cover games is a key responsibility of the team physician. Physicians should be involved with coaches and school administrators in preseason planning. Proper protective equipment must be available on the sidelines, as should appropriate means for transporting an injured athlete to the hospital. Communication among all members of the sideline team is critical, particularly with the transport team and the hospital receiving the injured athlete.

SUMMARY POINTS

- Before the start of the athletic season, school authorities must make it clear that the team physician has total authority in determining the fitness of any athlete to play.

- The team physician must be knowledgeable about all aspects of sports medicine, dedicated, and available for games as well as for midweek visits to check injuries.

- The team physician must take responsibility for the organization of equipment and personnel on the sidelines.

- The team physician's medical bag should contain essential supplies for dealing with an emergency until help arrives.

SUGGESTED READING

Johnson R. Herpes gladiatorum and other skin diseases. *Clin Sports Med.* 2004;23:473-484.

Johnson R. The unique ethics of sports medicine. *Clin Sports Med.* 2004;23:175-182.

McKeag DB, Hough DO, Zemper ED, eds. *Primary Care Sports Medicine.* Dubuque, IA: Brown & Benchmark; 1993:191-200.

Mellion MB, Walsh W. The team physician. In: Mellion MB, ed. *Sports Medicine Secrets.* Philadelphia, PA: Hanley & Belfus; 1994:1-4.

Puffer JC. Organizational aspects. In: Cantu RC, Micheli LJ, eds. *ACSM's Guidelines for the Team Physician.* Philadelphia, PA: Lea & Febiger; 1991:95-100.

Rubin A. Emergency equipment: what to keep on the sidelines. *Phys Sportsmed.* 1993;21:47-54.

CHAPTER 16

Female Athletes

Mimi D. Johnson, MD

Adolescent girls constitute the fastest-growing segment of young people participating in organized team sports—from 300,000 participants in 1972 to 2.3 million today. For the most part, this tremendous increase in female sports participation results from the passage by the US Congress of Title IX of the Educational Amendment Act of 1972. This amendment mandated equal athletic facilities for both women and men attending any college or university receiving federal financial assistance. This opportunity for college women filtered down to the high school level, resulting in improved equipment, coaching, and training for girls. Sports participation is now considered normal for girls, and it can be a good way to encourage regular exercise in this population. High school females active in sports have been found to have fewer pregnancies, a higher rate of graduation, and greater self-esteem than those not active in sports. Given the prevalence of girls and female adolescents involved in sports and the importance of keeping this population physically active, this chapter reviews a variety of sports medicine issues specifically from the perspective of treating the female athlete.

GENDER DIFFERENCES

Before puberty, boys and girls are comparable in exercise capacity and strength. Gender differences become apparent after puberty.

Strength

Strength in the female adolescent improves linearly with age through 15 years, but does not increase significantly with pubertal development, as it does in boys. After puberty, male adolescents are stronger than female adolescents in most measures of strength, although females are stronger in lower extremity strength per unit of lean body weight.

Female adolescents experience similar relative strength gains (percentage of improvement) as male adolescents under similar strength training conditions.

Training Effects

Adolescent females have reduced oxygen-carrying capacity compared with males during endurance training. When expressed per kilogram of lean body weight, the difference in absolute maximal oxygen consumption is less than 10%. There is no gender difference in percentage of $\dot{V}o_2max$ sustained during exercise or in the ability to improve $\dot{V}o_2max$ through training.

Skeletal Differences

Compared with adolescent males, adolescent females have narrower shoulders, a wider pelvis, and an increased Q-angle of the knee. The trunk length of the adolescent female makes up a slightly greater proportion of her total height, resulting in a shorter stride length than that of an adolescent male of the same height.

Body Composition

Lean muscle mass is greater in postpubertal males than in postpubertal females. Percentage of body fat is greater in postpubertal females than in postpubertal males. The reference adolescent's body fat ranges from 12.7% to 17.2% for males and 21.5% to 25.4% for females. Low fat is 10% to 13% body fat for males and 17% to 20% body fat for females.

MUSCULOSKELETAL INJURIES

Injury rates for conditioned athletes are similar for adolescent males and females, and injuries tend to be sport specific. However, some injury types and patterns occur more frequently in adolescent girls as compared with adolescent boys.

Anterior Cruciate Ligament Tears

There is an increased incidence of anterior cruciate ligament tears in female athletes compared with male athletes in the same sport, particularly basketball, volleyball, and soccer. The cause appears to be multifactorial, involving muscular strength, function, and recruitment; core strength; training (how the female athlete plants and cuts, or how she lands a jump); biomechanics; and balance. Prevention programs addressing some of these factors can reduce the risk of injury.

Anterior Knee Pain

Anterior knee pain, due to lateral patellar tracking, is more common in female athletes than in male athletes. This is most likely due to structural malalignment leading to increased valgus angulation of the knees and imbalance of muscle-tendon units around the patella. In addition, patellar subluxation and dislocation occur more frequently in girls.

Shoulder Pain

Decreased upper body strength and increased glenohumeral joint laxity may place the female athlete at increased risk for overuse injuries of the shoulder.

Wrist Injuries

Young gymnasts may develop distal radial physeal injuries from the repetitive compressive forces of bearing weight on the hands. This can result in premature growth arrest and positive ulnar variance.

Foot and Ankle Injuries

Anatomic malalignment and potential increased laxity of the ankles can contribute to the development of overuse injuries of the foot and ankle. It has been reported that female athletes have a greater risk of grade I ankle sprains than do male athletes. Bunion formation is more common in girls than in boys.

Spondylolysis

Girls participate in gymnastics and dance more frequently than boys, and these sports place them at a higher risk for stress fracture of the pars interarticularis, or spondylolysis.

PSYCHOSOCIAL ISSUES

It has been reported that apparel wear influences media attention, and that female athletes receive more negative comments from the media about appearance than do male athletes. This can influence self-esteem and may result in abnormal eating patterns. The incidence of sexual abuse and harassment by coaches is reported to be higher among female athletes.

MEDICAL CONCERNS

Anemia

There is a greater incidence of iron deficiency with and without anemia in female athletes than in male athletes. The greatest risk factors include menstrual loss and inadequate dietary intake. The US recommended daily allowance for adolescent girls is 15 mg of iron. To obtain 15 mg of iron, an adolescent girl needs to consume 2500 calories a day, and many female athletes consume less than 2000 calories a day. In addition, many female athletes eat a vegetarian diet without considering alternative sources of iron.

Iron Deficiency without Anemia Iron deficiency without anemia is characterized by a ferritin level between 12 ug/L and 20 ug/L and a normal hemoglobin level (although a hemoglobin level within the normal range may actually be low relative to the athlete's normal baseline). There is uncertainty as to whether iron deficiency without anemia affects performance, but it is a precursor to iron deficiency with anemia. The treatment is 50 to 100 mg of elemental iron a day (preferably taken with a source of vitamin C, such as orange juice, on an empty stomach), which needs to be continued for several months until the ferritin level is greater than 20 ug/L.

Iron Deficiency with Anemia Iron deficiency with anemia is characterized by hemoglobin and ferritin levels of less than 12 ug/L. Even mild anemia can have adverse effects on performance, particularly during endurance events. Treatment is 50 to 100 mg of elemental iron 3 times daily (preferably taken with a source of vitamin C on an empty stomach). A gradual progression of the dose from once daily to 3 times daily can reduce adverse gastrointestinal effects. The diagnosis can be confirmed by a rise of 1 g/dL of hemoglobin after 4 to 6 weeks of treatment. Treatment should continue for approximately 6 months, or until iron stores are replenished and ferritin levels are restored.

GYNECOLOGIC CONSIDERATIONS

Breast Support

Nipple abrasion resulting from excess friction (typically in running and jumping sports) can be alleviated by the use of lubricants, adhesive bandages applied over the nipples, and a sports bra. A good sports bra is soft and firm, is made mostly of nonelastic material with few seams and fasteners, and has good absorptive qualities.

Menstrual Cycle, Oral Contraceptive Use, and Sports Performance

World records have been set by athletes in all phases of menstruation. There is no statistically significant effect of menstrual phase or use of triphasic or low-dose oral contraceptives on physiologic variables during exercise. A small, statistically insignificant decrease in $\dot{V}o_2max$ has been shown during the luteal phase and while receiving oral contraceptives.

Exercise can help alleviate menstrual symptoms such as cramping, lower back pain, headache, and fatigue.

Stress Urinary Incontinence

Stress urinary incontinence typically occurs in athletes who run, jump, and perform high-impact landings. It has been reported that up to a quarter of female collegiate athletes experience stress urinary incontinence with sports. High-risk sports include field events, gymnastics, basketball, volleyball, bodybuilding, equestrian events, and martial arts, while moderate-risk sports include jogging, tennis, skiing, and skating. Sneezing and coughing may also cause incontinence in these athletes. Treatment involves performing Kegel exercises of both short and long duration (strength and endurance work). If specialized care is needed, referral to a physical therapist who specializes in pelvic floor dysfunction may be warranted. Prevention involves teaching children during toilet training that muscles help control urine flow, teaching pelvic floor exercises to athletes involved in high-impact sports, and teaching athletes to use those muscles on impact.

FEMALE ATHLETE TRIAD

The female athlete triad refers to the interrelationship among low energy availability/disordered eating, menstrual dysfunction, and decreased bone mineral density (BMD) in physically active girls and women. Energy availability is the amount of dietary energy remaining for all physiologic functions after subtracting energy expenditure from exercise. Low energy availability can result from increasing exercise energy (caloric) expenditure without increasing dietary energy (caloric) intake, from reducing dietary energy intake without reducing exercise energy expenditure, or both. This low energy availability results in a variety of hormonal alterations that cause menstrual dysfunction and may lead to decreased BMD.

Low Energy Availability/Disordered Eating

Disordered eating behavior leads to low energy availability in the female athlete. Disordered eating behavior may be unintentional, resulting from inadequate replenishment of the energy demands of training, or it may be intentional, a conscious attempt to lose weight or body fat to improve appearance or performance.

Unintentional Disordered Eating Unintentional or inadvertent disordered eating occurs in an athlete who does not recognize the need to increase her energy intake as she increases her training activity, and she subsequently develops oligomenorrhea or amenorrhea. This commonly occurs in the high school cross-country runner. This athlete is not aware of the energy demands of her sport and needs to be educated in optimizing her nutritional intake. Once educated, such athletes can make the changes required with little difficulty. They do not have psychological issues or concerns that interfere with their ability to increase food intake.

Intentional Disordered Eating Intentional disordered eating is more common than unintentional disordered eating. The athlete with intentional disordered eating typically restricts caloric and fat intake in an attempt to improve appearance or athletic performance. She may also develop other disordered eating behaviors, such as binge eating, or purging by vomiting or using laxatives, diuretics, and diet pills. She may compulsively exercise, or exercise excessively in addition to her normal training regimen. This can be difficult to detect; the athlete may simply appear to be training hard.

There is a spectrum of disordered eating behavior, ranging from mild (slight restriction of food intake or occasional binge eating and purging) to severe (significant restriction of food intake or regular binge eating and purging). Some athletes will meet the criteria for anorexia or bulimia nervosa.

Development of Disordered Eating Athletes of any sport may develop disordered eating behavior, but some sports place athletes at higher risk. These include sports that emphasize leanness, such as gymnastics, dance, diving, figure skating, long-distance running, and cross-country skiing, or sports that use weight classifications, such as martial arts and rowing.

A variety of factors may contribute to the development of disordered eating patterns in the young athlete: pressure to optimize performance or meet weight or body fat goals required by a coach; early initiation of sport-specific training; the idealization of thinness in society; unhealthy family dynamics; abuse; injury; and psychological factors such as inability to cope with stress in a healthy manner, decreased assertiveness, and low self-esteem. The personality traits that are associated with good athletes—perfectionism, compulsiveness, high achievement expectations—are the same traits that can increase the risk for disordered eating behavior.

Risks Involved in Disordered Eating In addition to menstrual dysfunction and potentially irreversible bone loss, disordered eating behavior can result in psychological and other medical complications, including depression; fluid and electrolyte imbalance; and changes in the cardiovascular, endocrine, gastrointestinal, and thermoregulatory systems. Some of these complications can be fatal.

Menstrual Dysfunction

The absence of regular monthly menstrual periods in a female athlete who is postmenarchal or older than 15 is not normal and signifies low energy availability or some other pathologic process.

Definitions The American Society of Reproductive Medicine has recently reduced the defining age for primary amenorrhea (absence of menses) from 16 years to 15 years of age due to the earlier occurrence of menarche.

Secondary amenorrhea is the persistent absence of menstrual cycles for more than 3 months after menarche has occurred. Even during the first several years after menarche has begun, it is unusual for menses to occur less often than every 3 months.

Oligomenorrhea refers to menstrual periods that occur at intervals longer than every 35 days. This may be common the first 2 years after menarche, but it is not normal after that time or after regular cycles have begun.

Energy Availability and Menstrual Function Luteinizing hormone (LH) pulsatility, and therefore normal menstrual function, depends on energy availability. Low energy availability results in altered concentrations of a number of metabolic hormones (growth hormone, insulin, cortisol, insulinlike growth factor [IGF]-1, leptin) and substrates (glucose, fatty acids, ketones), which may play a role in disrupting gonadotropin-releasing hormone (GnRH) pulsatility, and therefore LH pulsatility.

Consequences of Menstrual Dysfunction Estrogen production restrains bone resorption. Therefore, the hypoestrogenism associated with menstrual dysfunction may contribute to the loss of BMD. Other consequences of hypoestrogenism include impaired arterial vasodilation, impaired skeletal muscle oxidative metabolism, and high levels of low-density lipoprotein cholesterol.

Decreased Bone Mineral Density

Adequate energy and nutrient intake, along with bone-loading activities, promote bone health. Low energy availability may increase bone resorption and suppress bone formation. Current research suggests that decreased BMD may not only be a result of increased bone resorption due to decreased levels of estradiol, it may also be a result of decreased bone formation, resulting from changes in insulin, T_3, IGF-1, and perhaps cortisol and leptin. Because genetics, childhood nutrition and exercise, type of sport (high-impact sports appear to offset the negative effects of amenorrhea on bone), and other factors play a role in BMD, how much BMD an athlete with low energy availability/menstrual dysfunction will lose is variable. BMD is lower in amenorrheic athletes than in eumenorrheic athletes, and it declines with the total number of menstrual periods missed. Girls who begin menarche at a later age and have a lower weight during adolescence have the lowest BMD when compared with their peers. Disordered eating has been associated with low BMD, even in eumenorrheic athletes. In the athlete with disordered eating, increased energy availability, the resumption of menses, and weight gain result in increased BMD, although BMD may never be normalized.

Stress Fracture Stress fractures occur more commonly in female athletes and soldiers who have low BMD and/or menstrual irregularities. The risk for stress fracture in amenorrheic athletes is 2 to 4 times greater than that of regularly menstruating athletes.

Clinical Evaluation

The athlete with low energy availability or disordered eating may seek care from a health care provider for a sports preparticipation examination; for evaluation of menstrual dysfunction; for stress fracture; or because signs of disordered eating were recognized by parents, coaches, teammates, trainers, or the school nurse.

Most athletes with these conditions have low energy availability; however, other diagnoses must be considered and excluded. **Table 16.1** outlines the differential diagnoses for an eating disorder, menstrual dysfunction, and osteoporosis.

History During the preparticipation examination of the female athlete, an additional history can be obtained that will provide clues about energy availability (**Table 16.2**). If the initial screen is positive for disordered eating or low energy availability, an expanded medical history would be appropriate (**Table 16.3**).

Physical Examination In addition to the routine sports physical examination, it is appropriate to obtain the athlete's weight for height for age, which should preferably be at or above the 25th percentile by National Center for Health Statistics (NCHS) guidelines (see Appendix at the end of this chapter). The body mass index (BMI), if calculated, should be between the 25th and 75th percentiles for age

TABLE 16.1

Differential Diagnoses for Components of the Female Athlete Triad

Weight Loss/Eating Disorder
- Metabolic disease
- Malignancy
- Inflammatory bowel disease
- Achalasia
- Infection
- Mental illness (major depressive disorder, anxiety disorders, substance abuse disorders)

Menstrual Dysfunction
- Pregnancy
- Pituitary tumors (especially prolactinomas)
- Thyroid disease
- Polycystic ovary disease
- Premature ovarian failure
- Chronic illness
- Hypothalamic amenorrhea

Osteoporosis
- Metabolic disease
- Glucocorticoid induced

TABLE 16.2

Preparticipation Screening for the Female Athlete

- At what age did you begin menstrual periods?
- How often do you have a menstrual period?
- How long do your periods last?
- When was your last menstrual period?
- Have you ever taken birth control pills, and when?
- How many meals and snacks do you average each day?
- List the foods and drinks you had yesterday.
- List the foods and drinks you try to avoid.
- Do you eat or drink milk, calcium-fortified orange juice, yogurt, or cheese? How much each day?
- What has been your highest weight, and when?
- What has been your lowest weight in the past 2 years?
- Are you happy with your current weight?
- What do you feel your ideal weight would be?
- Have you ever tried to control your weight by dieting? Vomiting? Laxative use? Diuretics? Exercise?
- What sports do you participate in?
- How much time do you spend training for your sport each week?
- How much time do you spend exercising in addition to your sports workout (ie, extra running, calisthenics, StairMaster)?
- Have you ever had a stress fracture? When?

(the higher the lean muscle mass, the higher the BMI). Observation for Tanner stage, lean muscle mass, and body fat should be made.

If components of the female athlete triad are suspected, the physician should perform an expanded physical examination, including evaluation for signs of food restriction such as bradycardia, lanugo, and cold, discolored hands and feet, as well as signs of purging such as calluses on the dorsum of the hand and parotid gland enlargement (**Table 16.4**). The athlete should be evaluated for signs of androgen excess and enlargement of the thyroid gland. A pelvic examination may be indicated.

Laboratory Evaluation Laboratory evaluation should be performed to look for signs of infection, inflammatory process, chronic illness, and endocrine disease (**Table 16.5**).

Bone Mineral Density Evaluation

Dual energy x-ray absorptiometry (DEXA) should be considered in the athlete with a significant history of disordered eating or eating disorder, amenorrhea for 6 months or longer, prolonged oligomenorrhea, and/or a history of stress fracture or fracture from minimal trauma.

Treatment

Nutritional counseling may be all that is required for the athlete with inadvertent disordered eating. If she is able to increase her food intake as requested, and if she subsequently resumes menses, no further follow-up is needed. If she is unable to increase her food intake, it may safely be assumed that she has psychological issues that are making it difficult for her to do so. She should then be referred to an interdisciplinary team.

For the athlete who purposefully engages in disordered eating behavior and who is unable to make changes with nutritional counseling alone, it is best to institute an interdisciplinary team approach. Team members include a physician with expertise in treating eating disorders, a nutritionist, and a mental health practitioner, all of whom should have some understanding of sports. The family usually needs to be involved in treatment, and, on occasion, the coach and trainer may need to be involved.

Physician The physician monitors medical status and the athlete's ability to participate safely in sports. The physician

TABLE 16.3

Expanded Medical History for Disordered Eating

- Menstrual history
- Nutritional screening, including supplement use
- Weight history
- Exercise history
- Bone history (history of stress fracture)
- Family history (osteoporosis, weight history of family members, age of mother's menarche, polycystic ovarian syndrome and other causes of endocrine disease, mental illness)
- Medical history (chronic disease, infection, previous surgery, medication use)
- Sexual activity
- Symptoms of androgen excess, including facial, chest, or abdominal hair; acne; temporal balding
- Symptoms associated with menstrual dysfunction, including galactorrhea, headaches, decreased sense of smell
- Symptoms associated with restrictive eating and binge/purge behavior
  - Cold intolerance
  - Light-headedness, dizziness
  - Fatigue
  - Diarrhea/constipation
  - Abdominal bloating/discomfort
  - Decreased ability to concentrate
  - Sore throat/chest pain
  - Face/extremity edema
  - Depression

TABLE 16.4

Physical Examination for the Female Athlete Triad

- Height, weight, Tanner stage, general physical examination
- Signs of food restriction
  - Dry skin, brittle hair and nails
  - Decreased subcutaneous fat and muscle
  - Hypothermia
  - Bradycardia
  - Lanugo
  - Orthostatic blood pressure changes
  - Cold and discolored hands and feet
- Signs of purging
  - Parotid gland enlargement
  - Erosion of dental enamel
  - Calluses on dorsum of hand (Russell sign)
  - Orthostatic blood pressure changes
- Signs of androgen excess
  - Hirsutism
  - Obesity
  - Male pattern baldness
- Thyroid gland examination.
- Pelvic examination, if indicated.

may also coordinate care among the team members. It is often helpful to approach the athlete from the standpoint of her having low energy availability rather than from a subjective standpoint of her having an eating problem. With input from other team members, the physician may need to institute a contract for increasing energy availability and weight gain. This could involve allowing increased physical activity as energy intake and weight increases (**Figure 16.1**).

In many cases, the athlete's weight at the time of her last menstrual period is the weight she will need to attain before menses will resume. This may vary, depending on how much physical activity she is doing and whether or how much she has grown since her last menstrual period. A goal of healthy body composition measurements (lean muscle mass >25% by skinfold measurements), healthy weight range (>25% weight for height for age by NCHS

TABLE 16.5

Laboratory Evaluation for the Female Athlete Triad

- Urinalysis (pH often increased in disordered eating; specific gravity; signs of infection)
- Complete blood count and sedimentation rate
- Chemistry panel
- Pregnancy test, if indicated
- Thyroid function tests
- Prolactin
- Follicle-stimulating hormone
- Luteinizing hormone, testosterone, DHEA-S, and 17-hydroxyprogesterone if there are signs of androgen excess or concerns about polycystic ovaries

This contract is designed to help the athlete restore weight in a gradual manner in order to attain and maintain physical health, and return to an active lifestyle. This 16-year-old 5'4" gymnast's healthy weight range is between 106 and 128 pounds (25%–75% weight/height/age by National Center for Health Statistics guidelines [see Appendix]).

Basic rules:

- Athlete will be weighed once weekly, after voiding.
- She is to have no food or drink within 1 hour before being weighed.
- She will weigh in wearing a tank top and shorts.
- Parents will not discuss food and/or weight with athlete outside of clinical setting.
- Parents will support contract and ensure athlete remains in treatment.
- Athlete is expected to gain ½ pound per week.
- She may not perform any exercise until she has gained the appropriate amount of weight (see below).
- If weight loss persists, other activity restrictions may be necessary in order to conserve energy, ie, limit extracurricular activity.
- Hospitalization will be considered in the case of continued weight loss or inability to gain weight, and maintaining a very low weight, after a considerable period of time.

Guidelines as to what activities athlete can participate in at the corresponding weight follow:

- <94 pounds: May perform stretching only.
- 94 pounds: May perform light weight-training or calisthenics (25 repetitions, low weight) every other day, 3 days a week, for 15 minutes.
- 96 pounds: May perform beam and floor dance.
- 98 pounds: May perform bars.
- 100 pounds: May perform vault.
- 102 pounds: May perform floor (tumbling).
- 105 pounds: May begin aerobic activity (ie, elliptical trainer, bike) 10 minutes every other day.

At this point, body composition will be evaluated, along with energy intake, and advancing workouts will be determined. Athlete will need to increase caloric intake and continue to gain weight until menses have resumed.

Athlete's final healthy weight range will be determined once her vital signs have returned to normal, her body fat and lean muscle mass are adequate for a healthy athlete, and she has resumed regular menstrual periods of a normal length and pattern.

FIGURE 16.1 Sample contract for a competitive high school gymnast's return to activity.

guidelines [see Appendix at the end of this chapter] or BMI between the 25th and 75th percentiles for age), and resumption of regular menses can determine "healthy physical status" and allow a gradual return to full competition (**Table 16.6**).

Nutritionist The nutritionist provides guidance about meeting energy needs and encourages the athlete to make gradual changes in her food intake. The nutritionist can inform the athlete that weight is not an adequate measure of what the body is made of, that measurements of lean muscle mass and, perhaps, body fat can be more helpful. Many athletes have tried to eliminate fat and/or carbohydrate from their diets and need to be educated about the importance of these nutrients and encouraged to gradually add them back into their diets. A nutritionist with sports experience can encourage eating to promote health, as well as eating that will support sports performance.

Mental Health Practitioner The mental health practitioner helps the athlete address the psychological issues involved. Family therapy is almost always needed.

Treating Menstrual Dysfunction and Decreased BMD

Energy Availability The goal of treatment for menstrual dysfunction and decreased BMD is to increase energy availability. This can be accomplished by either increasing dietary energy intake, reducing exercise energy expenditure, or both. In many young athletes, it is most helpful to reduce exercise activity to a minimum until they are making good strides in increasing dietary energy intake. If weight has been lost, it is often helpful to regain most of the weight before beginning any aerobic activity.

Oral Contraceptives Hormonal treatment should never be substituted for correcting the fundamental deficit in energy intake or addressing the primary problem with eating. If the athlete is recalcitrant to increase dietary energy intake and/or has decreased BMD, consideration can be given to the use of

gonadal steroid hormones in the form of oral contraceptive pills (OCPs) or hormone replacement with the hope of minimizing bone loss. OCPs may be helpful for increasing BMD and preventing further bone loss, although the results of clinical studies are inconsistent. There are no established guidelines as to when or whether OCPs should be used in the amenorrheic adolescent younger than 15 years because of concerns about premature closure of growth plates and lack of research supporting therapy in this age group. Restoring regular menses by use of OCPs will not normalize the metabolic factors that impair bone formation and is unlikely to fully reverse the low BMD. If OCPs are considered, doses of more than 25 μg of ethinyl estradiol or its equivalent have been shown to have the best effects on BMD.

Other Pharmaceutical Agents The bisphosphonates are contraindicated in the young athlete of childbearing age, except in cases of glucocorticoid-induced osteoporosis or severe metabolic diseases of bone. All currently available pharmaceutical agents for osteoporosis are antiresorptive and do not increase bone formation, so they will not be completely efficacious in treating bone loss in athletes with amenorrhea.

Nutrition Bone-building nutrients have not been shown to reverse or improve low BMD in adolescent females. However, protein, vitamin D (400-800 IU/d), vitamin K, and calcium are recommended in women with low BMD who do not meet their dietary requirements or have little sun exposure. Dietary calcium should be increased to 1500 mg/d, which is equivalent to 5 servings of dairy. A serving of dairy includes a cup of milk or calcium-fortified orange juice, a cup of yogurt, or an ounce of cheese.

Prevention

Exercise and sports participation should be promoted in girls and adolescents for health and enjoyment. Prevention of the female athlete triad is important. Education needs to be provided to athletes, parents, and coaches regarding low energy availability/disordered eating and its related consequences. Parents and athletes should be informed about adequate energy and nutrient intake needed to meet energy requirements and provide for growth and development.

An athlete should never be asked to attain a specific weight and amount of body fat; instead, the athlete should be given a range of values. It is inappropriate to define an ideal level of weight or body fat for each sport. Athletes need to be taught that weight is not an accurate measure of fitness or fatness and that body composition measurements can better indicate what weight is made of. When weight is lost, fat and muscle are also lost.

TABLE 16.6

Determination of Healthy Physical Status in Female Athletes With Low Energy Availability

- 25%-75% weight for height for age by National Center for Health Statistics guidelines (see Appendix)
- 25%-75% body mass index for age
- Lean muscle mass ≥25% by skinfold measurement
- Regular monthly menstrual periods of normal length and pattern

Athletes, parents, and coaches need to know that amenorrhea is never a normal response to exercise.

Dietary practices, exercise practices, and menstrual history should be reviewed every year during the preparticipation physical examination because they may change from one year to the next.

SUMMARY POINTS

- Injuries in the female athlete are sport specific, although some injury types may occur more frequently in girls compared with boys.

- Iron deficiency, with and without anemia, is more common in the female athlete than in the male athlete.

- Girls involved in high-impact sports should be asked about stress urinary incontinence.

- The female athlete triad refers to the interrelationship among low energy availability/disordered eating, menstrual dysfunction, and decreased BMD in physically active girls and women.

- The development of low energy availability or disordered eating may be unintentional, resulting from inadequate replenishment of the energy demands of training, or it may be intentional, a conscious attempt to lose weight or body fat to improve appearance or performance.

- Amenorrhea in the young female athlete is never normal and should be evaluated and addressed.

- Low energy availability, with resulting hypoestrogenism and changes in other hormonal and substrate levels, can result in decreased accretion of BMD or BMD loss, even in the absence or amenorrhea.

- The mainstay of treatment for menstrual dysfunction and decreased BMD that result from low energy availability is to increase energy availability by decreasing exercise, increasing energy intake, or both.

SUGGESTED READING

AAP Committee on Sports Medicine and Fitness. Medical concerns in the female athlete. *Pediatrics.* 2000;106:610-613.

Drinkwater BL, Bruemner B, Chesnut CH 3rd. Menstrual history as a determinant of current bone density in young athletes. *JAMA.* 1990;263:545-548.

Ilhe R, Loucks AB. Dose-response relationships between energy availability and bone turnover in young exercising women. *J Bone Miner Res.* 2004;19:1231-1240.

International Olympic Committee. Position stand on the female athlete triad. IOC Medical Commission Working Group Women in Sport, 2005. http://multimedia.olympic.org/pdf/en_report_917.pdf. Accessed June 3, 2008.

Ireland ML, Nattiv A. *The Female Athlete.* Philadelphia, PA: WB Saunders; 2002.

Johnson MD, Martin TJ. Promotion of healthy weight-control practices in young athletes. AAP Committee on Sports Medicine and Fitness. *Pediatrics.* 2005;116:1557-1564.

Loucks AB, Thuma JR. Luteinizing hormone pulsatility is disrupted at a threshold of energy availability in regularly menstruating women. *J Clin Endocrinol Metab.* 2003;88:297-311.

Nattiv A, Loucks AB, Manore MM, Sanborn CF, Sundgot-Borgen J, Warren MP. American College of Sports Medicine position stand on the female athlete triad. *Med Sci Sports Exerc.* 2007;39(10):1867-1882.

Torstveit MK, Sundgot-Borgen J. The female athlete triad exists in both elite athletes and controls. *Med Sci Sports Exerc.* 2005;37:1449-1459.

APPENDIX: NATIONAL CENTER FOR HEALTH STATISTICS GUIDELINES: 25%-75% PERCENTILES FOR WEIGHT FOR HEIGHT FOR AGE

TABLE 16.A

Weight in Pounds of Youths Aged 12 Years at Last Birthday by Sex and Height Group in Inches: Selected Percentiles, United States, 1966-1970

Sex and height	Percentile						
	5th	10th	25th	50th	75th	90th	95th
Male							
Under 51.18 in.	*	*	*	*	*	*	*
51.18-53.15 in.	*	*	*	*	*	*	*
53.15-55.12 in.	54.6	60.8	66.6	69.7	76.5	83.1	86.9
55.12-57.09 in.	61.9	66.1	70.1	75.2	80.5	85.1	89.7
57.09-59.06 in.	70.8	73.2	78.7	84.2	90.2	101.6	115.7
59.06-61.02 in.	76.9	79.6	84.2	92.8	101.4	113.8	124.1
61.02-62.99 in.	84.4	86.9	92.4	101.9	111.3	126.5	136.5
62.99-64.96 in.	92.8	94.1	99.0	106.7	123.5	134.7	147.9
64.96-66.93 in.	95.5	102.3	108.0	199.9	132.1	150.6	168.9
66.93-68.90 in.	119.0	128.1	132.5	134.5	145.5	152.3	153.2
68.90-70.87 in.	*	*	*	*	*	*	*
70.87-72.83 in.	*	*	*	*	*	*	*
72.83-74.80 in.	–	–	–	–	–	–	–
74.80-76.77 in.	–	–	–	–	–	–	–
76.77 and over	–	–	–	–	–	–	–
Female							
Under 51.18 in.	–	–	–	–	–	–	–
51.18-53.15 in.	*	*	*	*	*	*	*
53.15-55.12 in.	55.1	55.1	58.2	63.7	70.8	75.2	75.4
55.12-57.09 in.	63.5	67.5	73.4	81.1	91.3	108.5	121.5
57.09-59.06 in.	70.1	72.3	78.3	78.9	94.4	106.5	111.6
59.06-61.02 in.	75.8	78.9	85.8	94.4	104.5	116.6	126.5
61.02-62.99 in.	83.6	86.4	94.8	103.2	118.6	133.8	140.0
62.99-64.96 in.	93.7	96.8	104.1	112.7	126.1	144.6	153.4
64.96-66.93 in.	96.8	103.8	111.1	117.1	131.6	142.2	157.2
66.93-68.90 in.	107.4	110.5	112.0	125.0	181.2	189.6	189.8
68.90-70.87 in.	–	–	–	–	–	–	–
70.87-72.83 in.	–	–	–	–	–	–	–
72.83-74.80 in.	–	–	–	–	–	–	–
74.80-76.77 in.	–	–	–	–	–	–	–
76.77 and over	–	–	–	–	–	–	–

From: Height and Weight of Youths Aged 12-17 Years, Vital and Health Statistics, Series 11, Number 24. Data from the National Health Survey, DHEW, 1973.

TABLE 16.B

Weight in Pounds of Youths Aged 13 Years at Last Birthday by Sex and Height Group in Inches: Selected Percentiles, United States, 1966-1970

Sex and height	Percentile						
	5th	10th	25th	50th	75th	90th	95th
Male							
Under 51.18 in.	–	–	–	–	–	–	–
51.18-53.15 in.	*	*	*	*	8	*	*
53.15-55.12 in.	60.0	60.8	63.7	68.3	76.9	95.0	95.2
55.12-57.09 in.	66.1	67.2	70.8	79.6	86.4	91.9	117.3
57.09-59.06 in.	71.4	74.7	79.6	83.6	90.8	98.1	102.3
59.06-61.02 in.	76.7	79.8	83.6	90.4	100.3	108.9	134.5
61.02-62.99 in.	83.3	86.4	91.9	101.0	112.7	129.4	136.0
62.99-64.96 in.	91.5	96.3	103.4	111.1	128.3	142.0	159.8
64.96-66.93 in.	102.1	104.7	108.7	118.2	131.0	152.1	165.3
66.93-68.90 in.	112.9	113.8	118.4	132.5	147.7	167.6	187.4
68.90-70.87 in.	124.1	127.6	132.5	139.6	155.0	194.7	196.2
70.87-72.83 in.	*	*	*	*	*	*	*
72.83-74.80 in.	–	–	–	–	–	–	–
74.80-76.77 in.	–	–	–	–	–	–	–
76.77 and over	–	–	–	–	–	–	–
Female							
Under 51.18 in.	–	–	–	–	–	–	–
51.18-53.15 in.	*	*	*	*	*	*	*
53.15-55.12 in.	–	–	–	–	–	–	–
55.12-57.09 in.	58.6	60.6	67.2	80.9	88.4	98.1	123.7
57.09-59.06 in.	76.5	78.5	84.2	89.3	97.4	118.2	127.0
59.06-61.02 in.	78.7	80.5	86.4	94.6	104.3	118.4	127.6
61.02-62.99 in.	86.2	88.0	96.6	106.7	118.6	134.5	145.3
62.99-64.96 in.	90.8	96.8	105.2	115.1	125.7	140.7	151.0
64.96-66.93 in.	101.9	104.5	115.1	128.1	135.6	152.8	168.0
66.93-68.90 in.	101.9	103.8	106.7	116.6	144.0	151.2	213.4
68.90-70.87 in.	*	*	*	*	*	*	*
70.87-72.83 in.	–	–	–	–	–	–	–
72.83-74.80 in.	–	–	–	–	–	–	–
74.80-76.77 in.	–	–	–	–	–	–	–
76.77 and over	–	–	–	–	–	–	–

From: Height and Weight of Youths Aged 12-17 Years, Vital and Health Statistics, Series 11, Number 24. Data from the National Health Survey, DHEW, 1973.

TABLE 16.C

Weight in Pounds of Youths Aged 14 Years at Last Birthday by Sex and Height Group in Inches: Selected Percentiles, United States, 1966-1970

				Percentile			
Sex and height	5th	10th	25th	50th	75th	90th	95th
Male							
Under 51.18 in.	–	–	–	–	–	–	–
51.18-53.15 in.	–	–	–	–	–	–	–
53.15-55.12 in.	*	*	*	*	*	*	*
55.12-57.09 in.	*	*	*	*	*	*	*
57.09-59.06 in.	81.4	85.1	87.3	89.5	92.6	87.3	94.1
59.06-61.02 in.	79.8	81.6	86.0	91.3	81.6	86.0	121.9
61.02-62.99 in.	83.1	85.3	92.2	101.6	85.3	92.2	138.2
62.99-64.96 in.	93.7	97.0	104.7	114.9	97.0	135.6	143.5
64.96-66.93 in.	105.2	108.7	113.8	122.1	108.7	155.6	166.9
66.93-68.90 in.	109.6	112.4	121.3	131.0	112.4	174.6	190.3
68.90-70.87 in.	112.2	121.5	129.0	142.6	121.5	164.2	185.2
70.87-72.83 in.	131.4	132.3	143.5	153.0	132.3	183.0	207.9
72.83-74.80 in.	*	*	*	*	*	*	*
74.80-76.77 in.	*	*	*	*	*	*	*
76.77 and over	–	–	–	–	–	–	–
Female							
Under 51.18 in.	–	–	–	–	–	–	–
51.18-53.15 in.	–	–	–	–	–	–	–
53.15-55.12 in.	*	*	*	*	*	*	*
55.12-57.09 in.	*	*	*	*	*	*	*
57.09-59.06 in.	70.5	77.8	80.0	93.3	104.7	109.1	112.7
59.06-61.02 in.	83.1	86.4	93.7	105.6	117.5	123.2	129.6
61.02-62.99 in.	90.8	95.7	102.1	109.3	122.6	137.1	141.8
62.99-64.96 in.	94.8	99.2	106.7	116.8	131.6	147.0	155.0
64.96-66.93 in.	101.2	104.7	114.9	125.2	136.2	155.4	168.4
66.93-68.90 in.	108.5	114.9	123.9	131.8	155.4	160.7	219.1
68.90-70.87 in.	114.0	114.6	127.2	131.8	142.4	154.8	155.6
70.87-72.83 in.	*	*	*	*	*	*	*
72.83-74.80 in.	–	–	–	–	–	–	–
74.80-76.77 in.	–	–	–	–	–	–	–
76.77 and over	–	–	–	–	–	–	–

From: Height and Weight of Youths Aged 12-17 Years, Vital and Health Statistics, Series 11, Number 24. Data from the National Health Survey, DHEW, 1973.

TABLE 16.D

Weight in Pounds of Youths Aged 15 Years at Last Birthday by Sex and Height Group in Inches: Selected Percentiles, United States, 1966-1970

				Percentile			
Sex and height	5th	10th	25th	50th	75th	90th	95th
Male							
Under 51.18 in.	–	–	–	–	–	–	–
51.18-53.15 in.	–	–	–	–	–	–	–
53.15-55.12 in.	–	–	–	–	–	–	–
55.12-57.09 in.	–	–	–	–	–	–	–
57.09-59.06 in.	*	*	*	*	*	*	*
59.06-61.02 in.	78.7	86.4	93.9	98.5	101.4	107.4	167.8
61.02-62.99 in.	88.8	95.0	103.0	108.5	125.0	153.4	168.2
62.99-64.96 in.	94.1	97.2	103.4	113.5	124.1	144.0	151.7
64.96-66.93 in.	105.8	107.6	117.1	124.3	135.1	147.9	161.6
66.93-68.90 in.	113.8	117.7	125.0	136.5	148.2	160.7	172.2
68.90-70.87 in.	117.1	122.6	131.6	141.8	153.2	176.8	196.7
70.87-72.83 in.	120.4	132.9	142.0	154.8	172.8	186.1	213.0
72.83-74.80 in.	128.5	129.0	138.7	155.9	186.5	203.7	244.3
74.80-76.77 in.	146.4	147.0	153.4	162.7	227.1	233.0	234.1
76.77 and over	–	–	–	–	–	–	–
Female							
Under 51.18 in.	–	–	–	–	–	–	–
51.18-53.15 in.	–	–	–	–	–	–	–
53.15-55.12 in.	–	–	–	–	–	–	–
55.12-57.09 in.	*	*	*	*	*	*	*
57.09-59.06 in.	79.4	86.9	92.8	100.1	116.2	122.8	146.2
59.06-61.02 in.	86.2	89.5	97.7	106.0	116.4	133.4	150.6
61.02-62.99 in.	91.3	95.9	102.1	112.0	121.5	131.8	143.7
62.99-64.96 in.	99.4	104.3	110.7	121.3	132.7	158.1	171.3
64.96-66.93 in.	104.7	108.7	121.5	128.8	144.8	163.4	178.6
66.93-68.90 in.	109.6	118.2	126.1	134.9	157.9	188.1	190.5
68.90-70.87 in.	109.6	110.0	118.6	137.6	156.1	158.5	174.6
70.87-72.83 in.	*	*	*	*	*	*	*
72.83-74.80 in.	*	*	*	*	*	*	*
74.80-76.77 in.	–	–	–	–	–	–	–
76.77 and over	–	–	–	–	–	–	–

From: Height and Weight of Youths Aged 12-17 Years, Vital and Health Statistics, Series 11, Number 24. Data from the National Health Survey, DHEW, 1973.

TABLE 16.E

Weight in Pounds of Youths Aged 16 Years at Last Birthday by Sex and Height Group in Inches: Selected Percentiles, United States, 1966-1970

				Percentile			
Sex and height	5th	10th	25th	50th	75th	90th	95th
Males							
Under 51.18 in.	–	–	–	–	–	–	–
51.18-53.15 in.	–	–	–	–	–	–	–
53.15-55.12 in.	–	–	–	–	–	–	–
55.12-57.09 in.	–	–	–	–	–	–	–
57.09-59.06 in.	*	*	*	*	*	*	*
59.06-61.02 in.	*	*	*	*	*	*	*
61.02-62.99 in.	92.6	93.0	98.5	103.2	119.9	131.8	148.2
62.99-64.96 in.	97.4	99.0	106.3	113.3	127.9	134.3	145.7
64.96-66.93 in.	106.9	109.8	116.2	127.9	140.9	152.8	167.3
66.93-68.90 in.	113.8	118.6	126.8	135.8	147.9	161.2	172.2
68.90-70.87 in.	124.1	128.3	134.5	144.2	159.8	176.6	184.7
70.87-72.83 in.	128.5	130.7	142.0	151.9	168.7	198.9	213.6
72.83-74.80 in.	140.4	146.8	153.7	172.8	199.1	213.8	245.6
74.80-76.77 in.	*	*	*	*	*	*	*
76.77 and over	*	*	*	*	*	*	*
Females							
Under 51.18 in.	–	–	–	–	–	–	–
51.18-53.15 in.	–	–	–	–	–	–	–
53.15-55.12 in.	–	–	–	–	–	–	–
55.12-57.09 in.	*	*	*	*	*	*	*
57.09-59.06 in.	96.8	97.2	99.0	112.4	120.2	158.7	158.9
59.06-61.02 in.	91.3	92.6	101.0	107.8	119.3	135.6	183.6
61.02-62.99 in.	97.0	100.5	106.7	113.8	124.3	136.5	152.1
62.99-64.96 in.	101.6	104.3	113.5	122.4	134.9	153.2	165.6
64.96-66.93 in.	103.8	107.6	117.5	130.3	148.4	173.5	191.1
66.93-68.90 in.	116.6	118.6	128.1	136.9	147.3	173.7	185.6
68.90-70.87 in.	129.2	129.6	136.0	145.3	177.7	218.5	232.6
70.87-72.83 in.	*	*	*	*	*	*	*
72.83-74.80 in.	–	–	–	–	–	–	–
74.80-76.77 in.	–	–	–	–	–	–	–
76.77 and over	–	–	–	–	–	–	–

From: Height and Weight of Youths Aged 12-17 Years, Vital and Health Statistics, Series 11, Number 24. Data from the National Health Survey, DHEW, 1973.

TABLE 16.F

Weight in Pounds of Youths Aged 17 Years at Last Birthday by Sex and Height Group in Inches: Selected Percentiles, United States, 1966-1970

	Percentile						
Sex and height	5th	10th	25th	50th	75th	90th	95th
Males							
Under 51.18 in.	–	–	–	–	–	–	–
51.18-53.15 in.	–	–	–	–	–	–	–
53.15-55.12 in.	–	–	–	–	–	–	–
55.12-57.09 in.	–	–	–	–	–	–	–
57.09-59.06 in.	–	–	–	–	–	–	–
59.06-61.02 in.	*	*	*	*	*	*	*
61.02-62.99 in.	96.6	102.3	106.3	109.6	127.4	154.1	161.4
62.99-64.96 in.	109.6	112.7	115.37	125.4	135.8	154.5	156.1
64.96-66.93 in.	110.7	117.3	124.3	135.6	147.5	160.3	170.4
66.93-68.90 in.	117.5	122.4	131.2	142.4	158.5	178.4	202.2
68.90-70.87 in.	125.4	129.9	135.6	146.6	162.3	175.0	194.9
70.87-72.83 in.	131.4	134.5	143.5	157.0	172.8	202.4	226.4
72.83-74.80 in.	137.6	146.2	155.4	166.0	178.1	199.1	204.8
74.80-76.77 in.	138.7	138.7	149.5	192.5	199.1	199.7	199.7
76.77 and over	–	–	–	–	–	–	–
Females							
Under 51.18 in.	–	–	–	–	–	–	–
51.18-53.15 in.	–	–	–	–	–	–	–
53.15-55.12 in.	–	–	–	–	–	–	–
55.12-57.09 in.	*	*	*	*	*	*	*
57.09-59.06 in.	85.1	85.5	88.4	99.4	100.8	112.7	112.9
59.06-61.02 in.	91.7	93.3	98.3	107.8	117.9	130.5	141.3
61.02-62.99 in.	97.9	100.3	107.4	117.3	127.2	135.8	168.0
62.99-64.96 in.	103.2	105.8	110.7	122.1	127.2	159.4	181.4
64.96-66.93 in.	105.6	110.9	121.5	130.7	143.5	153.0	157.9
66.93-68.90 in.	111.6	116.6	122.4	132.7	144.8	167.8	182.3
68.90-70.87 in.	121.0	125.0	132.5	136.0	165.8	167.3	183.0
70.87-72.83 in.	*	*	*	*	*	*	*
72.83-74.80 in.	–	–	–	–	–	–	–
74.80-76.77 in.	–	–	–	–	–	–	–
76.77 and over	–	–	–	–	–	–	–

From: Height and Weight of Youths Aged 12-17 Years, Vital and Health Statistics, Series 11, Number 24. Data from the National Health Survey, DHEW, 1973.

TABLE 16.G

Weight in Pounds of Adults Aged 18-24 Years at Last Birthday by Sex and Height Group in Inches: Selected Percentiles, United States, 1966-1970

	Percentile						
Sex and height	5th	10th	25th	50th	75th	90th	95th
Males							
62 in.	*	*	*	*	*	*	*
63 in.	*	*	*	*	*	*	*
64 in.	118	120	133	145	151	186	187
65 in.	111	112	121	134	145	164	193
66 in.	116	125	146	155	165	172	179
67 in.	121	131	140	153	173	187	203
68 in.	124	132	142	153	168	180	195
69 in.	133	139	147	161	182	208	224
70 in.	129	137	146	162	179	195	213
71 in.	141	146	157	170	187	202	228
72 in.	140	147	155	168	185	214	228
73 in.	132	157	164	180	201	229	247
74 in.	134	148	159	197	218	228	234
75 in.	*	*	*	*	*	*	*
76 in.	*	*	*	*	*	*	*
Females							
57 in.	*	*	*	*	*	*	*
58 in.	87	90	106	112	131	155	157
59 in.	95	98	107	112	132	145	162
60 in.	93	96	107	115	132	154	179
61 in.	97	101	109	118	132	150	182
62 in.	97	99	109	119	133	150	166
63 in.	101	106	114	129	142	162	188
64 in.	104	108	116	130	142	165	179
65 in.	104	110	119	130	143	162	190
66 in.	112	114	121	131	154	174	190
67 in.	112	115	129	138	151	164	187
68 in.	117	119	127	140	150	161	168
69 in.	104	119	130	134	142	152	170
70 in.	*	*	*	*	*	*	*

From: Height and Weight of Adults Aged 18-24, Vital and Health Statistics, Series 11, Number 24. Data from the National Health Survey, DHEW, 1973.

CHAPTER 17

Physically Disabled Athletes

Frank M. Chang, MD

Children with disabilities currently have the best opportunity ever to participate in sports and athletic activities. Strong voices advocating for the disabled, increased awareness in the lay community, and legislation such as the Americans with Disabilities Act have resulted in significant changes in attitude among children, parents, and school boards. These children are being mainstreamed into the classroom and given the opportunity to participate in academic and athletic opportunities with their able-bodied peers. Children with physical disabilities who are encouraged to participate in sports will improve their health, endurance, and flexibility, as well as their self-esteem and confidence—perhaps even more than their able-bodied peers.

SELF-CONCEPTS OF PHYSICALLY DISABLED ATHLETES

Self-concept is a term used to describe a person's own perception of himself or herself. Participation in programs like the Special Olympics has been shown to be directly related to improvements in self-concept. Studies comparing self-concepts of physically disabled athletes with able-bodied counterparts have shown that the scores of the physically disabled athletes fell within or close to the scores of able-bodied athletes. College wheelchair basketball players have been shown to have better mental health profiles than able-bodied college basketball players. A similar study comparing the mental health of college wheelchair basketball players with wheelchair nonathletes found that athletes experienced far less depression, emphasizing sports participation as a means of improving mood states in the physically disabled.

The term *physically disabled* refers to individuals with chronic musculoskeletal or neurologic disabilities that can be classified as congenital or acquired. **Table 17.1** and **Table 17.2** describe many common disabilities and the appropriateness for participation in specific sports. Many organizations such as the US Paralympic Committee and the Special Olympics classify athletes into groups on the basis of disability and functional level. This ensures that athletes are competing against functionally similar athletes. Athletes must be classified correctly to give them the best opportunity to succeed and to make the competitions fair. **Table 17.3** summarizes specific concerns for athletes with various disabilities.

GUIDELINES BASED ON SPECIFIC ABILITY/ DISABILITY

Amputations

Amputations are congenital or acquired. Acquired amputations can be traumatic or therapeutic, where part of a limb may be removed out of necessity because of a malignancy or vascular insufficiency. Amputations are further classified by the functional level that remains: in the lower extremity (eg, ankle, below knee, above knee, hip disarticulation) or in the upper extremity (eg, wrist, below elbow, above elbow, shoulder disarticulation). Determining the proper functional level is important because it helps ensure that athletes will compete against others with similar abilities.

Children with congenital deficiencies of the lower extremities usually lack the corresponding muscles and associated soft tissues attached to the missing skeletal

TABLE 17.1

Participation Possibility Chart for Individual Sports

Disorder	Archery	Bicycling	Tricycling	Bowling	Canoeing/Kayaking	Diving	Fencing	Field Events[a]	Fishing	Golf	Horseback Riding	Rifle Shooting
Amputation												
Upper extremity	RA	R	R	R	RA	R	R	R	R	RA	R	RA
Lower extremity (above knee)	R	R	R	R	R	R	—	R	R	R	R	R
Lower extremity (below knee)	R	R	R	R	R	R	R	R	R	R	R	R
Cerebral palsy												
Ambulatory	R	R	R	R	R	R	—	R	R	R	R	R
Wheelchair	R	—	—	R	R	—	—	—	R	—	—	R
Spinal cord disruption												
Cervical	RA		R	R	RA			—	R		X	RA
High thoracic: T1-T5	R		R	R	R		RA	R	R	RA	—	R
Low thoracolumbar: T6-L3	R		R	R	R		RA	R	R	RA	R	R
Lumbosacral: L4-sacral	R	R	R	R	R	R	R	R	R	R	R	R
Neuromuscular disorder												
Muscular dystrophy	RA		R	R	IA			—	R		X	RA
Spinal muscular atrophy	RA	—	R	R	—	—		R	R	R	—	RA
Charcot-Marie-Tooth	R	R	R	R	R	R	R	R	R	R	R	R
Ataxias	R	—	—	R	—	—		R	R	—	—	R
Other												
Osteogenesis imperfecta	R	—	R	R	R	—	R	R	R	R	—	R
Arthrogryposis	R	—	—	R	R	—	—	R	R	—	R	R
Juvenile rheumatoid arthritis	RA	—	—	RA	R	—	—	—	R	—	—	R
Hemophilia	RA	R	R	R	R	R	R	R	R	R	R	R
Skeletal dysplasia	R	R	R	R	R	R	R	R	R	R	R	R

TABLE 17.1—cont'd

Participation Possibility Chart for Individual Sports

Disorder	Sailing	Scuba Diving	Skating: Roller/Ice	Skiing: Downhill	Skiing: Cross-Country	Swimming	Table Tennis	Tennis	Tennis: Wheelchair	Track[a]	Track: Wheelchair	Weight Lifting
Amputation												
Upper extremity	R	R	R	R	R	R	R	R		R		R
Lower extremity (above knee)	R	R	I	RA	RA	R	R	I	R		R	R
Lower extremity (below knee)	R	R	R	R	R	R	R	R	I	R	I	R
Cerebral palsy												
Ambulatory	IR	R	R	RA	RA	R	R	R		R		R
Wheelchair	R					I	R		R	I	I	R
Spinal cord disruption												
Cervical	R			IA	IA	R	RA		IA		R	
High thoracic: T1-T5	R	R		IA	IA	R	RA		IA		R	
Low thoracolumbar: T6-L3	R	R		RA	RA	R	R		R		R	R
Lumbosacral: L4-sacral	R	I	R	R	R	R	R	R		R		R
Neuromuscular disorder												
Muscular dystrophy	R			IA	IA	R	RA		IA		R	
Spinal muscular atrophy	R	I		—	—	R	R		I		—	
Charcot-Marie-Tooth	R	R	R	R	R	R	R	R	R	R		R
Ataxias	R	I	I	—	R	R	R	R	R	—	R	—
Other												
Osteogenesis imperfecta	R	—	—	—	R	R	R	R	R	R	R	—
Arthrogryposis	R	—	—	—	R	R	R	R		R	X	—
Juvenile rheumatoid arthritis	R	—	—	—	—	R	R	—		—	—	—
Hemophilia	R	R	—	R	R	R	R	—		R	—	—
Skeletal dysplasia	R	R	R	R	R	R	R	R		R		—

a Club throw, discus, javelin, shot.

R indicates recommended; A, adapted; X, not recommended; I, individualized; and blank, no information or not available.

Adapted with permission from Chang FM. The disabled athlete. In: Stanitski CL, DeLee JC, Drez D Jr, eds. *Pediatric and Adolescent Sports Medicine*. Philadelphia, PA: WB Saunders; 1994:3;48-76. Copyright Elsevier.

TABLE 17.2

Participation Possibility Chart for Team Sports

Disorder	Baseball	Softball	Basketball	Basketball: Wheelchair	Football: Tackle	Football: Touch	Football: Wheelchair	Ice Hockey	Sledge Hockey	Soccer	Soccer: Wheelchair	Volleyball
Amputation												
Upper extremity	R	R	R	R	R	R		R	R	R	R	R
Lower extremity (above knee)	RA	RA			I	I	R			I	R	R
Lower extremity (below knee)	R	R	R	R	R	R		R		R		R
Cerebral palsy												
Ambulatory	R	R	I							R	R	R
Wheelchair	I	I					R				R	I
Spinal cord disruption												
Cervical												IA
High thoracic: T1-T5	RA	RA		R			R		R		R	RA
Low thoracolumbar: T6-L3	RA	RA		R			R		R		R	RA
Lumbosacral: L4-sacral	R	R	R					I		R		R
Neuromuscular disorder												
Muscular dystrophy	—	—	—	—	—	—	—	—	—	—	—	—
Spinal muscular atrophy	—	—	—	—	—	—	—	—	—	—	—	—
Charcot-Marie-Tooth	R	R	R	—	R	R	—	—	—	R	R	R
Ataxias	I	I	—	R	—	—	—	—	—	—	—	—
Other												
Osteogenesis imperfecta	—	—	—	R	X	—	—	X	X	X	R	—
Arthrogryposis	R	R	R	—	X	R	—	—	—	—	—	R
Juvenile rheumatoid arthritis	—	—	—	I	—	—	—	—	—	—	—	—
Hemophilia	I	R	R	—	X	—	—	X	—	I	—	R
Skeletal dysplasia	R	R	R	—	I	R	—	R	—	R	—	R

R indicates recommended; A, adapted; X, not recommended; and I, individual.

Adapted with permission from Chang FM. The disabled athlete. In: Stanitski CL, DeLee JC, Drez D Jr, eds. *Pediatric and Adolescent Sports Medicine*. Philadelphia, PA: WB Saunders; 1994:3:48-76. Copyright Elsevier.

TABLE 17.3

Concerns for Athletes with Disabilities

Disability	Specific Concerns
Amputation	• Skin and soft tissue irritation at prosthetic interface
	• Bony overgrowth of stump in skeletally immature children
	• Ligamentous knee injuries with below-knee prostheses
Cerebral palsy	• Altered motor control/coordination
	• Muscle strains due to contractures
	• Patellar overload/patella alta
	• Spasticity altering posture; may be painful
	• Coxa valga, femoral anteversion, acetabular dysplasia, subluxation of hip joint
	• Possible cognitive impairment
	• Seizures
Head injury	• Similar to cerebral palsy
	• Visual field defects
	• Possible cognitive impairment
	• Seizures
Meningomyelocele	• Altered motor function and sensation below involved level
	• Impaired bowel and bladder function
	• Presence of hydrocephalus that may affect cognitive function
	• Functional level and severity of hydrocephalus
	• Pressure sores and skin breakdown in wheelchairs
	• Difficulty with thermoregulation
	• Susceptibility to fractures that result from osteopenia
	• Muscle strains due to weakness, tightness, and imbalance
Spinal cord injury	• Similar to meningomyelocele
	• Skin irritation, blisters, breakdown, osteomyelitis from shoes, orthotics, or wheelchairs
	• Thermoregulation
	• Autonomic dysreflexia for injuries above T8
Down syndrome	• Atlantoaxial instability
	• Hypermobility of joints due to ligamentous laxity
	• Patellofemoral joint instability
	• Hip instability
	• Flat feet
Hearing impairment	• Compromised communication with other participants and sports personnel
	• Affected balance
Visual impairment	• Blind spots or complete blindness, making many sports difficult

elements, and they may also be missing other, less obvious soft tissue structures. Children with congenital short femurs or proximal focal femoral deficiencies usually also have an associated anterior cruciate deficient knee manifested by positive drawer and Lachman signs. This condition must not be mistaken for an acute rupture of the anterior cruciate ligament. Many of these patients are fitted with a below-knee prosthesis. The rigid prosthesis has less flexibility and elasticity than a normal lower leg and will also increase the risk of injury to the remaining knee ligaments. When a child is participating in sports with significant potential for knee injuries, a second prosthesis with medial and lateral hinges and a thigh lacer for additional support and suspension should be considered to protect the knee. Further research needs to be done to evaluate the protective value of these braces.

Children wearing prosthetic limbs are at increased risk for skin problems. With prosthetic lower limbs, the weight-bearing forces must be transferred to the skeleton through the skin and underlying soft tissues. Some amputation levels pose more difficulty for the prosthetist to transfer these forces successfully. For any lower extremity amputation above the level of the ankle, the skin and soft tissues transferring the weight-bearing forces are more susceptible to breakdown and pressure necrosis.

As children with amputations grow, stump overgrowth is a constant problem (**Figure 17.1**). This occurs most

frequently in the fibula, followed by the tibia, humerus, radius, ulna, and femur. During this process, the bone grows through whatever soft tissues the surgeon left to cushion the end of the stump. As the child runs and jumps, the skin may break down. To prevent this from occurring, the child, parents, coaches, and physical education teachers should know about the potential problem. If the end of the stump begins to feel bonier, or if erythema and skin irritation manifest, the child should be evaluated for stump overgrowth. The overgrown stump should be revised surgically to prevent the potential complications. In a young child, several stump revisions may be necessary at 2- to 3-year intervals before skeletal maturity is attained. Techniques of capping the end of the stump with transplanted cartilaginous caps have been effective in reducing the number of reoperations and sometimes provide a better end-bearing stump.

Cerebral Palsy

Cerebral palsy is an insult to the immature central nervous system (CNS) that results in a nonprogressive condition present around the time of birth. Many clinicians extend the diagnosis to include children with CNS injuries until 2 years of age. The CNS insult can be either physical or genetic. In children with cerebral palsy, muscle spasticity and poor tone result in inadequate motor control and lack of coordination, which are considered more significant

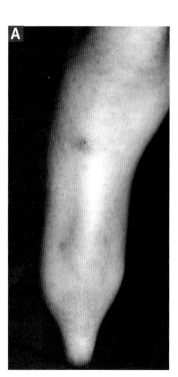
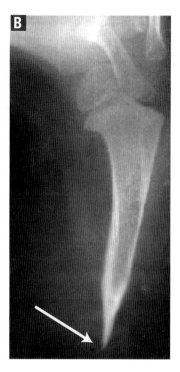

FIGURE 17.1 Stump overgrowth. (A) Clinical photograph showing bony overgrowth of the tibia in a below-knee amputee. (B) Radiograph showing bony spike that impales the skin and interferes with wearing a prosthetic.

limitations while participating in sports than susceptibility to injuries. Impaired hand-eye coordination results in difficulty controlling equipment like racquets, bats, or golf clubs. Difficulty catching and throwing and perceptual problems, such as judging the speed of a ball, are considered challenges but not insurmountable obstacles. Running with speed is more difficult. However, these deficiencies in coordination can be improved with practice.

Children with cerebral palsy are susceptible to overuse symptoms and are at increased risk of muscle strains because of muscle tightness. These children are frequently less active, so their muscles do not have the opportunity to stretch regularly or frequently. Muscle imbalance magnifies the problem, resulting in tightness and contractures of major muscle groups. The spastic muscles are usually an agonistic group of muscles. For example, the triceps surae group of muscles attached to the Achilles tendon is frequently spastic, overactive, and tight compared with the antagonistic ankle dorsiflexors, resulting in an equinus gait pattern.

The tightly contracted muscles result in joint stress. Patellar overload is common and will frequently evolve into true chondromalacia. Both growth and spasticity result in progressive tightening of the hamstrings and quadriceps muscles, causing a shortened stride length and increased pressure across the patellofemoral joint. In more severe cases, the tight hamstrings in conjunction with weakening ankle plantarflexors result in a crouched or flexed knee gait. This gait pattern contributes to the development of patella alta, or proximal migration of the patella. The increased pressure at the patello-femoral articulation gradually results in increased wear and damage to the articular surface of the patella. The symptoms are the same as in able-bodied children with patellar overload symptoms, but the problem is accentuated and more resistant to treatment. In addition, the tension on the quadriceps mechanism due to spasticity and contractures can produce a syndrome similar to Osgood-Schlatter, or jumper's knee. The constant pull of the patellar tendon can result in fragmentation of the lower pole of the patella visible radiographically, correlating with pain and tenderness clinically (**Figure 17.2**). Often, children experiencing knee pain may in fact have a hip injury that manifests as knee pain. The hips should be evaluated for injury when knee pain is the presenting complaint.

Muscle tightness and imbalance across the hip joint will gradually affect the normal development of the hip joint, and in more severe cases, the hip joint will subluxate and eventually dislocate. Coxa valga, femoral anteversion, and acetabular dysplasia may develop, and acetabular dysplasia may become symptomatic as the joint undergoes degenerative arthritic

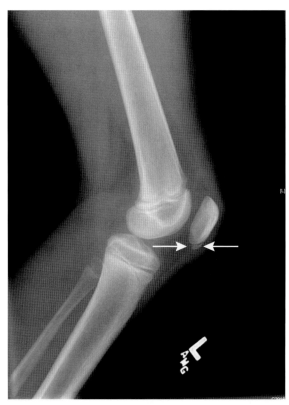

FIGURE 17.2 Lateral radiograph showing fragmentation of the distal end of the patella.

changes. As these changes occur, increased activity such as running and jumping will result in hip pain.

Head Injuries

Children with head injuries are functionally similar to children with cerebral palsy; however, neurologic function may improve in these children as the injured tissue recovers. Visual field defects, present in some children with head injuries, increase the potential for injuries and can cause problems if an object, such as a ball, passes through the child's blind spot.

Children with cerebral palsy or head injuries may be prone to seizures. Children with a history of seizures should be identified so appropriate precautions can be taken to minimize the risk of injury if a seizure occurs. For example, with skiers, a safety strap should be attached to the chair so if a seizure occurs on a chairlift, the strap will prevent a fall. Swimmers who are at risk should be supervised closely.

Meningomyelocele

Children with meningomyelocele have a congenital defect in the spinal cord and an associated defect in the arches of the vertebrae, which results in an inadequately protected spinal cord. The patient has altered motor function and sensation below the involved level. The sensory level usually corresponds to the motor level, and the involvement may be asymmetrical. In addition to motor and sensory deficits, bowel and bladder functions are impaired. Hydrocephalus is present in most children with spina bifida, requiring a ventriculoperitoneal shunt. In addition, cognitive difficulties, including nonverbal learning disorders, perceptual motor abnormalities, and visual spatial abnormalities, are common. This condition also increases the risk for seizures.

Sports participation for these children depends on several factors, the 2 most important being the child's neurologic functional level and the severity of hydrocephalus. The functional level of the spinal cord will affect the motor function of the lower extremities, and the severity of hydrocephalus will determine the degree of cognitive impairment and spasticity. Classification of children with meningomyelocele is based on their functional level (ie, the lowest nerve root level that is functioning). For example, if the child can actively dorsiflex the ankle but has no active plantar flexion, he or she is functioning at the L5 level—that is, the fifth lumbar nerve root is functioning, but there is no function below that level. The varying degrees of intellectual compromise from the hydrocephalus may result in the child having difficulty understanding the rules of the sport or may result in perceptual problems that could affect performance. Children with severe hydrocephalus should wear adequate head protection to prevent head injury and shunt damage.

Children with low lumbar and sacral level involvement can function almost normally; however, patients with low lumbar involvement may require orthoses to stabilize the foot and ankle. Children with involvement at the midlumbar level also may require braces to stabilize the knee. Those with higher-level involvement function best in a seated position, and those with midlumbar level involvement may perform physical athletic activities better in a wheelchair compared with ambulation in braces.

Children who wear braces and participate in sports may develop pressure sores and skin breakdown; therefore, lack of sensation is a concern. Children sitting in wheelchairs for prolonged periods of time are also susceptible to pressure sores and skin breakdown from the seat of the wheelchair. Individuals with normal sensation who experience discomfort will automatically shift positions as the pressure increases or as the tissues become ischemic, but children with impaired sensation do not have these same protective mechanisms. To avoid these problems, the child, parents, and coaches must inspect the skin frequently until skin pressure tolerances can be determined. Children must be taught to shift their weight frequently and to use their upper extremities to lift themselves off their seats. To decrease excessive pressure for children sitting in wheelchairs, specially designed cushioned seats are available to evenly distribute the weight and dissipate pressure. In addition, children with meningomyelocele have problems with thermoregulation.

Because weight-bearing and normal muscle activity stimulates skeletal development, children with meningomyelocele are more susceptible to fractures that result from osteopenia. When the muscles are not functioning and the skelton is not stressed by weight bearing, the bones receive less stimulation, and the skeletal elements become osteopenic.

Fractures in these children are more difficult to diagnose. Individuals with altered or absent sensation may not experience associated pain. The injured area may appear locally inflamed, so a fracture can easily be mistaken for an infection with swelling, erythema, increased local temperature, and a low-grade fever. Immobilization of a fractured extremity results in the bone becoming even more osteoporotic and susceptible to refracture when immobilization is completed. Minimizing the time of immobilization and non–weight bearing will decrease the incidence of refracture. Gradual, progressive weight-bearing after a fracture or recent operation and the use of functional braces can help prevent a refracture.

Children with meningomyelocele are also susceptible to muscle strains. Even the muscles at the lowest spinal level of function usually have less than 100% normal strength. Because children with spinal defects are less active, the overall motor power is not as well developed. Some muscles are also tighter than normal and prone to strains because of muscle imbalance and decreased flexibility.

Spinal Cord Injuries

Spinal cord injuries can be categorized as either complete or incomplete lesions. Incomplete lesions have varied motor and sensory involvement. Although spinal cord injuries in children are uncommon, they account for 13% to 15% of all spinal cord injuries, with boys affected twice as often as girls. Spinal cord injuries are typically traumatic and are associated with spinal fractures, but they may also be acquired nontraumatically as a result of conditions such as tumors, infection, inflammation of the spinal cord, arthritis, or disk degeneration. Younger children may have spinal cord injuries with no associated fractures because of their increased generalized ligamentous laxity.

The problems experienced in association with spinal cord injury are similar to meningomyelocele. Spinal cord injuries, except in special circumstances such as Brown-Sequard lesions, are typically transverse lesions with symmetric involvement. Spinal cord injuries can involve the cervical spinal levels and compromise upper extremity function. Intellectual function is usually intact unless the child experienced an associated head injury.

In children with insensate skin, shoes, orthotics, and wheelchairs can cause excessive localized pressure that leads to skin irritation, blisters, skin breakdown, soft tissue infections, and osteomyelitis. In addition to educating children to be aware of their skin and the interface with their braces, wheelchairs, and footwear, coaches, physical education instructors, and parents should also be aware of the potential problems and should periodically check the child's skin for redness, calluses, and blisters. Even if the child has no history of skin problems associated with a brace, the added stress of competitive sports can cause excessive skin pressure. In addition, children are constantly growing. With growth, the brace fit will change, eventually leading to altered pressure sites.

In children with spinal cord lesions proximal to T8, thermoregulation is a problem. Maintenance of body temperature depends on heat dissipation and heat production (see Chapter 8). Heat production mechanisms, such as shivering, and heat dissipation mechanisms, such as perspiration, are absent below the level of the spinal cord injury. The more proximal the neurologic level, the more difficult it is for the patient to compensate for changes in ambient temperature. Children with meningomyelocele have similar problems with thermoregulation. Precautions must be taken when participating in winter sports, and the children must be closely observed in hot environments. About half of athletes participating in track and field events may experience hyperthermia as a problem during competition, and 9% of those competing in swimming may experience hypothermia.

Children with spinal cord injuries above T8 are at risk of autonomic dysreflexia, a problem unique to the spinal cord injury population. It is a neurologic response triggered by a noxious stimulus and is characterized by a number of symptoms, including an increase in blood pressure, headache, sweating, piloerection, and bradycardia.

Autonomic dysreflexia is a medical emergency that requires immediate treatment. However, athletes have purposefully triggered autonomic dysreflexia to enhance their athletic performace. This practice is referred to as boosting and can be triggered by plugging catheter tubes, overdistending the bladder, sticking needles or other sharp objects into the skin, or wearing tight attire or leg straps. Boosting, a sympathetic spinal reflex, leads to a higher

release of catecholamines during exercise. Norepinephrine and epinephrine levels, as well as peak performance (watts), heart rate, and peak oxygen consumption, have been shown to rise in a boosted state, enhancing athletic activity. Boosting is dangerous and is banned by the governing bodies of wheelchair sports.

Down Syndrome

The abnormal collagen produced in association with Down syndrome results in generalized ligamentous laxity and decreased muscle tone. The ligamentous laxity causes hypermobility of joints and related problems, such as flexible flat feet and joint instability with associated subluxations and dislocations. Judgment may also be impaired because of intellectual compromise, and this may be compounded by the fact that children with Down syndrome frequently do not report discomfort or pain and may continue to participate despite the presence of symptoms.

Atlantoaxial Subluxation Atlantoaxial instability (AAI) and occipitocervical instability have been reported intermittently since 1965. Atlantoaxial subluxation affects approximately 15% of children with Down syndrome and is potentially the most devastating problem associated with this condition. The subluxation is caused by laxity of the annular ligament of C1 and is magnified by the generalized hypotonia. This results in excessive mobility between C1 and C2. The space available for the spinal cord consequently diminishes (**Figure 17.3**). As C1 displaces on C2, the odontoid can impinge on the spinal cord from the front, or the posterior ring can impinge on the spinal cord from behind. Excessive motion at this level can result in permanent damage to the spinal cord. If the motor tracks are injured, the patient is left a quadriplegic or quadriparetic with respiratory compromise.

Beginning in 1983, the Special Olympics has required athletes with Down syndrome to be screened for AAI before they can participate in any sport that places excessive stress on the head or neck, including sports such as tumbling, gymnastics, diving, soccer, high jump, football, butterfly and breaststroke in swimming, skiing, pentathlon, and warm-up exercises that place undue stress on the head and neck muscles. This requirement has raised awareness of the problem, and many school districts also now require screening before participation in physical education.

Atlantoaxial subluxation is best detected with lateral views of the cervical spine in maximum flexion and extension. Flexion-extension views are then compared to assess the atlanto-dens interval (ADI) (**Figure 17.4**). Statistically, the development of neurologic symptoms is greatest between

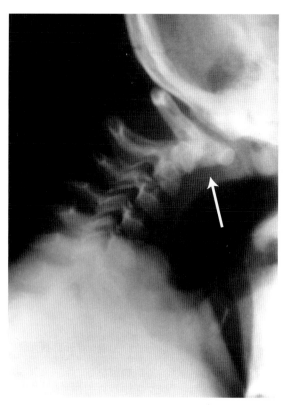

FIGURE 17.3 Flexion radiograph showing forward displacement of C1 on C2.

ages 5 and 10 years. Neurologic symptoms include neck pain, stiff neck, torticollis, progressive weakness or change in sensation in any extremity, decreasing endurance, loss of bowel or bladder control or a change in bowel habits, increased clumsiness, or a change in gait pattern.

The ADI is normally less than 2.5 mm, but the highest acceptable value is 4.5 mm in a child with Down syndrome. In an asymptomatic child with an ADI of more than 4.5 mm, activities that increase risk to the cervical spine should be restricted. If the ADI is excessive (>6.0 mm) or if the child has neurologic symptoms, the child is a candidate for a cervical surgical stabilization. Screening is recommended by some organizations and should be done before enrolling the child in any high-risk activities, when the school year begins, or in the presence of neurologic symptoms. Although some physicians still recommend follow-up screening at 3- to 5-year intervals until skeletal maturity, this is controversial because there is no set standard and the progression of AAI is difficult to track. Lateral radiographs of the cervical spine as a screening procedure for otherwise asymptomatic patients has potential but unproven value

in preventing spinal cord injury in young athletes with Down syndrome.

Knee and Hip Problems Other joints may cause problems in children with Down syndrome. The patellofemoral joint may be unstable and acutely or chronically subluxate or dislocate, and occasionally the hip joint may become unstable. Patellofemoral joint laxity can intensify any anatomic abnormalities, such as genu valgus, patella alta, or a hypoplastic medial femoral condyle, and can increase the instability. Recurrent subluxations and acute dislocations may not produce reports of pain in a child with Down syndrome. Treatment is more difficult because in addition to ligamentous laxity, the children are also relatively hypotonic, and nonoperative management frequently fails. Surgical realignment of the extensor mechanism may be necessary in more severe cases.

Hip instability is an even more difficult problem to treat. Excessive joint laxity can result in a hypermobile hip capsule that allows the hip to dislocate. Parents will describe audible clunking or popping sounds, usually with little evidence of symptoms. Some children with Down syndrome will even purposefully dislocate their hip for attention or self-stimulation. Nonoperative measures, such as temporary casting or prolonged abduction bracing, produce inconsistent results. Even surgical correction with femoral or pelvic osteotomies, combined with capsulorrhaphy and prolonged postoperative casting, do not always ensure permanent hip stability. Although hip damage and eventual degenerative changes do occur, the natural history of this problem is not well documented. The instability seems to diminish with progressive growth and development.

Foot Problems Because of ligamentous laxity, children with Down syndrome normally have flexible flat feet; however, most are asymptomatic. If planovalgus foot deformities are symptomatic, orthotics may help to minimize symptoms and excessive shoe wear.

HEARING IMPAIRMENT

Hearing-impaired children are not predisposed to any specific injuries and can participate in all sports, but they are at a disadvantage because communication with other participants and sports personnel is compromised. Not only can they not hear someone giving instruction, but often their speech is impaired. They also lack the ability to receive auditory cues. Because they do not have any visible physical disabilities, these children tend to play with other able-bodied children, leaving them at some disadvantage. Because the inner ear is connected to the vestibular apparatus, balance may be affected.

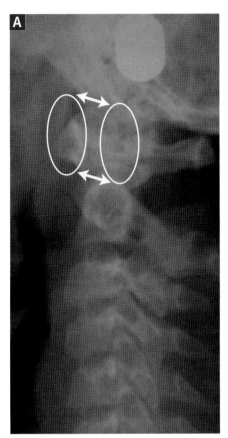
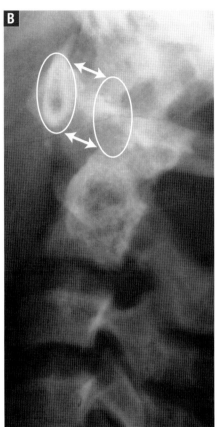
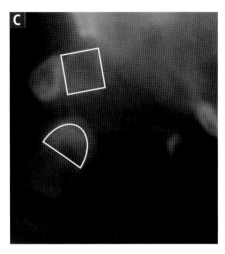

FIGURE 17.4 Atlantoaxial subluxation. (A) Lateral view of cervical spine in neutral position. (B) Lateral view in flexion shows displacement of C1 on C2. (C) Tomogram showing that the odontoid is a separate ossicle (os odontoideum).

Hearing aids are useful for some children. Lip reading and signing will facilitate communications but have obvious disadvantages during the heat of competition, especially in sports involving other team members or other competitors. For hearing-impaired children to experience maximum success in sports, they may elect to participate in individual activities like tennis, skiing, and running. Many swimming competitions have a starting light for hearing-impaired swimmers in addition to the traditional auditory stimulus.

VISUAL IMPAIRMENT

Participation without eyesight in sports is difficult at best. Occasionally, auditory cues can be substituted during some sports such as skiing, and special programs have been developed at a few ski resorts. As the proficiency and skills of the skier increase, the individual can ski faster and on more difficult terrain.

Other sports have been successfully adapted to the visually impaired. Speed skating, tandem bicycling, and competitive swimming are all gaining in popularity with visually impaired athletes. The Paralympic Games offer judo and Goalball for visually impaired athletes. Goal ball is a team sport designed for blind athletes. Participants compete in teams of three and try to throw a ball that has bells embedded in it into the opponents' goal. Beep baseball is a popular adaptive version of baseball that uses auditory cues from the ball and bases to allow visually impaired players the opportunity to participate. Rock climbing has become popular and gained international recognition when Erik Weihenmayer, a blind climber, successfully reached the summit of Mount Everest in May 2001.

Children with head injuries or those who have experienced strokes may also have limitations in their field of vision, depending on the anatomic location of the lesion. Awareness of the location of the visual field defect is important for safety and for choosing a sport in which the child's blind spot will not significantly impair his or her performance.

INTERNATIONAL COMPETITION

Special Olympics

The Special Olympics is an international organization that promotes physical fitness, well-being, and enjoyment through physical activity and athletic competition for children and adults with cognitive disabilities. Besides improving physical fitness and motor skills, the Special Olympics fosters friendships, an improved sense of self-confidence, and opportunities to grow. With more than 200 programs in 150 countries worldwide, the Special Olympics offers 26 sports, ranging from alpine skiing to golf (**Table 17.4**). Participants compete in different divisions on the basis of age and ability. Local, regional, and national competitions are held annually, with an Olympic-style international competition held every 4 years. Anyone with an intellectual disability or cognitive delay can participate in the Special Olympics. Children with Down syndrome must be screened before participating in some sports.

Paralympics

The International Paralympic Committee (IPC) is the international governing body of sports for athletes with a physical disability. It comprises more than 160 national Paralympic committees and 5 international disability sports federations. The Paralympics are organized in a similar fashion to the Olympics, with summer and winter games. The first international Paralympic Games were held in Rome in 1960, drawing 400 athletes from 23 countries, and since that time the games have evolved and grown, with almost 4000 athletes from 140 countries participating in the 2004 Paralympic Games in Athens, Greece. At the 2006 Winter Games in Torino, Italy, 1300 athletes, trainers, and guides from 40 countries competed for 58 gold medals. Athletes are grouped for competition according to their disability. The Paralympic Games are held at the same venues as the regular Olympic Games, with world and regional competitions held between Olympic seasons. The Summer Paralympic Games offer 26 sports, most of which are equivalents to the better-known Olympic sports (**Table 17.5**). Paralympians perform and compete at elite levels, with some Paralympians holding records that surpass those of their able-bodied counterparts. The IPC is developing sporting opportunities in all parts of the world at all levels to give more athletes the opportunity to perform.

ADAPTIVE EQUIPMENT

To make more sports available to children with disabilities, adaptive equipment is available to help them participate. An ankle-foot orthosis can be a simple solution to help

TABLE 17.4

Special Olympics Sports

- Alpine skiing
- Aquatics
- Athletics
- Badminton
- Basketball
- Bocce
- Bowling
- Cross-country skiing
- Cycling
- Equestrian
- Figure skating
- Floor hockey
- Football (soccer)
- Golf
- Gymnastics
- Power lifting
- Roller skating
- Sailing
- Snowboarding
- Snowshoeing
- Softball
- Speed skating
- Table tennis
- Team handball
- Tennis
- Volleyball

stabilize the ankle. However, sophisticated terminal devices for prosthetics are available for different activities. Wheelchair athletes may obtain low-profile, lightweight sports chairs for competitive activities such as basketball, tennis, racing, or rugby. Specialized hand-crank road and mountain bicycles have been developed for various terrains and purposes. Upper extremity prostheses are available with interchangeable terminal devices that can adapt to hold bats, hockey sticks, golf clubs, racquets, and ski poles. New technology has provided energy-storing materials for lower limb prostheses that can enhance athletic performance. Many prosthetists can help create individualized prosthetics for various athletic endeavors, such as swimming and scuba diving.

TABLE 17.5

Paralympic Sports Programs

Athens 2004

- Archery
- Athletics
- Boccia
- Cycling
- Equestrian
- Football (soccer), 5 players a side
- Football (soccer), 7 players a side
- Goalball
- Judo
- Power lifting
- Sailing
- Shooting
- Swimming
- Table tennis
- Volleyball
- Wheelchair basketball
- Wheelchair fencing
- Wheelchair rugby
- Wheelchair tennis

Torino 2006

- Alpine skiing
- Biathlon
- Ice sledge hockey
- Nordic skiing
- Wheelchair curling

South African racer Ernst Van Dyk posted 1:18.27 at the 2004 Boston Marathon. Court sports, such as tennis, basketball, and rugby, require lightweight, maneuverable chairs for quickness around the court (**Figure 7.6**). Wheelchairs have become specialized, depending on the demands for different sports. Wings or bumpers on the frame are helpful for sports like basketball or rugby, in which contact with other chairs is inevitable. These wings extend around the base to protect the footrest and help prevent chairs from locking up with other chairs. Antitip bars help stabilize the chair while the athlete leans forward or back. Wheelchair rugby was made popular by the documentary film *Murderball*. In this sport, the chairs are designed much like a basketball chair but with slight modifications. Covers are placed over the spokes of the wheels to prevent a hand getting caught. The players are harnessed in so that when the chair gets tipped, the player goes with it. Chairs are outfitted with a front bumper or a pick bar, which is used to spin, tip, or ram opponents' chairs. Tennis wheelchairs are similar to basketball or rugby chairs, but they are characterized by more freedom in design because it is unlikely that they will collide with another player. Quickness and maneuverability are paramount, and different 3- and 4-wheel designs are available to suit the individual preference of the tennis player. Many beginning wheelchair athletes will want to experiment with different chairs and adjustments within their chair to optimize balance, performance, and comfort.

Adaptive equipment for skiing has become much more common around the country since many ski resorts have developed adaptive ski programs. Skiers are evaluated to determine which adaptive equipment is necessary to

Just as technology for terminal devices has become more sophisticated, adaptive equipment for various sports is equally as advanced. Wheelchairs are no longer simply for community ambulation. Wheelchairs are designed with specific sports in mind. Sport wheelchairs have been greatly influenced by revolutions in cycling technology. Lighter, stronger wheels found in bicycles are used in wheelchairs as well. Racing wheelchairs have cambered wheel alignment to provide a wider base of support (**Figure 7.5**). The athlete is seated lower to the ground to lower the center of gravity. A third, front wheel extends the frame horizontally a few feet in front of the chair to make the chair more aerodynamic and to increase the base of support for greater stability. Many wheelchair racers post good marathon times:

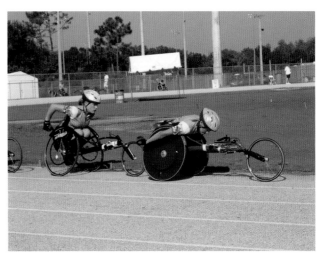

FIGURE 17.5 Wheelchair racers.

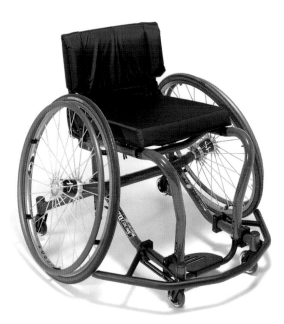

FIGURE 17.6 Court wheelchair. Reproduced with permission of sunrisemedical.com

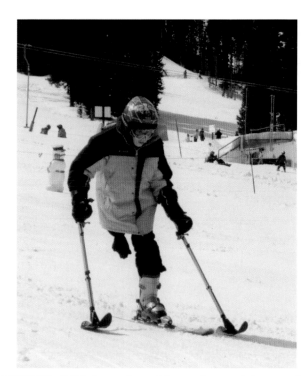

FIGURE 17.7 Amputee skier using outriggers for lateral support.

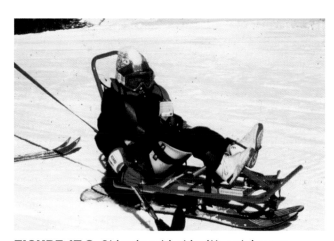

FIGURE 17.8 Skier in a bi-ski with outriggers.

optimize their performance. Devices such as outriggers help provide lateral support and timing to amputee skiers and others who need augmented lateral support (**Figure 7.7**). Ski bras and bungee cords can be used for skiers with poor muscle control or weakness in the hips to provide a stable platform and control the tips of the skis. Wheelchair ambulators, or children with a high lumbar-level or thoracic-level spina bifida or spinal cord injury, may ski in a modified sled device or a sit-ski (**Figure 7.8**). Beginners usually learn to sit-ski on a bi-ski, which has 2 skis underneath the seat to provide a wider base of support and to help turn. As the skier progresses, more competitive sit-skiers will advance to a monoski, which is lighter, faster, and more maneuverable. A monoski is good for independence and higher speeds on a mountain. Many monoskiers can load themselves onto the chairlift without help. Adaptive skiing has become widespread and can be adapted for many different types and levels of disability.

THERAPEUTIC DANCE AND MUSIC

Many recreational activities are available for the disabled, including dance. Dance programs have emerged around the United States and in Canada that adapt dance classes for people with disabilities. Be it ballet or wheelchair folk dance, dancing can provide many of the same benefits as sports. The movements necessary for dancing can help

improve strength, endurance, flexibility, and motor control, and the social and self-esteem benefits stemming from a shared experience like dancing can be equally great.

Certain music classes are available for physically and developmentally disabled children. Playing a musical instrument with specific rhythms and patterns in mind requires the use of different muscles, so children can improve their motor control in the process. When fine motor control is difficult, percussion instruments are a good musical option. The rhythms, melodies, and patterns inherent in playing a musical instrument can affect the patient's neurologic structures. The brain processes music in both hemispheres, which can stimulate cognitive function. The teamwork necessary to play instruments in a group provides social engagement. Music is a powerful therapy tool that can be adapted and individualized for each child's disability to achieve maximum benefit.

CONCLUSIONS

Every child, able-bodied or disabled, deserves the opportunity to participate in sporting activities, be they recreational or competitive. Sports provide a way to increase physical ability, and the pure joy of participating can produce great emotional rewards. Awareness and promotion of sports programs for people with disabilities opens the door for even more children around the world. Despite their physical disabilities, these athletes continue to push their limits and perform at elite levels. Accomplishing their athletic goals is a fulfilling experience, not only for the athlete but also for everyone involved in the program. Children should be encouraged to participate at all levels and strive to do their best, but most important, to have fun doing it.

SUMMARY POINTS

- Participation in athletics is a good way for children with physical disabilities to improve physical fitness and self-esteem.

- Participation of health care providers in adaptive sports can be rewarding for the providers and participants.

- Patients and coaches should be aware of different disabilities and the potential medical risks of sports participation.

- The interface between the adaptive equipment and the athlete should be monitored for proper fit and overuse.

- The best technique for detecting atlantoaxial instability is using lateral flexion and extension views of the cervical spine in conjunction with the monitoring of neurologic symptoms; however, the efficacy of this technique is still being debated.

- There are organizations in many communities that arrange sporting events for athletes with disabilities.

- The benefits of participation in sporting activities are numerous and can be obtained by engaging in both recreational and competitive activities.

SUGGESTED READING

American Academy of Orthopaedic Surgeons. Sports and recreational programs for the child and young adult with physical disability. In: *Proceedings of the Winter Park Seminar, Winter Park, CO.* Chicago, IL: American Academy of Orthopaedic Surgeons; 1983.

American Academy of Pediatrics Council on Children with Disabilities. Promoting the Participation of Children With Disabilities in Sports, Recreaction, and Physical Activities. *Pediatrics.* 2008;121(5):1057-1061.

Burnham R, Wheeler G, Bhanbhani Y, et al. Intentional induction of autonomic dysreflexia among quadriplegic athletes for performance enhancement: efficiency, safety and mechanism of action. *Clin J Sport Med.* 1994;4:1-10.

Chang FM. The disabled athlete. In: Stanitski CL, DeLee JC, Drez D Jr, eds. *Pediatric and Adolescent Sports Medicine.* Philadelphia, PA: WB Saunders; 1994:3:48-76.

Chang FM. Sports programs for the child with a limb deficiency. In: Herring JA, Birch JG, eds. *The Child with a Limb Deficiency.* Rosemont, IL: American Academy of Orthopaedic Surgeons; 1998:361-377.

Deaf Sports Federation Web site. http://www.usadsf.org/. Accessed June 3, 2008.

Dec KL, Sparrow JS, McKeag DB. The physically-challenged athlete: medical issues and assessment. *Sports Med.* 2000;19:821-834.

DeLee JC, Drez D Jr., Miller M, eds. *DeLee and Drez's Orthopaedic Sports Medicine: Principles and Practice.* 2nd ed. Philadelphia, PA: WB Saunders; 2003.

Disabled Sports USA Web site. http://www.dsusa.org/. Accessed June 3, 2008.

International Paralympic Committee Web site. http://www.paralympic.org/. Accessed June 3, 2008.

National Disability Sports Alliance Web site. http://www.ndsaonline.org/. Accessed June 3, 2008.

National Sports Center for the Disabled. http://www.nscd.org/. Accessed June 3, 2008.

Paulsen P, French R, Sherrill C. Comparison of mood states of college able-bodied and wheelchair basketball players. *Percept Mot Skills.* 1991;73:396-398.

Paulsen P, French R, Sherrill C. Comparison of wheelchair athletes and nonathletes on selected mood states. *Percept Mot Skills.* 1990;71(3 pt 2):1160-1162.

Pfiel J, Marquardt E, Holtz T, Niethard FU, Schneider E, Carstens C. The stump capping procedure to prevent or treat terminal osseous overgrowth. *Prosthet Orthot Int.* 1991;15:96-99.

Schmid A, Schmidt-Trucksa A, Huonker M, et al. Catecholamines response of high performance wheelchair athletes at rest and during exercise with autonomic dysreflexia. *Int J Sports Med.* 2001;22:2-7.

Sherrill C, Hinson M, Gench B, Kennedy SO, Low L. Self-concepts of disabled youth athletes. *Percept Mot Skills.* 1990;70(3 pt 2):1093-1098.

Special Olympics Web site. http://www.specialolympics. org/. Accessed June 3, 2008.

Sussman MD, ed. *The Diplegic Child.* Rosemont, IL: American Academy of Orthopaedic Surgeons; 1992.

Tenholder M, Davids JR, Gruber HE, Blackhurst DW. Surgical management of juvenile amputation overgrowth with a synthetic cap. *J Pediatr Orthop.* 2004;24:218-226.

United States Association of Blind Athletes Web site. http://www.usaba.org/. Accessed June 3, 2008.

United States Cerebral Palsy Athletic Association Web site. http://www.uscpaa.org/. Accessed June 3, 2008.

United States Olympic Committee Web site. http://www.usoc.org/. Accessed June 3, 2008.

Weihenmayer E. *Touch the Top of the World: A Blind Man's Journey to Climb Farther Than the Eye Can See.* New York, NY: Plume; 2002.

Weiss J, Diamond T, Demark J, Lovald B. Involvement in Special Olympics and its relations to self-concept and actually competency in participants with developmental disabilities. *Res Dev Disabil.* 2003;24:281-305.

Wheelchair Sports USA Web site. http://www.wsusa.org/. Accessed June 3, 2008

Wilson PE. Exercise and sports for children who have disabilities. *Phys Med Rehabil Clin N Am.* 2002; 13:907-923.

CHAPTER 18

Complementary and Alternative Medicine

Cora Collette Breuner, MD, MPH

Complementary and alternative medicine (CAM), also known as integrative, holistic, or natural care, includes a number of therapeutic modalities and practices that may not be fundamental to the traditional health care system.

Expenditures for visits to alternative medicine providers are considerable. In 1997, an estimated $25–30 billion was spent in the United States, $12.2 billion of which was paid out of pocket. Nearly 1 in 5 individuals taking prescription medicines was also taking herbs or high-dose vitamin supplements. The Centers for Disease Control and Prevention's National Center for Health Statistics found that 36% of US adults used some form of CAM (excluding prayer) for their health.

Because of CAM's widespread use and its potential to affect traditional health care delivery, all patients should be asked about their use not only of herbals and supplements but also of forms of complementary or integrative interventions, including homeopathy, chiropractic, massage, or acupuncture, as well as any treatment that may be considered nontraditional or alternative.

NATUROPATHY

Naturopathy is a system of healing that views disease as a manifestation of alterations in the processes by which the body naturally heals itself. It emphasizes health restoration as well as disease treatment. Today, naturopathy, or naturopathic medicine, is practiced throughout Europe, Australia, New Zealand, Canada, and the United States. The 6 principles of naturopathic practice in North America are listed in **Table 18.1**.

Core modalities include diet modification and nutritional supplements, herbal medicine, acupuncture and Chinese medicine, hydrotherapy, massage and joint manipulation, and lifestyle counseling. Treatment protocols combine what the practitioner deems to be the most suitable therapies for the individual patient.

HERBALS

Herbals are summarized in **Table 18.2**.

Caffeine

Caffeine is used to enhance sports performance and increase energy.

Mechanism of action: Caffeine acts by indirectly increasing the levels of norepinephrine, epinephrine, and dopamine and stimulating α- and β-adrenoreceptors. Caffeine also inhibits phosphodiesterase and antagonizes adenosine receptors, which appears to be its key physiologic effect. Caffeine can also antagonize benzodiazepine receptors.

Potential benefits: Caffeine may help reduce accidents at work. Caffeine supplementation may have an ergogenic effect.

Side effects: Side effects may include increased blood pressure, insomnia palpitations, tachycardia, chest pain, and coronary vasospasm; caffeine may cause diuresis, increase urinary calcium, and increase core temperature.

Ephedra

Ephedra (ma huang, *Ephedra sinica*) products are used to aid weight loss, enhance sports performance, and increase energy.

TABLE 18.1

Six Principles of Naturopathy

- The healing power of nature
- Identification and treatment of the cause of disease
- The concept of "first, do no harm"
- The doctor as teacher
- Treatment of the whole person
- Prevention

Mechanism of action: Ephedra, like caffeine, acts by increasing the levels of norepinephrine, epinephrine, and dopamine and stimulating α- and β-adrenoreceptors.

Potential benefits: Ephedra may promote modest short-term weight loss.

Side effects: In 2004, the US Food and Drug Administration banned the sale of dietary supplements containing ephedra because of its serious adverse effects, including tachycardia, palpitations, and death.

St. John's Wort

St John's wort (*Hypericum perforatum*) is used to treat depression.

Mechanism of action: Hypericin and hyperforin are the 2 active ingredients, which inhibit the reuptake of serotonin, norepinephrine, and dopamine and in vitro inhibit monoamine oxidase (MAO).

Potential benefits: St. John's wort is prescribed for the treatment of depression and may be more effective than placebo and as effective as standard antidepressants for mild to moderate depression. Minimal effects are seen for major depression.

TABLE 18.2

Herbs Relevant to the Young Athlete

Substance or Common Name	Latin Name	Uses	Mechanism of Action	Dose	Side Effects
Caffeine	…	Performance enhancement	Increases dopamine	Not recommended in children and adolescents	Increased urinary calcium, decreased perceived exertion, tachycardia, palpitations
Ephedra	*Ephedra sinica*	Energy booster, weight loss	Increases norepinephrine and epinephrine	Banned by the US Food and Drug Administration in 2004	Tachycardia, palpitations, death
St. John's wort	*Hypericum perforatum*	Depression	SSRI, MAO inhibitor	300 mg tid	Induces cytochrome P-450 system and can increase metabolism of drugs metabolized by this system
Echinacea	*Echinacea*	Immune booster	T cell activator; stimulates alternate complement pathway	6-9 mL juice tid with URI symptoms	Rash
Ginseng	*Panax ginseng*	Energy booster, enhance quality of life	May affect the hypothalamus-pituitary-adrenal axis	200 mg daily	Agitation, insomnia, nausea
Kava	*Piper methysticum*	Sedative	Binds to GABA receptors	60 mg daily	Oversedation, liver damage
Peppermint	*Agonis flexuosa*	Irritable bowel syndrome	Decreases smooth muscle spasm	0.2 mL tid	May cause GERD
Valerian	*Valeriana officinalis*	Sleep aid	Depresses some centers of the central nervous system	400 mg HS	Paradoxical stimulation
Chamomile	*Matricaria recutita*	Anxiolytic, peptic ulcer disease	Includes chamazulene (antispasmodic), apigenin (anxiolytic), bisoprolol (anti-inflammatory)	Tea tid	Mild allergic reaction
Ginger	*Zingiber officinale*	Antiemetic, anti-inflammatory, analgesic	Pharmacologically active components of the oleoresin include gingerols	2-4 g fresh gingerroot daily	Mild heartburn; may decrease platelet aggregation

GABA indicates γ-aminobutyric acid; GERD, gastroesophageal reflux disease; MAO, monoamine oxidase; and SSRI, selective serotonin reuptake inhibitor.

Side effects: St. John's wort may cause gastrointestinal (GI) symptoms, dizziness, and confusion. St. John's wort can induce the cytochrome P-450 metabolic pathway. It may interact with cyclosporine, certain antiretroviral agents (including indinavir), anticoagulants, and oral contraceptives. Serotonin syndrome may occur with its simultaneous use with selective serotonin reuptake inhibitors (SSRIs).

Echinacea

Echinacea (*Echinacea angustifola, E pallida, E purpurea*) has been used by Native Americans for hundreds of years for upper respiratory infections. Its use is popular in Europe, where it is taken to support and stimulate the immune system.

Mechanism of action: Echinacea works by stimulating the alternate complement pathway and can promote T cell activation. Echinacea may have immune-modulating effects. Components of this herb can inhibit viral replication and enhance killer cell activity.

Potential benefits: Echinacea preparations were not found to be better than placebo for the treatment or prevention of upper respiratory symptoms.

Side effects: Adverse effects are usually mild and may include skin rash, GI upset, and diarrhea. Echinacea should not be used in patients who are immunocompromised, who have an autoimmune disease, or who are allergic to the plant.

Ginseng

Ginseng may strengthen both mental and physical capacity. It is purported to be an energy booster, to improve glycemic control, and to enhance quality of life. It has also been used as an aphrodisiac.

Mechanism of action: The main active agents in *Panax ginseng* are ginsenosides, which are triterpene saponins. *Panax ginseng* may affect the hypothalamus-pituitary-adrenal axis and the immune system and may also improve tissue insulin sensitivity.

Potential benefits: Studies investigating ginseng's effects on physical performance have had mixed outcomes. Some reports showed no difference between ginseng and placebo; in others, a significant decrease in heart rate and an increase in maximal oxygen uptake were noted.

Side effects: Ginseng may cause vaginal bleeding and hypoglycemia. Those with diabetes should be cautioned. Cardiovascular effects include tachycardia and palpitations.

Kava

Kava (*Piper methysticum*) is important in cultural ceremonies in the South Pacific, where it has traditionally been used as a ritual drink. It is used for its sedating and calming effects.

Mechanism of action: Kava may increase the number of γ-aminobutyric acid (GABA) receptor binding sites and may act as a dopamine agonist.

Potential benefits: Kava reduces participant study scores on anxiety scales when compared with placebo.

Side effects: Kava dermopathy, or yellowing and flaking of the skin, may occur. A risk of elevated liver enzymes, acute hepatitis, and extrapyramidal-like dystonic reactions have been observed. Oversedation may occur when kava is combined with sedatives or alcohol.

Peppermint

Peppermint (*Agonis flexuosa*) is used to treat irritable bowel syndrome, colic, nausea, congestion, and cough. In addition, it is an anxiolytic and is used as a topical analgesic for headache and myalgia.

Potential benefits: Studies support the use of peppermint oil to treat irritable bowel syndrome and dyspepsia pain.

Side effects: In infants, apnea may result when it is applied under or in the nose. In all ages, gastroesophageal reflux, heartburn, and mild rectal burning may occur.

Valerian

Valerian (*Valeriana officinalis*) has been used as a sedative agent and sleep aid.

Mechanism of action: Valerian root affects GABA receptors, which results in a combination of direct relaxation of the smooth muscle and a depression of some centers of the central nervous system.

Potential benefits: Studies of the effect of valerian on sleep found no significant difference between its use and placebo.

Side effects: Valerian use may result in paradoxical anxiety and restlessness, as well as heart palpitations. It may potentiate the effect of barbiturates. With long-term use, its abrupt withdrawal can trigger delirium and cardiac arrhythmias.

Chamomile

Historically, chamomile (*Matricaria recutita*) has been used for GI discomfort, peptic ulcer disease, colic, and mild anxiety.

Mechanism of action: Chamomile has 3 active ingredients: chamazulene, an antispasmodic; apigenin, an anxiolytic; and bisoprolol, an anti-inflammatory.

Potential benefits: Chamomile may be effective as a mouthwash for mucositis associated with chemotherapy. It may be effective in treating colic.

Side effects: Few people are sensitive to chamomile or develop allergic reactions. People sensitive to ragweed and chrysanthemums or other members of the Compositae family are the most likely to develop contact allergies to chamomile.

Ginger

Ginger (*Zingiber officinale*) has been used to aid digestion and treat stomach upset, diarrhea, and nausea. Since ancient times, ginger has also been used to help treat arthritis, colic, diarrhea, and heart conditions.

Mechanism of action: Ginger contains antiemetic, anti-inflammatory, and analgesic properties. Ginger promotes the flow of bile into the intestine through contraction of the gallbladder. Pharmacologically active components of the oleoresin include gingerols.

Potential benefits: Ginger has been found to be effective in treating pregnancy-induced morning sickness. In addition, in people with osteoarthritis of the knee, ginger lessened their pain, resulting in the need for fewer painkillers.

Side effects: Side effects may include mild heartburn and a decrease in platelet aggregation.

Training and Licensure Requirements

Only 4 schools in the United States and 2 in Canada offer an accredited program toward a doctorate in naturopathic medicine. The 4-year curriculum, like that of conventional medical schools, begins with a wide range of courses in basic science and normal physiology. A national licensing examination, NPLEX (Naturopathic Physicians Licensing Examination), has been in place since 1999. Fourteen states plus Washington, DC, Puerto Rico, and the US Virgin Islands currently license naturopathic physicians.

HOMEOPATHIC MEDICINE

Overview

Homeopathy is a medical discipline that was first promoted in the late 18th century by Samuel Hahnemann. Homeopathic medicine sales have greatly increased recently. In some European countries, up to 40% of physicians use homeopathy in their practice.

Theory

Homeopathy is one of the most controversial CAM therapies. The philosophy of homeopathic medicine includes finding a substance that causes a particular response, then using a highly dilute preparation of this substance in the patient. The theory "like cures like" is that a homeopathic remedy can promote healing in patients with similar symptoms. Many health care providers do not believe that substances diluted infinitesimally preserve their biological effects. Others believe that homeopathic remedies are an allowable therapy for many medical problems.

The preparation of homeopathic remedies requires serial dilution (for example, "30C potency" is a remedy that has been diluted 1:100, 30 successive times) and shaking.

In clinical studies, homeopathy has been found to be more effective than placebo for symptomatic seasonal allergies and postoperative ileus. However, no significant effect in small trials was found in the treatment of respiratory tract infections, gynecological problems, and musculoskeletal disorders.

One of the most common homeopathic preparations used after an injury is that of the flower head of the leopard's bane plant (*Arnica montana*), which is used to treat bruises and muscle strains. The sesquiterpene lactones of *Arnica* can produce anti-inflammatory and analgesic effects. It should not be used on dry or broken skin.

Other homeopathic remedies that may be used in athletes include the daisy (*Bellis perennis*) and St. John's wort (*Hypericum*) for contusions, strains, and sprains. Overuse injuries may be treated with wild rosemary (*Rhododendron tomentosum,* formerly *Ledum palustre*) or rue (*Ruta graveolens*). Sarcolactic acid may be used for overexertion and its resulting muscle soreness and fatigue. Arthritis pain may be relieved by poison ivy (*Rhus toxicodendron*), bryony (*Bryonia alba*), apis (made from honeybee venom), and wild rosemary. A homeopathic remedy for gout is autumn crocus (*Colchicum autumnal*).

Complications

Complications of homeopathic medicine may include a temporary provocation of symptoms. Toxicity is generally not a complication because of the dilute nature of the remedies.

Training and Licensure Requirements

There are many homeopathic schools in the United States. They offer 2- to 4-year programs, although a diploma or certificate does not provide a license to practice. Qualification for licensure generally requires applicants to have at least 300 to 500 hours of homeopathic training, and they must pass oral and written examinations. Many health professionals, including medical doctors, osteopathic physicians, chiropractors, acupuncturists, nurse practitioners, and veterinarians, obtain licensure. Homeopathy is included within the scope of practice of naturopathic doctors (NDs), currently licensed in 14 states.

ACUPUNCTURE

Theory

The ancient Chinese art of acupuncture is based on the premise that energy (*qi* or *chi*) flows through the body along meridians connected by acupuncture points. *Qi* flow is modified when fine needles are inserted at acupuncture points. Acupuncture's use in the United States has increased and incorporates techniques from China, Japan, Korea, and other countries. It is one of the most frequently suggested CAM therapies.

The acupuncturist takes a history from the patient; examines the tongue to assess its shape, color, and coating; and takes a pulse to assess the force, flow, and character of the radial pulse. Treatment includes placement of a solid sterile needle, acupressure, cupping, or moxibustion (the practice of burning dried herbs over the acupuncture needles). The mechanism of action of acupuncture is not well understood, but it may be due to inhibition of pain impulses at the local site of needle stimulation or due to the body's release of opioid peptides and other neurotransmitters.

Clinical trials did not find sufficient evidence to promote or contraindicate acupuncture in the treatment of lateral elbow pain, although it may be of some short-term benefit. There is clinical evidence of benefits for dental pain, postoperative nausea and vomiting, and chemotherapy-related nausea and vomiting. Its use is possibly beneficial in the treatment of migraine or tension headaches, osteoarthritis of the knee, chronic low back pain, shoulder pain dysmenorrhea, and substance abuse.

Complications

Serious adverse events from acupuncture, although extremely rare, include pneumothorax, angina, septic sacroiliitis, epidural abscess, and temporomandibular abscess.

Training and Licensure

Licensed Acupuncture Approximately 40 states have established training standards for acupuncture certification, with different requirements for obtaining a licensure. Up to 4000 hours of course work and instruction may be required to sit for a particular state's certification examination.
Medical Acupuncture To perform medical acupuncture, one must have graduated from an accredited allopathic or osteopathic medical school in the United States or Canada or possess final certification by the Educational Commission for Foreign Medical Graduates (ECFMG). The provider must complete a minimum of 300 hours of systematic acupuncture education and pass the licensure examination.

YOGA

Yoga comes from the Sanskrit word *yuga*, "to join," "to yoke oneself," or "to harness to a discipline or a way of life." Yoga includes meditation; relaxation; control of breathing; and various physical postures, known as asanas. Yoga may be an effective intervention for overweight adults, and it also may strengthen and increase muscle tone in patients with eating disorders.

Research, although sparse, on the physiological effects of yoga indicates that it results in a lower heart rate during and after yoga practice; blood pressure is not altered. Practitioners of yoga report higher satisfaction with life and better temperaments.

Yoga may help healthy people develop strength and flexibility. Meditation, controlled breathing, and stretches may be an important adjunct treatment for sports performance anxiety, hypertension, heart disease, depression, lower back pain, and headache.

Table 18.3 summarizes the recommendations of the American Academy of Orthopaedic Surgeons regarding yoga.

Complications

If a joint is pushed beyond anatomic limits, injuries may occur. For example, hyperflexion of the knee could cause, or aggravate, a meniscus injury. Patients with lumbar disk injuries should be careful with yoga poses that involve extreme forward bending. Wrist pain may be associated with hand weight-bearing poses. Serious complications from yoga are rare but have been reported, and include pneumomediastinum with a vigorous Valsalva.

TABLE 18.3

Yoga Recommendations from the American Academy of Orthopaedic Surgeons

- Speak to a physician before participating in yoga if you have any preexisting injuries or conditions.
- Work with a qualified yoga instructor. Inquire about experience and credentials.
- Warm up well because cold muscles, tendons, and ligaments are vulnerable.
- Wear clothing that allows for proper movement.
- Start slowly while you learn the basics, such as proper breathing, before you see how far you can stretch.
- Ask questions if you are unsure of a pose or movement.
- Know your limits. Do not go beyond your experience or comfort level.
- Drink plenty of fluids, especially if participating in Bikram, or hot, yoga.
- Listen to your body. Stop or take a break if you experience pain. If pain persists, consult a medical professional.

Reproduced with permission from: Tips to prevent yoga injuries, in Mosely CF (ed): Your orthopaedic connection. Rosemont, IL: American Academy of Orthopaedic Surgeons, 2007. Available at http://orthoinfo.aaos.org.

Training and Licensure Requirements

Many different schools of yoga exist, with curricula varying depending on the type of yoga being taught. Training may include techniques, anatomy and physiology, diet, philosophy, methodology, and personal practice. Specialized yoga training is available.

No license is required to teach yoga. The Yoga Alliance (http://www.yogaalliance.org) has attempted to bring standardization to yoga teachers. To become a registered Yoga Alliance teacher requires study of technique, teaching methods, anatomy and physiology, philosophy, ethics, and lifestyle, as well as practical experience.

MASSAGE

Theory

There are 5 forms of massage therapy. The first, and most common, is traditional European or Swedish massage, which is performed with the patient on a table or in a special massage chair; its focus is on relaxing the muscles and improving circulation. Sports massage is a deep muscle or deep tissue therapy. Bodywork is a form of structural massage that uses deep tissue massage to correct posture problems and movement imbalances. The Oriental method, acupressure or shiatsu, is the fourth form of massage. Reflexology, the fifth form of massage, is an energy massage in which the focus is primarily on the hands, feet, and ears.

There is insufficient clinical evidence to promote the effects of massage on sports performance. There has been research on lactate clearance, delayed onset of muscle soreness, muscle fatigue, the psychological effect of massage, and injury prevention and treatment. Further research is needed to determine how massage affects tissue healing, lymphatic drainage, and flexibility, as well as its psychological effects. Research has shown that massage as an intervention is effective particularly when provided in combination with exercise and education. Massage has also been found to be beneficial in patients with chronic lower back pain, with long-term benefits continuing after cessation of treatment.

Complications

No complications have been reported with massage, but side effects include temporary pain or discomfort, bruising, and swelling. Some patients may be sensitive to or allergic to massage oils. Patients with deep vein thrombosis, coagulopathy, fractures, or open or healing wounds should not undergo massage therapy.

Training and Licensure Requirements

Thirty-three states and the District of Columbia offer credentialing to professionals in massage and bodywork. Massage therapists must receive at least 600 hours of instruction to take the massage national certification examination.

CHIROPRACTIC

Overview

Patients see chiropractors more frequently than any other providers of CAM in the United States. Chiropractors may treat lower back pain, cervical pain, headache, dysmenorrhea, or carpal tunnel syndrome. Back and neck problems are the most common reasons that patients seek treatment from chiropractors.

Theory

Chiropractic is a system of health care concerned with the diagnosis, treatment, and prevention of musculoskeletal disorders, with resultant effects on general health. Chiropractors emphasize clinical interventions that support the natural ability of the body to self-heal, using manipulation and mobilization of the spine, rehabilitation and exercise programs, patient education, and lifestyle modification. Malaligned bones in the spinal column, called subluxations, may lead to the entrapment of spinal nerves, with production of disease resulting from suboptimal functioning of tissues and organs. Manipulation frees the recuperative power inherent to the body, and the body heals itself. Physical adjustment of the spine restores proper alignment of the spine by relieving nerve entrapments.

Adjustments should not be performed until all contraindications to care are reviewed. In lower back pain in children, chiropractic resulted in improvement, although patients who experienced chronic lower back pain were less likely to respond to therapy.

Complications

Complications of chiropractic manipulation, although rare, may occur. These include strokes, myelopathies, and radiculopathies. These are more likely to take place with upper cervical spine manipulation, incorrect diagnosis, bleeding dyscrasia, herniated disk, or improper technique. Neurologic and vertebrobasilar events may occur, although rarely; these include serious adverse events (eg, subarachnoidal hemorrhage, paraplegia), moderately adverse events that require medical attention (eg, severe headache), and minor adverse events (eg, midback soreness). Chiropractic has been linked to delayed diagnosis of conditions like diabetes and neuroblastoma, and occasionally, spinal manipulation may be inappropriately used to treat serious medical conditions.

Training and Licensure

Prechiropractic education requires at least 3 years of college-level course work. Four years of chiropractic training follow this; 2 years of basic sciences are required. Chiropractors must then successfully complete a 4-part national board examination. A 1-year internship at a college clinic is also required to become a licensed chiropractor. Osteopathic schools provide required courses on manipulation. Some osteopaths may incorporate manipulation into their daily practice.

CONCLUSION

Injured children or adolescents and their families have many options for treatment, both conventional and alternative. An integrated approach is the most effective. This requires common sense. The provider, the patient, and the patient's family must have an honest, nonjudgmental conversation about alternative care. Time, expense, and safety should be discussed. Our CAM colleagues can provide invaluable assistance in treating athletes, and they can help bring holistic and integrated health care to this population.

SUMMARY POINTS

- CAM is an important therapeutic option athletes may turn to for injury prevention and healing.
- Many herbal and homeopathic remedies are helpful in the young athlete.
- Acupuncture, chiropractic, and massage have been shown to effectively alleviate pain.
- Many excellent resources are available to learn about collaborating with integrative health care providers.

SUGGESTED READING

AAP Web site on CAM. http://www.aap.org/sections/CHIM.

American Association of Naturopathic Physicians Web site. http://www.naturopathic.org/. Accessed December 28, 2008.

American Board of Medical Acupuncture Web site. http://www.dabma.org. Accessed December 28, 2008.

American Massage Therapy Association Web site. http://www.amtamassage.org. Accessed December 28, 2008.

Associated Bodywork & Massage Professionals Web site. http://www.abmp.com. Accessed December 28, 2008.

Barnes PM, Powell-Griner E, McFann K, Nahin RL. Complementary and alternative medicine use among adults: United States, 2002. *CDC Advance Data Report #343.* 2004. http://nccam.nih.gov/news/report.pdf. Accessed November 28, 2007.

Berman BM, Lao L, Langenberg P, Lee WL, Gilpin AMK, Hochberg MC. Effectiveness of acupuncture as adjunctive therapy in osteoarthritis of the knee: a randomized, controlled trial. *Ann Intern Med.* 2004;141:901-910.

Breuner CC. Complementary medicine in pediatrics: a review of acupuncture, homeopathy, massage and chiropractic therapies. *Curr Prob Pediatr Adolesc Health Care.* 2002;32:347-384.

Chirobase Web site. http://www.chirobase.org/. Accessed December 28, 2008.

ConsumerLab.com. http://www.consumerlab.com. Accessed December 28, 2008.

Coulter ID, Hurwitz EL, Adams AH, Genovese BJ, Hays R, Shekelle PG. Patients using chiropractors in North America: who are they, and why are they in chiropractic care? *Spine.* 2002;27:291-296.

Council for Homeopathic Certification Web site. http://www.homeopathicdirectory.com. Accessed June 9, 2008.

Dantes F, Rampes H. Do homeopathic medicines provoke adverse effects? A systematic review. *Br Homeopath J.* 2000;89:S35-S38.

Eisenberg DM, Davis RB, Ettner SL, et al. Trends in alternative medicine use in the United States, 1990-1997. *JAMA.* 1998;280:1569-1575.

Ernst E. Prospective studies of the safety of acupuncture: a systematic review. *Am J Med.* 2001;110:481-485.

Furlan AD, Brosseau L, Imamura M, Irvin E. Massage for low-back pain. *Cochrane Database Syst Rev.* 2002;(2): CD001929.

Green S, Buchbinder R, Barnsley L, et al. Acupuncture for lateral elbow pain. *Cochrane Database Syst Rev.* 2002;(1): CD003527.

Gupta N, Khera S, Vempati RP, Sharma R, Bijlani RL. Effect of yoga based lifestyle intervention on state and trait anxiety. *Indian J Physiol Pharmacol.* 2006;50:41-47.

Hayden JA, Mior SA, Verhoef MJ. Evaluation of chiropractic management of pediatric patients with low back pain: a prospective cohort study. *J Manipulative Physiol Ther.* 2003;26:(1):1-8.

HerbMed database. http://www.herbmed.org. Accessed December 28, 2008.

Integrative Yoga Therapy Web site. http://www.iytyogatherapy.com. Accessed December 28, 2008.

Kashyap AS, Anand KP, Kashyap S. Complications of yoga. *Emer Med J.* 2007;24(3):231.

Lee AC, Li DH, Kemper KJ. Chiropractic care of children. *Arch Pediatr Adolesc Med.* 2000;154:401-407.

Lee KP, Carlini WG, McCormick GF, Albers GW. Neurologic complications following chiropractic manipulation: a survey of California neurologists. *Neurology.* 1995;45:1213-1215.

Lyss G, Schmidt TJ, Merfort I, Pahl HL. Helenalin, an anti-inflammatory sesquiterpene lactone from Arnica, selectively inhibits transcription factor NF kappa B. *Biol Chem.* 1997;378:951-961.

Martin NA, Zoeller RF, Robertson RJ, Lephart SM. The comparative effects of sports massage, active recovery, and rest in promoting blood lactate clearance after supramaximal leg exercise. *J Athl Train.* 1998;33:30-35.

Meeker WC, Haldeman S. Chiropractic: a profession at the crossroads of mainstream and alternative medicine. *Ann Intern Med.* 2002;136:216-227.

Morasaka A. Sports massage: a comprehensive review. *J Sports Med Phys Fitness.* 2005;45:370-380.

National Center for Complementary and Alternative Medicine Web site. http://nccam.nih.gov/health/acupuncture. Accessed December 28, 2008.

National Center for Homeopathy Web site. http://www.homeopathic.org/law.htm. Accessed December 28, 2008.

National Certification Commission for Acupuncture and Oriental Medicine Web site. http://www.nccaom.org. Accessed December 28, 2008.

Natural Medicines Comprehensive Database. http://www.naturaldatabase.com. Accessed December 28, 2008.

Pomerantz B, Chiu D. Naloxone blockade of acupuncture analgesia: endorphin implicated. *Life Sci.* 1976;1757.

Richardson WH, Stone CM, Michels JE. Herbal drugs of abuse: an emerging problem. *Emerg Med Clin North Am.* 2007; 25(2):435-457.

Rogers NL, Dinges DF. Caffeine: implications for alertness in athletes. *Clin Sports Med.* 2005;24(2):e1-13.

Schell E, Allolio B, Schonecke W. Physiological and psychological effects of hatha-yoga exercise in healthy women. *Int J Eating Disord.* 1993;41:46-52.

Shang A, Huwiler-Muntener KH, Juni P, et al. Are the clinical effects of homeopathy placebo effects? Comparative study of placebo controlled trials of homeopathy and allopathy. *Lancet.* 2005;366:726.

Sherman KJ, Cherkin, DC, Erro, J, Miglioretti DL, Deyo RA. Comparing yoga, exercise, and a self-care book for chronic low back pain. *Ann Intern Med.* 2005;143(2): 849-856.

Thien V, Thomas A, Markin D, Birmingham C. Pilot study of a graded exercise program for the treatment of anorexia nervosa. *Int J Eat Disord.* 2000;28(1):101-106.

Triano J. Biomechanical mechanism of chiropractic. In: Rakel DP, Faass N, eds. *Complementary Medicine in Clinical Practice.* Sudbury, MA: Jones and Bartlett; 2006:363-371.

Vohra S, Johnston BC, Cramer K, Humphreys K. Adverse events associated with pediatric spinal manipulation: a systematic review. *Pediatrics.* 2007;119:e275-e283.

Weerapong P, Hume PA, Kolt GS. The mechanisms of massage and effects on performance, muscle recovery and injury prevention. *Sports Med.* 2005;35(3):235-256.

SECTION 4

Medical Conditions

CHAPTER 19

Cardiac Conditions

Reginald L. Washington, MD

Cardiac conditions such as dysrhythmias, hypertension, and heart disease can affect a child's ability to safely participate in sports. Signs and symptoms such as murmurs, syncope, and chest pain may also affect a child's ability to be physically active. It is important to establish the safety of physical activity for these children and to encourage them to participate at levels that are appropriate for their specific condition. Most of these children can participate in physical activities without limitations, but there are exceptions. All children with cardiac conditions should be evaluated individually to determine their physical limitations before they increase their physical activity. Before any increase in physical activity, children should undergo a preparticipation physical evaluation (PPE). This chapter highlights the cardiovascular components of the PPE and reviews the most common cardiovascular disorders in children. Children with known congenital defects require specialty evaluation that is beyond the scope of this chapter.

MURMURS

Heart murmurs are commonly encountered in children, and by some estimates, up to 85% of young athletes have audible heart murmurs detected during screening examinations. Most heart murmurs are considered functional or innocent. Often, heart murmurs are first identified during the PPE. Once they are detected, further evaluation should seek to answer these questions: Is the murmur functional or organic? If the murmur is organic, should participation in physical activity be limited? What type of evaluation should be completed before participation in physical activity is allowed?

Functional Murmurs

Still's Murmur The most common type of murmur in children is Still's murmur, which is characterized by a medium- to high-pitched, slightly vibratory or moaning murmur heard only during systole. It is easiest to hear along the lower left side of the sternum, although it radiates widely from the apex of the heart to the upper left side of the sternum. The child should lie in a supine position during auscultation because the sound decreases dramatically when the child is sitting or standing (**Table 19.1**). These murmurs are usually intermittent and become louder when cardiac output increases—for example, with anxiety, fever, or exercise.

Venous Hum Another common functional murmur is the venous hum. This continuous blowing or humming murmur is best heard above or below the clavicles on either side when the child is sitting. However, it is generally inaudible when the child is supine or when the return of venous blood from the neck to the heart is obstructed by gently compressing the jugular vein. If the murmur persists despite performing these maneuvers and continues to be heard when the child is supine, the differential diagnosis must include a patent ductus arteriosus (PDA). A child with a suspected PDA should be examined by a cardiologist before increasing physical activity.

Organic Murmurs

Organic murmurs are generally characterized by their harshness rather than by their intensity. Organic murmurs are not vibratory in nature, but they are audible with the child in any position. Organic murmurs may be caused by minor defects in the atrial or ventricular septa or by more complex cardiovascular problems such as narrowing of the aortic or pulmonary valves or cyanotic heart disease. If

TABLE 19.1

Common Heart Murmurs Affected by Positional Changes

Murmur	Increased	Decreased
Still's murmur	Supine	Sitting, standing
Venous hum	Sitting	Supine
Hypertrophic cardiomyopathy	Standing, Valsalva	Sitting, supine

TABLE 19.2

Evaluation of Heart Murmurs

History
- Family history
- Syncope or near syncope
- Chest pain
- Palpitations
- Exercise tolerance

Physical Examination
- Auscultation
- Peripheral pulses
- Blood pressure in the arms and legs

Selective Diagnostic Tests
- Chest radiograph
- Electrocardiogram
- Echocardiogram
- Exercise stress test

there is any suspicion of such problems, the child should be referred to a cardiologist.

Evaluation of Heart Murmurs

A complete evaluation consists of a thorough history and physical examination, an electrocardiogram (ECG), a radiograph of the chest, and often, an echocardiogram (**Table 19.2**). An assessment for heart murmurs should begin with a thorough history of the child and the immediate family members. The history should also document any adverse responses to exercise or activity and relevant symptoms, such as near syncope, syncope, chest pain, palpitations, or decreased exercise tolerance. The physical examination should include a thorough evaluation of the cardiovascular system, including peripheral pulses, auscultation, and blood pressure in the arms and the legs. Ordinarily the pressure recorded in the legs is about 10 mm Hg higher than in the arms. An ECG, a chest radiograph, an echocardiogram, or an exercise stress test may provide additional information. However, these tests should be selected and interpreted by someone experienced in diagnosing and treating congenital heart disease.

The presence of an organic murmur alone does not preclude physical activity or sports participation. Many children with organic murmurs have good cardiovascular function and are capable of full, active involvement in all physical activities. Guidelines for advising these children about participating in sports are contained in the proceedings from the 36th Bethesda Conference on Cardiovascular Abnormalities in the Athlete.

DYSRHYTHMIAS

A variety of tests can be used to diagnose and characterize dysrhythmias. Particularly important, however, is obtaining a thorough patient and family history (**Table 19.3**). An ECG and occasionally long-term recording devices (24-hour Holter monitor or activity monitors) also provide useful information.

TABLE 19.3

Elements of History When Assessing Patient for Dysrhythmias

Questions about Patient History
- Number, frequency, and duration of episodes
- Time of day when episodes occur
- Relationship of episodes to meals or exercise
- Severity of symptoms
- Recent use of medications, caffeine, or illicit substances
- Associated symptoms, including headache, nausea, vomiting, tingling of the extremities, loss of vision, or syncope

Questions about Family History
- Sudden death
- Syncope
- Near syncope or dizziness
- Seizures
- Supraventricular tachycardia
- Prolonged QT syndrome
- Hypertrophic cardiomyopathy
- Congestive cardiomyopathy
- Arrhythmogenic right ventricular dysplasia

Not all children with dysrhythmias require medical treatment or restrictions from physical activities. For instance, dysrhythmias originating from wandering atrial pacemakers or the sinus node are usually benign and do not require treatment. A child with these conditions may participate in athletic activities without any restrictions.

Children with premature ventricular contractions (PVCs) may report that their heart is skipping beats. An ECG will reveal an irregular rate originating from the ventricle. The rhythm is irregular, and the extra beat is followed by a compensatory pause. The next beat after the compensatory pause is more forceful and is perceived by the patient as a skipped beat. No treatment is required if the PVCs are uniform, appear singly (not in couplets), and disappear when the heart rate exceeds 140 beats/minute. However, if these criteria are not met, further evaluation by a cardiologist is warranted before athletic participation can be allowed.

Supraventricular tachycardia (SVT) is also known as paroxysmal atrial tachycardia. In this dysrhythmia, abnormally rapid conduction of an atrial impulse into the ventricle causes episodic increases in the heart rate. A child with SVT requires further evaluation and perhaps medical treatment before participation in sports is approved.

Children who have complete heart blocks or complex dysrhythmias (atrial flutter, atrial fibrillation, junctional tachycardia, or ventricular tachycardia) should be evaluated and treated as necessary by a cardiologist before participating in athletic activities.

NEAR SYNCOPE AND SYNCOPE

Children who experience episodes of near syncope report dizziness and light-headedness, either with or without exercise. They often feel cold, clammy, and sweaty and have thready peripheral pulses and low blood pressure. With syncope, however, these symptoms are followed by loss of muscle tone and loss of consciousness. Syncope and near syncope may be associated with underlying cardiac conditions, including vasodepressor syncope (fainting), primary and secondary cardiovascular syncope, vascular syncope, and noncardiovascular syncope (**Table 19.4**).

Vasodepressor syncope is a loss of consciousness caused by a sudden decrease in blood pressure. Associated signs and symptoms may include dizziness, light-headedness, pallor, diaphoresis, nausea, hyperventilation, and tachycardia. This type of syncope can be triggered by anxiety or fear in response to the sight of blood, loud noises, or other environmental stimuli. Typically, the syncopal episode lasts less than

TABLE 19.4	
Causes of Near Syncope and Syncope	
Syncope	**Cause**
Vasodepressor syncope	Sudden decrease in blood pressure and loss of consciousness, often triggered by anxiety or fear in response to sight of blood, loud noises, or other environmental stimuli
Cardiovascular syncope	Congenital heart conditions causing low cardiac output or dysrhythmia
Vascular syncope (orthostatic or neurogenic)	Hypotension and/or bradycardia due to blood pooling in legs; characterized by abnormal tilt test
Noncardiovascular syncope	Hypoxia, hypoglycemia, hyperventilation, seizures, vertigo, hysteria, severe migraines

1 minute and is preceded by prodromal symptoms. If the environmental stimulus is identified and eliminated, participation in sports may continue. If the episodes persist, continued participation in sports is not recommended until the athlete is evaluated by a cardiologist.

Primary and secondary cardiovascular syncope may result from congenital heart problems that cause low cardiac output or dysrhythmia. Patients with syncope should thus be evaluated for underlying congenital heart problems before participating in sports.

Vascular syncope (also known as orthostatic or neurocardiogenic syncope) occurs when blood pools in the lower parts of the body, reducing the amount of blood returning to fill the left ventricle. During a tilt test examination, children with this type of syncope will demonstrate a normal increase in heart rate, followed by a precipitous fall in heart rate and/or blood pressure. Often, severe problems, such as seizures, develop. These children often require medication before being allowed to participate in athletic activities and should be examined by a cardiologist.

Noncardiovascular syncope is caused by hypoxia, hypoglycemia, hyperventilation, seizures, vertigo, hysteria, or severe migraines. The history and physical examination will help determine which tests or specialty consultations should be obtained before sports participation. Activity restrictions should be determined individually and depend on the cause of the syncope. Syncope must be properly diagnosed and treated, if necessary, before the child participates in athletic activities.

CHEST PAIN

Young athletes rarely complain of chest pain. However, when they do, cardiovascular causes must be ruled out first. To make this determination, an evaluation of the characteristics of chest pain will help determine its cause (**Table 19.5**). Such factors include duration and quality of the pain, factors that provoke and relieve the pain, and the location and radiation of the pain. Chest pain can be caused by injury to the musculoskeletal system or can originate from conditions affecting the lungs, pleura, mediastinum, myocardium, or pericardium. Musculoskeletal pain is usually related to a specific episode of trauma and is characterized by localized pain and tenderness that occurs with specific movements or activities. Some common causes of chest wall pain include contusions or fractures of the ribs or sternum, strains of the pectoralis or intercostal muscles, costochondritis, and costosternitis.

Nonmusculoskeletal pain or pain from abnormalities of the heart or lungs occurs without antecedent trauma, is less well localized, and is less clearly related to specific movements or activities. Chest pain may be associated with inflammation or infection of the pleura or pericardium. Chest pain is also frequently reported as a component of asthma.

Cardiac causes of chest pain tend to produce symptoms that are worse with stress on the cardiovascular system. Pain from myocardial ischemia can occur with hypertrophic cardiomyopathy or aortic stenosis. A history of near syncope, syncope, palpitations, or exercise intolerance raises concern for these conditions. Echocardiography is recommended for patients with features of Marfan or Turner syndrome and chest pain because of the possibility of dissection of the aorta.

Fortunately, chest pain in children is rare. However, because of the potential for serious underlying conditions, each case of chest pain needs to be satisfactorily explained before the child is cleared to participate in athletic activities.

SYSTEMIC HYPERTENSION

Blood pressure measurements should be interpreted on the basis of sex-, age-, and height-specific norms available from the National Heart, Lung, and Blood Institute. Evaluation of blood pressure requires the use of appropriately sized cuffs. Appropriately fitting cuffs should cover approximately two-thirds of the upper arm. A cuff that is too small will result in falsely high readings. Larger athletes often require a thigh cuff for use on the arm. If blood pressure is initially high, repeat measurements should be taken after a few minutes and, if necessary, after the athlete lies down for several minutes. If the blood pressure is still high, the athlete should be questioned about the use of stimulants (caffeine, nicotine, cold or cough medications) and anabolic or corticosteroids, which can increase blood pressure. If signs and symptoms of systemic hypertension persist, the athlete should be evaluated for target-organ damage such as retinal changes (determined by ophthalmoscope examination), increased left ventricular mass (by echocardiography), and renal damage (analysis of blood and urine, and perhaps imaging studies). Children with target-organ damage may need to be restricted

TABLE 19.5

Causes and Character of Chest Pain

Musculoskeletal Causes
- Contusions or fractures of ribs or sternum
- Pectoralis or intercostal muscle strains
- Costochondritis
- Costosternitis

History of Trauma
- Localized pain and tenderness
- Aggravated by specific movements or activities

Nonmusculoskeletal Causes
- Pleuritis
- Pericarditis
- Asthma
- Cardiac conditions
  - Hypertrophic cardiomyopathy
  - Aortic stenosis (myocardial ischemia)
  - Aortic rupture (Marfan or Turner syndrome)

No History of Trauma
- Poorly localized
- No tenderness
- Not clearly related to specific movements or activities

from isometric exercises or some high-contact dynamic sports.

Children with severe, untreated, or unresponsive hypertension should avoid sports that involve prolonged periods of isometric exercises or stress and high-contact sports that might directly damage organs. If a child has interest in a sport that involves a high isometric component, prolonged handgrip stress testing should be performed before sports participation is approved.

ACQUIRED HEART DISEASE

Some children may have acquired heart disease. For instance, rheumatic fever can damage the aortic and mitral valves. Therefore, children who have had rheumatic fever should be evaluated by a cardiologist before beginning an athletic activity.

Individuals who have had Kawasaki disease without cardiovascular complications may participate in all activities. However, if the child has arteritis or coronary artery aneurysms, approval by a cardiologist should be obtained before participation is allowed.

Mitral valve prolapse is present in approximately 8% of children, but most of them can participate in physical activities. Children with mitral valve prolapse and a history of syncope, chest pain that is intensified by exercise, dysrhythmias, significant mitral insufficiency, or a family history of sudden death should be examined by a cardiologist before participating in vigorous physical activities.

CONGENITAL HEART DISEASE

Congenital heart diseases include a number of specific conditions and occur at a rate of 8 per 1000 live births. It is impractical to define the same limits for all children with congenital heart disease because some may have only minor defects, whereas others may have complex, inoperable defects. Furthermore, children who have undergone corrective or palliative surgery may not have achieved successful results. Because of these factors, children with congenital heart conditions need to be evaluated individually according to the guidelines established by the Bethesda Conference.

SUDDEN CARDIAC DEATH

The incidence of sudden cardiac death in children is estimated to be 7.5 per million per year of participation in boys and 1.5 per million per year of participation in girls. This accounts for between 10 and 25 cases of sudden death reported each year. Most of these studies, however, do not include a death that may occur during physical education classes, intramural sports, or casual recreational sports.

The most common cardiac causes of sudden death include hypertrophic cardiomyopathy, congenital coronary artery anomalies, aortic stenosis, myocarditis, dilated cardiomyopathy, mitral valve prolapse, and dysrhythmias (Table 19.6).

Screening echocardiograms have been suggested to identify some of the causes of sudden death. Most experts believe that in most settings, screening echocardiograms are not indicated because of the high cost of the procedure and the low frequency of disorders that are detected.

The role of automated external defibrillators (AEDs) in response to a cardiac arrest in children is not clear. The availability of an AED at a sporting event should not be construed as absolute protection against death resulting from cardiac arrest. Nor should it supersede restrictions based on underlying cardiac abnormalities against participation in competitive sports.

Cardiac Causes of Sudden Death

Most patients who die suddenly have hypertrophic cardiomyopathy and have had prodromal symptoms, although it is believed they may have kept these symptoms to themselves. These athletes frequently will have had

TABLE 19.6	
Common Causes of Sudden Cardiac Death and Warning Signs	
Cause	**Warning Signs**
Hypertrophic cardiomyopathy	• Prodromal symptoms common (chest pain, palpitations, presyncope, or syncope)
	• Systolic murmur
	• Abnormal electrocardiogram
	• Family history
Anomalies of the left coronary artery	• Infrequent prodromal symptoms
	• Often normal physical examination, family history, and electrocardiogram
Aortic stenosis	• Characteristic heart murmur
Mitral valve prolapse	• Characteristic heart murmur
Aortic rupture	• Physical stigmata of Marfan or Turner syndrome
Acute myocarditis	• Febrile illness followed by prolonged fatigue
Dysrhythmias	• Abnormal electrocardiogram

presyncope or syncope with or without exercise before the fatal event. They may also have experienced chest pain and palpitations during exercise. It is important to emphasize, however, that some of these athletes may have been asymptomatic for years. A systolic murmur will often be found, but only when the athlete is standing or with a Valsalva maneuver, and these murmurs are often very soft. Therefore, it is important during a PPE to examine the athlete in several positions and to do so in a quiet room. An ECG may show left ventricular hypertrophy. If this diagnosis is suspected, the athlete should be referred to a cardiologist before participation is allowed.

Anomalies of the left coronary artery are also frequently mentioned as a cause of sudden cardiac death. These athletes may or may not have had symptoms of syncope associated with activity or chest pain. This is a difficult diagnosis to make when the athlete has a negative family history, a normal physical examination, and a normal ECG. However, if symptoms lead to the suspicion of this diagnosis, activity should be restricted and the athlete should undergo evaluation of the coronary arteries immediately.

Athletes with aortic stenosis and mitral valve prolapse will have heart murmurs or abnormal auscultatory findings that should lead to the suspected diagnosis. Athletes who have the physical characteristics of Marfan syndrome should be screened to exclude the possibility of a dilated aorta. Athletes who have an acute febrile illness followed by prolonged fatigue may have acute myocarditis that also may lead to an acute cardiac death.

Although the incidence of sudden cardiac death is rare in this age group, a high index of suspicion should prevent some cases from occurring.

SUMMARY POINTS

- Before participating in any sports, children should undergo a complete physical examination that includes a thorough personal and family history of any cardiac conditions.

- Most athletes who experience cardiac symptoms during physical activity will not appear to have cardiac disease during their initial assessment, so specific laboratory tests may be necessary to evaluate them further.

- Most children with cardiovascular conditions can participate in most, if not all, physical activities.

- The most common cardiac causes of sudden death include hypertrophic cardiomyopathy, congenital coronary artery anomalies, aortic stenosis, myocarditis, dilated cardiomyopathy, mitral valve prolapse, and dysrhythmias.

- It is the primary responsibility of a child's health care provider to evaluate that child's individual cardiovascular problems and set individual limits on physical activity, with appropriate consultation with a cardiologist.

SUGGESTED READING

AHA Scientific Statement. Recommendations of physical activity and recreational sports participation for young patients with genetic cardiovascular diseases. *Circulation* 2004:109:2807-2816.

American Academy of Pediatrics, Committee on Sports Medicine and Fitness. Cardiac dysrhythmias and sports. *Pediatrics.* 1995;95:786-788.

American Academy of Pediatrics, Council on Sports Medicine and Fitness. Medical conditions affecting sports participation. *Pediatrics* 2008;121:841-848.

36th Bethesda Conference. Eligibility recommendations for competitive athletes with cardiovascular abnormalities. *J Am Coll Cardiol.* 2005;45:1313-1377.

National High Blood Pressure Education Working Group on High Blood Pressure in Children and Adolescents: A Pocket Guide to Blood Pressure Measurement in Children. US Department of Health and Human Services, National Institutes of Health, National Heart, Lung, and Blood Institute. MIH Publication 07-5268, May, 2007. http://www.nhlbi.nih.gov/health/public/heart/hbp/bp_child_pocket/bp_child_pocket.pdf.

Pelliccia A, Di Paolo FM, Quattrini FM, et al. Outcomes in athletes with marked ECG repolarization abnormalities. *N Engl J Med.* 2008;358:152-161.

Samson RA, Berg RA, Bingham R. Use of automated external defibrillators for children: an update—an advisory statement from the pediatric advanced life support task force. International Liaison Committee on Resuscitation. *Pediatrics.* 2003;112:163-168.

Washington RL. Children with heart disease. In: Skinner JS, ed. *Exercise Testing and Exercise Prescription for Special Cases.* Baltimore, MD: Lippincott, Williams, and Wilkins; 2005;337-348.

CHAPTER 20

Head Injuries

Bryan W. Smith, MD, PhD

Although head injuries can range from catastrophic to uncomplicated, they are never simple. Hundreds of thousands of head injuries occur annually during organized athletic activity. Although collision sports such as boxing, football, and ice hockey are associated with a high risk of head injury, sports such as basketball, soccer, lacrosse, baseball, and wrestling also pose significant risk. Unorganized activities like biking, in-line skating, and skateboarding also result in emergency visits for head injuries.

For years, the medical community has debated treatment guidelines for concussions, the most common head injury in sports. Although many guidelines have been developed, none has received universal acceptance. This chapter reviews the differential diagnosis and pathophysiology for athletic head injury, outlines the symptoms of concussion, discusses the evaluation of the athlete with a head injury, and presents management and return-to-play decisions.

DIFFERENTIAL DIAGNOSIS AND PATHOPHYSIOLOGY

The most common types of head injury due to sports are summarized in Table 20.1.

Epidural Hematoma

Epidural hematomas usually occur from damage to the middle meningeal artery via a temporal skull fracture. Most often, the mechanism of injury involves a high-impact event, such as being struck by a baseball. Typically, the injured athlete will experience a lucid period followed by a severe headache. Prompt recognition and subsequent treatment at a trauma center can prevent brain injury and save the athlete's life.

Subdural Hematoma

High-impact trauma to the skull can injure venous structures beneath the dura mater, resulting in a subdural hematoma. Falls or high-speed collisions are the usual mechanism of injury. With a concomitant skull fracture, symptoms can evolve over minutes. However, without a fracture, the symptoms may take days to occur. Usually the athlete is rendered unconscious for some period of time. Even in the best of circumstances, significant morbidity can occur as a result of brain damage.

Second-Impact Syndrome

Second-impact syndrome is a rare condition. It is believed to be caused by a loss of autoregulation of the vascular components of the brain, and it may occur when an athlete experiences a second head trauma before fully recovering from a previous one. Resultant massive cerebral edema occurs over seconds to minutes, frequently progressing to death. It is most common in boxers and football players younger than 21. Typically, these events occur in the first 2 weeks after the first head injury. Although debate exists about whether this syndrome actually occurred in many of the reported cases, it has been a driving factor in the development of most concussion scales and return-to-play guidelines.

Malignant Brain Edema Syndrome

Malignant brain edema syndrome is rare and poorly understood. It can occur in young children after a single head trauma. The pathophysiology resembles the second-impact syndrome with loss of vascular autoregulation and resulting diffuse cerebral hyperemia. Neurologic decline to coma and death may take minutes to hours, so prompt recognition and treatment at a trauma center are essential.

TABLE 20.1

Types of Head Injury

Condition	Pathophysiology	Cause	Symptoms
Epidural hematoma	Damage to middle meningeal artery via temporal skull fracture	High-impact event	Lucid period followed by severe headache
Subdural hematoma	Injury to venous structures beneath the dura mater	Falls or high-speed collisions	Evolves over minutes to days; usually associated with loss of consciousness
Second-impact syndrome	Loss of autoregulation of the vascular components of the brain, causing massive cerebral edema	Second episode of head trauma before recovery from an initial head injury	Evolves over seconds to minutes, frequently progressing to death
Malignant brain edema syndrome	Loss of vascular autoregulation and persistent cerebral hyperemia	Follows single episode of head trauma	Neurologic decline to coma or death in minutes to hours
Cerebral concussion	Transient traumatic disruption of neural function	Mild to severe head trauma	Neurologic impairment that usually resolves spontaneously after a sequential course

Cerebral Concussion

A cerebral concussion is a transient, traumatic disruption of neural function. This neuronal insult causes an increased demand for glucose intracellularly. A transient mismatch in glucose delivery and utilization occurs. This mismatch is believed to alter cerebral blood flow regulation. In animal studies, this can last a few weeks. How long and to what extent this occurs in humans after a concussion is not known but is likely variable. Structural changes in the brain are not typically seen on neuroimaging studies. Neurologic impairment usually resolves spontaneously and follows a sequential course.

The signs and symptoms reported in athletes who have experienced a concussion are provided in **Table 20.2**. There is no precise correlation of symptomatology to the length of time the brain is injured intracellularly. However, symptoms are variable in their occurrence and resolution. Even a minor concussion can result in symptoms that last for several days. Younger individuals (high school athletes and younger) whose brains are still developing may take longer to recover from a concussion than adults.

Loss of consciousness and amnesia are symptoms that have formed the basis for most concussion grading scales. Most athletes who experience a concussion do not lose consciousness. The degree of amnesia varies greatly; some individuals do not have evidence of amnesia. More than 20 concussion grading schemes exist to help the practitioner determine the severity of insult. The symptom variability complicates the grading of the injury. All the grading scales are based on anecdotal experience. Recently there has been a movement by experts to abandon grading scales.

TABLE 20.2

Signs and Symptoms of Concussion

- Headache
- Sleep disturbance
- Dizziness
- Confusion
- Nausea
- Unsteadiness
- Concentration difficulty
- Disorientation
- Amnesia
  - Posttraumatic
  - Retrograde
- Loss of consciousness
- Irritability
- Hyperexcitability
- Vomiting
- Visual disturbance
- Tinnitus
- Light-headedness
- Fatigue
- Performance impairment
- Impact seizure

Some have recommended categorizing concussions as simple or complex.

Simple concussions typically resolve spontaneously in 10 or fewer days. No complications or sequelae persist, and the athlete may return to play when appropriate. Complex concussions are less defined and incorporate either persistent symptoms or specific sequelae, such as convulsions or prolonged loss of consciousness. An athlete with past concussions may have future concussions classified as complex if it takes less insult to cause an injury or if the symptoms persist for a longer period of time.

Postconcussion Syndrome

Postconcussion syndrome is a variant of a complex concussion that consists of varying degrees of headache, irritability, concentration and memory impairment, dizziness, sleep disturbance, and fatigue. Although its incidence is unknown, this syndrome may be more common than recognized. It is defined by concussion symptoms that persist beyond a month, but symptoms may last weeks to months. Although the cause of postconcussion syndrome is poorly understood, it is probably the result of alterations in neurotransmitter function. In most cases, a concussion in which symptoms persist for more than 10 days and do not appear to resolve should be evaluated by a computed tomography (CT) scan or magnetic resonance imaging (MRI) to rule out gross trauma. Neuropsychological testing may be useful to document the degree of suspected cognitive dysfunction. Neurologic referral should be considered in protracted cases. Return to play should be permitted once symptoms have fully resolved and diagnostic studies are normal.

CLINICAL EVALUATION AND MANAGEMENT

Preparticipation Examination

Asking the athlete about past head injuries during the preparticipation examination can be informative. Having previous head injuries may place future ones in a complex category, and at the time of injury, the athlete often cannot remember the number of previous injuries. The preparticipation examination also provides an opportunity to perform any screening tests for baseline purposes and permits review of available options for protective equipment.

Acute Injury Evaluation and Management

Initial evaluation and management depend on the athlete's state of consciousness. If the athlete is unconscious, the neck must be immobilized to prevent possible catastrophic damage to the cervical spine. Next, the airway must be established and adequate ventilation ensured. This may require intubation. During this period, circulation needs to be monitored and established if necessary. Before the athlete is transported to a trauma center, the cervical spine must be stabilized. If there are signs of neurologic deterioration such as posturing or pupillary changes, moderate hyperventilation should be initiated if the athlete can be intubated. If conditions and time permit, a Glasgow Coma Scale value should be obtained.

Initially, the conscious or rapidly awakening athlete should be managed the same way as the unconscious athlete, beginning with an evaluation for cervical spine injury. After medical personnel have determined that it is appropriate to move the athlete, he or she should be escorted off the playing field, and any abnormality of the athlete's gait, balance, and orientation should be noted. It is best to take the athlete to a quiet place. For the unconscious athlete, prompt transport to a trauma center that has neuroimaging and subspecialists should be considered.

History

The athlete should be questioned about the mechanism of injury and any symptoms he or she is experiencing (**Table 20.1**). These symptoms can be quantified by using a symptom checklist. The patient's affect is important. It is not uncommon for the athlete to be hyperexcitable, irritable, sullen, or moody after a concussion. If the athlete avoids answering the questions, it is possible that he or she cannot answer because of the injury. The athlete usually wants to return to play and thus may attempt to deceive the examiner to hide his or her injuries.

Physical Examination

During the physical examination, the athlete's orientation needs to be evaluated (**Table 20.3**). The athlete should be questioned about person, place, and time. For example, the athlete should be asked to identify his or her school, opponent, and position played, and the current score. (The scoreboard should be blocked from the athlete's view.) The answers are important, as is the manner in which they are given: the care provider should check for slurred speech. Memory is assessed by asking the athlete to recall the mechanism of injury and the events before the injury (eg, menu for pregame meal, the score at halftime). Both short-term and long-term memory can be evaluated by giving the athlete 3 to 5 words to recall immediately and at the end of the examination.

The next part of the evaluation consists of a cranial nerve assessment, gross visual field examination, pupillary and funduscopic examination, otoscopic examination of

TABLE 20.3

Physical Examination for Evaluation of Concussion

Component	Practical Examples
Orientation	• Ask about school, opponent, position played, score.
Speech	• Is speech slurred?
Memory	• Test recall of injury and events before the injury.
	• Have athlete recall 3-5 words.
Cranial nerve assessment	...
Gross visual field assessment	...
Pupillary and funduscopic examination	...
Otoscopic examination of tympanic membranes	• Rule out blood in the middle ear.
Generalized examination for strength and sensation	...
Deep tendon reflexes	...
Concentration	• Have athlete recite months of the year backward.
	• Have athlete recite a string of 3-6 numbers backward.
	• Have athlete perform serial 7s test–starts at 100 and subtracts 7 repeatedly.
Coordination	• Observe gait.
	• Administer Romberg or pronator drift test.

each tympanic membrane for blood in the middle ear, a generalized examination for strength and sensation, and a check of deep tendon reflexes. Positive findings on these tests are rare in the athlete with concussion. When they are present, however, prompt transport of the athlete to a trauma center is often warranted. The absence of these signs does not exclude a potentially serious brain injury.

The last phase of the evaluation involves testing concentration and coordination. The concussed athlete usually demonstrates abnormalities of concentration and/or coordination. To assess concentration, the athlete should be asked to recite the months of the year backward. It is important to note the speed as well as the accuracy. A second test is recitation of a string of numbers backward, starting with 3 numbers and progressing to 6 numbers. For a third test, the serial 7s test, the athlete begins at 100 and

subtracts 7 repeatedly, ending at 2. Although accuracy is important, the clinician should note whether the athlete becomes frustrated or confused or takes an inordinate amount of time to complete the task. Some athletes may be unable to complete either test, particularly the serial 7s test, even under normal conditions. Preseason baseline testing for comparison may be useful. Coordination is assessed by observing the athlete's gait walking toward and away from the examiner and by having the athlete perform a Romberg test or a pronator drift test. The pronator drift test involves holding the arms out in front in a supinated position and closing the eyes. A positive test involves dropping an arm, moving the arms away from midline, or pronating an arm. The neurologic examination ends with a request that the athlete recall the words given to him or her to remember earlier in the examination.

The athlete should be reevaluated 15 minutes later to see if the symptoms or signs have resolved. If the athlete stays on the bench and does not return to play, it is a good idea to have someone stay on the bench with him or her. With football players, the athlete's helmet should be taken from him to keep him from returning to the field without medical clearance.

Diagnostic Tests

Standardized Assessment of Concussion (SAC) The Standardized Assessment of Concussion (SAC) is a diagnostic tool designed to objectively assess orientation, immediate memory, concentration, and delayed recall. It takes approximately 5 minutes to administer and has been designed for use on the field by physicians, athletic trainers, and coaches. There are multiple versions of the SAC, so different ones can be administered to minimize practice effects when the athlete repeats the test. This test is most useful if the athlete has been pretested during the preparticipation examination to provide a baseline value. The SAC is valid and reliable for children older than 5 years.

Sport Concussion Assessment Test (SCAT) The Sport Concussion Assessment Test (SCAT), developed by the Prague Concussion Consensus Panel, incorporates a symptom checklist and a medical evaluation assessing memory, concentration, orientation, recall, and neurologic screening. It provides return-to-play criteria.

Balance Error Scoring System (BESS) The Balance Error Scoring System (BESS) is a test of balance and coordination. The BESS tests for postural sway and uses 3 stance positions (double leg, single leg, and tandem) on both firm and foam surfaces. It has been shown to have good validity and reliability in determining balance deficits in concussed individuals.

Imaging Studies

Imaging studies may provide useful diagnostic information if symptoms worsen or fail to resolve within a reasonable time. Usually CT is more readily available. It is adequate to evaluate for gross blood in the cranium and evidence of skull fracture. All athletes do not require imaging. The length of time the athlete was unconscious, concomitant focal symptoms, and the physician's experience in evaluating head injuries must be considered when ordering an imaging study. More subtle pathology, such as vascular malformations and small bleeds, can be identified by MRI, so MRI is preferred in protracted cases—typically if symptoms fail to resolve by 1 week. Functional imaging modalities such as positron emission tomography, single-photon emission computed tomography, and functional MRI hold future promise in defining concussion recovery.

Neuropsychological Testing

Many neuropsychological tests exist to evaluate various cognitive skills. Their use in children younger than the late teens is limited as a result of the child's cognitive maturation. In the past, these tests were usually performed by neuropsychologists alone, but now they are available on a variety of computer platforms so that others can administer them. This has permitted health care providers to obtain baseline values for large numbers of athletes, which is essential for the testing to be useful in making return-to-play decisions. In some concussed athletes, these tests have demonstrated abnormalities even after the athlete's symptoms resolved. The reverse has also been shown. Although these tests have been a major step forward in the assessment of the concussed athlete, there is still a lack of consensus regarding their routine use when assessing concussion. Questions still remain regarding their clinical validity and use. The use of these tests for assessing a simple concussion should be based on the level of experience of the clinician in managing concussions and the clinician's underlying background knowledge of the patient. In cases of complex concussion or persistent symptomatology, neuropsychological tests have a more defined role in providing objective information to assist the clinician in making return-to-play decisions. Neuropsychological tests are often performed shortly after the time of injury and followed sequentially to monitor injury resolution. Learning effects can bias this process of repetitive testing. The most useful time to perform testing is after symptoms resolve, in order to determine if the athlete is ready to be cleared to resume playing and in order to establish a new baseline as a reference point for future testing if a subsequent injury occurs.

TREATMENT

Standard treatment for most concussions is rest and observation for as long as the athlete is symptomatic. Most concussions resolve without sequelae. Athletes can usually be managed at home by a responsible caregiver who is able to watch the athlete. All athletes should be observed closely for 24 hours if rendered unconscious, and hospitalization may be necessary. There is no defined role for analgesics in the acute treatment of concussion. Any analgesic that may increase bleeding should be avoided. The athlete is allowed to eat and to sleep but should be awakened every 2 to 3 hours if he or she has any significant symptoms before going to sleep. Worsening symptoms, new symptoms, or deteriorating neurologic signs warrant urgent physician reexamination. These instructions need to be conveyed in writing to the caregiver. Transport to a trauma center for imaging studies and neurosurgical consultation may be necessary in these rare instances.

While the athlete recovers and is still symptomatic, daily follow-up by a physician is preferred. In the young symptomatic athlete, activities of daily living should be appropriately modified to permit sufficient cognitive rest. School activities, such as class workload and homework, may need to be altered. Tests should be delayed or postponed, and the athlete should be excused from physical education. The athlete may need to return home to rest during the course of the school day.

RETURN TO PLAY

Many factors influence the decision to return the athlete to play after a head injury. Current recommendations in the literature are based on anecdotal clinical experiences rather than scientific research. Adherence to even the most conservative guidelines is no guarantee against an undesirable outcome.

The athlete who is symptomatic or demonstrates signs of concussion should not be allowed to return to any physical activity that may result in another head trauma. In many situations, this decision requires trusting the athlete to honestly answer questions about the resolution of symptoms. It is important to establish a rapport with the athlete and to inform him or her of the magnitude of the situation. But this approach is often impractical, particularly in young athletes, in which case the athlete should be managed conservatively. Sometimes athletes' responses cannot be trusted because they want to return to play, and they cannot appreciate the consequences.

In the past, if the athlete had not been rendered unconscious, was asymptomatic, and demonstrated no neurologic signs of change in mental or physical status 15 minutes from the time of concussion, he or she could return to activity if this was the first concussion. However, this scenario usually resulted in the athlete admitting to symptoms after the game. It is prudent to not allow athletes of high school age or younger back into the game or practice if they have had any symptoms or sign of a concussion.

Returning the athlete to play after a concussion is a clinical judgment for the physician. There is no consensus for the exact number of days needed to recover from a concussion. The severity of the concussion, number of previous concussions, the risk for further injury, and the athlete's understanding and acceptance of the potential for risk and complications must be taken into account when deciding to return the athlete to play. Each concussion places the athlete at greater risk for subsequent insult. Established return-to-play guidelines are based on anecdotal experience and suggest restrictions ranging from taking 1 week off to pulling the player from play to the end of the season, depending on the degree of injury and the number of previous concussions. Because second-impact syndrome has been reported primarily in teenage athletes, it could be postulated that the autoregulatory control in a developing brain is not as mature in this age group as in adults. Therefore, conservative management is prudent when considering returning young athletes back to activity.

Guidelines currently in practice should not be viewed as fixed standards of care but as starting points in the decision-making process. Grading scales may be inaccurate, thus putting athletes at increased risk for harm when they return to play or unnecessarily restricting the athlete from return to play. In clinical practice, return-to-play decisions should be made on an individual basis.

A stepwise, graduated approach to return to play takes into account recovery, resolution of symptoms, and the athlete's performance on subsequent physical examinations at rest and after a series of progressively harder physical activity challenges (**Table 20.4**). Progression to the next stage depends on completing the current stage in an asymptomatic condition. If symptoms recur, the athlete should drop back to the previous level and wait 24 hours before considering progressing to the next level.

PROTECTIVE EQUIPMENT/PREVENTION

Helmets were not designed to prevent concussions. However, helmets help prevent other head traumas. In activities such as biking and in-line skating, helmets greatly reduce the risk of serious head injury. Current research in football

TABLE 20.4

Stepwise Approach Model to Return to Play

A. Symptomatic
  1. No physical activity (eg, sports, physical education class, driving, biking)
  2. Cognitive rest
    a. Modify academic activities, advance as tolerated
    b. Avoid bright lights, loud noise
    c. Encourage sleep
B. Asymptomatic at rest (daily progression to next step if asymptomatic; return to previous step if symptomatic)
  Step 1. Advance cognitive activities to full (if not already)
  Step 2. Stationary biking, calisthenics, jogging advance to sprinting
  Step 3. Noncontact, sport-specific drills
  Step 4. Contact, sport-specific drills advance to full participation

uses sensors in the helmet to record the location and severity of head trauma. This may be a first step to designing a football helmet that can help prevent concussion. Mouth guards prevent damage to the teeth but not concussion.

There is debate about whether protective equipment actually increases the risk of injury: if players feel they are invincible, they may play more aggressively. These issues can be addressed by good coaching and officiating. Game skills or techniques, such as heading a soccer ball, should be taught when the athlete has the necessary strength, coordination, and understanding to safely master the technique. Heading a soccer ball in an appropriate manner has not been found to cause concussion. If protective equipment is worn, it must be properly fitted and maintained. It should be appropriate for the age and size of the athlete. The same maintenance recommendations go for game equipment.

SUMMARY POINTS

- Athletes frequently suffer head injuries, and because of the potential for a catastrophic outcome, all head injuries should be considered serious.

- All individuals involved in sports (eg, athletes, coaches, parents, teachers, athletic trainers, team physicians) should recognize the signs and symptoms of a head injury and understand the need to seek prompt medical attention in the event of such injury.

- All medical personnel should be reminded that any unconscious athlete should be considered to have a cervical spine injury unless it is proved otherwise.

- Established grading scales and return-to-play guidelines may help in the clinical decision-making process for a concussion but should not substitute for the clinical judgment of the examining physician.

- Athletes should not be allowed to return to practice or competition while displaying signs of a concussion.

- In the young concussed athlete, activities of daily living should be appropriately modified to permit sufficient cognitive recovery.

- Return-to-play decisions should be made on an individual basis following a stepwise progression to full, unrestricted activity.

- If protective equipment is worn, it must be properly fitted and maintained.

- Game equipment should be the appropriate size for the athlete and properly maintained.

SUGGESTED READING

Aubry M, Cantu R, Dvorak J, et al. Summary and agreement statement of the First International Conference on Concussion in Sport, Vienna 2001. *Clin J Sport Med.* 2002:12:6-12.

Centers for Disease Control and Prevention. Heads up: concussion in high school sports. Atlanta, GA: US Department of Health and Human Services, CDC; 2005. Available at http://www.cdc.gov/ncipc/tbi/coaches_tool_kit.htm.

Concussion (mild traumatic brain injury) and the team physician: a consensus statement. *Med Sci Sports Exerc.* 2006;38:395-399.

Guskiewicz KM, Bruce SL, Cantu RC, et al. National Athletic Trainers' Association position statement: management of sport-related concussion. *J Athl Train.* 2004;39:280-297.

Kirkwood MW, Yeates KO, Wilson PE. Pediatric sport-related concussion: a review of the clinical management of an oft-neglected population. *Pediatrics.* 2006;117: 1359-1371.

McCrory P, Johnston K, Meeuwisse WH, et al. Summary and agreement statement of the Second International Conference on Concussion in Sport, Prague 2004. *Clin J Sport Med.* 2005;15:48-55.

Meehan MP III, Bachur RG. Sport-related concussion. *Pediatrics* 2009;123:114-123.

Quality Standards Subcommittee, American Academy of Neurology. Practice parameter: the management of concussion in sports. *Neurology.* 1997;48:581-585.

For Information on Specific Diagnostic Tests

BESS

Guskiewizc KM. Postural stability assessment follwing concussion: one piece of the puzzle. *Clin J Sport Med.* 2001;11(3):182-189. www.csmfoundation.org

BESS and SAC

McLeod TCV, Perrin DH, Guskiewicz KM, et al. Serial administration of clinical concussion assessments and learning effects in healthy young athletes. *Clin J Sports Med.* 2004;14(5):287-295.

McLeod TCV, Barr WB, McCrea M, Guskiewicz KM. Psychometric and measurement properties of concussion assessment tools in youth sports. *J Athletic Training.* 2006;41(4):399-409.

SAC

McCrea M. Standardized mental status assessment of sports concussion. Clin J Sports Med. 2001;11(3):16-181. www.csmisolutions.com

SCAT

McCrory P, Johnston K, Meeuwisse W, et al. Summary and Agreement Statement of the 2nd International Conference on Concussion in Sport, Prague 2004. *Clin J Sports Med* 2005;15(2):48-55. www.multimedia.olympic.org

CHAPTER 21

Eye Injuries

John B. Jeffers, DVM, MD

Most coaches tell their young athletes, "Keep your eye on the ball." Many sports require athletes to wear protective equipment for every part of the body except the eyes. The American Academy of Pediatrics and the American Academy of Ophthalmology strongly recommend the use of protective eyewear for all athletes for all sports and recreational activities. During childhood and adolescence, muscle coordination and reaction time are still developing, making young athletes particularly vulnerable to eye injuries. If young athletes become comfortable with wearing eye protectors early on, they may develop the habit of wearing them throughout their athletic careers, thus greatly decreasing the overall incidence of severe eye injuries later. Sport-appropriate, properly fitting eye protectors have been found to reduce the risk of significant eye injury by at least 90%.

PREPARTICIPATION PHYSICAL EVALUATION

Ideally, the preparticipation physical evaluation should include a complete eye examination. However, most athletic programs use only a table-top visual screening device to measure acuity, muscle balance, and stereoacuity. Whether or not a complete examination or screening is performed, it is important to obtain pertinent past ocular history by asking questions outlined in **Table 21.1**.

SPORTS-RELATED EYE INJURIES

Every year, many sports- and recreation-related eye injuries are treated in hospital emergency departments in the United States. In 2006, basketball was associated with the most injuries with 5902, followed by baseball and softball together with 2829, then football (1965), soccer (1954), racquet sports (1527), and golf (1444). In all these sports, the highest percentage of injuries occurs in the age group of 5 to 14 years, with the exception of basketball, in which a slightly higher percentage of injuries are experienced in the 15- to 24-year age group. In basketball, most eye injuries are the result of trauma from fingers and elbows. In the past, baseball and softball injuries occurred while participants were batting, but experience indicates that being hit by misjudged balls—fly balls, bad-hop grounders, and line drives—is now the most common cause of eye injury.

For most types of bodily injury, risk of injury is related to the nature of the sport. Contact or collision sports have a greater potential for causing injury compared with noncontact or noncollision sports. However, eye injuries can occur even in noncontact sports. For example, although racquetball is classified as a noncontact sport, balls or racquets travel at high speeds, and impact with an eye can cause potentially devastating injuries. A general rule of thumb is that the more intraocular damage there is, the less orbital damage, and vice versa. The force of the impact has to be dissipated somewhere in the tissues.

Signs and symptoms of serious eye injury are listed in **Table 21.2**. The risk of eye injury in many common sports is categorized in **Table 21.3**. Boxing and full-contact martial arts are considered high-risk sports because protection is not available or permitted. Wrestling was considered a high-risk sport in the past; however, the National Collegiate Athletic Association now allows the use of eye protectors, which were previously prohibited, as long as there are no sharp edges on the protector.

TABLE 21.1

Questions to Ask at the Preparticipation Physical Evaluation

Question	Comment
Is the athlete wearing glasses or contact lenses (rigid or nonrigid)?	Severe myopia (nearsightedness) increases the risk for retinal detachment.
Has the athlete had refractive surgery?	Trauma to the eye may cause a rupture of the globe, particularly after radial keratotomy, or dislodgement of a corneal flap after LASIK surgery.
Has the athlete had previous eye trauma or intraocular surgery?	Scarred or weakened tissue that results from a previous injury or surgical procedure, such as cornea transplant surgery, can predispose the athlete to eye injuries.
Does the athlete have amblyopia, or lazy eye?	Athletes with this condition are functionally 1-eyed, and severe injury to the good eye would be a tragedy.

LASIK indicates laser-assisted in situ keratomileusis.

TABLE 21.2

Signs and Symptoms of Serious Eye Injury

- Sudden complete or partial loss of vision
- Complete or partial loss of visual field
- Pain, with or without eye movement
- Photophobia (light sensitivity)
- Diplopia (double vision)
- Protrusion of 1 eye
- Posttraumatic flashing lights or perception of large floaters
- Irregularly shaped pupil
- Foreign body sensation
- Red eye
- Blood in the anterior chamber
- Halos around lights (indicative of corneal edema)

TABLE 21.3

Categories of Sports Eye-Injury Risk to the Unprotected Player

High Risk	Moderate Risk	Low Risk	Eye Safe
Small, fast projectiles	• Tennis	• Swimming	• Track and field[a]
• Air rifle	• Badminton	• Diving	• Gymnastics
• BB gun	• Soccer	• Skiing (snow and water)	
• Paintball	• Volleyball	• Noncontact martial arts	
Hard projectiles, "sticks," close contact	• Water polo	• Wrestling	
• Basketball	• Football	• Bicycling	
• Baseball, softball	• Fishing		
• Cricket	• Golf		
• Lacrosse (men's and women's)			
• Hockey (field and ice)			
• Squash			
• Racquetball			
• Fencing			
Intentional injury			
• Boxing			
• Full-contact martial arts			

Reprinted with permission from Vinger PF. A practical guide for sports eye protection. *Phys Sports Med.* 2000;28(6). http://www.physsportsmed.com/issues/2000/06_00/vinger.htm. Accessed September 25, 2007.
[a] Javelin and discus have a small but definite potential for injury. However, good field supervision can reduce the extremely low risk of injury to nearly negligible.

PROTECTIVE EYEWEAR

Approximately 90% of sports-related eye injuries are preventable with the use of appropriate eye protectors. Protective eyewear is usually made of polycarbonate because it is a strong, shatterproof, lightweight, and highly impact-resistant plastic that can withstand impact from a 22-caliber gunshot or a ball or other object traveling at 90 mph. It is also capable of absorbing ultraviolet light and is available in prescription and nonprescription lenses. TriVex is a newer material that is comparable to polycarbonate as a protective lens material. Contact lenses offer no protection, and street-wear glasses (corrective eyeglasses or sunglasses) are not only inadequate to protect against eye injuries but also may make the injury more severe.

Because many children's sports leagues, schools, and teams do not require protective eyewear, parents and health care providers should encourage its use. **Table 21.4** lists general specifications for eye protectors. Eye protectors can take the form of polycarbonate or TriVex glasses or goggles (soccer, basketball, baseball or softball fielders, racquet sports), polycarbonate or TriVex face guards attached to a helmet (youth baseball or softball batters, and base runners), polycarbonate or TriVex shields attached to a helmet-mounted wire face guard (football), wire or polycarbonate or TriVex mask on helmet (ice hockey, boy's lacrosse), and wire cage covering the eyes (girl's lacrosse, field hockey). Protective eyewear for specific sports should conform to the standards of the American Society for Testing and Materials (ASTM) (**Table 21.5**).

TYPES OF EYE INJURY

Sharp Injury

Eye injuries may be caused by contact with blunt or sharp objects. For example, sharp objects include fingers, which can poke an eye, or fingernails, which can lacerate the eyelid, cornea, or sclera. In addition, nonprotective eyewear can shatter and lacerate the eye and eyelid.

Blunt Injury

More often, eye injuries are caused by blunt objects that strike the eye. Common injuries of this type include edema and ecchymosis of the lids, orbital fracture, corneal abrasion, traumatic iritis, traumatic hyphema, traumatic cataract, retinal detachment, and edema or bleeding in the retina or vitreous. When a blunt force strikes the eye, the anteroposterior diameter suddenly decreases and the equatorial diameter suddenly increases, like a round balloon pressed between the palms (**Figure 21.1**). This distortion of the globe often causes the intraocular or intraorbital tissues to tear and hemorrhage or orbital bones to fracture.

Fractures

Orbital fractures occur frequently as a result of sports injuries. As intraorbital pressure increases, the thinner walls of the floor and medial aspect of the orbit often fracture,

---

TABLE 21.4

Specifications for Eye Protectors

- Regular glasses and contact lenses do not protect the eyes from injury. Additional eye protection should be worn by athletes who wear contact lenses and those who do not need corrective lenses. Athletes requiring corrective lenses should wear prescription polycarbonate or TriVex lenses.

- For most sports, polycarbonate or TriVex lenses that are 3 mm thick at the center offer the best protection. For sports that pose low risks of eye injury, polycarbonate or TriVex lenses that are 2 mm thick at the center are acceptable.

- For specific sports, eye protectors should meet the standards of the American Society for Testing and Materials (ASTM).

- All eye protectors should be made with sturdy polycarbonate or TriVex frames with molded temples. Glasses that are hinged at the temple tend to bend when struck. Some sports eye protectors have neon-colored cushions at the nose and temple that young athletes like and are more likely to wear.

- Lenses of eye protectors should be treated to resist fogging.

- Eye protectors should be fitted by an experienced ophthalmologist, optometrist, or optician. Most complaints about wearing eye protectors concern poor fit.

- Face protectors (shields or cages) attached to helmets may be made of polycarbonate, TriVex, or wire. Most collision sports, such as hockey, lacrosse, and football, require the use of face protectors. Female lacrosse players wear a wire cage covering the eyes. Eye protection for baseball includes face guards attached to the helmet and sports goggles that can include a corrective lens for children who wear glasses. The helmet must fit properly and be secured with a chin strap for maximum protection.

TABLE 21.5

Recommended Eye Protectors for Selected Sports

Sport	Minimum Eye Protector	Comment
Baseball/softball (youth batter and base runner)	ASTM standard F910	Face guard attached to helmet
Baseball/softball (fielder)	ASTM standard F803 for baseball	ASTM specifies age ranges
Basketball	ASTM standard F803 for basketball	ASTM specifies age ranges
Bicycling	Helmet plus street-wear/fashion eyewear	...
Boxing	None available; not permitted in the sport	Contraindicated for functionally 1-eyed athletes
Fencing	Protector with neck bib	...
Field hockey (men and women)	ASTM standard F803 for women's lacrosse (goalie: full face mask)	Protectors that pass for women's lacrosse also pass for field hockey
Football	Polycarbonate eye shield attached to helmet-mounted wire face mask	...
Full-contact martial arts	None available; not permitted in the sport	Contraindicated for functionally 1-eyed athletes
Ice hockey	ASTM standard F513 face mask on helmet (goal tenders: ASTM standard F1587)	HECC- OR CSA- certified full-face shield
Lacrosse (men)	Face mask attached to lacrosse helmet	...
Lacrosse (women)	ASTM standard F803 for women's lacrosse	Should have option to wear helmet
Paintball	ASTM standard F1776 for paintball	...
Racquet sports (badminton, tennis, paddle tennis, handball, squash, and racquetball)	ASTM standard F803 for selected sport	...
Soccer	ASTM standard F803 for selected sport	...
Street hockey	ASTM standard 513 face mask on helmet	Must be HECC or CSA certified
Track and field	Street wear with polycarbonate lenses/fashion eyewear[a]	...
Water polo/swimming	Swim goggles with polycarbonate lenses	...
Wrestling	No standard available	Custom protective eyewear can be made

American Academy of Pediatrics Committee on Sports Medicine and Fitness. Protective eyewear for young athletes. *Pediatrics*. 2004;113:619-622.
ASTM indicates American Society for Testing and Materials; HECC indicates Hockey Equipment Certification Council; and CSA indicates Canadian Standards Association.
[a] Eyewear that passes ASTM standard F803 is safer than street-wear eyewear for all sports activities with impact potential.

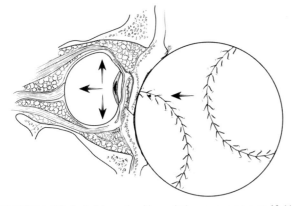

FIGURE 21.1 A blow to the globe may occur if the ball is small enough to fit inside the bony orbit or if a larger ball filled with air, like a kicked soccer ball, is funneled into the orbit. Forces are transmitted to suddenly decrease the anteroposterior diameter of the eye and increase the equatorial diameter.

causing a so-called blowout fracture (**Figure 21.2**). Another mechanism for a floor fracture is a strong impact on the inferior rim of the orbit that causes the bone to buckle. Extraocular tissues may become entrapped in the fracture sites and limit movement of the eye, resulting in double vision. In large floor fractures, when the orbital edema and hemorrhage subside, periocular tissue sinks into the sinus cavity and causes enophthalmos, or sunken eye. Because the roof of the orbit is also the floor of the brain, a forceful blow to the superior orbital rim can fracture the roof and introduce an infection. If an orbital fracture is suspected, athletes should be instructed not to blow their nose to prevent the introduction of air into the orbit and to decrease the risk of organisms residing in the sinus and gaining access to the orbit, causing a secondary infection.

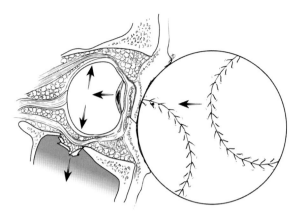

FIGURE 21.2 If sufficient force is transmitted to the globe, it may increase intraorbital pressure sufficient to fracture the thin floor or medial wall of the orbit, causing a blowout fracture.

TABLE 21.6

Emergency Kit for Sports-Related Eye Injuries

- Card to test near vision
- Penlight with blue filter
- Fluorescein strips
- Sterile eyewash (saline) in a plastic squeeze bottle
- Plastic or metal eye shields
- Topical anesthesia, such as proparacaine hydrochloride 0.5%
- Cotton applicator sticks for removal of foreign bodies
- Soft plastic sandwich bags to make ice packs or moist chambers
- Tape
- Topical ophthalmic antibacterial solution, such as polymyxin B and trimethoprim or sulfacetamide 10%
- Topical ophthalmic antibacterial ointment, such as erythromycin or bacitracin
- Topical cycloplegic solution, such as tropicamide 1%

CLINICAL EVALUATION

Before conducting their evaluations, examiners must wash their hands. If water is not available, alcohol wipes may be used instead. A list of equipment for conducting emergency eye examinations is provided in **Table 21.6**. First, the mechanism of injury is identified, and the examiner determines the direction and magnitude of the injuring force. For example, was the athlete struck by a slow ground ball or a 90-mph pitch? This information may suggest the extent of potential injuries. Second, a topical anesthetic should be applied to control pain because a comfortable athlete will be more cooperative. However, topical anesthesia should not be used to mask pain so that the athlete can continue playing. Third, baseline visual acuity should be measured before the eyes are manipulated or examined with hands or a penlight. Later, any improvement or worsening can be measured against this baseline. To test baseline visual acuity, a card (or any printed material) designed to measure near vision should be held 14 inches from the eye and the size of the smallest print (in centimeters) that the athlete can read should be measured. If the card is held closer than 14 inches, this distance should be recorded. If the athlete is unable to read any print, the examiner should hold up a few fingers at a distance and ask the athlete to count them, then document the distance and acuity. Athletes with poorer vision may be tested by hand movements. Light perception—whether the athlete can determine the presence and direction of light—is a test for minimal vision. With no light perception, all vision is lost.

In the case of chemical or particle exposure (eg, exposure to field markings or dust from artificial turf), the initial test for visual acuity may be skipped. Instead, the affected eye should immediately be gently flushed with large amounts of clean water from a shower or hose or any potable solution, such as milk or juice, for 15 to 30 minutes, depending on the amount and concentration of chemical or particles involved. Physiologic saline or eyewashes in plastic squeeze bottles also work well. Contact lenses are best left in place during the initial irrigation. They may be removed later.

Next, the examiner should check eye movements in all directions and note any limitations; pupillary response to light should also be assessed. Dilation of the pupil when a flashlight is shined on that eye may indicate an afferent pupillary defect. After the initial examination and first aid treatment, the injured eye should be protected with a metal or plastic eye shield. A simple eye shield can be made from the bottom of a Styrofoam cup or milk carton, making certain the shield does not put any pressure on the eye. Depending on the severity of the injury, the athlete may require a repeat evaluation before returning to play. If there is any doubt about the diagnosis or the severity of the injury, the athlete should be referred to an ophthalmologist.

TREATMENT

Edema and Ecchymosis of the Eyelids

To treat edema and ecchymosis of the eyelids, a small amount of crushed ice—about the size of a golf ball—is placed in a soft plastic sandwich bag, the bag wrapped in gauze, the top secured, and the bag applied to the injured area. Little weight should be placed on the injured eye. The bag may be taped to the forehead to help keep it in place and to avoid pressure against the eye. This is best done while the athlete is sitting.

Protruding Edematous Conjunctiva

When left exposed, a protruding edematous conjunctiva tends to become dry and infected. Instead of applying an antibiotic ointment (which makes reexamination difficult), a moist chamber should be created to prevent the tissues from drying by taping a piece of plastic wrap or one side of a soft plastic sandwich bag tightly around the orbit and nose. Medicated eye solution may then be applied.

Lacerations of the Eyelid or Eyeball

In the case of lacerated eyelids or eyeballs, visual acuity should be measured. The injured eye should be covered with an eye shield. The examiner should refer the athlete to an ophthalmologist. Any avulsed tissue should be saved in saline and sent along with the athlete.

Corneal Abrasions

To treat corneal abrasions, topical antibiotic ointment or drops should be applied. Cycloplegic drops are not necessary to treat a corneal abrasion but can be considered if needed for discomfort. However, ointment and dilation blur vision, so the athlete may not be able to return to play immediately (**Figure 21.3**). Abrasions should be treated without patching the eye, especially for patients who wear contact lenses or if an organic mechanism of injury is suspected, because of the risk of trapping bacteria or fungal elements behind the patch. If a foreign body is suspected, copious irrigation should be performed first.

Traumatic Iritis

When the iris is contused, an acute, painful iritis with photophobia results. Vision is blurred, and the pupil may be small on the affected side. Topical corticosteroid and cycloplegic drops should be applied, although topical corticosteroid drops should not be used if a corneal abrasion is also present. An athlete with this injury should be examined by an ophthalmologist.

Traumatic Cataract

Traumatic cataract is most commonly characterized by a foreign body that penetrates the lens, which causes immediate blurred vision, an opaque lens, and sometimes intraocular hemorrhage. A severe, forceful blow to the eye often results in a cataract. The examiner should use an eye shield to protect the eye with a traumatic cataract, with or without subluxation or luxation of the lens, and refer the athlete to an ophthalmologist.

Orbital Fracture

In the case of a suspected orbital fracture, athletes should be advised against blowing their nose. Oral antibiotics and a decongestant nasal drop or spray may be prescribed (**Figure 21.4**). This injury also requires prompt examination by an ophthalmologist.

Traumatic Hyphema

A hyphema is a contusion to the iris that causes tearing of tissue and bleeding in the anterior chamber of the eye (**Figure 21.5**). The signs and symptoms may be identical to that of traumatic iritis, but with a penlight with magnifying loupes, a layer of blood can be appreciated over the lower iris. Immediate management consists of measuring visual acuity, covering the injured eye with an eye shield, and

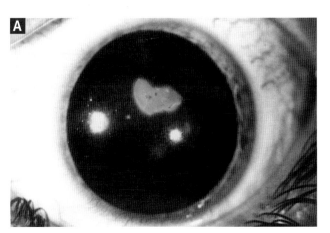 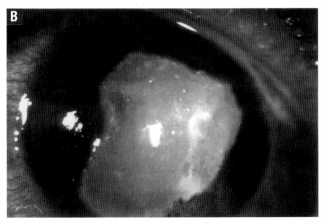

FIGURE 21.3 (A) Small corneal abrasion. (B) Large corneal abrasion.

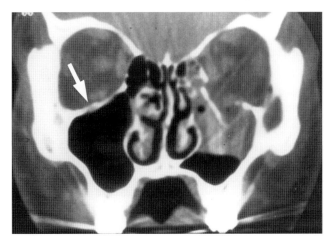

FIGURE 21.4 Computed tomography scan showing blood in the maxillary sinus as a result of a left orbit fracture.

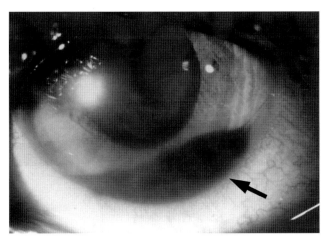

FIGURE 21.5 A layer of blood is visible over the lower iris when viewed with a penlight with magnifying loupes.

keeping the athlete's head elevated. This injury also requires immediate examination by an ophthalmologist.

RETURN-TO-PLAY GUIDELINES

Depending on the injury and on the physician's evaluation, an injured athlete may return to play immediately. However, an athlete who has received a topical anesthetic in the eye should not be permitted to return to play.

A recovering athlete may return to play when an ophthalmologist has determined that the ocular tissue has had sufficient time to heal. Especially in the case of a traumatic hyphema, the athlete may experience another blow to the body that could trigger a Valsalva maneuver, which increases the pressure inside the eye and causes

rebleeding. In addition, the injured eye must be free of pain and discomfort and have adequate recovery of vision. For all athletes, the use of sport-appropriate, well-fitting protective eyewear is strongly recommended.

FUNCTIONALLY 1-EYED ATHLETES

Functionally 1-eyed athletes must be identified during the preparticipation physical evaluation. By definition, the athlete's weaker eye has a best-corrected visual acuity worse than 20/40, whereas the stronger eye has a best-corrected visual acuity of 20/40 or better. The most common cause of this condition is amblyopia, or lazy eye. However, previous trauma, serious eye disease, or intraocular surgery may cause scarring and decrease the vision in the eye.

This athlete must take special precautions to protect the better eye from sports-related injuries that could have serious consequences in the athlete's lifestyle. The functionally 1-eyed athlete may participate in most sports as long as appropriate, well-fitted protective eyewear is worn. When a helmet is required, both an eye protector and the face shield or cage should be worn. The athlete should not be allowed to participate in sports that pose high risks of eye injury, such as boxing and full-contact martial arts. Athletes should always wear eye protectors during sporting events, but it is also strongly recommended that they wear glasses with polycarbonate or TriVex lenses during all waking hours. These individuals will be unable to obtain an unrestricted driver's license in many states if they lose vision in the better eye.

SUMMARY POINTS

- Injury of the eye that results in significant pain or change in visual acuity requires evaluation by an ophthalmologist.

- The young athlete is developing muscle coordination and improving reaction time and therefore is at increased risk for eye injuries.

- All young athletes should be encouraged to wear appropriate protective eyewear. Because many children's sports leagues, schools, and teams do not require protective eyewear, parents and health care providers should encourage its use.

- Protective eyewear should be mandatory for functionally 1-eyed athletes for all sports, recreational, and work-related activities.

- If young athletes become comfortable wearing protective eyewear when they are young, they may develop the habit of wearing the protector as they get older.

SUGGESTED READING

American Academy of Pediatrics Committee on Sports Medicine and Fitness. Protective eyewear for young athletes. *Pediatrics.* 2004;113:619-622.

American Society for Testing and Materials. *Annual Book of ASTM Standards: Vol. 15.07. Sports Equipment; Safety and Traction for Footwear; Amusement Rides; Consumer Products.* West Conshohocken, PA: American Society for Testing and Materials; 2003.

Jeffers JB. An on-going tragedy: pediatric sports-related eye injuries. *Semin Ophthalmol.* 1990;5:216-223.

Larrison WI, Hersh PS, Kunzweiler T, Shingleton BJ. Sports-related ocular trauma. *Ophthalmology.* 1990;97:1265-1269.

Turriff T. *Product Summary Report—Eye Injuries Only—Calendar Year 1997.* Chicago, IL: Prevent Blindness America; 1998.

US Consumer Product Safety Commission. *Sports and Recreational Eye Injuries.* Washington, DC: US Consumer Product Safety Commission; 2000.

Vinger PF. Athletic eye injuries and appropriate protection. In: *Focal Points: Clinical Modules for Ophthalmologists.* San Francisco, CA: American Academy of Ophthalmology; 1997;15:1-14.

Vinger PF. The eye and sports medicine. In: Duane TD, Tasman W, Jaeger EA, eds. *Duane's Clinical Ophthalmology on CD-ROM. 2005 Edition.* Vol 5. Philadelphia, PA: Lippincott Williams & Wilkins; 2005: chap 45.

Vinger PF. A practical guide for sports eye protection. *Phys Sports Med.* 2000;28(6). http://www.physsportsmed.com/issues/2000/06_00/vinger.htm. Accessed September 25, 2007.

CHAPTER 22

Maxillofacial Injuries

Steven M. Sullivan, DDS

Many sports-related injuries involve the maxillofacial, or face and jaw, region. The use of face masks and mouth guards has greatly reduced the number of injuries in many sports, but injuries still occur and are even more prevalent in contact sports without mandatory protection.

Most maxillofacial injuries occur in children between the ages of 8 and 15 years. Boys experience 2 to 3 times as many injuries as girls as the result of the larger number of male participants in sports and the kinds of sport boys tend to select. Changes in the craniofacial skeleton during development may predispose children to certain types of maxillofacial injuries. With dental injuries, the anterior teeth, especially the maxillary central incisors, are most frequently injured. Children are also predisposed to contact injuries of the lower jaw because the emerging permanent teeth are proportionately large compared with the other facial structures. Although crown fractures are the most common injuries to the permanent teeth, the primary teeth tend to be displaced.

Time from injury is one of the most critical concerns with injuries such as root fracture, displacement, and tooth avulsion. Treatment must be provided as quickly as possible because delays can markedly affect outcome and contribute to root resorption, posttraumatic infection, or delayed tooth loss. A dentist should evaluate almost any athlete who experiences a dental injury.

INITIAL EVALUATION OF MAXILLOFACIAL INJURIES

The clinical evaluation should include inspection of both the hard tissues, which include teeth and supporting bone, and the soft tissues of the oral cavity (**Figure 22.1**). Any lacerations to the soft tissues should be examined carefully, especially if tooth fractures are evident. Tooth fragments that have become embedded in the soft tissues may not be apparent. All teeth and tooth fragments should be located, and if there is any suspicion of ingestion or aspiration of the teeth, radiographs of the chest and abdomen may help find them (**Figure 22.2**). Any trauma that causes a fracture of a tooth or alveolus can also cause a fracture of basal bone; therefore, the occlusion and temporomandibular joints should also be evaluated. The temporomandibular joints can easily be evaluated by assessing the range of motion and identifying whether the mouth opens in a normal, straight manner. Deviations to one side could indicate a fracture of the condylar process. Another possible sign of an injury is a malocclusion (**Figure 22.3**), which may be caused by a fracture of the mandible or maxilla.

COMMON INJURIES OF TEETH

Common injuries of teeth, in increasing order of severity, include crown fracture, dentin injury, pulp injury, displacement, intrusion, and avulsion (**Table 22.1**). Appropriate initial treatment is important to prevent permanent damage.

If the initial clinical evaluation performed on the playing field reveals injuries beyond simple superficial chips of the crown, the patient should be immediately taken to an oral and maxillofacial surgeon or emergency department for a more thorough evaluation and appropriate treatment.

Fractures of the Tooth Crown

When a crown fracture occurs, the first and most important task is to protect the neurovascular components, or the pulp, within the central portion of the tooth (**Figure 22.4**). Aesthetics at this point are not the main concern and can be dealt with later. If exposed, the pulp can become contaminated and possibly destroy the tooth. These injuries could require further invasive treatment, such as endodontic therapy, in addition to restoration of the fractured crown.

TABLE 22.1

Common Injuries of Teeth

Injury	Diagnosis	Treatment	Caution
Crown fracture	Fracture of enamel structure only	Aesthetic treatment	Ensure no further damage to pulp or dentin
Dentin injury	Cream- or yellow-colored dentin exposed under enamel; painful	Restorative materials placed on tooth in dental office emergently; evaluate for pulp injury	Can cause permanent disfigurement if not addressed promptly
Pulp injury	Neurovascular structures exposed in central part of tooth; may be pink or bleeding	Endodontic and aesthetic treatment in dental office emergently	Protect exposed pulp immediately
Displacement	Tooth is mobile, but alveolar process is stable when structures are palpated	Reposition tooth immediately (within 90 minutes) with good results if <1 mm mobility; splint tooth for 7-10 days if >1 mm mobility	Ensure that alveolar process is not fractured; refer to dentist for splinting
Intrusion	Crown appears shorter than adjacent teeth	Permanent teeth require orthodontic or surgical repositioning with or without endodontic therapy; teeth may reerupt passively in children	Immediate referral necessary to evaluate for further injury
Avulsion	Tooth is completely knocked out of socket	Immediate replantation and stabilization; store tooth in tooth-preserving medium	Do not touch or clean root to avoid further damage

Crown fractures typically involve fractures of the enamel structure, which are usually only superficial chips (**Figure 22.5**). Fractures into the dentin, however, are more serious. They not only produce discomfort and disfigurement but also can compromise the pulp. At clinical inspection, these fractures expose the outer enamel component and the cream- to yellow-colored dentin underneath (**Figure 22.6**). Fractures of the crown that involve the pulp chamber are identified by exposed pink or bleeding pulp (**Figure 22.7**). This type of fracture requires immediate attention.

Emergency treatment of fractured teeth by the dentist includes emplacing a calcium hydroxide base and restoring the tooth with acid-etched composite restoration material. Ideally, the team physician should have these materials on hand (**Table 22.2**) to temporarily treat the fracture until definitive treatment can be provided (**Figure 22.8**). The athlete's dentist or specialist should provide timely follow-up.

Tooth Displacement Injuries

Injuries caused by high-velocity impact and injuries experienced at the alveolar level may displace or completely avulse the teeth and fracture the supporting alveolar bone. The upper and lower front teeth are most often displaced. With all displacement injuries, it is important to determine whether the tooth or the entire alveolar process has been displaced. This is accomplished by cleaning the oral cavity and then palpating the alveolar process to identify which components move. If the teeth alone move, they may be readily repositioned into the socket. If the teeth and alveolar process both move, there is a more serious fracture. Although this step is uncomfortable for the athlete, it is one

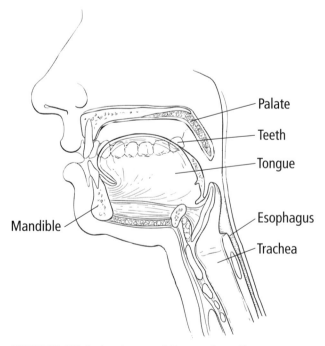

FIGURE 22.1 Anatomy of the oral cavity.

Palate

Teeth

Tongue

Esophagus

Trachea

Mandible

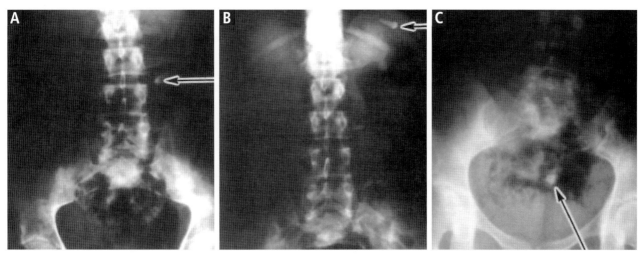

FIGURE 22.2 Aspirated teeth often appear on radiographs. (A) Premolar tooth in stomach. (B) Premolar tooth in lower thorax. (C) Premolar tooth in the abdomen. Reproduced with permission from the Academy of General Dentistry. Prevention and management of ingested foreign bodies. *Gen Dent*. 1993;41:422-444.

of the most important steps in the initial management of the injury. Teeth that show minor mobility (<1 mm) typically will not require any further stabilization, although further injury must be avoided. Teeth that move more than 1 mm require splinting for 7 to 10 days. Splints should be applied by a dentist in a controlled environment where the teeth and jaws can be positioned properly and the splinting material can be applied in a dry field.

Early treatment of a more severe displacement injury (>1-2 mm) (**Figure 22.9**) involves repositioning and stabilizing the tooth, followed by further evaluation and management. With all displacement injuries, time is crucial.

TABLE 22.2

Suggestions for the Contents of the Dental Emergency Kit

• Elastic bandages	• Hydrogen peroxide
• Adhesive tape	• Masks
• Ammonia inhalers	• Mouth mirror
• Anesthetics (local, topical)	• Mixing pad
• Ball burnisher dental instrument	• Needles (long, short)
• Biohazard bags	• Plugger dental instrument
• Butane torch	• Pocket flashlight
• Cotton rolls	• Save-A-Tooth (tooth-preserving system)
• Cotton-tip applicators	• Scissors
• Dental floss	• Spatula
• Dycal (calcium hydroxide paste system)	• Spoon excavator dental instrument
• Explorer (dental pick)	• Syringe (aspirating)
• Gauze (2 × 2)	• Tongue depressors
• Gloves (latex, nonallergenic)	• Tongue depressors (taped)
• Hemostat	• Zinc oxide and eugenol

Table modified with permission from Ranalli DN, Demas PN. Orofacial injuries from sport. Preventive measures for sports medicine. *Sports Med*. 2002;32:409-418.

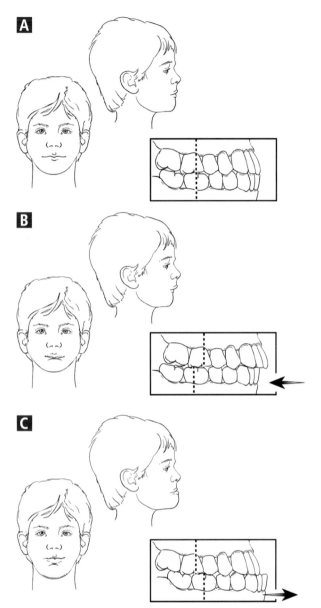

FIGURE 22.3 Evaluation of the temporomandibular joint should include assessment of possible malocclusion. (A) Normal bite. (B) Overbite. (C) Underbite.

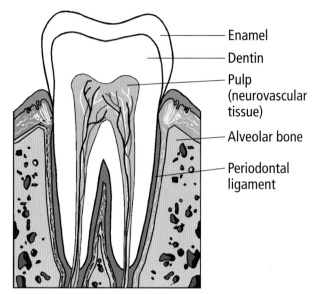

Enamel

Dentin

Pulp (neurovascular tissue)

Alveolar bone

Periodontal ligament

FIGURE 22.4 Anatomy of a tooth.

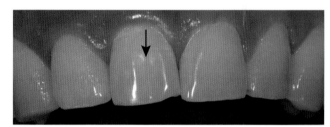

FIGURE 22.5 Central incisor with a superficial enamel fracture.

If the displaced teeth are repositioned within 90 minutes of injury, fewer problems ensue, including loss of the tooth or root resorption. In nearly 50% of patients, displacement injuries may proceed to necrosis of the pulp, so close observation and follow-up by a dentist or endodontist is necessary.

Some of the more severe displacement injuries are intrusive displacement injuries in which the normal crown appears shorter than those of adjacent teeth or appears in

FIGURE 22.6 Injured central incisor with involvement of the deeper dentin layer. Reprinted with permission from Andreasen JO. *Traumatic Injuries of the Teeth*. 2nd ed. Copenhagen, Denmark: Munksgaard; Philadelphia, PA: WB Saunders; 1981.

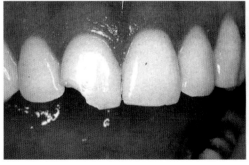
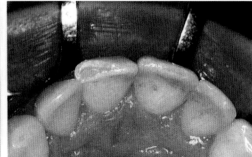

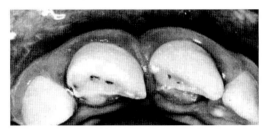

FIGURE 22.7 Frank pulp exposure of injured central incisors. Reprinted with permission from Andreasen JO. *Traumatic Injuries of the Teeth*. 2nd ed. Copenhagen, Denmark: Munksgaard; Philadelphia, PA: WB Saunders; 1981.

infraocclusion, as if it failed to erupt (**Figure 22.10**). These injuries occur most often with teeth that have fully formed roots. In children aged 6 to 8 years, teeth that intrude minimally will often reerupt passively because the roots of their teeth have not yet completely formed. Intruded permanent teeth require either orthodontic or surgical repositioning and endodontic therapy. In any case, immediate treatment by a dentist should be arranged.

Tooth Avulsion Injuries

Avulsions of the maxillary central incisors are some of the most common dental injuries in children because these teeth have recently or are in the process of erupting and have loosely structured periodontal ligaments. The ideal treatment of an avulsed tooth is early replantation and stabilization. Once again, time is critical. If immediate replantation is not possible, the tooth should be stored in a container with an appropriate medium that will nourish the cellular components of the root surface. The best transport media is Hank's balanced salt solution, followed by, in descending order, milk, saline, or the athlete's own saliva. Tap water should not be used. The tooth should not be placed for transport in the mouth because of the risk of damage to the tooth, swallowing, or aspiration. The root surface should not be cleaned or touched (ie, the tooth should be picked up by the crown only), except to

gently remove any superficial contaminants. Often, the storage medium passively washes away the debris. Any attempts to clean the root surface can harm periodontal membrane cells and prevent successful replantation.

PREVENTION OF DENTAL INJURIES

One of the most important preventive measures for dental injuries is the use of mouth guards and face masks. The National Collegiate Athletic Association estimates that 200 000 dental injuries per year can be prevented by this simple measure alone. Since the introduction of mandatory mouth guards and padded helmets with face masks, the incidence of dental injuries in football has been reduced from 10% to approximately 0.40%. Mouth guards should cover all tooth surfaces and should also include occlusal coverage to prevent vertical crown fractures.

Mouth guards offer a substantial degree of protection to the teeth and oral soft tissue, and they also protect athletes from concussion. The characteristics of an ideal mouth guard are listed in **Table 22.3**. The 3 types of mouth guards commercially available are the stock mouth guard, mouth-formed mouth guard, and custom-made protectors. Stock mouth guards are preformed, sold over the counter, and are worn as manufactured. They are inexpensive, but they are bulky and must be held in place by clenching the teeth, which tends to interfere with breathing and speech. Mouth-formed protectors are usually thermoplastic and reasonably priced. They are placed in boiling water to soften, briefly dipped in cold water, and then placed over the maxillary arch and under the upper lip using a constant pressure upward and backward for about 30 seconds to form it to the teeth. Custom-formed (vacuum) mouth guards are fabricated over a dental cast with a vacuum-formed material. They are the most comfortable and interfere least with breathing and speech. However, they are also the most expensive because they require at least 2 visits to the dentist for proper fitting. Mouth-formed protectors offer the best compromise between fit and cost for

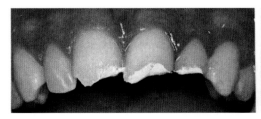
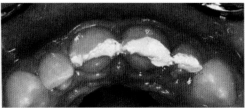

FIGURE 22.8 Treatment of fractured teeth with Dycal calcium hydroxide. Reprinted with permission from Andreasen JO. *Traumatic Injuries of the Teeth*. 2nd ed. Copenhagen, Denmark: Munksgaard; Philadelphia, PA: WB Saunders; 1981.

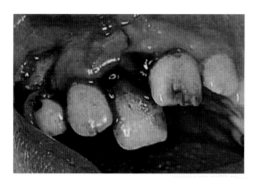

FIGURE 22.9 Severe displacement (lateral luxation and extrusion) of right central incisor. Reprinted with permission from Andreasen, JO. *Traumatic Injuries of the teeth.* 2nd. ed. Copenhagen, Denmark: Munksgaard; Philadelphia, PA: WB Saunders; 1981.

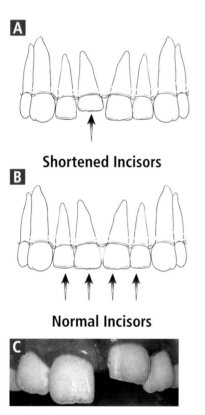

A

Shortened Incisors

B

Normal Incisors

C

FIGURE 22.10 With severe displacement injuries, the normal crown can appear shorter (A) than those of the normal adjacent teeth (B). (C) Intruded left central incisor. Reprinted with permission from Andreasen, JO. *Traumatic Injuries of the Teeth.* 2nd. ed. Copenhagen, Denmark: Munksgaard; Philadelphia, PA: WB Saunders; 1981.

most young athletes. Athletes must be cautioned to avoid excessively trimming the mouth guard because this will reduce its protective effect. Nervous chewing of the mouth guard also reduces fit and protection. Damaged mouth guards should be replaced.

TABLE 22.3

Characteristics of the Ideal Mouth Guard

- Soft and comfortable, but firm enough to withstand trauma
- Fabricated easily at low cost
- Adaptable over dental appliances
- Does not interfere with speech or breathing
- Does not deteriorate after prolonged use
- Does not have an offensive odor or taste
- Nontoxic

COMMON FACIAL INJURIES

Common facial injuries include fractures of the mandible, nasal bones, zygomatic complex, and maxilla, as well as soft tissue lacerations (**Table 22.4**). Immediate recognition of these conditions is necessary to ensure appropriate treatment.

Mandible Fractures

The most common mandible fracture involves the condylar process, followed by fractures of the mandibular angle (**Figure 22.11**). As tooth follicles develop near the mandibular angle and ramus, the bone quantity in that area diminishes and predisposes the posterior mandible to fractures. Approximately 50% of all mandible fractures occur in areas posterior to the teeth; the remaining 50% are distributed among the mandibular body, anterior mandible, and dentoalveolar components.

An athlete who is believed to have a mandible fracture should be evaluated to ensure that the airway is open. The oral cavity should be inspected to identify whether there are loose or missing teeth, to find these teeth, and to ensure that the airway is patent. With mandible fractures, the most common finding is malocclusion, which is easily assessed by asking the patient if his or her teeth meet differently now than they did before the incident. Gross malocclusions indicate mandible fractures, whereas minor malocclusions suggest greenstick fractures or effusions into the temporomandibular joints (**Figure 22.12**). Additional signs and symptoms of mandible fractures include bruising in the mouth, mucosal tears, crepitus at the fracture sites, palpable irregularities along the bone surfaces if bones are markedly displaced, and numbness of the lower lip and chin on the side of the fracture if it crosses the mandibular canal. Significant edema can develop; sometimes profuse bleeding develops if the inferior alveolar artery is cut by severely displaced bones.

TABLE 22.4

Common Facial Injuries

Type	Diagnosis	Treatment	Caution
Mandible fracture	• Malocclusion; bruised mouth or mucosal tears; crepitus at fracture site; numbness of lip and chin	• Fully immobilize until C spine evaluation • Simple closed reduction with wires or open reduction with rigid internal fixation within 7-10 days • Temporary stabilization with elastic bandages wrapped from chin to crown of head to keep mouth closed	• Search mouth for loose or fractured teeth; ensure airway is patent • Open fractures require immediate surgical care
Nasal fracture	• Nasal septum tender when moved; obvious deviation of nasal bones on either side; epistaxis is common	• Constant direct pressure for epistaxis with or without ice packs • Reduction managed by specialist within 4 days for children, 10-12 days for adolescents; internal packing for 48 hours; possibly external nasal splints	• Nasal septal hematomas require prompt aspiration
Zygomatic fracture	• Palpate adjacent bones for step defects (ie, temporal, frontal, maxilla) • Epistaxis may occur	• Patient should not blow nose until evaluated by surgeon and computed tomography scans • Displaced fractures require open reduction and rigid fixation	• Evaluate for any eye injury at the scene and send for ophthalmologic evaluation • Uncommon in children because of immature air cells
Maxillary fracture	• Malocclusion or open-bite malocclusion; examine carefully for dental injuries or loose teeth	• Emergent treatment by specialist • Closed or open surgical techniques	• Periorbital swelling, diplopia, epistaxis, step defects of zygomatic buttress, or facial lengthening may occur • Uncommon in children
Soft tissue laceration	• Inspect mouth for lacerations from teeth	• On-site application of gauze pressure dressings to control bleeding • Suture lacerations >5 mm in length; lacerations penetrating through the lip require layered closure	• Inspect mouth and laceration for foreign bodies • Provide tetanus booster for contaminated lacerations

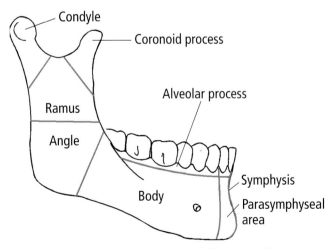

FIGURE 22.11 Bony anatomy of the mandible.

Any athlete who experiences a mandible fracture should be fully immobilized, including the head and neck, and evaluated for injury to the cervical spine. Open mandible fractures require immediate care by an oral and maxillofacial surgeon. The mandible may be stabilized temporarily by wrapping elastic bandages around the head, beginning under the chin and going over the top of the head to hold the mouth closed (**Figure 22.13**). The mandible can also be stabilized with wires, but only individuals who have been trained to do so should perform this procedure. Inappropriately placed wires can dislodge teeth and result in their eventual loss.

Patients with mandible fractures should receive definitive treatment as quickly as possible—certainly no later than 7 to 10 days after the injury. Treatment includes simple closed reduction by wiring the jaws together and open reduction with rigid internal fixation. Typically, in 6 to 8 weeks, the mandible will regain 75% of its preinjury strength.

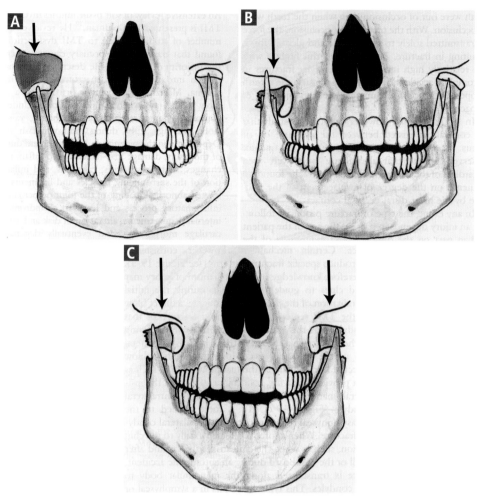

FIGURE 22.12 Common condylar injury patterns. (A) Joint effusion-hemarthrosis. (B) Unilateral condylar fracture. (C) Bilateral condylar dislocation fracture with anterior apertognathia (open bite). Reprinted with permission from Fonseca RJ, Walker RV, Betts NJ. *Oral and Maxillofacial Trauma*. 3rd ed. Philadelphia, PA: WB Saunders; 2004: 529.

Nasal Fractures

The most common midfacial fracture in young athletes is a nasal fracture. The nose, a prominent structure on the face, is vulnerable to injury, especially when helmets and face masks are not worn. Nasal fractures should be evaluated, and epistaxis, if present, should be controlled with constant direct pressure to the nose with the athlete in a sitting position. If a bag of crushed ice is available, pressure can be applied with it to facilitate vasoconstriction and reduce bleeding.

Nasal fractures involving the nasal septum are easily diagnosed by exerting an upward pressure on the columella. Typically, the nasal septum will be extremely tender when moved slightly, which suggests possible separation of the septum from the maxillary crest. Deviations of the nose or saddle-nose deformities suggest displacement of the nasal

bones on either side (**Figure 22.14**). Nasal septal hematomas must be identified and aspirated promptly to avoid septal necrosis.

Nasal fractures can usually be managed on an outpatient basis. Nasal reduction should be managed by a specialist, and it is ideally performed immediately before swelling develops or within 4 days for children and 10 to 12 days for adolescents. Treatment, administered under local or intravenous sedation, includes manipulating and elevating the nose, packing it for internal support, and splinting it for external support. The internal packing generally remains in place for approximately 24 to 48 hours to prevent septal hematomas from forming; it also provides outward support for the nasal bones. External nasal splints are generally worn for 7 to 10 days. Suggestions about returning to play

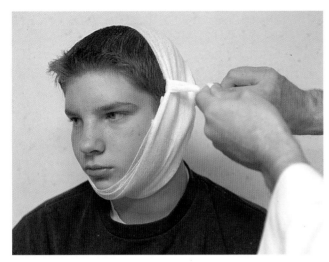

FIGURE 22.13 The mandible may be temporarily stabilized by wrapping elastic bandages under the chin and over the head.

will depend on the extent of the injury, the stability of the fracture, the options for protective headgear, and the risk of further injury or potential injury. The patient should not participate in athletic activity without protective facial equipment for 4 to 6 weeks to allow the injury to heal completely and also to avoid reinjury.

Zygomatic Fractures

Fractures of the zygomatic complex often occur in contact sports in which protective headgear is not worn. Fortunately, because children have not yet developed air cells in their bones, fractures of the zygomatic complex are not common in children younger than age 10 or 12 years. The zygoma articulates with 4 other bones: the temporal, the frontal, the maxillae, and the greater wing of the sphenoid (**Figure 22.15**). Therefore, a fracture of the zygomatic

complex can be evaluated by palpating several areas: at the temples near the brow bone, along the rim below the eye, and inside the mouth along the roof under the cheekbones (**Figure 22.16**). Typically, step defects will be noted, and the zygoma may move. However, it is not uncommon for the zygoma to become impacted, posteriorly and medially, into the maxillary sinus, and therefore seem stable, even though it is displaced. Epistaxis is also a fairly common finding. Blood from the maxillary sinus will ultimately drain through the nose. The patient may also have periorbital ecchymosis, diplopia, and numbness over the cheek.

All fractures of the zygomatic complex should immediately raise concern about eye injuries, which are true emergencies. It is important to examine baseline visual acuity (eg, the ability to read a newspaper at arm's length) to evaluate the pupil, to assess whether structures passing through the superior orbital fissure have been compromised, and to evaluate the extraocular movements. A consultation with an ophthalmologist is mandatory to reassess visual acuity and to check for occult eye injury. After a clinical evaluation for any eye injuries, the patient should be instructed to avoid blowing the nose and to follow up immediately with a maxillofacial surgeon so that axial and coronal computed tomography scans can be performed to ascertain the degree of displacement. Displaced fractures require surgery, including open reduction and stabilization with rigid fixation. These fractures typically heal in approximately 6 weeks, and athletes may be allowed to return to play afterward.

Maxillary Fractures

Maxillary fractures in children are rare and account for only a tiny percentage of all facial fractures for several reasons. First, the bones of the maxilla are fairly elastic. Second, the maxilla is buttressed by adjacent facial bones

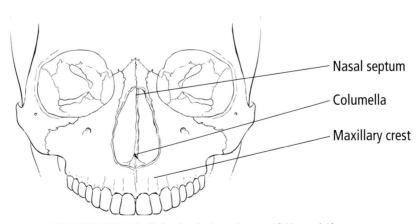

Nasal septum

Columella

Maxillary crest

FIGURE 22.14 Principal structures of the midface.

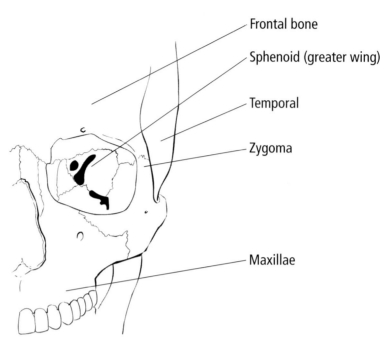

FIGURE 22.15 Bony anatomy of the zygomatic complex.

Frontal bone

Sphenoid (greater wing)

Temporal

Zygoma

Maxillae

and deciduous teeth. Third, the maxillary sinuses have not yet developed air cavities. All of these factors result in a structure that is difficult to fracture under normal conditions.

Athletes with suspected maxillary fractures require careful examination for dental injuries as well, and any loose or missing teeth should be located. The most obvious clinical finding in a maxillary fracture is a malocclusion. Often, patients will notice that the teeth do not come together as they did before the injury. Sometimes, an open-bite malocclusion, seen when the upper teeth do not overlap or touch the lower teeth, will be evident. Along with the malocclusion, step defects at the zygomatic buttress, bruising, periorbital swelling, diplopia, facial lengthening, and/or epistaxis may also suggest a maxillary fracture. These athletes require examination at the emergency department and consultation with the appropriate specialist.

Typically, maxillary fractures in children can be treated surgically with closed techniques. In the operating room, the occlusion will be reestablished and a functional reduction accomplished. Maxillary fractures are usually stabilized for 4 to 6 weeks, with or without the use of maxillomandibular wiring. In general, open reduction with internal fixation is contraindicated in patients with multiple unerupted permanent teeth. For these patients, closed reductions can achieve good results as well. The use of protective headgear, such as face masks, reduces the incidence of maxillary fractures.

Soft Tissue Lacerations

Most lacerations of the maxillofacial region are associated with or are a direct result of injuries to the teeth. Lacerations of the lips and mouth are fairly common. Inside the mouth, lacerations of the mucosa that are less than 5 mm in length do not require suturing. However, lacerations longer than 5 mm that penetrate through the lip, for example, require layered closure to prevent unsightly scarring.

Lacerations that require surgical repair should first be debrided and cleansed, then covered with pressure dressings to control hemorrhaging until the patient can be transported for definitive treatment. Fortunately, the vessels of the facial structures are fairly elastic, and direct pressure will adequately stop the bleeding. Extremely large or unstable lacerations may need to be tacked temporarily with a 3-0 or 4-0 silk suture after infiltration with a local anesthetic into the vestibules of the corner of the mouth. With tongue lacerations, untrained clinicians may find it more difficult to effect local anesthesia. However, in urgent situations when temporary tacking sutures are required, injection of the anesthetic agent into the tongue itself, although uncomfortable, will often suffice. Small, resorbable sutures are preferred for tongue lacerations. Typically, a 4-0 or 5-0 suture applied in a layered fashion achieves good results.

Lacerations outside the mouth, like any cutaneous injury, require immediate care beginning with control of

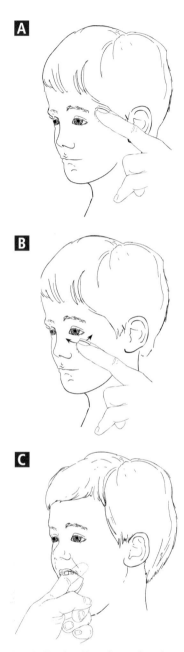

FIGURE 22.16 Evaluation for a fracture of the zygomatic complex. The examiner should palpate (A) the temples near the brow, (B) along the orbital rim below the eye, and (C) inside the mouth under the cheekbones.

bleeding, primary cleansing of the wound, inspection for foreign bodies, and application of gauze pressure bandages. Any patient with a laceration that has been contaminated by soil may require a tetanus booster.

After lacerations are repaired, guidelines for returning to play should be established on the basis of the extent of the injury, its location, and the likelihood of reinjury. Whenever possible, the injured area should be protected.

SUMMARY POINTS

- Use of protective gear such as mouth guards and face masks is one of the most important preventive measures for avoiding dental injuries.

- Fractures into the dentin or of the crown that involve the pulp chamber (exposed pink or bleeding pulp) require immediate attention.

- Typically, teeth that move more than 1 mm require splinting for 7 to 10 days.

- If immediate replantation is not possible, the tooth should be stored in a container with an appropriate medium (in order of preference, Hank's balanced salt solution, milk, saline, or saliva, but not tap water) that will nourish the cellular components of the root surface. The tooth should not be placed for transport in the mouth.

- Athletes with on-field injuries that are more serious than a simple crown chip should be immediately referred to an oral and maxillofacial surgeon or to the emergency department for a more thorough evaluation.

- Ideally, reduction of a nasal fracture is performed immediately, before swelling develops. However, within 4 days for children and 10 to 12 days for older adolescents is acceptable.

SUGGESTED READING

Andreasen JO. *Traumatic Injuries of the Teeth.* 2nd ed. Copenhagen, Denmark: Munksgaard; Philadelphia, PA: WB Saunders; 1981.

Fonseca RJ, Walker RV, Betts NJ, Barber HD, Powers MP. *Oral and Maxillofacial Trauma* "3rd ed." Philadelphia, PA: WB Saunders; 2004.

McTigue DJ. Evaluation and management of dental injuries in children. http://www.uptodate.com/patients/content/topic.do?topicKey=ped_oral/4310

Nowak A, Slayton R. Trauma to the primary teeth: setting a steady management course for the office. *Contemp Pediatr.* 2002;11:99.

Online Sports Dentistry Web site. http://www.sportsdentistry.com/. Accessed June 10, 2008.

Posnick JC. Management of facial fractures in children and adolescents. *Annals Plastic Surg.* 1994;33:4.

Ranalli DN, Demas PN. Orofacial injuries from sport. Preventive measures for sports medicine. *Sports Med.* 2002;32:409-418.

Treating and preventing facial injury. American Association of Oral and Maxillofacial Surgeons. http://www.aaoms. org/public/Pamphlets/PIP.FaceInjury.pdf. Accessed June 10, 2008.

Treatment of injuries to the primary dentition. American Dental Association. http://www.ada.org/prof/resources/pubs/jada/patient/patient_07.pdf. Accessed June 10, 2008.

CHAPTER 23

Chest and Abdominal Injuries

P. Cameron Mantor, MD
David W. Tuggle, MD

Although serious injuries to the lungs, liver, spleen, and other organs are uncommon, they can occur in young athletes, particularly in those who participate in contact sports. Coaches, athletic trainers, and physicians should all be aware of the potential thoracic and abdominal injuries that occur in the young athlete.

The most common bony injuries to the chest are rib fractures, costochondral separations, clavicle fractures, and sternoclavicular dislocations. Fractures of the scapula or sternum are rare. These injuries are usually associated with collisions between athletes or between an athlete and a fixed object. Stress fractures of the bones of the thorax are not uncommon, especially from repetitive throwing or in athletes who participate in contact sports.

Abdominal injuries also occur when children participate in contact sports. The extent of injury is directly related to the amount of force involved. Injuries to abdominal organs can lead to significant morbidity and even permanent impairment. The organs most vulnerable to injury are the spleen and liver, followed by the kidney, pancreas, and gastrointestinal tract. Children with known liver or spleen enlargement are at higher risk of injury.

ANATOMY AND BIOMECHANICS OF THE CHEST

The thorax is a flexible cage. Each rib articulates posteriorly with the vertebral column, and the first 7 ribs articulate with the sternum (**Figure 23.1**). Ribs 8, 9, and 10 articulate with the cartilage superior to them, and the 11th and 12th cartilages are free. The tip of the 12th rib is at the level of the second lumbar vertebra, and the 10th rib is the lowest anterior rib. The clavicle lies anterior to the first rib, making the first rib difficult to feel. The second rib is easy to locate because the costal cartilage articulates at the junction of the manubrium of the body of the sternum. The sternal angle is opposite the second costal cartilage and is a key landmark in the chest that is used when counting the ribs. The scapula protects the posterior ribs and vertebral column and is encased in muscle and fascia.

The bony thorax is flexible in young children. However, as children get older, the bones of the thorax become more rigid and are more prone to fracture. Children assume adult bone physiology at about age 8 years. The flexibility of the bony thorax is important to the young athlete. Most sports injuries to the thorax impair the athlete's performance because of the pain associated with the injury.

CLINICAL EVALUATION

History

Identifying the mechanism of injury is crucial in diagnosing the injury. It is also important to know whether the force came from another player or from a fixed structure. Blows of great force can be delivered over a small surface area, resulting in significant damage.

The most common symptom of all thoracic injuries is pain, which may be difficult to localize and may be associated with shortness of breath.

Physical Examination

The examination should start with observation of the athlete's respirations. Viewing the quality and rate of respirations provides valuable clues about the severity of injury. Gentle palpation of the chest wall may localize the

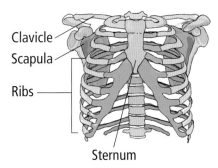

FIGURE 23.1 Bony anatomy of thoracic cage.

area of injury. Pain and swelling can be a sign of muscle injury or fracture. Rib fracture is the most common injury, and significant displacement of a fractured edge of a rib (**Figure 23.2**) could cause a pneumothorax. Palpation of the neck and supraclavicular area may reveal crepitus consistent with a pneumothorax with subcutaneous air caused by rib fractures. With multiple rib fractures, flail chest and subsequent respiratory distress are possible. An athlete who cannot move or use his or her arm may have a fracture of the clavicle on that side. Gentle palpation of the bone generally identifies the fracture. Sternal fractures are less common, although sternoclavicular dislocations can be seen. Auscultation of the chest may reveal decreased breath sounds on the injured side, which may be the result of splinting from pain and decreased ventilation or pneumothorax. Tympany to percussion also suggests pneumothorax.

Abdominal injuries typically affect soft tissues and viscera. Palpation may reveal tenderness, guarding, or rigidity. Bowel sounds should be present; their absence may indicate a possible bowel injury or peritonitis.

Imaging Studies

Radiographs of the chest are the single most useful test in identifying specific thoracic injuries. A rib series may be more useful in identifying obscure nondisplaced fractures. Anteroposterior views will best demonstrate clavicle fractures (**Figure 23.3**). Lateral views are most useful in evaluating the presence of a sternal fracture.

Radiographs of the abdomen are less helpful in detecting significant abdominal injuries. More frequently, an ultrasound and a computed tomography (CT) scan will be necessary.

TREATMENT

Definitive diagnosis and treatment of most chest injuries require transport to a hospital where appropriate studies can be performed.

Immobilization of rib fractures is impossible; however, taping or elastic bindings may alleviate the pain. Surgery is rarely indicated for sternal or scapula fractures. Most athletes simply require limited activity until the pain subsides.

Nonsteroidal anti-inflammatory drugs are typically recommended for pain management. Narcotics may be used in certain circumstances, but they promote respiratory depression in some patients and thus are of less benefit.

INTRATHORACIC INJURIES

Life-threatening chest injuries include pneumothorax, tension pneumothorax, hemothorax, cardiac contusion, pericardial tamponade, and pulmonary contusion (**Table 23.1**).

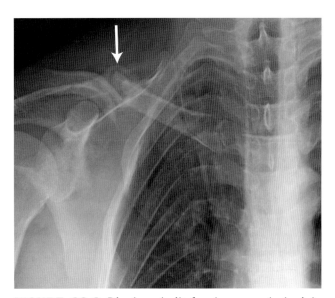

FIGURE 23.2 Displaced rib fractures and clavicle fracture.

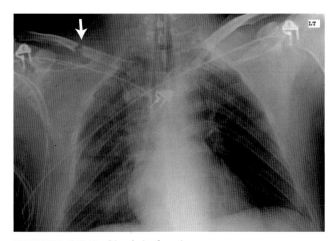

FIGURE 23.3 Clavicle fracture.

TABLE 23.1

Intrathoracic Injuries

Condition	Cause	Diagnostic Test	Treatment
Pneumothorax	Air enters pleural space, usually due to rib fracture	Chest x-ray	Probable chest tube
Tension pneumothorax	Air continues to accumulate in the pleural space, causing progressive lung collapse and shifting of mediastinum	Chest x-ray	Emergency needle decompression followed by chest tube
Hemothorax	Blood accumulates in pleural space due to blunt or penetrating trauma	Chest x-ray	Chest tube
Cardiac contusion	Direct trauma to anterior chest wall or sternum	Electrocardiogram	Treatment of associated arrhythmias
Pericardial tamponade	Accumulation of fluid within the pericardial sac due to penetrating or blunt trauma	Cardiac ultrasound	Needle decompression; probable surgery
Pulmonary contusion	External chest trauma due to blow to chest wall, causing accumulation of fluid and/or blood within the pulmonary parenchyma	Chest x-ray	Supplemental oxygen; possible intubation and mechanical ventilation
Commotio cordis	Sudden death as a result of significant impact to the chest from a baseball or helmet	None	Resuscitation rarely successful

Simple Pneumothorax

A pneumothorax develops when air enters the pleural space but cannot escape (**Figure 23.4**). A rib fracture usually causes direct injury to the lung parenchyma. This injury can occur when a football player is forcefully tackled or a bicyclist falls during a high-speed race. Air accumulates and compresses the lung on the affected side, causing a ventilation-perfusion mismatch. Characteristic signs and symptoms include chest pain and difficulty breathing. Auscultation of the chest reveals decreased breath sounds, and percussion reveals

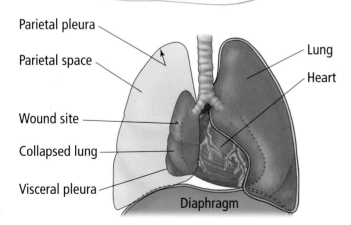

FIGURE 23.4 Pneumothorax occurs when air leaks into the pleural space from an opening in the chest wall or surface of the lung. The lung collapses as air fills the pleural space, and the 2 pleural surfaces are no longer in contact.

hyperresonance. Palpation of the anterior neck and supraclavicular region may reveal crepitus consistent with a pneumothorax with subcutaneous air. Radiographs confirm the diagnosis (**Figure 23.5**).

Athletes should be taken to the emergency department for examination and probable chest tube placement. Simple pneumothorax does not require needle decompression. If rib fractures are present, complete return to unrestricted activity may take up to 6 weeks.

Tension Pneumothorax

The cause of a tension pneumothorax is similar to that of a simple pneumothorax, but it differs clinically in that air continues to accumulate within the pleural space. The entrapped air causes progressive collapse of the lung on the affected side (**Figure 23.6**). Shifting of the mediastinum may decrease cardiac output and compromise lung function on the opposite side. A tension pneumothorax is a medical emergency that must be promptly recognized and treated. Patients have severe dyspnea and tachypnea. If left untreated, this injury will lead to respiratory arrest. In addition to decreased breath sounds and hyperresonance, signs of tension pneumothorax include tracheal deviation away from the side of injury and distention of the jugular veins. Immediate intervention includes needle decompression with a 14-gauge angiocatheter placed anteriorly in the second intercostal space. This procedure relieves the tension pneumothorax, but the athlete must be transported to the emergency department for placement of a chest tube.

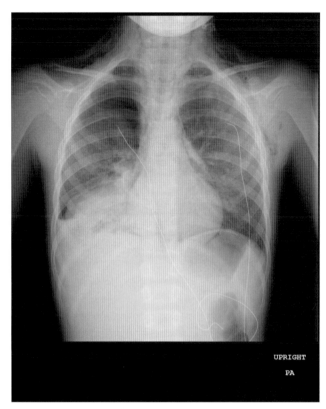

FIGURE 23.5 Radiograph of the chest showing pneumothorax on the right side with subcutaneous air.

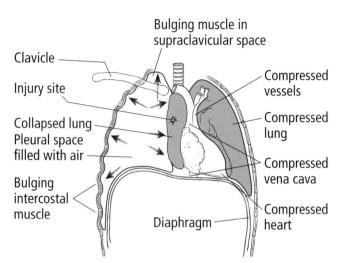

FIGURE 23.6 Tension pneumothorax can develop if a penetrating chest wound is bandaged too tightly and air from a damaged lung cannot escape.

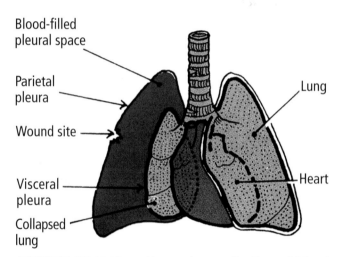

FIGURE 23.7 Hemothorax is a collection of blood in the pleural space produced by lacerated blood vessels in the chest.

Hemothorax

A hemothorax occurs when blood accumulates within the pleural space after either blunt or penetrating trauma, with resulting injury to the lung parenchyma or an intercostal vessel (**Figure 23.7**). Bleeding is usually self-limited and rarely requires surgical intervention; however, the blood must be removed from the chest cavity to prevent complications, such as infection, empyema, or chronic atelectasis of the lung.

The clinical significance of this injury depends on the amount of blood lost and the extent to which the fluid itself impairs respiratory function. Symptoms such as dyspnea and tachypnea are related to the amount of ventilatory compromise. Auscultation of the chest reveals decreased breath sounds, and percussion reveals dullness on the affected side. Radiographs confirm the diagnosis (**Figure 23.8**). The athlete should be immediately transported to the emergency department for placement of a chest tube.

Cardiac Contusion

A cardiac contusion is caused by direct trauma to the anterior chest wall or sternum, which may occur in any contact sport. Athletes typically report chest discomfort related to trauma but may be otherwise asymptomatic. The clinically important

consequences of this condition are arrhythmias, which, if severe, can lead to an abrupt cardiac collapse. Definitive diagnosis outside of the emergency department is difficult. An ECG is mandatory if cardiac contusion is suspected. The focus of management is to identify arrhythmias and initiate prompt pharmacologic therapy. Once resolved, further risk of sudden dysrhythmia is low. Long-term medical therapy is rarely necessary, and prompt return to full physical activity can be expected.

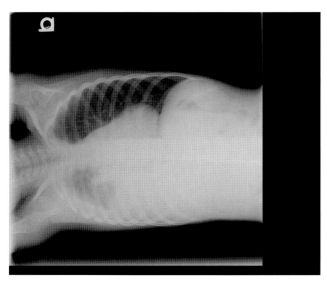

FIGURE 23.8 Radiograph of the chest showing hemothorax on the right side.

Pericardial Tamponade

Pericardial tamponade is an accumulation of fluid within the pericardial sac. Although it is most frequently associated with penetrating injuries, blunt injuries, such as an unprotected blow to the sternum, can also cause this injury. The pericardial sac is firm and fibrous, so the accumulation of fluid can lead to significant hemodynamic compromise. This is caused by the inability of the heart to fill, which severely reduces cardiac output and leads to shock. The hallmark signs and symptoms of cardiac tamponade, called the Beck triad, include jugular vein distention, hypotension, and muffled heart tones. Differentiating cardiac tamponade from a tension pneumothorax can be difficult. If this injury is suspected, the athlete should be transported to the emergency department immediately. Cardiac ultrasonography is an excellent tool to use in diagnosing this injury. Once diagnosed, therapy includes volume resuscitation, needle decompression of the pericardial sac, and possibly surgical intervention.

Pulmonary Contusion

A pulmonary contusion is a common and potentially life-threatening injury associated with significant external chest trauma from sports such as football or hockey. This type of contusion can occur after a significant blow to the chest wall, with or without associated rib injuries. The significance of the underlying pulmonary injury is related to the amount of force imparted to the chest wall and the amount of fluid and blood accumulated within the pulmonary parenchyma. The degree of ventilation-perfusion mismatch is also related to the severity of illness. Symptoms range from mild tachypnea requiring minimal therapy to complete respiratory failure, which may require mechanical ventilation. Diagnosis is based on radiographic evidence of pulmonary injury.

Treatment includes supplemental oxygen and judicious use of analgesics. If hypoxemia persists, intubation and mechanical ventilation may be necessary. All patients with pulmonary contusions must be observed for signs and symptoms of pneumonia, including a cough, fever, high white blood cell count, and the presence of infiltrate on chest radiograph. Prompt treatment with pulmonary physiotherapy and antibiotics is necessary if pneumonia is present. If the patient's respiratory status continues to deteriorate, acute respiratory distress syndrome may develop. Referral to a critical care facility is usually necessary at this point because mortality can reach 50%.

Commotio Cordis

Sudden death as a result of a significant impact to the chest is known as commotio cordis. Nonpenetrating injury such as the impact from a fast-pitch baseball or a helmet blow in football or hockey is the usual cause. Young boys between the age of 6 and 16 years are most affected. Recognition and resuscitation are rarely successful, and death is instantaneous.

Return to Play

Most thoracic injuries are bony in nature. Typically, with thoracic injuries such as rib fractures, return to play may take 6 weeks or longer, depending on the number of ribs fractured. Some authorities recommend 3 months of recovery before organized contact sports are resumed. Chest protectors are available to protect previously injured ribs. Return to play for other diagnoses varies and should be deferred to the athlete's treating physician.

ABDOMINAL INJURIES

Table 23.2 summarizes the cause, diagnostic tests, and treatment for various abdominal injuries.

Contusion to the Abdominal Wall

Contusions to the abdominal wall can occur from a forceful hit in any athletic event. Findings that include bruising and pain over the affected area associated with muscular contraction aid in establishing a diagnosis. Treatment usually requires little more than icing the affected area for 12 to 24 hours. The athlete can return to play as soon as the pain has resolved or no longer limits activity. Occasionally, enough force is imparted to the abdominal muscles to cause bleeding and formation of a hematoma. Treatment is the same as for contusion, but recovery may take weeks.

TABLE 23.2

Abdominal Injuries

Condition	Cause	Diagnostic Test	Treatment
Abdominal wall contusion	Forceful hit	Physical examination	Icing; symptomatic treatment
Muscle strain	Vigorous stretching of muscle fibers during contraction or as a result of overuse	Physical examination	Icing; symptomatic treatment; muscle stretching and strengthening
Splenic rupture	Blunt trauma left upper quadrant	CT	Management of intra-abdominal bleeding; intravenous fluids; blood transfusion; possible surgery
Liver contusions, lacerations, fractures	Blunt trauma right upper quadrant	CT	Management of intra-abdominal bleeding; intravenous fluids; blood transfusion; possible surgery
Pancreas injuries	Direct blow with fist, ski pole, bicycle handlebar to the body of the pancreas as it overlies the vertebral column	Ultrasound or CT; serum amylase and lipase	Usually resolves spontaneously
Kidney contusions, fractures	Blow to posterior lower rib cage or lumbar region	Abdominal CT with contrast	Management of associated retroperitoneal hemorrhage; usually nonoperative
Gastrointestinal tract injuries	Direct blows to the abdomen that force the bowel against the spine or peritoneum	Clinical examination most relevant; upright KUB x-ray to rule out free air	Supportive management of possible ileus; surgical resection if associated perforation

CT indicates computed tomography.

Muscle Strain

Muscle strains can also occur in sporting events. Fast, vigorous stretching of the muscle fibers during contraction leads to acute discomfort and muscle spasm. The discomfort is aggravated by the continued use of the strained muscle. Return to play is delayed with this injury. Muscle strain may also result from overuse of the muscles, such as that which occurs with weight lifting. In these instances, the discomfort is mild at first and becomes more severe with continued injury to the muscles. Patients with abdominal muscle strain should discontinue the activity that caused the injury and follow gradual rehabilitation until recovery is complete.

Injuries to the Spleen

Blunt trauma to the upper left quadrant of the abdomen or the lower rib cage often results in injury to the spleen. Snowboarders and boogie boarders are accounting for more and more of these injuries. The amount of abdominal discomfort may be minimal, despite the presence of a significant injury. On occasion, irritation of the diaphragm from bleeding, inflammation, or enlargement may cause referred pain to the left shoulder. If the injury causes significant intra-abdominal bleeding, systemic signs such as tachypnea, tachycardia, and hypotension may develop. Immediate treatment with intravenous fluid resuscitation

is necessary because patients with significant bleeding may progress to shock. Therefore, athletes with a suspected spleen injury require immediate transport to the emergency department. The most useful diagnostic test is an abdominal CT scan, although occasionally ultrasound is more readily available. These modalities are also useful after the patient's recovery.

Nonoperative management is appropriate for patients whose vital signs are stable and who have no other significant intra-abdominal injury that would require laparotomy; however, this course of management will then require close, continuous monitoring by the surgical staff. If blood transfusion requirements reach 40 mL/kg, then surgery is required.

For patients who remain stable, observation in an intensive care unit for up to 24 hours is adequate. Continued observation and bed rest for 3 days, with evaluation of hemoglobin levels, is necessary before discharge. Once discharged, these patients should remain at home for 3 weeks. If evaluation at this point reveals good recovery, and repeat ultrasound or CT scans document complete healing, patients may be released from the house but should be restricted from physical activity for another 3 months. Once evaluation reveals a completely healed spleen, athletes may return to full physical activity; however, they should be cautioned about the possibility of reinjury if they return before the spleen is completely healed. Although uncommon, delayed rupture of the spleen, usually as a consequence of a recurrent forceful blow to the same area, has been reported.

Surgical options, if necessary, include splenorrhaphy, or suturing the spleen, and splenectomy. If a splenectomy is indicated, immunizations and antibiotic prophylaxis should be considered as well. The management of splenic injuries has improved in recent years because of an increased awareness of postoperative sepsis. After surgery, patients will need 6 to 8 weeks to recover before resuming physical activity.

Injuries to the Liver

The causes of hepatic injuries are similar to those of splenic injuries. The liver, although larger than the spleen, is fairly well protected by the rib cage and abdominal wall muscula-ture. The hepatic capsule is also significantly stronger than that of the spleen. However, if the liver is enlarged as a result of a viral infection or for another reason, then it would be more susceptible to injury than normal.

Common injuries include contusions, lacerations, and fractures. The most common symptom is pain over the area of injury. Injuries that cause intra-abdominal bleeding will produce signs and symptoms of shock. Athletes should be transported to the emergency department to undergo a CT scan. Plain radiographs are of little help unless associated skeletal injuries are suspected.

Most athletes with hepatic injuries can be treated with-out surgery. Indications for surgery include hemodynamic instability and the need for blood transfusions of 40 mL/kg or more. Hepatic resection is rare. Follow-up care is similar to that for splenic injuries. Return to full physical activity will take 6 to 8 weeks.

Injuries to the Pancreas

The pancreas is a relatively protected organ located in a ret-roperitoneal position in the middle of the epigastrium. A direct blow, as with a fist, a ski pole, or a bicycle handlebar, to the body of the pancreas as it overlies the vertebral col-umn is the usual mechanism of injury. Signs and symptoms include diffuse, nondescript abdominal pain with occa-sional vomiting. Most cases of pancreatic contusion resolve spontaneously unless there is a significant injury to the parenchyma or the main pancreatic duct. Diagnosis of pancreatic injury includes testing for serum amylase and lipase, as well as radiologic evaluation with either an ultrasound or CT scan.

Nonoperative treatment is most often indicated; how-ever, significant injuries to the parenchyma or main duct may require surgical intervention.

Injuries to the Kidneys

The kidneys are located deep in the retroperitoneal space, where they are protected by the lumbar musculature and the lower rib cage. Significant blows to this area can cause injuries that vary from simple contusions to fractures through the capsule that carry the potential for significant hemorrhage into the retroperitoneal space. Signs and symptoms include mild to moderate discomfort in the re-gion of the kidney, along with microscopic or macroscopic hematuria. Diagnostic imaging should include an abdomi-nal CT scan with contrast.

Nearly all renal injuries can be managed without surgery. Complete healing, as evidenced by CT scan, should occur within 3 months. Once healed, athletes should be able to return to full activity.

Injuries to the Gastrointestinal Tract

Intestinal injuries are caused by direct blows to the abdomen that force the bowel against the spine or the firm retroperito-neum. Signs and symptoms of bowel injury may be absent if the bowel sustains only simple contusions. Athletes typically seek medical care only if a transmural injury has occurred. In the absence of a perforation, the patient may have diffuse pain from the physical injury and nausea caused by an ileus. Diagnosis is difficult, and therapy is supportive, with cessa-tion of oral intake and intravenous fluid therapy. If a major injury results in perforation, then fever, diffuse pain, and peritonitis will be present, and surgical resection is indicated. This injury can occur anywhere from the duodenum to the colon, with injuries to the latter being less common. Once athletes have physically recovered from the laparotomy, usually within 6 weeks, they can return to physical activity.

SUMMARY POINTS

- Although uncommon, serious injuries to the lungs, liver, spleen, and other organs can occur in young athletes.

- The most common symptom of all thoracic injuries is pain, which may be difficult to localize and may be associated with shortness of breath.

- Radiographs of the chest are the single most useful test in identifying specific thoracic injuries.

- Sudden, severe impact to the chest can lead to sudden death called commotio cordis.

- Blunt trauma to the abdomen most commonly causes injury to the spleen and liver. The pancreas, kidneys, and gastrointestinal tract can also be injured.

- Snowboarding and boogie boarding are fast becoming a significant source of abdominal injuries.

- Prevention of abdominal and rib injuries includes the use of rib protectors or proper padding for sports such as football, hockey, and fencing.

SUGGESTED READING

Barrett GR, Shelton WR, Miles JW. First rib fractures in football players: a case report and literature review. *Am J Sports Med.* 1988;16:674-676.

Billups D, Martin D, Swain RA. Training room evaluation of chest pain in the adolescent athlete. *South Med J.* 1995;88:667-672.

Emery CA. Risk factors for injury in child and adolescent sport: a systematic review of the literature. *Clin J Sport Med.* 2003;4:256-268.

Galan G, Penalver JC, Paris F, et al. Blunt chest injuries in 1,696 patients. *Eur J Cardiothorac Surg.* 1992;6:284-287.

Link MS, Wang PJ, Maron BJ. What is commotio cordis? *Cardiol Rev.* 1999;5:265-269.

CHAPTER 24

Exercise, Asthma, and Anaphylaxis

David M. Orenstein, MD
Gregory L. Landry, MD

Asthma, one of the most common chronic medical conditions of childhood, affects up to 15% of all children. Nearly all people with asthma have symptoms triggered by or exacerbated by exercise. Asthma induced by exercise, or exercise-induced asthma (EIA), affects patients with asthma, as well as people without previously recognized asthma. As many as 10% of high school and college athletes have been diagnosed with EIA. Asthma and EIA remain underdiagnosed in part because symptoms of EIA often manifest after, not during, exercise and may resolve spontaneously. Further, athletes with EIA might not wheeze, the classic sign of asthma, but rather cough or report chest tightness, shortness of breath, or even chest pain.

Exercise can also produce urticaria, angioedema, and anaphylaxis, all of which may occur individually or together in the same syndrome. Urticaria is characterized by localized nonpitting edema of the superficial dermis. Usually there are well-circumscribed wheals that often coalesce to form larger wheals. Angioedema is well-demarcated localized edema that involves deeper layers of skin and subcutaneous tissue. Anaphylaxis is a life-threatening illness that usually involves upper airway distress and/or hypotension in previously sensitized individuals. Signs and symptoms of asthma can occur with these entities but are rare.

Because asthma and anaphylaxis are 2 distinct clinical entities, they will be discussed separately.

EXERCISE-INDUCED ASTHMA

Pathophysiology

The pathophysiology of EIA is related to the function of the airways to humidify and warm inspired air to body temperature before it reaches the intrathoracic airways. These functions are handled efficiently when ambient air is already warm and humidified or minute ventilation is low. However, when ambient air is extremely cold or dry, or when minute ventilation is increased with exercise, warming and humidifying is incomplete. The cool, dry air that reaches the bronchi is a major stimulus for EIA. The resultant bronchospasm and airway inflammation cause airway constriction and produce coughing, chest tightness, and shortness of breath. If inflammation already exists, EIA is even more likely to occur. Particles and toxic components of polluted air worsen the signs and symptoms.

The exact sequence of cellular events leading to airway narrowing is not fully known, but mediators of inflammation derived from mast cells may be partly to blame. Support for this theory comes from an observed refractory period in almost half of patients with EIA. In these individuals, the asthma response to successive exercise challenges will diminish. This observation is consistent with a depletion of inflammatory mediators from mast cells where replenishment is incomplete if the interval between exercise challenges is 1 hour or less. Further support for the role of inflammatory mediators comes from the protective effect of leukotriene inhibitors.

Clinical Evaluation

History EIA is most likely to occur with, or especially after, a period of relatively intense exercise of at least 6 to 8 minutes' duration. If the ambient air is cold and dry, the likelihood of an episode is increased. Exercise bouts that are shorter or longer than 6 to 8 minutes are less likely to prompt EIA, with the possible exception of extremely intense brief bursts, which may also provoke bronchoconstriction. For reasons that are not yet clear, swimming is less likely than other sports to stimulate EIA, although it is thought to be related to the high humidity in most swimming pools. Signs and symptoms can include any one or a combination of coughing, wheezing, chest tightness, difficulty breathing, or chest pain. Symptoms typically last from 10 to 60 minutes and resolve spontaneously. Inhalation of a β-agonist bronchodilator, such as albuterol, can hasten resolution of symptoms. Outdoor sporting events, especially those held in cold weather, are more likely to produce symptoms of asthma than indoor events. Skiers (especially cross-country), skaters, and swimmers competing at an elite level are more likely to have EIA than their less active peers, likely because of their hours of inhaling large volumes of air that is cold and dry (skiers and skaters) or laden with chlorine (swimmers).

Physical Examination The athlete with EIA will often have a normal physical examination between episodes. Careful attention to the nose and sinuses may reveal abnormalities because of the association among asthma, allergic rhinitis, and sinusitis. Auscultation of the lungs may reveal unilateral adventitious sounds, which suggest a foreign body, pneumonia, or a mass.

Children with asthma may not take deep breaths because these cause coughing. However, athletes must be encouraged to take deep breaths. Forced expiration may produce coughing, wheezing, or rhonchi, which suggest asthma but are not specific findings for this diagnosis.

A careful examination of the heart is also necessary because cardiac disease may produce exercise-induced cough and intolerance.

Diagnostic Testing Diagnosing EIA is usually relatively straightforward. An athlete who coughs and wheezes, who reports chest tightness, and who experiences difficulty breathing or chest pain during or after exercise is likely to have EIA. If the athlete is known to have asthma, he or she can expect increased symptoms of asthma with exercise, and formal testing is seldom needed. In athletes not previously known to have asthma, diagnosis of EIA can often be established by a therapeutic trial of β-agonist inhalation (eg, 2 puffs of albuterol) 15 minutes before exercise. If this approach is not successful, pulmonary function testing can help identify individuals with obstruction of large and small airways. However, athletes with exercise-related airway obstruction may have normal baseline pulmonary function. In these individuals, a bronchial provocation test can be performed by using exercise, cold air, methacholine, or histamine. A newer test, the eucapnic voluntary hyperventilation challenge, appears to be more sensitive than sport-specific and laboratory-based challenges and remains under investigation.

With an exercise challenge, pulmonary function testing is performed before exercise and every 3 to 5 minutes after exercise for 15 or 20 minutes. The exercise challenge should last 6 to 8 minutes and should raise the athlete's heart rate to 180 beats/minute. Typically, in an athlete with EIA, forced expired volume in 1 second (FEV_1, a measure of large airway function) or midexpiratory flow (sometimes called FEF_{25-75}, a measure of small airway function) will decrease. Traditionally, decreases of 15% to 20% are required to confirm the diagnosis, although lower decreases may be clinically significant. False-negative tests are common.

Athletes occasionally have signs and symptoms of EIA but do not meet the diagnostic criteria for EIA when given a bronchial provocation test. This may occur because the athlete exercises in cold, dry air, or other aspects of the test do not re-create the environment (including the intense setting of competition) that provokes the symptoms. In these instances, empiric treatment may still be prudent.

Differential Diagnosis

Few conditions are confused with EIA. The condition that is most difficult to distinguish from EIA is vocal cord dysfunction (VCD). This adduction of the vocal cords had been thought to be unusual and confined to elite female athletes. It is now recognized more widely. It probably has a psychogenic basis. VCD produces symptoms that are similar to EIA, but it is not responsive to bronchodilators. Diagnosis is made with either formal pulmonary function tests before and after exercise (in which the inspiratory loop of the flow-volume curve is flattened, while FEV_{25-75} and FEV_1 are preserved) or with direct visualization of the adducted vocal cords by flexible fiber-optic laryngoscopy after exercise. Flow-volume loops must be specifically requested because they are not routinely performed as part of an exercise provocation study. The diagnosis can be suggested by history, with VCD commonly occurring earlier in exercise than EIA and often giving the sensation of throat blockage (patients frequently point to their throat when asked about their symptoms).

Other conditions that mimic EIA include viral or bacterial lung infections that can produce coughing or shortness of breath that worsens with exercise, and trauma to the larynx or chest that causes pain or difficulty breathing that is more pronounced with the deep breathing associated with exercise. Gastroesophageal reflux should also be considered as a potential trigger for EIA. Cardiac causes of chest pain and cough should be considered in the differential diagnosis.

Treatment and Prevention

EIA is usually easy to treat and prevent (**Figure 24.1**). If EIA occurs, 2 puffs of a β-agonist bronchodilator such as albuterol will almost always reverse the airway obstruction and relieve the symptoms. Prevention is also possible and should be the preferred method of treatment instead of relying on rescue treatment once symptoms appear. The first step in prevention is taking 2 puffs of a β-agonist bronchodilator 15 minutes before exercise. If a β-agonist is not tolerated,

then cromolyn sodium or nedocrimil can be used in the same way. If these medications, used independently, do not prevent EIA, then both may be administered together before exercise. If necessary, the athlete may double the number of puffs of both agents. Some of the oral leukotriene inhibitors, such as montelukast, also help prevent EIA, but they are not typically used for treatment of simple EIA.

If treatment with these agents does not prevent EIA, the athlete should be asked to demonstrate the proper technique for using the inhaler. Other considerations include

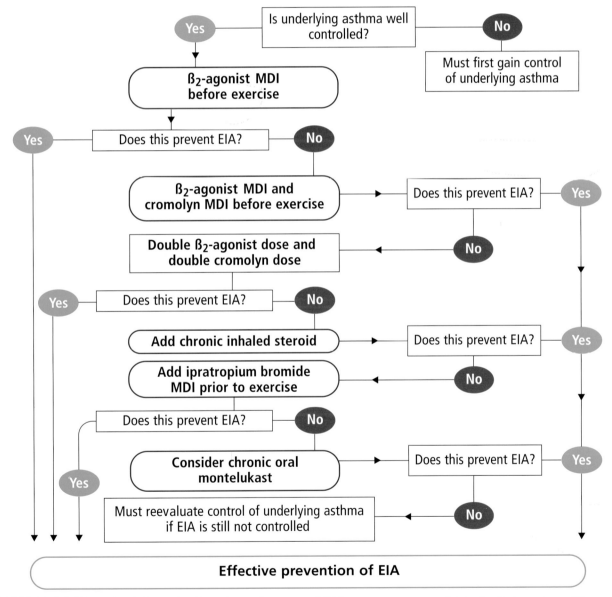

FIGURE 24.1 Flow chart for selecting drugs to prevent EIA. Adapted from Morton A, Fitch K. Asthmatic drugs and competitive sports . An update. *Sports Med*. 1992;14:228-242.

the possibility that the inhaler canister is empty or the medication has expired. If these causes have been explored, the diagnosis should be questioned, and referral to an asthma specialist is indicated. In most patients, the diagnosis of EIA is correct, but the athlete has underlying asthma, with chronic, inadequately controlled airway inflammation. Pulmonary function testing will show baseline airway obstruction with incomplete response to an inhaled bronchodilator. This inflammation must be controlled. Long-term treatment with an inhaled anti-inflammatory agent, such as inhaled corticosteroids or cromolyn sodium, will usually reduce inflammation.

Most of the drugs now in use for treating and preventing asthma are legal for use in scholastic, collegiate, and international competition (**Table 24.1**). In international competition, the athlete will need to apply for a therapeutic use exemption.

Nonpharmacologic treatment may help some athletes with EIA. For example, a scarf may be tied around the nose and mouth to help warm and humidify inspired air. Sometimes, warm-up exercises before practice or competition can induce a refractory period (in about half of patients with asthma) and thus make the competition less likely to invoke EIA. To induce a refractory period, the athlete need not exercise long enough and with enough intensity to actually induce some bronchospasm. There are no universal warm-up exercises, and routines will likely vary among athletes; however, 10 to

TABLE 24.1

Drugs Commonly Used for Exercise-Induced Asthma (EIA)

Medication	Route of Administration	Effectiveness in EIA	Legal or Banned[a]	Use
Cromolyn sodium	Aerosol	Good	Legal	P
Leukotriene modifiers				
Montelukast	Oral	Good	Legal	P, T
Zafirlukast	Oral	Good	Legal	P, T
β_2-Agonists				
Albuterol[b]	Aerosol	Excellent	Legal	P, T
Albuterol[b]	Oral	Fair	Banned	P, T
Terbutaline	Aerosol	Excellent	Legal	P, T
Terbutaline	Oral	Fair	Banned	P, T
Orciprenaline	Aerosol	Excellent	Legal	P, T
Salmeterol	Aerosol	Excellent	Legal	P, T
Clenbuterol	Aerosol	Excellent	Banned	P, T
Formoterol	Aerosol or dry powder inhaler	Excellent	Legal	P, T
Theophylline	Oral	Good	Banned	P, T
Ipratropium bromide	Aerosol	Fair	Legal	T
Corticosteroids				
Beclomethasone	Aerosol	Unknown	Legal	P, T
Budesonide	Aerosol	Fair	Legal	P, T
Fluticasone	Aerosol	Fair	Legal	P, T
Mometasone	Aerosol	Fair	Legal	P, T
Prednisone	Oral	Unknown	Banned	T
Prednisolone	Oral	Unknown	Banned	T

Adapted from Hebestreit H, Bar-Or O (editors). *The Young Athlete*. Volume XIII in *The Encyclopedia of Sports Medicine*, an IOC Medical Commission Publication in collaboration with the International Federation of Sports Medicine. Blackwell Publishing, 2008.

P indicates prophylaxis; T, therapeutic.

[a] Most of the legal medications require a therapeutic use exemption to be used legally in international competition. The World Anti-Doping Agency Web site contains more information (http://www.wada-ama.org/).

[b] Albuterol is called "Salbutamol" outside the United States.

15 minutes of exercise is usually sufficient to induce a refractory period. If the athlete has a refractory period, subsequent exercise bouts will be less likely to induce symptoms for about 2 hours. For high school and college athletes, the suggestion of changing sports may not be practical, but parents of younger children may be advised to help their children select lower-risk sports. However, because pharmacologic treatment is so effective, few athletes will have to abandon their sport of choice, and no young person with EIA should be excluded from sports or physical activity.

Most athletes with asthma respond well to exercise training. Many professional and Olympic athletes with asthma have attained high levels of sports performance. Youngsters with asthma should be encouraged to exercise and participate in sports.

EXERCISE-INDUCED ANAPHYLAXIS

Pathophysiology

Exercise can produce urticaria, angioedema, and anaphylaxis separately or together in the same syndrome. Classic exercise-induced anaphylaxis (EIAna) was first described 20 years ago. Since then, hundreds of patients have described a similar pattern of initial signs and symptoms of EIAna.

In more than half of patients with classic EIAna, food or drugs are a coprecipitant with exercise. The food that triggers EINna most often is celery, followed by the more common food allergens such as shellfish and wheat. EIAna has also been reported after ingestion of a variety of medications. Jogging is the most common precipitating type of exercise, but EIAna has also been associated with other types of exercise.

Clinical Evaluation

History Athletes often report the same pattern of initial signs and symptoms, including fatigue, generalized warmth, pruritus, and erythema. Information about an athlete's last meal and medication regimen in relationship to beginning exercise is important. Some athletes may report that symptoms develop if they exercise too soon after eating.

A serious episode is characterized by a variety of airway problems, including choking, stridor, and dysphagia, and abdominal pain and vomiting. Symptoms typically last between 30 minutes and 4 hours. About one-third of patients experience syncope in association with EIAna, but only one death has been reported.

Physical Examination Soon after the initial signs and symptoms develop, large urticaria (1-2.5 cm) develop with angioedema. However, in some athletes, only small punc-

tate (2-4 mm) urticaria develop. This is called cholinergic urticaria because it is thought to be triggered by cholinergic response in the skin as the result of temperature changes. This form of urticaria, called variant EIAna, is rarely associated with angioedema, bronchospasm, or hypotension. **Treatment and Prevention** Epinephrine is the treatment of choice. However, as with any anaphylactic reaction, intravenous fluids, antihistamines, and oxygen are helpful if epinephrine does not resolve the symptoms. Some athletes will improve spontaneously if they stop exercising.

For most athletes, the key to treatment is prevention. All athletes with EIAna should be referred to an allergy specialist because of the high association of this condition with food allergies. Athletes who are food sensitive should undergo skin testing and should be encouraged to keep a food diary to help better identify offending foods. Some athletes may be able to safely exercise only in the morning after an overnight fast.

Prophylactic antihistamines are helpful for some athletes. Diphenhydramine and hydroxyzine are regarded as the most effective, but their strong sedative effects may limit their use in some individuals. Any of the nonsedating antihistamines may be beneficial. Athletes should be counseled to use antihistamines liberally until more is known about the precipitating factors in their case. Some athletes will always require pretreatment to be able to exercise free of symptoms. These athletes should not exercise alone and should carry an emergency epinephrine kit with them at all times.

Coaches and physicians should also keep an emergency epinephrine kit in the first aid kit or medical bag. The kit must be kept out of heat and light, and its expiration date should be checked frequently.

URTICARIA

There are stimuli other than exercise that can cause urticaria. An athlete who notices small 2- to 4-mm wheals associated with exercise and passive warming likely has cholinergic urticaria (CU). (Passive warming will not cause CU in the patient with variant EIAna.) Warming an extremity with a heating pad or immersing an extremity in hot water (40°C-42°C) to raise the body core temperature 0.5°C to 1.5°C will usually trigger CU. Intradermal injection of acetyl methylcholine chloride will usually produce 2- to 4-mm urticaria in patients with CU but not in patients with variant EIAna. These tests for CU are very specific but not particularly sensitive. Treatment of CU consists of an antihistamine such as hydroxyzine or cetirizine, but not all athletes will find their CU severe enough to warrant treatment.

Cold urticaria occurs on cold-exposed skin. There are several reports of this phenomenon in athletes who use ice to treat injuries. Occasionally cold urticaria induces a systemic reaction with headache, flushing, faintness, and, rarely, collapse. The reaction can be severe if the entire body is immersed in cold water. This makes any activities in water risky for individuals who are prone to this condition. Treatment consists of awareness, avoidance of cold, and use of antihistamines such as hydroxyzine or cetirizine. In severe cases, corticosteroids must be used.

VENOM ALLERGIES

Another cause of anaphylaxis is an allergic reaction after a sting from a venomous insect, most commonly yellow jackets, honeybees, wasps, hornets, and ants. Reactions to these bites are responsible for about 50 deaths in the United States each year. Most systemic reactions are immediate and produce symptoms of anaphylaxis.

Epinephrine must be immediately administered, followed by transport to the emergency department. Large local reactions to stings produce induration and erythema within 24 to 72 hours. In these instances, a severe systemic reaction is not likely. However, athletes who experience this type of large reaction may be at risk for a systemic reaction in the future, and they should carry an emergency epinephrine kit with them at all times. Most allergy specialists do not recommend immunotherapy for these individuals.

Athletes who have experienced an anaphylactic reaction to a sting should be referred to an allergy specialist to identify the specific venom allergy and to discuss immunotherapy. This type of therapy has been shown to significantly reduce reactions to subsequent stings in most patients. These athletes must carry an emergency epinephrine kit at all times.

SUMMARY POINTS

- EIA is common but underdiagnosed because signs and symptoms may not include wheezing and may occur mostly after exercise.

- EIA is most likely to occur with endurance exercise in cool, dry air.

- In most athletes, EIA is readily prevented by taking 2 puffs of inhaled albuterol, cromolyn sodium, or nedocrimil before exercise.

- Once it is recognized and treated, EIA should not prevent athletes from enjoying a full athletic career.

- EIAna can produce urticaria, angioedema, and anaphylaxis either separately or together.

- Most athletes with EIAna have a related food or medication allergy.

- Injection of epinephrine usually resolves EIAna symptoms, but treatment is largely preventive.

- Referral to an allergy specialist and liberal use of prophylactic antihistamines are recommended for athletes with EIAna.

- Athletes who are allergic to venomous insect stings should carry an emergency epinephrine kit with them everywhere.

SUGGESTED READING

DuBaske LM, Horan RF, Sheffer Brigham, AL, et al. Exercise-induced allergy syndromes. In: Weiler JM, ed. *Allergic and Respiratory Disease in Sports Medicine.* New York, NY: Marcel Dekker; 1997:253-278.

Graft DF, Valentine MD. Insect sting allergy. In: Kaplan AP, Kersey R, eds. *Allergy.* 2nd ed. Philadelphia, PA: WB Saunders; 1997:652-663.

Morton A, Fitch K. Asthmatic drugs and competitive sports. An update. *Sports Med.* 1992;14:228-242.

National Collegiate Athletic Association Web site. http://www.ncaa.org/. Accessed June 3, 2008.

Parsons JP, Mastronarde JG. Exercise-induced bronchoconstriction in athletes. *Chest.* 2005;128:3966-3974.

United States Olympic Committee Drug Control Program hotline. (800) 233-0393.

Volcheck GW, Li JT. Exercise-induced urticaria and anaphylaxis. *Mayo Clin Proc.* 1997;72:140-147.

Weiler JM, Malloy C. Asthma and athletes. *Clin Rev Allergy Immunol.* 2005;29:139-149.

World Anti-Doping Agency Web site. http://www.wada-ama.org/. Accessed June 3, 2008.

CHAPTER 25

Acute Illnesses and Youth Sports

Paul R. Stricker, MD

Whether children join an organized sport, play during school recess, or are active in their backyard, exercise and physical activity are important to their overall health and well-being. Like other children, young athletes can become ill from a variety of infections that may affect their ability to participate. Team sports in particular place children in close contact with each other for extended lengths of time and may increase a child's risk of contracting an infection.

Physicians should be aware of the potential implications of a sick young athlete. Important considerations include the relationship between exercise and the immune system, the severity of the illness and its effect on the ability of the athlete to either continue participating or to require a period of rest, the type of illness and the risks for serious sequelae, the danger of contagion to other individuals or team members, treatment options and their effects on performance, and suggestions for a gradual return to exercise activity.

EXERCISE, IMMUNITY, AND INFECTION

The effects of exercise on the immune system continue to be actively investigated. Researchers seek to understand how exercise induces changes in the immune system because exercise affects the quantitative and functional aspects of various immune markers. Studies investigate the short- and long-term effects of exercise on those quantitative and functional measures of the immune system, including neutrophils, lymphocytes, and immunoglobulins. Interpretation of research in this area has been complicated by inconsistencies and differences in protocols. In addition, there is an imbalance between the many laboratory studies of short-term exercise and the fewer number of studies that assess the

effects of intense exercise over long periods of time. Furthermore, translating changes in immune markers into clinical significance remains difficult. However, some important trends require notice. Research studies define short-term exercise as physical effort that is performed on a treadmill, stationary bicycle, or arm ergometer for short bursts of activity. Long-term exercise includes consistent aerobic activity several times a week at levels at or above 75% of the maximum oxygen uptake ($\dot{V}o_2max$), as well as high-intensity or endurance sports such as long-distance running, cross-country skiing, swimming, and competitive cycling.

During physical activity, many physiologic changes occur, and changes in one body system (eg, hormonal changes) can affect other systems. For example, with exercise, levels of epinephrine and cortisol rise. Epinephrine peaks during exercise and then diminishes during recovery, while cortisol rises more steadily and remains increased for a longer period of time. Quantitative changes in immune components include increases in neutrophils and lymphocytes with rising epinephrine levels mostly from demargination, as well as delayed increases in neutrophils and decreases in lymphocytes corresponding to the rise in cortisol, with a return to baseline in a few hours. This decrease in lymphocytes includes a change in lymphocyte subsets such as the decreased ratio of CD4 cells to CD8 cells. In long-term exercisers, cortisol levels often remain high even at rest, and large increases in cortisol appear in many overtrained athletes. The catabolic nature of prolonged increase of cortisol and its effects on lymphocytes may contribute to the susceptibility to infection. Even though numbers of white blood cells (WBCs) increase with each bout of exercise and then return to baseline, those long-term and intense exercise regimens tend to have much lower WBC counts over time.

Functional assessment of immune components also reveals changes with exercise. Neutrophil chemotaxis and phagocytosis are diminished with exercise and even suppressed below baseline with long-term, high-intensity training. Salivary immunoglobulin A concentration is decreased with short-term exercise and is even suppressed below baseline levels with long-term, high-intensity training. Natural killer cell activity actually increases, but then decreases during recovery back to baseline. In general, exercise affects the quantity and activity of many immune system components, and these changes raise concern about the athlete's ability to ward off pathogens during periods of recovery from intense exercise. These effects of exercise on the immune system are summarized in **Table 25.1**.

Researchers agree that, in general, individuals who exercise at a moderate level (<60% $\dot{V}O_2$max) actually enhance their immune function and may experience shorter duration of illness compared with those who do not exercise. However, an increasing body of evidence supports the idea that elite athletes may be at greater risk for infections than those who exercise at a more moderate level. Increased training volume and intensity (>80% $\dot{V}O_2$max) can increase the risk of upper respiratory infections, and individuals who exercise during infections with certain viruses such as coxsackie virus, adenovirus, or influenza may be at increased risk for myocarditis.

UPPER RESPIRATORY INFECTIONS

Although viral upper respiratory infections (URIs) can affect anyone at any time of the year, rates of infection in the general public usually peak in the fall and winter, when many viruses are predominant. During these times,

youngsters are in school, attend classes, play together, and participate in team training in close proximity with many other children, so infectious agents are shared. All athletes and active youngsters should be reminded to maintain good personal hygiene by washing their hands frequently and by not sharing water bottles or towels. Topical hand antiseptic gels can be helpful if used correctly. Over-the-counter medications may help subdue certain symptoms, but antihistamines and decongestants should be used with some caution. These medications increase the risk of dehydration, tax the cardiovascular system, and affect the body's ability to regulate temperature. Children should remain well hydrated and refrain from strenuous exercise, especially in the heat.

Such techniques may help reduce the spread of infections, yet an athlete engaged in high-intensity exercise may still be at an increased risk for URI. For example, the risk of URI is higher in long-distance runners when they increase their training mileage and also during the 2 weeks after a race. Other data demonstrate that the risk of URI increases with longer periods of training and with a higher intensity of effort. Many athletes report that they contract more infections during various times in the competitive season when they train intensely, and also during and after major competitions, which are stressful both physically and emotionally.

Oxidative Stress

Recent research has started to elucidate the negative effects of oxidative stress on the body. Oxidative stress increases with emotional stress, the stress of exercise, and with obesity and overweight. By-products of oxidative stress include lipid peroxides and free radicals, and along with

TABLE 25.1

Effects of Exercise on the Immune System

Short-term Exercise		Long-term Exercise	
Increases:	Decreases:	Increases:	Decreases:
• Number of WBCs	• Number of CD4 cells	• Number of neutrophils	• Number of WBCs
• WBC adhesion	• CD4/CD8 ratio	• WBC adhesion	• CD4/CD8 ratio
• Number of neutrophils	• Serum IgG		• Serum IgG
• Number of NK cells	• Salivary IgA		• Salivary IgA
• Number of lymphocytes	• Neutrophil activity		• Neutrophil activity
• Number of CD8 cells	• Lymphocyte proliferation		• Number of NK cells
• NK activity			• Number of lymphocytes

WBC indicates white blood cell; NK, natural killer; and Ig, immunoglobulin.

increased cortisol levels and temporary exercise-induced suppression of immune function, they may negatively affect the immune system. Other variables such as fatigue, psychological stress, and inadequate recovery time also are contributing factors. These potential negative effects can be fought by allowing the body enough rest to to recover and by reducing psychological stress. Oxidative stress can be staved off by eating foods high in antioxidant value. There is evidence that synthetic vitamins do not have a significant protective effect and may even be harmful in some cases. However, natural sources of phytochemicals and antioxidants, such as vitamin C, vitamin E, and β-carotene found in fruits and vegetables, exert a significant antioxidant effect as a result of their high bioavailability.

The effects of exercise on the risk of URI remain a complicated issue because it is difficult to isolate the effects of exercise from those of the psychological stress associated with such things as training and competition, environmental and weather conditions, exposure to individuals who are ill, and inadequate nutrition. The best prevention strategy is to eat a well-balanced diet, drink plenty of fluids, get enough rest, and avoid overtraining.

ROLE OF ANTIBIOTICS

Athletes intent on training through an illness may ask for an antibiotic at the first sign of a runny nose. If this is the case, the physician should reassure the athlete, describe the course of viral infections, and explain that they are unresponsive to antibiotics. If a medication needs to be prescribed to reduce symptoms, it should not interfere with drug-testing policies or cause side effects such as excessive drowsiness.

Conversely, athletes who resist antibiotic therapy to treat a true bacterial infection should also be reassured that the antibiotic is necessary for proper treatment and resolution of illness. Antibiotics such as ampicillin, amoxicillin, tetracycline, and trimethoprim-sulfamethoxazole have not been shown to adversely affect aerobic capacity or strength. However, an antibiotic should be selected carefully to avoid problems such as nausea, diarrhea, photosensitivity, and allergic reaction.

EFFECTS OF INFECTIONS ON TRAINING

Few well-designed studies examine the effects of illness on the body's response to exercise, and those that exist show varying results. Some studies of subclinical viral infections and exercise did not show a decrease in performance, whereas others showed decreases in endurance and isometric strength. Still, some generalizations can be made. Active infections and illnesses that cause fever can be detrimental to athletes. Fever, which is due to a disturbance of hypothalamic thermoregulatory function, can affect the body's ability to regulate body temperature for up to 12 weeks, thus increasing the risk of heat exhaustion and heatstroke. Fever may also worsen dehydration, especially if the athlete is also losing fluids from diarrhea or vomiting, and even small amounts of dehydration can negatively affect endurance. Acute febrile illnesses affect performance from a combination of decreased exercise tolerance, dehydration, fatigue, increased cardiac output, and direct viral effects on muscle tissue as evidenced by myalgias. Once the fever has resolved, exercise tolerance must be regained before the body is stressed by significant energy requirements; this reduces the risk of injury and suboptimal performance.

Some illnesses may not produce clinically important fevers or threats to thermoregulation, but they warrant concern in that they may be contagious to other team members. In such cases, the athletes need to be educated regarding ways to reduce the spread of disease. URIs with a significant cough, viral gastroenteritis with diarrhea, and varicella are examples. Other contagious illnesses like mumps, influenza, meningitis, and hepatitis are less likely to be a problem with consistent immunization practices.

Infectious Mononucleosis

Infectious mononucleosis carries with it the risk of contagion. Although splenic rupture associated with splenomegaly can occur, it is rare. Rupture of the spleen most frequently occurs during the first 4 to 21 days after symptoms appear. An athlete may usually return to activity 3 to 4 weeks after the onset of the illness if other symptoms are greatly diminished and if the young athlete feels able to begin moderate exercise. Determining splenomegaly by palpation is unreliable, and ultrasonographic measurements are variable even among the normal athlete population. Without baseline measurements before illness, it is difficult to determine the status of the spleen unless serial measurements confirm a decrease in size over time. Variability of symptoms and type of sport involvement make it necessary to individualize a gradual return to training for an athlete recovering from mononucleosis.

CONCLUSION

Research investigating the response of various immune markers is ongoing. Moderate exercise tends to enhance immune function, whereas prolonged and intense exercise may compromise immunity and increase the risk of URI. Athletes often want to continue to train and compete despite an illness, and the physician is regularly faced with decisions regarding return to play. In general, if symptoms are confined above the neck, such as a runny nose or nasal congestion, athletes may continue at a level they can tolerate. However, athletes with systemic symptoms such as fever, myalgias, and high resting heart rate should refrain from intense exercise. Risks of serious sequelae including dehydration, heat exhaustion, prolonged illness, and myocarditis may preclude a rapid return to physical activity and competition. Return to play depends on the absence of fever, fewer symptoms, adequate hydration, and a return to normal resting heart rate, which may require 7 to 14 days of rest and/or limited activity.

Exercise during certain viral illnesses may have potentially serious complications, but significant infections are less frequent than the common cold. Evaluation of the athlete is important to assess whether the illness is confined locally or is manifesting systemic symptoms, and to plan treatment with appropriate return to activity. Treatment should focus on allowing activity levels to gradually increase and on relieving symptoms without producing other undesirable effects.

Progressive return to activity involves relative rest—that is, allowing the athlete to safely continue certain aspects of his or her sport. The focus is usually on nonstrenuous skills and technique, while gradually increasing intensity and effort as energy levels and recovery permit.

SUMMARY POINTS

- Moderate exercise tends to enhance immune function, whereas prolonged, intense exercise may have a negative effect on immunity and requires close attention to eating properly, getting enough rest, and avoiding overtraining.

- The risk of URI increases with longer periods of training and higher intensity of effort.

- Good hygiene practices should be encouraged in schools and among teammates who come into close contact; these practices should include washing hands frequently and not sharing water bottles or towels.

- Symptoms above the neck are probably mild enough to allow activities as tolerated, but over-the-counter medications should be used cautiously because of the risks of dehydration and increased cardiac output.

- Youngsters should not exercise, compete, or participate while experiencing systemic total body symptoms, especially with a fever, because dehydration, risk of heat exhaustion or heatstroke, myocarditis, increased cardiac demand, risk of injury, and poor performance may result.

- Fever causes impaired thermoregulation for up to 12 weeks.

- While the illness resolves, the athlete should rest and remain hydrated while gradually increasing activity. Relative rest permits athletes to remain involved in their sport without overexerting themselves.

SUGGESTED READING

American Academy of Pediatrics Council on Sports Medicine and Fitness. Medical conditions affecting sports participation. *Pediatrics*. 2008;121:841-848.

Bloomer R, Goldfarb A, McKenzie M. Oxidative stress response to aerobic exercise: comparison of antioxidant supplements. *Med Sci Sports Exerc*. 2006;38:1098-1105.

Burstein R, Hourvitz A, Epstein Y, et al. The relationship between short-term antibiotic treatments and fatigue in healthy individuals. *Eur J Appl Physiol*. 1993;66:372-375.

Fitzgerald L. Overtraining increases the susceptibility to infection. *Int J Sports Med*. 1991;12:5-8.

Green K, Rowbottom D, Mackinnon L. Acute exercise and T-lymphocyte expression of the early activation marker CD69. *Med Sci Sports Exerc*. 2003;35:582-588.

Hinton J, Rowbottom D, Keast D, et al. Acute intensive interval training and in vitro T-lymphocyte function. *Int J Sports Med*. 1997;18:130-135.

Hosey R, Mattacola C, Kriss V, et al. Ultrasound assessment of spleen size in collegiate athletes. *Br J Sports Med*. 2006;40:251-254.

Hosey R, Rodenberg R. Training room management of medical conditions. *Clin Sports Med*. 2005;24:477-506.

Illback N, Fohlman J, Friman G. Exercise in coxsackie B3 myocarditis: effects on heart lymphocyte subpopulations and the inflammatory reaction. *Am Heart J*. 1989;117:1298-1302.

Mackinnon L. Chronic exercise training effects on immune function. *Med Sci Sports Exerc.* 2000;32:369-376.

Nieman D. Exercise, upper respiratory tract infection, and the immune system. *Med Sci Sports Exerc.* 1994;26:128-139.

Novas A, Rowbottom D, Jenkins D. Tennis, incidence of URTI and salivary IgA. *Int J Sports Med.* 2003;24:223-229.

Rowbottom D, Green K. Acute exercise effects on the immune system. *Med Sci Sports Exerc.* 2000;32:369-376.

Samman S, Sivarajah G, Man J, et al. A mixed fruit and vegetable concentrate increases plasma antioxidant vitamins and folate and lowers plasma homocysteine in men. *J Nutr.* 2003;133:2188-2193.

Waninger K, Harcke H. Determination of safe return to play for athletes recovering from infectious mononucleosis: a review of the literature. *Clin J Sports Med.* 2005;15:410-416.

Weber T. Environmental and infectious conditions in sports. *Clin Sports Med.* 2003;22:181-196.

CHAPTER 26

Chronic Conditions

Claire M. A. LeBlanc, MD

Children with chronic medical conditions face unique risks when they participate in sports. These risks depend not only on the specific disease but also on the severity of the illness and on the sport, environment, coaching, supervision, training regimen, and level of competition. Despite the challenges, children or adolescents with a chronic condition may also benefit from becoming more physically active because most can experience many of the same benefits as their healthy peers. These include improved fitness and motor coordination, as well as psychological benefits, such as improved self-esteem, body image, social development, and concentration. Other advantages are more disease specific, and in fact, physical activity may be part of the suggested treatment regimen. Finally, an active child may be more likely than an inactive one to adopt a habit of lifetime physical activity that may translate into reduced cardiovascular morbidity and mortality in adulthood. The extent to which children with chronic health conditions can exercise should be based on the demands of the activity or sport, the effect of the disease on performance, and the potential for acute or chronic worsening of the child's illness as a result of participation (**Table 26.1**). Thus, each child must be considered individually and regularly reevaluated.

INSULIN-DEPENDENT DIABETES MELLITUS

Insulin-dependent diabetes mellitus (IDDM), or type 1 diabetes, is an autoimmune disease that results in the destruction of pancreatic β cells leading to severe insulinopenia. Long-term complications include retinopathy, microalbuminuria, and peripheral neuropathy in children who have had this illness for at least 5 years, as well as a higher incidence of chronic renal failure and cardiovascular disease in adulthood. Intensified therapy and improved

glycemic control greatly decrease the development and progression of these complications, but more frequent and severe hypoglycemic episodes may result. This is especially of concern in childhood, so the American Diabetic Association (ADA) currently recommends the achievement of good metabolic control through individualized diabetes care provided by a pediatric multidisciplinary team. Nutrition, activity, and insulin replacement are the pillars of management, and a change to any one of these requires adjustments to the others. Regular self-monitoring of blood glucose before meals, at bedtime, and during and after exercise is important. This allows individualized adjustments of insulin and dietary intake that permit safe participation in most sports.

Risks of Exercise

During exercise, many integrated neural, cardiovascular, and hormonal responses occur to ensure the delivery of oxygen and metabolic fuels (glucose, fatty acids) to working muscles. Activation of the sympathetic nervous system allows redistribution of blood flow to exercising muscles. Catecholamines suppress insulin secretion and stimulate lipolysis and glycogenolysis in liver and muscle tissue. Increases in glucagon augment hepatic gluconeogenesis. High growth hormone and cortisol levels antagonize insulin action and limit glucose utilization in nonexercising tissue. Despite these exercise-related changes, blood glucose levels fluctuate minimally in healthy individuals; however, this may not be the case in athletes with diabetes.

In IDDM, plasma insulin concentrations do not decrease with exercise and may actually increase. Higher insulin levels are more likely to occur when short-acting insulin is injected subcutaneously into an exercising limb just before a workout. This may be because of local increases in temperature, hyperemia, or greater lymph flow. Sustained insulin

TABLE 26.1

Risks and Benefits of Exercise in Children With Chronic Health Conditions

Condition	Risks of Exercise	Benefits of Exercise
Insulin-dependent diabetes mellitus	• Hypoglycemia • Ketoacidosis	• Increased physical fitness • Improved overall health • Increased sensitivity to insulin • Possibly fewer long-term complications
Type 2 diabetes	• Ketoacidosis • Heat illness	• Weight loss • Lower visceral and body fat • Increased insulin sensitivity • Fewer long-term complications
Cystic fibrosis	• Dehydration • Arterial oxygen desaturation • Hypoglycemia[a] • Ketoacidosis[a] • Possibly worsening of cor pulmonale	• Increased physical fitness • Improved self-esteem • Improved overall health • Possibly, decreased morbidity and mortality
Epilepsy	• Seizures	• Increased physical fitness • Improved self-esteem • Improved overall health
Cerebral palsy	• Overuse injuries • Dehydration • Seizures	• Increased physical fitness • Improved self-esteem • Improved muscle strength
Muscular dystrophy	• Cardiopulmonary complications (late stages of disease)	• Increased physical fitness • Improved self-esteem • Improved muscle strength
Chronic renal failure	• Dehydration, electrolyte imbalance • Muscle cramps, seizures, syncope • Hypertension, cardiac arrhythmias • Fractures • Trauma to transplanted kidney	• Increased physical fitness • Improved self-esteem
Chronic anemia	• Cardiopulmonary complications • Splenic rupture • Risk of sudden death in sickle cell (heat, dehydration, altitude, chilling)	• Increased physical fitness • Improved self-esteem
Hemophilia	• Bleeding (into joints, muscles, and other organs)	• Increased physical fitness • Increased levels of factor VIII • Increased strength in muscles and ligaments • Improved hemarthropathy outcome
Cancer	• Cardiopulmonary complications of chemotherapy • Damage to solitary organ	• Increased physical fitness • Improved self-esteem • Improved quality of life • Improved bone mineral density • Reduced risk of breast cancer

[a] Children with cystic fibrosis-related diabetes mellitus.

levels during exercise result in a marked suppression of hepatic glucose production and greater muscle glucose utilization, resulting in a faster decline in blood sugar. A blunted response of the counterregulatory hormones and catecholamines also occurs, especially in children with autonomic neuropathy, so the classic warning signs of hypoglycemia are not appreciated before severe manifestations occur. Patients with well-controlled IDDM may experience hypoglycemia up to 36 hours after exercise; this may relate to an insufficient replenishment of muscle and liver glycogen stores during recovery. The extent to which blood glucose drops with exercise depends mostly on the duration and intensity of the activity. Endurance events (those lasting 30 minutes or more) such as distance running, swimming, canoeing, or bicycling may precipitate larger drops in blood glucose.

High-intensity exercise is associated with excessive counterregulatory hormone production and insufficient insulin secretion so that hepatic glucose formation exceeds the rate of muscle glucose utilization, creating transient hyperglycemia. When exercise stops, insulin levels rapidly increase, and blood glucose normalizes in healthy individuals. This response does not occur in IDDM, so sustained postexercise hyperglycemia may result, especially if preexercise glucose levels are elevated. Some insulin-deprived children with poorly controlled IDDM may experience ketoacidosis with exercise. Although the uptake of ketones into muscle during exercise is high, increased glucagon and cortisol levels enhance lipolysis and hepatic ketogenesis. If left untreated, ketonemia and acidemia may cause extreme fatigue, coma, and eventually death.

Most children with IDDM are free of the long-term complications of their disease, but they should be screened for the presence of nephropathy, proliferative retinopathy, peripheral neuropathy, and autonomic neuropathy. Those with overt nephropathy and associated elevated blood pressure are at risk for hemodynamic compromise during high-intensity exercise. Activities that strain or jar the head may precipitate vitreous hemorrhage or retinal detachment in youth with diabetic retinopathy. Peripheral neuropathy may lead to a loss of protective sensation of the feet, increasing the risk of injury during exercise. Autonomic neuropathy may increase the risk of adverse cardiovascular events during exercise, including abnormal heart rat response, orthostatic hypotension, myocardial ischemia, and sudden death. These individuals may also have impaired thermoregulation.

Benefits of Exercise

Many studies have shown that participation in sports improves the physical fitness of patients with IDDM. Also, exercise may positively affect the disease process itself. For example, hypertension and serum lipid profiles improve with physical training. Furthermore, evidence suggests that high levels of physical activity may reduce the risk of long-term diabetic complications such as neuropathy and microangiopathy. An increased sense of well-being, improved self-esteem, and enhanced quality of life as a result of exercise may help affected children and youth cope better with their chronic disease. However, the effects of training programs on the long-term control of blood glucose in patients with IDDM have not yet been clearly determined.

Recommendations

Children with IDDM can take part in any physical activity or sport. To participate safely, affected children and their parents should be thoroughly educated in the skills of self-management and understand the principles of blood glucose regulation before, during, and after exercise. Although there are general guidelines for those who want to engage in sports, every child must be advised individually (**Table 26.2**). Prolonged aerobic exercise (eg, sporting events lasting 30 minutes or more) is more likely to be associated with hypoglycemia. Blood glucose levels should be monitored more closely; insulin reduced before exercise; and additional carbohydrate feedings taken before, during, and after the event. Teammates and coaches should be taught how to recognize the signs and symptoms of hypoglycemia. Ready sources of glucose or carbohydrates should be available on the sidelines. Hypoglycemia may be especially dangerous in situations requiring mental alertness, sustained effort, or neuromuscular coordination. Thus, scuba diving, hang gliding, rock climbing, skydiving, motor sports, and long-distance swimming or running are considered to be high-risk activities for competitors with diabetes, and appropriate training and support systems need to be in place. Special precautions should also be considered for those using an insulin pump. The pump should be removed or a waterproof device substituted during water sports. A sport guard case or protective pad should cover the device during contact sports, and extra layers of clothing should protect it from freezing in cold weather.

Children with diabetic retinopathy should avoid heavy lifting and excessive jarring of the head to avoid ocular injury. Those with peripheral neuropathy need to use proper footwear and monitor their feet for skin trauma, and those

TABLE 26.2

Suggestions for Children With Insulin-Dependent Diabetes Mellitus Who Want to Engage in Sports

- Always wear a diabetes identification bracelet or shoe tag and bring a glucometer, food, and fast-acting carbohydrates to the sporting venue.

- Inject insulin subcutaneously at least 1 hour before exercise at a site away from an exercising muscle (eg, the abdomen). Patients on multi-injections of short and intermediate insulin should decrease the dose before exercise by up to 30%-50%. Those on an insulin pump should omit or greatly reduce the basal infusion rate during exercise and decrease or skip premeal boluses. The magnitude of insulin reduction depends on the type, intensity, and duration of exercise and should be individualized. Postexercise insulin doses should be adjusted on the basis of glucose monitoring.

- Check blood glucose level before exercising and only exercise if it is 100-200 mg/dL. If the exercise continues for more than 30 minutes, perform blood glucose testing every 30 minutes during exercise and 15 minutes after exercising. Check blood glucose level again at bedtime and, if low, eat slow-release carbohydrates (eg, whole wheat bread with cheese or shredded wheat cereal with milk) and test blood glucose level once or twice during the night.

- Exercise only if metabolic control is good (ie, blood glucose levels are 100-250 mg/dL without ketonuria). If >250 mg/dL with ketosis or >300 mg/dL, delay exercise; if blood glucose level is <100 mg/dL, eat more carbohydrates and recheck blood glucose levels before exercise.

- Increase complex carbohydrate intake 1-3 hours before exercise, especially if the exercise session is unplanned. Drink carbohydrate solutions (eg, juice or commercially available sport drinks with 6%-8% glucose) every 30 minutes during prolonged exercise. Replenish carbohydrate stores after exercising.

- Remember that blood glucose levels may be low for more than 36 hours after prolonged exercise.

- Try not to exercise during peak times of insulin activity or within 1 hour of insulin injection.

with autonomic neuropathy should be monitored for cardiovascular risk factors and carefully maintain fluid and electrolyte balance during prolonged exercise in warm climates. If affected with overt nephropathy and hypertension, they should be restricted from weight lifting and high-static sports until hypertension is under adequate control, and should be promptly referred for evaluation by a specialist if symptomatic.

TYPE 2 DIABETES

In contrast with IDDM, patients with type 2 diabetes have normal to increased pancreatic insulin production, but tissue receptors are impaired. Although it was formerly considered to be a disease limited to adults (adult-onset diabetes), the incidence of type 2 diabetes in children and adolescents has dramatically increased over the past decade. Members of certain ethnic groups are especially vulnerable, including those of Native American, African, Hispanic, and Asian descent. Other risk factors include a family history of type 2 diabetes in a first- or second-degree relative, exposure to diabetes in utero, overweight, polycystic ovarian syndrome, acanthosis nigricans, hypertension, dyslipidemia, and impaired glucose tolerance. Adequate nutrition and increased physical activity are important elements in the prevention and treatment of this disorder.

Risks of Exercise

An active lifestyle is the first line of management for those with type 2 diabetes unless there is serious metabolic decompensation with severe symptomatic hyperglycemia and/or diabetic ketoacidosis at diagnosis. These individuals require immediate insulin therapy. Although this is less of a problem than in type 1 diabetes, individuals with type 2 diabetes who are on insulin therapy or are taking medications that stimulate insulin secretion are at risk for hypoglycemia with exercise. Although resistance training may be an effective and popular form of exercise for obese youth, this activity might exacerbate elevated blood pressures in children with marked, sustained hypertension. Obese individuals exercising in hot and humid climates also have a higher risk of heat illness. Those with associated microvascular disease (nephropathy, neuropathy, retinopathy) may be at risk for complications with exercise. Although the risk of retinopathy in youth with type 2 diabetes is lower than in those with type 1 diabetes, other complications, such as microalbuminuria, hypertension, and neuropathy occur more frequently. These individuals may be at greater risk for complications with exercise.

Benefits of Exercise

Physical training induces similar benefits to those described for obesity. These include weight loss, lower visceral fat, lower percentage of body fat, reduced resting blood pressure, better self-esteem and self-concept, and improved insulin sensitivity. The latter is short-lived and disappears when individuals assume a less active lifestyle. For optimal results, the patient's preferred physical activity should be fun and should incorporate large muscles moving the whole body over a distance. Emphasis should be placed on duration rather than intensity, water-based sports, and resistance training. Lifestyle modifications should also be made, including reducing sedentary activities, such as watching TV.

Recommendations

Current ADA guidelines suggest office-based screening by fasting glucose every 2 years for children 10 years of age or older who are overweight (body mass index >85th percentile for age) plus any 2 of the following: family history of type 2 diabetes in a first- or second-degree relative; Native American, African American, Latino, Asian American, or Pacific Islander race; presence of signs of or conditions associated with insulin resistance (acanthosis nigricans, hypertension, dyslipidemia, polycystic ovarian syndrome). Those who have or are at risk for type 2 diabetes should adopt an active, healthy lifestyle. Children with severe hyperglycemia or ketoacidosis require immediate medical attention and treatment with insulin. Severe hypertension (blood pressure >99th percentile for age + 5 mm Hg) is a contraindication for weight lifting and sports with a high static component, such as rock climbing and throwing. Acclimatization to hot and humid climates and adequate hydration are important for obese youth, who are at a higher risk of heat illness. The suggestions for IDDM patients with microangiopathic complications can be applied to this population.

CYSTIC FIBROSIS

Cystic fibrosis (CF) is the most common fatal autosomal recessive disease among whites, with a frequency of 1 in 2000 to 3000 live births. It is caused by mutations in the CF transmembrane conductance regulator (CFTR) protein, a complex chloride channel found in all exocrine tissues. Abnormal chloride transport leads to viscous secretions in the lungs, pancreas, liver, intestine, and reproductive tract, as well as greater salt loss in sweat. The severity of this disease varies with the type of genetic mutation and may include chronic sinopulmonary infections, obstructive lung disease, fat and protein malabsorption, reduced insulin secretion, focal biliary cirrhosis, bowel obstruction, and infertility. Pulmonary disease is the leading cause of morbidity and mortality, and in general, exercise tolerance is related to the severity of this complication. Fortunately,

most patients with CF can participate in sports; some have completed marathons and triathlons.

Risks of Exercise

During maximal exercise testing, the aerobic performance of healthy individuals is limited by cardiac output and the energy metabolism of exercising muscles. Although patients with severe CF (FEV_1 < 50%) may have reduced cardiac function, their exercise performance is most limited by a subnormal ventilatory capacity. This may be a consequence of airflow limitation with reduced alveolar ventilation, an inadequate lung diffusion capacity, malnutrition, reduced respiratory muscle strength, and impaired oxidative efficiency of working muscles. In these patients, desaturation of arterial oxygen may occur, reflecting significant ventilation-perfusion mismatching, intrapulmonary right to left shunting, or cor pulmonale with congestive right heart failure. Exposure to high altitude (eg, mountain climbing) facilitates these complications. During exercise, patients with CF may also develop severe coughing spells with or without hypoxemia. Although this may represent typical exertional or postexertional expulsion of respiratory mucus, some children with CF also have asthma. Individuals with CF, particularly those with bronchiectasis and bullae, are at risk for a pneumothorax if they should experience major intrapulmonary pressure changes during activities like scuba diving. CF patients also lose large quantities of sodium chloride in sweat, which may reduce their exercise tolerance, especially in hot climates. When CF patients exercise in the heat, serum sodium, chloride, and osmolality levels drop, impeding these patients' thirst perception and increasing the risk of dehydration. In CF patients who develop diabetes mellitus, prolonged exercise (more than 30 minutes) may result in hypoglycemia, and those with a high urine output may become dehydrated. Some children with CF have splenomegaly or liver dysfunction and may be at increased risk of organ damage if they engage in contact or collision sports.

Benefits Of Exercise

For patients with CF, participation in physical activity increases fitness and improves their self-esteem and well-being. Specific benefits include enhanced clearance of mucus from the airways, which may be a reflection of an inhibition of sodium channels in the respiratory endothelium, increasing water content and reducing the viscosity of respiratory mucus. Specific training (eg, inspiration against resistance) can be useful to increase the strength and endurance of respiratory muscles. Some programs, including home-based exercises, slow the rate of decline in pulmonary function. Improved exercise tolerance occurs with aerobic training, and strength exercises can increase muscle mass and power. Some evidence suggests that a high level of physical activity and aerobic fitness may decrease morbidity and mortality in patients with CF.

Recommendations

Patients with CF should be encouraged to exercise as much as is medically feasible. Those who have severe lung disease should undergo exercise testing with oximetry to determine the maximum suggested exercise intensity. Supplemental oxygen or bronchodilator therapy is required with physical activity in some cases. Those with exercise-induced hypoxemia should avoid high-altitude sports such as mountain climbing. CF patients with severe bronchiectasis should not scuba dive. To prevent hyponatremic dehydration, patients exercising in a hot or humid climate should be encouraged to gradually acclimatize to the environment and drink beverages containing about 50 mmol/L of sodium chloride every 15 to 20 minutes even if not feeling thirsty, and ingest salty foods during and after exercise. Salt tablets are contraindicated. Individuals with CF-related diabetes should increase carbohydrate and fluid intake before, during, and after sports. The few patients with an enlarged spleen or diseased liver should avoid contact or collision sports.

EPILEPSY

Epilepsy is a common neurologic disorder that occurs in 0.5% to 1% of children. It is manifested by randomly recurring unprovoked seizures. Epilepsy may be partial or generalized in nature with or without loss of consciousness. In some patients, epileptic seizures may be precipitated by flickering light, hyperventilation, inadequate sleep, alcohol, drugs, or sudden discontinuation of antiepileptic medication. Parents commonly impose heavy restrictions on sport participation for safety reasons, yet seizures are rarely triggered by physical activity.

Risks of Exercise

Children with well-controlled disease can take part in all sports. Little research is available addressing the issue of exercise-induced seizures, but most reports suggest that the risk is low in children with well-controlled disease. Prolonged exercise of moderate intensity, rather than intermittent exercise, appears to be more likely to trigger seizures. Contact sports are associated with higher rates of mild traumatic brain injury, but there are no reports of increased seizure frequency. Epileptics with poorly

controlled disease may injure themselves or others during participation in certain sports. Activities with potential for self-injury include cycling, rock climbing, water sports, weight lifting, and horseback riding; activities that may result in harm to others include motor vehicle racing, javelin, discus, archery, and shooting.

Benefits of Exercise

Some evidence suggests that physical activity and a high level of fitness may raise the seizure threshold. For a child with epilepsy, regular physical activity is important to maintain self-esteem and general well-being.

Recommendations

Children with epilepsy should be encouraged to live an active lifestyle. Before embarking in sports, they should be assessed by a neurologist. Individuals with well-controlled seizures may participate in all sports, even those that are considered strenuous or involve body contact, if they maintain fluid and electrolyte balance, wear proper safety equipment, and adhere to safe play guidelines. However, boxing is contraindicated, as it is in all children. If seizure control is suboptimal, the athlete requires individual assessment for collision and contact sports. Similarly, noncontact sports like archery, rifle shooting, swimming, scuba, weight lifting, strength training, and sports involving heights should be avoided. Motor sports are contraindicated because even the rare occurrence of seizures might result in catastrophic injury to the athlete and others. Each child and adolescent should be independently managed because other sports may cause seizures in certain individuals.

CEREBRAL PALSY

Cerebral palsy (CP) is a nonprogressive encephalopathy associated with gestational and perinatal insults to the brain that occurs in 4 out of 1000 live births. This disease may be classified according to the type of motor abnormality (eg, athetosis, ataxia, spasticity) or the extremities affected (eg, hemiplegia, diplegia, quadriplegia). There are many social barriers restricting children with CP from participation in sport and recreation, and as a result they are typically more deconditioned than their healthy peers. Their locomotion also comes at a high metabolic cost. This inefficient ambulation is a result of poor muscle endurance, power, and strength, which may relate to the uncoordinated actions of antagonistic muscles (coactivation of flexors-extensors of lower extremity) and an abnormal walking style (crouching, tiptoe walking). Despite these limitations, patients with CP can improve their physical fitness and walking ability with training and can enjoy participation in many sports.

Risks of Exercise

Because patients with CP generally have an imbalance of tone, strength training needs to be greater in the muscles with lower tone (eg, extensors of upper limbs in spastic CP) to avoid making this inequality worse. Muscle stretching to improve flexibility is important in these individuals, but it must be done carefully to avoid inadvertent tactile stimulation of muscles with high tone because this may create more spasticity. Severely affected patients have problems with swallowing and excessive drooling, which can lead to dehydration with exercise. Wheelchair athletes are at higher risk of serious shoulder (rotator cuff) injuries from overuse during sports. Those with associated seizure disorders require specific attention to this comorbidity.

Benefits of Exercise

Patients with CP are able to improve strength, fitness, and motor function with regular exercise training. However, these benefits are short-lived unless they train at least twice a week throughout the year. Regular training may also allow greater skill acquisition in the athlete's chosen sport. Team sports are additionally beneficial for developing and maintaining interactive social skills. Aquatic exercise may be preferable because more severely affected individuals can take part with less stress to their joints.

Recommendations

Children with CP should be encouraged to be physically active and maintain an upright gait as long as possible. Training exercises need to be tailored to the ability of the athlete. Exercises to improve endurance include walking, cycling, swimming, and wheelchair sprinting. Improvements in muscle strength should focus on training with free weights and exercise machines. Motor skills required for sport-specific participation might include ball throwing and catching and possibly dynamic balancing. For optimal benefit and compliance, the child should train at least twice a week, and recreation and fun should be emphasized. A wide variety of sports are available for participation at recreational and competitive levels. These include archery, boccia, bowling, track and field, cross-country events, cycling, equestrian, power lifting, slalom, soccer, swimming, table tennis, target shooting, wheelchair team handball, and several winter sports.

DUCHENNE MUSCULAR DYSTROPHY

Duchenne muscular dystrophy (DMD) is an X-linked recessive genetic disorder characterized by a complete lack of dystrophin, which is essential to the structural integrity of the muscle cell membrane. This condition occurs in about 1 of 3000 to 4000 live male births. It manifests as muscle weakness at 4 to 5 years of age and becomes progressively worse over time. Typically children remain ambulatory until 9 to 12 years of age, when a wheelchair becomes necessary. The move to a wheelchair may be the result of decreased residual muscle strength, joint contractures, and bed rest after procedures; worsening of balance with associated fear of falling; development of overweight; and parental preference to make it easier on the child. These patients later have severe complications including cardiomyopathy or respiratory failure, causing them to become bedridden by their early 20s. Children with DMD are less fit than their healthy peers. They have reduced muscle strength, peak power, and muscle endurance, and low aerobic power as a result of the small number of functional motor units in their muscles. Despite these issues, patients with DMD often have residual unaffected muscles (especially early in the disease) that are trainable. With such training, upright gait may be prolonged and progressive loss of strength slowed down.

Risks of Exercise

Although some concerns about activity-induced deterioration (overwork weakness) have been raised, these claims have been refuted. Children with DMD often have raised serum creatine kinase levels after exertion, but there is no proof that this reflects direct damage to their muscles. Training can also improve aerobic exercise performance without muscle function worsening. Specific respiratory muscle exercises may be helpful early in the disease, but if they are initiated in the later stages, it may add to the work of breathing.

Benefits of Exercise

Immobilization has been shown to quickly reduce fitness and motor function, so it should be minimized and regular physical activity encouraged. Mild to moderate physical activity appears to be safe for children with DMD and is associated with improved self-esteem, independence, and socialization. Stretching exercises can maintain joint range of motion. Training of the unaffected muscle tissue helps improve the strength and endurance of the residual motor units. Muscle strengthening exercises need to be combined with additional activities that encourage the patient to rise, stand, and walk to prolong the upright ambulatory period. This training can also improve aerobic fitness, which is critical to preventing and treating obesity. When these individuals become overweight, fat accumulates in the dystrophic muscles, which further impairs gait and also interferes with respiratory function. Specific exercises targeting respiratory muscles have been initiated in the attempt to improve pulmonary function. When performed early in the disease, these exercises may improve respiratory muscle endurance, as well as maximal inspiratory and expiratory pressures.

Recommendations

Participation in recreational activities for 20 to 30 minutes for 3 days per week at mild to moderate intensity seems to be safe for children with DMD. Each child needs to be assessed individually, and exercise should be adjusted according to the level of impairment. In general, children should be encouraged to increase their level of physical activity, but if pain or fatigue occurs, intensity and/or frequency should be decreased. Shorter duration of exercise and the incorporation of frequent rest breaks may be helpful. There is no need for preexercise fitness testing unless there are specific concerns regarding cardiac or pulmonary disease.

CHRONIC RENAL DISEASE

In addition to the excretion of nitrogenous waste products, healthy kidneys are vital in the maintenance of fluid, electrolyte, and acid-base balance. Other tasks include the secretion of hormones that participate in the regulation of systemic and renal hemodynamics (renin, prostaglandins, bradykinin), calcium, phosphorus, bone metabolism (1.25-dihydroxyvitamin D3), and red blood cell (RBC) production (erythropoietin). Chronic renal insufficiency, defined as an irreversible reduction (by at least 60%) in kidney function, occurs in about 1 per 100,000 children in the United States each year. Affected children may have abnormalities of urine output, hypertension, anemia, bone disease, edema, electrolyte and acid-base disturbances, and malnutrition and growth failure. Once renal function diminishes to less than 5% of normal, end-stage renal disease (ESRD) occurs, which requires dialysis (peritoneal, hemodialysis) or transplantation. Impaired exercise tolerance and sports performance are seen in children with renal failure, especially once ESRD develops. Muscle wasting (from protein malnutrition), anemia, hypertension, electrolyte and acid-base disturbances, metabolic deficiencies, impaired carbohydrate metabolism, mental health issues, and medication side effects work in combination to

impair cardiopulmonary function, oxygen transport, and skeletal muscle ability during physical activity. However, physical activity can be beneficial to children with renal failure as long as adequate attention is paid to these issues.

Risks of Exercise

Dehydration and electrolyte abnormalities are more likely to occur during exercise in children with renal insufficiency even before ESRD. Hyponatremia, hypocalcemia, and hyperkalemia may occur, which can cause muscle cramps, seizures, and syncope from cardiac dysrhythmias. Exercise can greatly worsen hypertension and increase the risk of fractures in those with renal osteodystrophy. Children on dialysis or children who have received transplants may experience trauma to the peritoneal or vascular access catheters, to an arteriovenous fistula, or to the new kidney that is more superficially located in the abdomen. Children with chronic renal disease are often self-conscious about their stunted growth and reduced muscle mass. Placing such individuals in sport or exercise programs requiring maximum bursts of energy; prolonged, intense exercise; or full-body contact may result in a failure to perform and lower self-esteem.

Benefits of Exercise

Exercise training programs have been shown in adults with chronic renal disease to improve aerobic fitness. The use of erythropoietin to correct the chronic anemia associated with renal failure can improve exercise tolerance in adults and children. Further gains in fitness may be limited by a diminished contractile reserve in patients with left ventricular hypertrophy and generalized reduction in muscle capillarity, which correlates with poor oxygen transport. Aerobic exercise is additionally useful to help lower blood pressure in those with hypertension and to improve physical performance and health-related quality of life. Resistance exercises have been shown in adult studies to improve muscle strength and physical functioning. Combined aerobic and strength training programs may be additionally beneficial. Bone mineral density can be enhanced by participation in weight-bearing physical activities. Adopting a healthy, active lifestyle may improve the serum lipid profile and reduce the threat of cardiovascular disease, which is the leading cause of mortality in adults with ESRD. Active children are also more likely to have better self-esteem and social confidence, which may be lacking in individuals with chronic renal failure.

Recommendations

Adopting an active lifestyle is an important goal for children with chronic renal insufficiency. The intensity of the exercise and types of sports suggested for these children need to be based on their level of fitness, the severity of disease, presence of dialysis catheters or transplanted kidney, and the nature of any disease complications. Affected children may benefit from exercise testing, which can be used to measure baseline fitness, dysrhythmias, and blood pressure responses to exertion. It is important to select an activity that the child prefers and that will lead to success. Sports such as swimming, cycling, aerobics, dance, running, tennis, baseball, and golf are suggested by most nephrologists. Weight lifting should be avoided because it may increase hypertension and cause abdominal hernias in those on peritoneal dialysis. Children with various dialysis tubing might be at increased risk of infection when they swim, especially in nonchlorinated water. Children with a transplanted kidney should avoid contact sports.

CHRONIC ANEMIA

To work efficiently during exercise, the muscles require an ongoing source of oxygen. The delivery of oxygen to the tissues (Vo_2) depends on blood flow (Q), hemoglobin concentration (Hb, which binds O_2 in RBCs), and oxygen saturation in blood (So_2), according to the Fick equation: $Vo_2 = 0.139 \times Q \times Hb \times S_AO_2 - S_VO_2$. The oxygen dissociation curve also plays a role. Accordingly, the amount of oxygen released in the tissues depends on local temperature and pH, as well as the affinity of hemoglobin for oxygen, which may vary with the type of anemia. There are many causes of chronic anemia, but all are due to either lack of bone marrow production, shortened survival of RBCs, or both. Normal individuals compensate for anemia during exercise by increasing plasma volume, stroke volume, and resultant cardiac output with or without compensatory left ventricular hypertrophy. They also increase the erythrocyte 2,3 diphosphoglycerate concentration, which reduces the oxygen affinity of hemoglobin, facilitating release in tissues. Yet those with chronic anemia may be unable to adequately compensate during exercise, and as a result oxygenation of the tissues is significantly reduced. Indeed, exercise performance may be impaired with even mild anemia. Studies of adults with varying degrees of iron deficiency have demonstrated a 20% reduction in exercise capacity when hemoglobin drops by as little as 1-2 g/dl.

Risks of Exercise

All anemias can adversely affect exercise tolerance, but the degree of impairment depends on the severity of the anemia and individual variations. There are other risks of exertion associated with specific types of anemia.

Children with sickle cell disease have excessive hemoglobin S, which causes the RBCs to change their shape, thus increasing mechanical fragility and leading to chronic hemolysis. Such children have higher cardiac output during exercise, often with left ventricular hypertrophy, which may be a reflection of microvascular occlusion in the coronary circulation and cardiomyopathy. Chronic hemolysis can also lead to iron overload, which may deposit in the myocardium, further impairing cardiac function. Painful crises and pulmonary infarction are more likely to occur when individuals work out at high altitudes or extremes of temperature because of greater sickling and hemolysis. Repeated pulmonary involvement can lead to chronic lung disease with impaired alveolar capillary perfusion, which also reduces exercise tolerance. Sickle cell trait is a milder condition that is not associated with anemia. Most affected individuals can take part in all sports without difficulty. However, during strenuous exercise in the heat or at high altitudes, dehydration and rare cases of severe rhabdomyolysis and death have been reported.

β-Thalassemia is an inherited hemoglobinopathy caused by a defect in hemoglobin synthesis that varies in clinical expression from mild (thalassemia minor) to severe (thalassemia major). Children with thalassemia minor may have a normal hemoglobin concentration and tolerate exercise well, whereas those with thalassemia major are more likely to have severe hemolytic anemia with significant hepatosplenomegaly requiring repeated blood transfusions. This results in damage to the liver and heart from chronic iron deposition. Exertion in those with severe thalassemia is poorly tolerated because of inadequately understood pulmonary function abnormalities, including restrictive and small airway obstructive defects, hyperinflation, and decreased maximal oxygen uptake, as well as cardiac malfunction. Myocardial hemosiderosis leads to arrhythmias (both supraventricular and ventricular) and end-stage restrictive cardiomyopathy, which in turn lead to heart failure.

Iron is essential to life, with the majority bound in heme proteins (hemoglobin and myoglobin). Low iron levels may occur, especially in adolescence, because of inadequate nutrition or excessive gastrointestinal or menstrual blood loss. Iron-deficiency anemia is associated with impaired exercise performance because of poor oxygen delivery and inadequate aerobic metabolism in muscle (iron plays a critical role in the action of several key enzymes of energy metabolism). Individuals with iron deficiency but normal hemoglobin levels may have less exercise tolerance, although the evidence is unclear.

Benefits of Exercise

There is no absolute level of hemoglobin at which exercise is contraindicated. Children with reasonably stable chronic anemia can develop a state of cardiovascular fitness appropriate to their individual degree of anemia. They can best achieve this through a graduated program of aerobic cardiovascular conditioning. Optimal muscle strength, flexibility, and body composition can also be attained. Physical activity can provide emotional benefits, such as an improved sense of well-being and accomplishment.

Recommendations

Exercise and sports for children and youth with chronic anemia need to be selected according to the severity and type of anemia, as well as the abilities of the individual. Athletes should be encouraged to choose attainable goals and avoid activities that might lead to complications of their disease. Children with stable sickle cell disease may take part in all sports except those with high exertion and collision or contact. Overheating, chilling, dehydration, and exercising at altitude must also be avoided. Those with sickle cell trait are not restricted from any sport, but they should be carefully conditioned, hydrated, and acclimatized to reduce any possible risk of rhabdomyolysis and sudden death. Although most individuals with mild thalassemia and near-normal hemoglobin levels can safely participate in all sports, those with more severe disease (cardiopulmonary disease and splenomegaly) are limited to low-intensity, noncontact aerobic exercise.

HEMOPHILIA

The 2 most common forms of hemophilia are types A and B, which result from the lack of adequate amounts of blood clotting factors VIII and IX, respectively. These are sex-linked recessive genetic disorders, so only boys have episodes of excessive bleeding. The magnitude of bleeding depends on the quantity of factor present in blood and varies from mild (up to 40% of normal) to severe (<1%-2% of normal) deficiencies. Bleeding is best treated with infusions of genetically engineered recombinant human factors VIII and IX because these do not carry the risk of blood-borne infection. Joint or muscle bleeding episodes require immediate factor replacement to achieve levels of 30% to 40%. More severe bleeding (intracranial, vital organs, airway) requires transportation to an emergency center for imaging, supportive care, and factor replacement to levels greater than 80% of normal. Prophylactic treatment with factor VIII or IX reduces spontaneous bleeding in severe hemophilia and can markedly decrease the risk of subsequent destructive hemophilic arthropathy. With

such improvements in treatment, many affected boys can enjoy physical activity and can participate more safely in a variety of sports. This is important, because studies show lower anaerobic power, fitness scores, and muscle strength in children affected with hemophilia.

Risks of Exercise

Hemophilia does not affect children's ability to play sports or their fitness. However, those with recurrent intra-articular bleeds can develop progressive joint destruction, limiting the strength, power, and work capacity of the affected extremity. Participation in collision and contact sports may result in life-threatening bleeding.

Benefits of Exercise

Exercise improves muscle strength and coordination, which may improve joint stability and reduce the risk of injury. This could decrease the incidence or improve the outcome of hemophilic hemarthropathy. Acute bouts of exercise may significantly increase factor VIII levels in the blood for up to 10 hours through β-adrenergic receptor stimulation. Involvement in team sports encourages psychosocial development and improved self-esteem.

Recommendations

As a general rule, children with hemophilia should be encouraged to be active, even if physical activity occasionally results in bleeding. The choice of sport should be based on the level of clotting factor, the preferences of the child, the stresses of the sport, and the cooperation of the coach. Generally, collision and contact sports (eg, boxing, ice hockey, football, rugby, wrestling) are contraindicated. However, swimming, golf, dance, and cycling may be well tolerated. Certain modifications of other sports are also suggested, including avoiding pitching and sliding in baseball, heading the ball in soccer, and jumping dismounts in gymnastics. At times of joint pain and swelling, it is best to avoid physical activity involving that joint until resolution.

Children with hemophilia who have not been treated with ultrapure or genetically engineered products are at greater risk for blood-borne infections such as hepatitis and HIV. Although this does not mean that they must be excluded from sports participation, universal precautions apply. This includes the use of latex gloves to clean and cover all wounds and to wash up spills with a 1:10 bleach-water solution. Teammates and coaches should be made aware that if a child with hemophilia engages in sports, an emergency plan to treat bleeding is required.

Whenever possible, the child should wear protective clothing and equipment. When bleeding occurs, the affected muscle or joint should be cooled with cold compresses or ice packs, and the deficient clotting factor should be replenished as soon as possible.

CANCER

Over 12 000 children and youth are diagnosed with a malignancy each year in the United States; the most common are leukemia and lymphoma. With recent advances in treatment, 80% of these children can be cured. However, many are not fit and have reduced bone mineral density that may persist years after treatment. Long-term survivors of childhood cancers have reduced physical performance and restricted participation in activities of daily living. Exercise may help improve the quality of life of these individuals.

Risks of Exercise

The ability of cancer patients to engage in strenuous exercise is determined by the type, grade, and stage of the neoplasm itself and also by the location of the tumor and the treatment regimen. In general, competitive sports should be avoided while cancer treatment is in progress, but physical activity should be encouraged as long as certain limitations are addressed. Central intravenous lines may be damaged by trauma or may become infected if the child goes swimming.

Cancer survivors also have risks with exercise. Leukemia survivors may experience reduced immune function when they exercise, and those with brain tumors frequently experience significant neurologic impairments that may limit sport selection. Children with Wilms' tumor are usually left with one hypertrophied kidney that may be more prone to injury during contact sports. Those with bone tumors (osteosarcoma, Ewing's sarcoma) may have to learn to ambulate with a deformed or amputated limb.

Various chemotherapeutic agents can have a direct impact on sport participation. Most suppress bone marrow growth and increase the risk for infection, but some drugs have specific toxicities related to exercise. Bleomycin can cause interstitial lung disease, limiting exercise tolerance. Vincristine and vinblastine sometimes cause peripheral neuropathies, leading to foot and wrist drop; cisplatinum and carboplatin may cause renal tubular dysfunction, resulting in electrolyte, calcium, and magnesium imbalances. Doxorubicin has been shown to be toxic to the myocardium during and beyond 15 years after treatment, and its use can lead to sudden death. A cardiologist should

thoroughly evaluate these patients before they engage in competitive sports.

Benefits of Exercise

Habitual physical activity has been demonstrated to reduce the risk of colon cancer during adult years. Teenage girls who are regularly physically active at a vigorous level and avoid weight gain as adults may reduce their risk of breast cancer. Adult and child cancer survivors who take part in exercise programs can improve fitness, percentage of body fat, bone mineral density, self-esteem, and quality of life.

Recommendations

All children with cancer should be encouraged to be physically active in the rehabilitative and remission phases. They should be evaluated for conditions specific to their cancer or treatment that might require exercise modification. Implanted intravenous devices should be protected from water and direct trauma. Those who have received doxorubicin or other potentially cardiotoxic therapies need a full evaluation by a cardiologist before they can be cleared for sports participation.

SUMMARY POINTS

- Despite the risks associated with chronic medical conditions, affected children should be encouraged to be physically active whenever possible.

- In many instances, the benefits of exercise will outweigh the risks.

- Exercise can increase a child's levels of strength, aerobic fitness, and overall health.

- Physical activity can improve children's emotional well-being.

- Participation in recreational or competitive sports may improve social interaction.

SUGGESTED READING

Adams GR, Vaziri NS. Skeletal muscle dysfunction in chronic renal failure: effects of exercise. *Am J Physiol Renal Physiol.* 2006;290:F753-F761.

American Academy of Pediatrics, Council on Sports Medicine and Fitness. Medical conditions affecting sports participation. *Pediatrics.*2008;121(4):841-848.

American Academy of Family Physicians, American Academy of Pediatrics, American College of Sports

Medicine, American Orthopedic Society of Sports Medicine, American Osteopathic Society of Sports Medicine. *Preparticipation Physical Evaluation.* 3rd ed. New York: McGraw-Hill Healthcare Information, 2004.

American Diabetes Association. Standards of medical care in diabetes. Position statement. *Diabetes Care.* 2006;29(suppl 1):1-85.

Bar-Or O. Pathophysiological factors which limit the exercise capacity of the sick child. *Med Sci Sports Exerc.* 1986;18:276-282.

Bar-Or O, Rowland TW. *Pediatric Exercise Medicine From Physiologic Principles to Health Care Application.* Champaign, IL: Human Kinetics; 2004.

Diabetes Research in Children Network Study Group. Impact of exercise on overnight glycemic control in children with type 1 diabetes mellitus. *J Pediatr.* 2005;147:528-534.

Dodd KJ, Taylor NF, Damiano DL. A systematic review of effectiveness of strength training programs for people with cerebral palsy. *Arch Phys Med Rehabil.* 2002;83:1157-1164.

Eppens MC, Craig ME, Cusumano J, Hing S, Chan AK, Howard NJ, Silink M, Donaghue KC. Prevalence of diabetes complications in adolescents with type 2 compared with type 1 diabetes. *Diabetes Care.* 2006;29(6):1300-1306.

Ginty F, Rennie KL, Mills L, Stear S, Jones S, Prentice A. Positive, site-specific associations between bone mineral status, fitness, and time spent at high-impact activities in 16- to 18-year-old boys. *Bone.* 2005;36:101-110.

Goldberg B, ed. *Sports and Exercise for Children With Chronic Health Conditions.* Champaign, IL: Human Kinetics; 1995.

Harris S, Boggio LN. Exercise may decrease further destruction in the adult haemophilic joint. *Haemophilia.* 2006;12:237-240.

Howard GM, Radloff M, Sevier TL. Epilepsy and sports participation. *Curr Sports Med Rep.* 2004;3:15-19.

Johansen KL. Exercise and chronic kidney disease. *Sports Med.* 2005;35:485-499.

Kelly M, Darrah J. Aquatic exercise for children with cerebral palsy. *Dev Med Child Neurol.* 2005;47:838-842.

Kriemler S, Boguslaw S, Schurer W, Wilson WM, Bar-Or O. Preventing dehydration in children with cystic fibrosis who exercise in the heat. *Med Sci Sports Exerc.* 1999;31:774-779.

Lucia A, Earnest C, Perez M. Cancer-related fatigue: can exercise physiology assist oncologists? *Lancet Oncol.* 2003;4:616-625.

Orenstein DM, Higgins LW. Update on the role of exercise in cystic fibrosis. *Curr Opin Pulm Med.* 2005;11:519-523.

Sherry P. Sickle cell trait and rhabdomyolysis: case report and review of the literature. *Mil Med.* 1990;155:59-61.

Topin N, Matecki S, LeBris S, et al. Dose-dependent effect of individualized respiratory muscle training in children with Duchenne muscular dystrophy. *Neuromuscul Disord.* 2002;12:576-583.

CHAPTER 27

Blood-Borne Pathogens

William L. Risser, MD, PhD

The risk of human immunodeficiency virus (HIV) infection, as well as infection by other blood-borne pathogens such as hepatitis B virus (HBV) and hepatitis C virus (HCV), is a major concern for many athletes, parents, and athletic programs. Immunization against HBV is an important protective measure for everyone involved with athletic programs, including the laundry and janitorial staff. This chapter discusses issues related to infection and transmission of blood-borne pathogens in young athletes. The precautions outlined in this chapter for the prevention of exposure to blood and other body fluids visibly contaminated with blood should help to minimize the chance of transmission of infection.

RISK OF TRANSMISSION AND SPORTS PARTICIPATION BY INFECTED ATHLETES

During athletic activity, children and adolescents may be exposed to blood that is contaminated with HIV, HBV, or HCV. Exposure is most likely to occur in sports such as wrestling, football, boxing, or rugby, in which close physical contact occurs and bleeding wounds are common. Exposure can also occur from contact with blood on equipment, clothing, playing surfaces, or locker room floors. A list of recommended supplies and equipment for sideline wound care is provided in **Table 27.1**.

Findings from studies of HIV transmission in health care settings are summarized in **Table 27.2**. No substantiated cases of HIV transmission have been documented in the athletic setting, although an unsubstantiated report alleges that a professional Italian soccer player infected another player during a collision.

The risk of HIV transmission between athletes is almost certainly much lower than the risk posed to health care workers who are stuck with contaminated needles.

Infection through mucous membranes or damaged skin appears to require prolonged exposure to large quantities of blood. These findings have led several sports medicine organizations to publish policy statements permitting sports participation for HIV-positive athletes, if their health allows. The risk of transmission of infection from HIV-positive athletes is thought to be extremely low, but it cannot be assumed to be nonexistent. The greatest risk of transmission continues to be through sexual activity or illicit intravenous drug use, including use of anabolic steroids. Thus, it is important to advise athletes to practice safe sex and to avoid injecting drugs.

The American Academy of Pediatrics, but no other expert body, suggests that athletes with HIV may be informed of the small risk that they pose to others so that these athletes can consider whether they want to participate in sports that pose the greatest risk of contact with blood, in particular wrestling. All experts agree that health care providers are not authorized to notify the athletic staff or other athletes that a specific athlete is HIV positive without the athlete's and his or her parents' informed consent. In addition to possible legal consequences, unauthorized disclosure of HIV status would probably cause the athlete to be excluded from participation. Furthermore, there are potential legal challenges to testing athletes for blood-borne pathogens solely as a condition or consequence of their sports participation.

Coaches and staff should inform athletes and their families that the athletic program has a policy of nondisclosure of the infection status of athletes, and that a small risk of transmission of HIV infection may exist in sports such as football and wrestling in which bleeding wounds and damaged skin are common. These guidelines also apply to athletes infected with HCV, although this condition is more easily transmitted than HIV.

TABLE 27.1

Recommended Supplies and Equipment for Sideline Wound Care

- Gloves, disposable vinyl or latex
- Soap and water, or alcohol-based antiseptic handwash
- Occlusive dressings
- Towels, disposable and nondisposable
- Bags for disposable blood-contaminated material
- Bags for nondisposable blood-contaminated material
- Basin for mixing bleach solution
- A ¼-cup container and a 1-quart container
- Clean uniforms
- Equipment for assisted ventilations
- Oral airways

TABLE 27.2

Routes of HIV Transmission in Health Care Settings

Type of Exposure	Infection Rate (95% Confidence Interval)
Needlesticks	0.2%-0.3% (0.1-0.5)
Exposure of mucous membranes or damaged skin	0.1% (0.01-0.5)
Exposure of intact skin	0% (0.0-0.1)

HBV presents a greater transmission risk than either HCV or HIV. In Japan, a chronically infected sumo wrestler infected several of his high school team members, apparently by skin-to-skin contact. In the United States, 11 of 65 members of a football team were infected by exposure to an asymptomatic carrier over a period of 19 months. In Sweden, an epidemic of infection was documented among orienteers. Though the mode of transmission was not clear, the source of infection may have been basins of water that were contaminated with blood when they were used to wash open wounds. In health care workers, the risk of infection from percutaneous exposure to HBV may be as great as 45% if the blood is HBV e-antigen positive.

Alone among expert bodies, the National Collegiate Athletic Association recommends that athletes acutely infected with HBV should be removed from close-contact, combative sports such as wrestling until they are no longer infectious. It also recommends that those chronically infected with HBV should be excluded from such sports, particularly if they are e-antigen positive.

PREVENTION OF INFECTION

A series of 3 vaccinations for HBV will protect almost all athletes from the small risk of acquiring infection during sports participation and the greater risk of acquiring infection during sexual activity or intravenous drug use. Health care providers and coaches should urge young athletes, both children and adolescents, to be immunized if they were not immunized when they were younger. In many areas of the country, free HBV vaccinations are available to indigent youths. Because immunization in infancy has become standard practice, in the next few years, most athletes will already have been vaccinated and will probably have lifelong immunity. Individuals who have had fewer than 3 hepatitis B immunizations do not have to start the series over. For example, if they have had 2 of 3, they just need the third. This vaccine provides long-lasting immunity; no booster doses are required.

Administrators and coaches should initiate measures to prevent athletes from being exposed to blood and to protect those who have been exposed. It is particularly important to protect athletes and staff who may be exposed repeatedly, such as adults who give first aid, laundry workers, and cleaners who may handle bloody clothing or equipment. Several organizations have published guidelines for athletic settings that are based on recommendations by the Centers for Disease Control and Prevention (CDC) for health care providers and public safety workers.

A summary of the American Academy of Pediatrics' recommendations for handling blood-borne pathogens in the athletic setting is provided in **Table 27-3**. These recommendations are consistent with those written by the American Medical Society for Sports Medicine, the American Orthopaedic Society for Sports Medicine, and the CDC. Implementation of these recommendations may require additional time and effort from the staff and administrators of athletic programs. However, the recommendations are not complex or demanding, and they may help protect staff and athletes from the small risk of contracting an infection with a blood-borne pathogen.

TABLE 27.3

Recommendations for Handling Blood-borne Pathogens

- Before and during participation, athletes and caregivers should cover damaged skin with an occlusive dressing that will remain intact during vigorous activity.

- Athletes should be instructed to report bleeding wounds immediately. Athletes who are bleeding should be removed from play, and their wounds should be cleaned with soap and water or another skin antiseptic and covered with a durable, occlusive dressing.

- Minor skin damage that is not bleeding may be cleaned and covered during scheduled breaks. During breaks, if an athlete's equipment or uniform is wet with blood, the equipment should be cleaned and disinfected and the uniform replaced.

- Those who treat injuries should wear disposable latex or vinyl gloves to avoid contact with blood or other body fluids visibly contaminated with blood and contaminated equipment or uniforms. After removing their gloves, medical personnel should wash their hands with soap and water or some other disinfectant.

- Equipment and playing surfaces contaminated with blood must be cleaned until all visible blood is gone, and then disinfected with a freshly made bleach solution containing 1 part bleach in 10 parts water. The contaminated equipment or area should be in contact with the bleach solution for at least 30 seconds. The area may be wiped with a disposable cloth after the minimum contact time or be allowed to air-dry.

- Bags used to assist with ventilation and oral airways should be available for use during resuscitation. Mouth-to-mouth resuscitation should be performed only if such equipment is not available.

- Equipment handlers and laundry and janitorial staff should be trained in proper procedures for cleaning bloody surfaces and equipment and for handling washable or disposable materials that are contaminated with blood.

- Depending on state regulations, school athletic programs may be required to comply with Occupational Safety and Health Administration (OSHA) guidelines or other guidelines for preventing infection. Even if it is not required, compliance with OSHA guidelines is a good way to protect the staff.

- Coaches and health care workers should educate athletes about the risks of transmission of blood-borne pathogens through sexual activity and needle sharing during the use of illegal drugs, including anabolic steroids. Athletes should be taught not to share personal items such as razors, nail clippers, and toothbrushes that might be contaminated with blood.

Adapted with permission from Committee on Sports Medicine and Fitness, American Academy of Pediatrics. Human immunodeficiency virus and other blood-borne viral pathogens in the athletic setting. *Pediatrics*. 1999;104:1400-1403.

EFFECTS OF INFECTION ON PERFORMANCE

Strenuous exercise does not appear to increase the risk that athletes with asymptomatic HIV infection will become symptomatic, or adversely affect asymptomatic athletes who have HBV or HCV infections. Young athletes are rarely ill enough from symptomatic HIV infection that they will need to limit their participation in sports. Athletes who are acutely ill with a hepatitis virus should not participate until the fever is gone and they are feeling well. This may take several weeks.

SUMMARY POINTS

- Athletes and athletic program staff may have a small risk of acquiring an HIV, HBV, or HCV infection.

- Experts state that athletes infected with HIV or HCV may be allowed to play all sports. However, there is some disagreement about the participation of athletes acutely or chronically infected with HBV, especially if they are e-antigen positive.

- Athletes are more likely to acquire HBV, HCV, and HIV through sexual activity and needle sharing than during athletic activity. They should be encouraged to practice safe sex and avoid injecting drugs, including anabolic steroids.

- All athletes and athletic program staff should complete the series of 3 immunizations against hepatitis B.

SUGGESTED READING

American Medical Society for Sports Medicine (AMSSM) and the American Orthopaedic Society for Sports Medicine. Human immunodeficiency virus and other blood-borne pathogens in sports. *Clin J Sport Med*. 1995;5:199-204. http://www.newamssm.org/hiv.html. Accessed June 3, 2008.

Committee on Sports Medicine and Fitness, American Academy of Pediatrics. Human immunodeficiency virus and other blood-borne viral pathogens in the athletic setting. *Pediatrics*. 1999;104:1400-1403.

Feller A, Flanigan TP. HIV-infected competitive athletes: what are the risks? What precautions should be taken? *J Gen Intern Med.* 1997;12:243-246.

Guidelines for prevention of transmission of human immunodeficiency virus and hepatitis B virus to health-care and public-safety workers. *MMWR Morb Mortal Wkly Rep.* 1989;38(suppl 6):1-37.

Kordi R, Wallace WA. Blood borne infections in sport: risks of transmission, methods of prevention, and recommendations for hepatitis B vaccination. *Br J Sports Med.* 2004;38:678-684.

Mast EE, Goodman RA, Bond WW, Favero MS, Drotman DP. Transmission of blood-borne pathogens during sports: risk and prevention. *Ann Intern Med.* 1995;122:283-285.

National Collegiate Athletic Association Guideline 21. Blood-borne pathogens and intercollegiate athletics. http://www.ncaa.org/library/sports_sciences/sports_med_handbook/2005-06/2005-06_sports_medicine_handbook.pdf, 54-60.

CHAPTER 28

Skin Conditions

Rodney S. W. Basler, MD

Although certain systems of the body—most notably the cardiovascular, pulmonary, and musculoskeletal systems—benefit directly from physical activity, the integumentary (skin) system, by outward appearances, does not. Because the skin has direct contact with the environment, it often bears the burden of sports-related injuries and infections. With ever-increasing numbers of young children participating in sports activities, sports-related skin conditions are becoming more common. In addition, some skin diseases occur specifically or manifest differently in children and adolescents. Many sports-related skin conditions can be prevented with good hygeine and simple interventions, as listed in **Table 28.1.**

INJURIES

Calluses and Corns

Common calluses are areas in which the stratum corneum, the outermost horny layer of the skin, becomes thickened with excess keratin (**Figure 28.1**). A corn is produced when the stratum corneum forms a conical mass that points up into the dermis, causing inflammation and pain. Calluses and corns are most commonly seen on the feet, although they can develop anywhere the skin is subjected to friction or direct pressure. Golfers, gymnasts, and competitors in racquet sports, for example, can develop prominent calluses on their hands.

Calluses lack the tender spots seen in corns; therefore, calluses, unlike corns, are not painful or irritating. Treatment is often directed toward the prevention of blisters, which can form beneath calluses. After the affected area is soaked, the callus or corn can be pared with a pumice stone,

file, or scalpel blade. Because this represents an area of friction, care should be taken to avoid removing too much excess stratum corneum. This could make the area even more tender. Friction in the area can be reduced by the use of thin padding or an orthotic, or by wearing different shoes.

Competitive athletes are prone to develop calluses, but simple measures such as wearing gloves and properly fitting shoes can often help prevent them.

Blisters

Blisters are tender vesicles that form at a site that is exposed to repetitive frictional or shearing forces (**Figure 28.2**). Nearly all sports expose the skin to these forces, so blisters are common. Any moist environment softens the skin and promotes their formation.

Blisters may be filled with clear fluid or blood, depending on their severity and the site where they occur. They are best treated by draining the fluid up to 3 times in the first 24 hours after their appearance. The epidermal roof of the blister should remain intact to protect the newly forming epidermis. However, if by accident the covering skin is removed, a nonadhesive, permeable sterile membrane (DuoDERM) may be used to cover the blister for 5 to 7 days. This dressing will protect the site and promote healing.

Blisters may be prevented in a number of ways, including use of properly fitting shoes and maintaining sports equipment such as racquet grips. Also, wearing athletic socks made of fabrics that wick moisture from the skin, and using petroleum jelly to lubricate pressure points or those parts of the foot that are in contact with the shoe, may help prevent blister formation.

TABLE 28.1

Prevention of Skin Conditions in Athletes

- Perform good skin hygiene (washing with soap and water)
- Dry skin creases well
- Change absorbent socks frequently
- Wash workout clothes daily
- Wear properly fitted shoes
- Wear shower shoes
- Apply petroleum jelly to bony prominences that are prone to blisters or calluses
- Apply petroleum jelly to opposing skin surfaces to minimize friction
- Soak and pare down calluses
- Wear insulated shoes and gloves (to prevent chilblains)
- Wash with benzoyl peroxide soap (to prevent pitted keratolysis)
- Wear loose-fitting cotton undergarments (to prevent tinea cruris)
- Use drying agents (to prevent tinea cruris)
- Change out of wet swimwear (to prevent occlusive folliculitis)
- Apply antifungal foot powders
- Disinfect floor mats and equipment
- Inspect the skin of athletes before contact sports (to prevent spread of contagious skin lesions)
- Provide occlusive coverage of open or contagious skin lesions

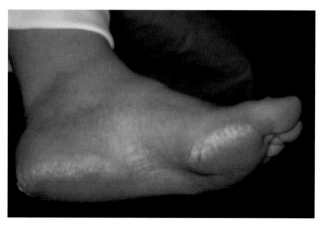

FIGURE 28.1 Callus.

Chafing

Chafing, or inflamed desquamation of the skin, occurs when opposing areas of the body, especially the inner thighs or the armpits, rub together. Chafing may also occur from fabric-to-skin or equipment-to-skin contact. Tennis players and athletes who compete in endurance sports such as bicycling and cross-country running are particularly

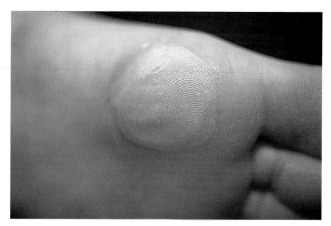

FIGURE 28.2 Blister.

prone to this injury because of sustained, repetitive motion involved with these sports. Although the inner thighs are more commonly involved, chafing can also occur on the skin of the armpits and on the lateral aspect of the neck. In male endurance runners, chafing and bleeding of nipples is common. Application of petroleum jelly to the nipples before running and wearing a loose shirt can help.

Acute chafing is treated by applying cool compresses to the irritated area for 15 to 20 minutes 3 times a day. When exudate is no longer weeping from the area, soothing ointments such as triple-antibiotic ointment or petroleum jelly can be applied to lubricate the skin. Often, this problem can be prevented by wearing longer shorts made of fabrics, such as nylon, that minimize friction. Tight-fitting briefs that extend to the midthigh can be worn, and ointments can be used to lubricate vulnerable areas. Body powders may also reduce friction. Finally, weight loss can eliminate excess subcutaneous fat that makes upper thighs larger, resulting in a smaller area of skin contact between this part of the leg.

Abrasions

Abrasions, also known as turf burn, mat burn, road rash, or strawberries, occur when the epidermis is scraped away by friction, causing punctate bleeding and exudate (**Figure 28.3**). Abrasions are localized to the area of skin that made contact with the friction-producing surface, such as artificial turf, the wooden floor of a basketball court, or a road surface.

Initial treatment should include cleansing the area with warm water and antibacterial soap or with hydrogen peroxide. Gravel or any other particulate matter should be débrided from the wound. A sterile, nonadhesive membrane may then be applied to the wound and changed daily for

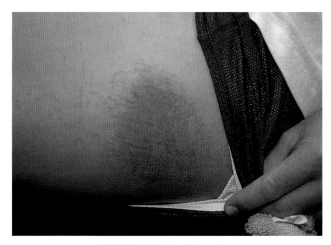

FIGURE 28.3 Abrasion.

several days. For deeper wounds, antibiotic cream or spray should be applied and then covered with a sterile nonadhesive membrane, which should be changed daily. Heavier ointments should be avoided because they hold in infectious bacteria. Careful débridement, cleansing, topical antibiotic prophylaxis, and use of sterile nonadhesive membranes minimize the risk of secondary infection. Elbows, knees, and other vulnerable areas should be protected with additional clothing and pads to prevent abrasions.

Cauliflower Ear

Cauliflower ear is the thickening and distortion of the normal auricular cartilage caused by bleeding into the soft tissue of the ear (**Figure 28.4**). The inflammatory response to the

blood causes destruction and scarring of the cartilage. Direct trauma or friction of the ear causes this injury, which occurs most commonly in wrestlers, rugby players, and boxers who fail to use protective headgear or who use headgear that does not fit properly. A hematoma of the ear should be drained within the first several days after the injury. Under sterile conditions, the blood can be aspirated with a syringe and small needle (23 or 21 gauge). A compression dressing should be applied to the ear to prevent rebleeding. For the compression dressing, a variety of materials have been used successfully, including sterile saline-soaked cotton, flexible collodion, silicone putty, or plaster of Paris. Anything that molds to the contour of the ear will work. Gauze or elastic wrap needs to be wrapped around the head to provide gentle compression to the ear and dressing for at least 24 hours. Athletes should be advised to seek medical attention at the first sign of infection. The longer the wrestler can stay off the mat, the less likely the ear will rebleed, and the better the cosmetic result. Plastic surgeons generally do not consider any reconstructive surgery of a deformed ear until a wrestler has completed his career. Use of properly fitting headgear will usually prevent the injury.

Black Heel and Black Palm

Black heel, also called talon noir, is characterized by blue-black spots on the back or side of the heel (**Figure 28.5**). For reasons that are not well understood, black heel primarily affects teenagers and young adults, especially basketball players. It is asymptomatic, and its palmar equivalent, black palm, affects weight lifters, golfers, and tennis players. Black heel requires no special diagnostic procedures or treatment, and as a rule, it resolves spontaneously at the end of the athletic season or when the athletic activity is stopped.

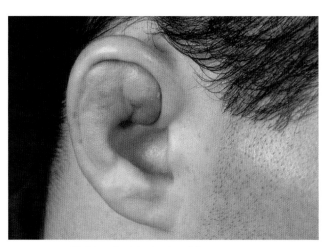

FIGURE 28.4 Cauliflower ear.

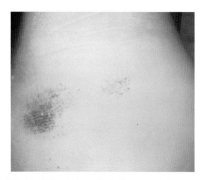

FIGURE 28.5 Black heel (talon noir). Reproduced with permission from Basler RSW, Garcia MA. Acing common skin problems in tennis players. Physician Sportsmed. 1998;26:38.

Acne Mechanica

The combined effects of heat, occlusion, pressure, and friction—especially that caused by football and hockey equipment—lead to the appearance of inflammatory papules and pustules on the skin (**Figure 28.6**). This condition, known as acne mechanica, may be a flare-up of preexisting acne in teenagers or a new condition in prepubertal boys. Acne mechanica tends to be localized under the areas of the body that support the weight of athletic equipment, such as the shoulders, forehead, and chin in football and hockey players; the shoulders and lateral back of golfers who carry their bags; and the center of the back in weight lifters, where it comes into contact with the weight bench. If left untreated, cystic lesions may develop.

Systemic antibiotics do not work as well for acne mechanica as they do in treating acne vulgaris. Therefore, the affected area should be cleansed thoroughly with a mildly abrasive cleanser and brush after each workout. Topical astringents or 10% benzoyl peroxide often helps. The acne lesions tend to greatly improve or completely resolve at the end of the athletic season when the athletes no longer wear the equipment.

Football and hockey players should be advised to wear clean, absorbent T-shirts under their pads to prevent acne mechanica. During the off-season, the underlying acne vulgaris can be controlled with aggressive systemic and topical therapy.

Hemorrhage Under the Toenails and Fingernails

Hemorrhage under the nails, which is sometimes proudly displayed by athletes as a kind of badge of courage, occurs in many sports, notably running, skiing, bicycling, and tennis. In this last group, it is referred to as tennis toe. In this type of injury, the nail bed separates from the nail plate when the toes are repeatedly jammed into the front of the shoe (**Figure 28.7**). Although the pressure of the blood collecting under the nail plate can cause severe pain and disfigurement, serious medical consequences are rare.

In disabling cases when the patient reports such severe pain that he or she cannot walk, the blood can be drained from under the nail with a cauterizing instrument or a red-hot paper clip. Care must be taken to avoid penetrating the nail bed. In most instances, however, these hemorrhages can be treated nonsurgically by soaking the foot in warm water. Prevention includes trimming the great toenails across in a straight line to a comfortable length. Athletic shoes must be fitted carefully for length and, more important, the height of the toe box.

Pernio (Chilblains)

Pernio, or chilblains, is an unusual injury to the skin caused by vasoconstriction in response to acute hypothermia. This condition is seen predominantly in teenage and young adult women for reasons that are not well understood, particularly in ice skaters and skiers. The distal segments of the toes, and occasionally the fingers, become blue or violet and are painful and exquisitely tender (**Figure 28.8**).

The simplest way to treat this condition is to advise the patient to wear heavy socks at all times, even while sleeping. Low-potency corticosteroid creams will help to eliminate inflammation without causing further vasoconstriction. In severe cases, a systemic vasodilator, such as infedipine, might be considered. To prevent pernio, the use of any tight-fitting clothing or equipment such as gloves or ski boots should be avoided. When outdoors in cold weather, athletes should be reminded to rewarm the extremities whenever possible.

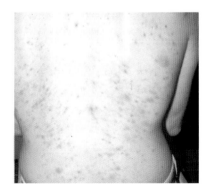

FIGURE 28.6 Acne mechanica. Reproduced with permission from Basler RSW, Garcia MA. Acing common skin problems in tennis players. Physician Sportsmed. 1998;26:43.

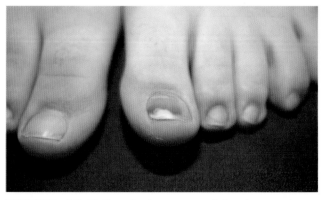

FIGURE 28.7 Tennis toe caused by hemorrhage under the nail.

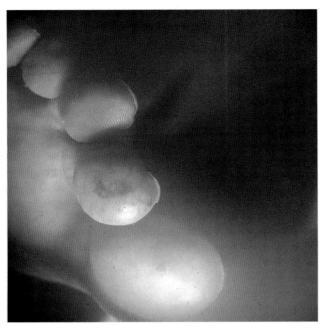

FIGURE 28.8 Pernio in young woman skier.

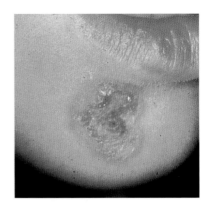

FIGURE 28.9 Impetigo.

INFECTIONS

Impetigo and Methicillin-Resistant *Staphylococcus aureus*

Superficial bacterial infections, referred to as impetigo or pyoderma, can develop in association with nearly all contact sports and may reach epidemic proportions in wrestlers. Virulent bacterial strains, especially staphylococcal and streptococcal species, may be spread by direct contact or fomites such as equipment and improperly sterilized mats. Community-acquired methicillin-resistant *Staphylococcus aureus* has become of special interest to sports medicine practitioners because of its fulminate course and the difficulty of completely eliminating the organism. Large abscesses that develop rapidly and that are extremely tender and inflamed should be surgically drained and should alert the provider to initiate therapy with a sulfa-based antibiotic while waiting for culture results. Other options include the oral antibiotic linezolid, which is appropriate for adolescents over age 16, or clindamycin if the strain is not resistant to those medications. Gymnasts are at risk for infection from abrasions received from gymnastic equipment, especially the pommel horse.

Impetigo manifests as pustules or small purulent bullae on exposed areas of skin, with predilection for those areas bordering mucous membranes, such as around the mouth and nose (**Figure 28.9**). These lesions rapidly progress to shallow erosions with a heavy yellow or honey-colored crust. Infected athletes should not come into direct contact with other athletes or equipment until evidence of infection, specifically purulent drainage, has resolved. Careful attention to sterilization of mats and equipment on a regular schedule is mandatory. Athletes should be strongly encouraged to shower with an antibacterial soap immediately after competition.

Treatment of small areas of impetigo can be carried out by gently scrubbing the involved area, followed by the application of triple-antibiotic or mupirocin cream 3 times a day. However, in most instances, appropriate systemic antibiotic therapy is advised to reduce contagion and to permit the athlete to return to competition as soon as possible.

Erythrasma

Another superficial dermatologic infection that is occasionally encountered in young athletes, most likely because of the heavy concentration of perspiration in the skin folds and increase in body heat during physical exertion, manifests as irregular, dry, scaling patches, pink to brown in color. This is referred to as erythrasma. The inguinal creases and toe webs are most commonly involved, but the condition may remain asymptomatic in the latter location. Persistent scratching leads to excoriations and lichenification, especially in the groin. The key to diagnosis is the demonstration of red-orange fluorescence under a Wood's lamp, a finding that is pathognomonic for the disease.

Treatment of erythrasma is usually confined to conservative measures, beginning with the use of an antibacterial soap, such as Cetaphil Antibacterial or Lever 2000. Topical acne-fighting preparations, particularly aqueous solutions of 2% erythromycin or 2% clindamycin, will usually eliminate the *Corynebacterium* species responsible for the infection. Systemic erythromycin administered over 2 to 3 weeks may be required for difficult cases. The problem will usually persist indefinitely if left untreated.

Occlusive Folliculitis

Occlusive folliculitis is a deep infection that is usually seen in the area under protective padding or swimsuits. It is similar in appearance to acne mechanica and produces more inflamed pustules (**Figure 28.10**). One of the more common examples of this condition is the so-called bikini bottom, which occurs in swimmers who wear their swimwear for long periods of time. The tender pustules may become cystic and appear in areas that coincide with the overlying clothing or equipment.

Although topical antibiotics such as clindamycin or erythromycin solutions may greatly improve mild cases, systemic antibiotics are often required. Prevention includes changing out of swimwear as soon as possible after workouts or during long days at the beach. Absorbent powder applied to the involved areas after showering may also help.

Pitted Keratolysis

Malodorous footwear and athletic socks are a nearly universal finding among young athletes, especially boys. With pitted keratolysis, however, a species of bacteria invades the epidermis and causes a particularly pungent foot odor. Besides the odor, the skin appears white and macerated with distinct pits and surrounding areas of faint erythema (**Figure 28.11**). Excessive sweating is almost always present.

Affected areas should be cleansed with an antibacterial soap and treated with an over-the-counter acne preparation such as 10% benzoyl peroxide gel. Topical prescription products such as clindamycin and erythromycin solutions are also effective. Prevention includes washing the feet with an antibacterial soap, drying them with a towel, and then allowing the feet to air-dry. Applying absorbent powder under socks is also helpful.

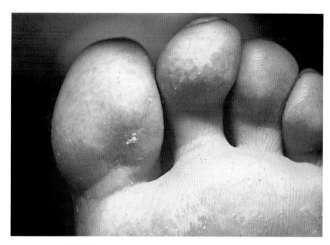

FIGURE 28.11 Pitted keratolysis.

Plantar Warts

Plantar warts are painful and tender hyperkeratotic papules that can erupt anywhere on the soles of the feet. The combination of the macerating effect of perspiration; exposure to the human papilloma virus; and the warm, moist environment of the locker room contribute to the development of plantar warts. In severe cases, symptoms can be nearly disabling, especially when the lesions occur over the weight-bearing areas of the foot. Small black dots, which are the tips of capillaries in the skin, help differentiate these lesions from corns and calluses (**Figure 28.12**). Confluence of individual papules over a large area of the foot may result in mosaic plantar warts.

Aggressive therapies to excise and desiccate the wart with electric currents or lasers carry significant risks of short- and long-term disability, including the inability to

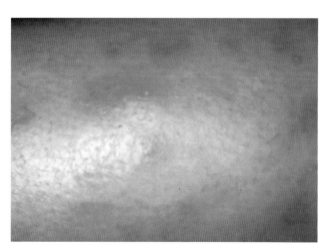

FIGURE 28.10 Occlusive folliculitis.

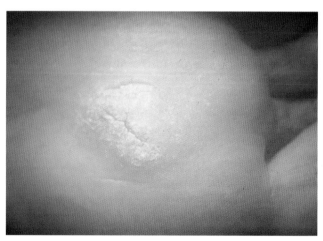

FIGURE 28.12 Plantar wart.

walk, and can leave permanent scarring. More conservative approaches generally permit the athlete to continue competition during treatment. The application of liquid nitrogen to warts on the sole is less advantageous than when it is used on verrucae in other locations because the thick plantar skin often does not cause a deep enough blister to encompass the root of the wart, even though the large blisters that form often cause significant pain and morbidity, especially in young athletes. Shaving the warts and applying cantharidin under occlusion for 2 to 3 days, or prescribing 40% salicylic acid plasters, changed daily, are preferred methods of treatment. The use of shower thongs in the locker room and foot powders or a topical 10% aluminum chloride solution can diminish maceration of the skin.

Molluscum Contagiosum

Molluscum contagiosum is an infection caused by a virus of the pox group that is common among children and adolescents, particularly among young wrestlers, who refer to them as wrestler's warts (**Figure 28.13**). This infection, which is also seen with some frequency in swimmers, is identified by its groups of small, waxy, fleshy papules that often have central depressions or pits.

A small number of mollusca can be removed easily by curettage, although this procedure causes superficial epidermal abrasions. Freezing the papules with liquid nitrogen or stripping them with a high-quality adhesive tape are simple techniques to treat the infection. Prevention consists primarily of avoiding infected competitors and aggressively removing lesions as soon as they appear to prevent self-inoculation. Infected wrestlers should not participate in practice or competition unless lesions are solitary or localized and clustered and can be covered with a gas-permeable membrane, followed by ProWrap and stretch tape.

Herpes Gladiatorum

Herpes gladiatorum, or wrestler's herpes, is a herpes simplex viral infection that most commonly affects the head, neck, and upper extremities. Its characteristic groups of vesicles appear on red, swollen, edematous skin (**Figure 28.14**).

Systemic antiviral medications similar to those used against other types of herpes infection, including acyclovir, valacyclovir, and famciclovir, are indicated. Specific suggestions for immediate initial therapy are listed in **Table 28.2**. To promote healing, the epidermal roof of individual vesicles can be removed, followed by application of benzoin to the base of the lesion and the intradermal injection of dilute triamcinolone under the infected areas. As with all of the skin infections in athletes, infected competitors should not wrestle until all the lesions are scabbed over, but noncontact conditioning is permissible. Contact with others must be avoided until the vesicles dry. In an athlete with a history of herpes infection, prophylaxis includes long-term, low-dose suppression therapy with acyclovir throughout the course of the season when the athlete may be exposed to infected individuals. Any wrestler with more than one outbreak in a season should be considered for suppression therapy.

General Fungal Infections

The intimate relationship between fungi and sports is evidenced by commonly used terms such as athlete's foot and jock itch. In nearly every instance, the increased incidence of the infection in athletes is due to the effect of perspiration, which breaks down the natural barrier

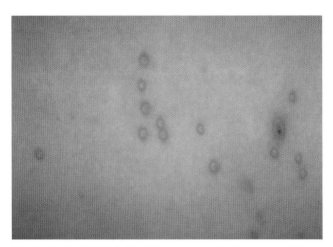

FIGURE 28.13 Molluscum contagiosum.

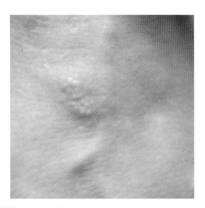

FIGURE 28.14 Herpes gladiatorum.

of a dry, intact epidermis and makes the skin vulnerable to invasion of fungal elements.

Tinea Versicolor and onychomycosis Some fungal infections, such as tinea versicolor and onychomycosis, have widespread distribution among human populations and are commonly seen in nonathletic patients. However, the fact that *Malassezia furfur,* the causative organism for tinea versicolor, has a natural predilection for sand contributes to a high risk of infection among participants of water sports and beach volleyball. Because repeated trauma to toenails may add to susceptibility for fungal infection, athletes may demonstrate increased potential for onychomycosis. The treatment for both of these conditions in athletes is the same as for the general population and is provided in **Table 28.2**.

Tinea Pedis The term *tinea pedis* refers specifically to dermatophyte infection of the foot; *athlete's foot* is a more generic term that may encompass bacterial and yeast infection, and may even extend to contact dermatitis and dyshidrotic eczema. Although all of these conditions share common characteristics such as erythema, scaling, and vesicle formation, tinea pedis usually originates in the toe webs, with the fourth toe web nearly always involved, and manifests with sharp margination, most often unilaterally.

The continuously damp environment of locker rooms, particularly showers, is often the source of infective fungal elements, combining a maximum concentration of organisms with a minimally resistant barrier represented by the macerated skin over the foot. Because of these causative factors, wearing shower thongs and using fungistatic powders such as Zeasorb-AF after carefully drying the feet are of definitive preventive benefit. Treatment suggestions are included in **Table 28.2**. Suppression of toe web fungus is important in diminishing the chance of its spreading to other areas of the body from this reservoir of infection.

Tinea Corporis and Cruris Fungal infections in susceptible areas of the body, especially the skin folds of the axilla and groin, are usually the result of organisms being transported from the toe webs, often by towel drying after a shower, and the feet need to be carefully examined when a diagnosis of tinea corporis or capitis is being entertained. The exception to this rule is the tinea gladiatorum infection, which is often seen in wrestlers as a result of direct-contact transmission. This specific entity is covered in detail in the following section dealing with skin problems in wrestlers.

Tinea cruris manifests as a sharply marginated erythema with some scaling centered in the inguinal crease. Unlike yeast infections, fungal infections will not involve the actual genitalia because of the fungistatic effect of scrotal and vulvar sebum. The diagnostic signs of tinea capitis are also discussed in detail in the section on wrestling, and treatment options are listed in **Table 28.2**.

Scabies

Although scabies is more correctly listed under the category of infestation rather than infection, it is another skin disease that can produce a miniepidemic among members of an athletic team. Intense itching is the hallmark of this disease, which is sometimes spread by towels, uniforms, or equipment. Affected individuals usually have excoriated papules or small vesicles appearing in lines, almost always on the webs of the fingers (**Figure 28.15**). Intensely pruritic papules on the skin of the penile shaft are characteristic signs of scabies.

Treatment of scabies must be aggressive and persistent. The drug of choice is 5% permethrin. One percent lindane lotion, the gold standard of treatment in the past, is no longer recommended because of neurologic concerns. Permethrin should be removed by bathing 8 to 14 hours after application. Individuals with scabietic eczema can use corticosteroid cream to treat pruritus. As with the other skin infections, any athlete who has a suspicious rash—especially one with pruritic papules on the back of the hand, wrist, or webs of the fingers—should not compete or practice. The athlete may return to competition after appropriate treatment.

Wrestling

Wrestlers represent a particularly difficult subset of young athletes in terms of prevention of infection because of the prevalence of organisms and the skin-to-skin contact. In addition, superficial abrasions, which are universally present in competitors, offer easy access to the deeper layers of the epidermis. **Table 28.3** lists National Collegiate Athletic Association guidelines for skin conditions and participation in wrestling.

Fungal infections are a special concern in wrestlers, with incidence rates as high as 77% among members of high school wrestling teams. The presentation of erythematous bull's-eye plaques with inflammation and scaling, from which the term ringworm derives, poses little diagnostic challenge, but unfortunately is rarely seen. The trichophyton species that usually causes tinea corporis in wrestlers tends to produce lesions that are nondescript, with mild erythema and fine scale (**Figure 28.16**). Initial scalp lesions are often difficult to differentiate from seborrheic eczema.

TABLE 28.2

Pharmacologic Treatment of Common Skin Conditions in Athletes

Condition	Treatment
Impetigo	• Mupirocin ointment 3 times a day for 10-14 days for minor cases
	• 10-day course of cephalosporin or penicillinase-resistant penicillin derivative
	• For suspected methicillin-resistant *Staphylococcus aureus*, 10-day course of sulfa-based antibiotic, clindamycin or linezolid
Erythrasma	• Antibacterial soap such as Cetaphil Antibacterial or Lever 2000
	• Topical 2% erythromycin gel or ointment twice a day for 10-14 days
	• Erythromycin 250 mg by mouth 4 times a day for 14 days
Occlusive folliculitis	• 1% clindamycin solution twice a day
	• Systemic antibiotics: cephalexin 500 mg twice a day for 2-4 weeks
Pitted keratolysis	• Topical 10% benzoyl peroxide twice a day for 2-4 weeks
Verrucae (warts)	• Keratolytic agents: salicylic acid solutions or tape
	• Liquid nitrogen
	• Cantharidin
	• Laser treatment
	• Surgical removal by curettage
Molluscum contagiosum	• Liquid nitrogen
	• Cantharidin
	• Curettage
	• Electrodesiccation
	• Imiquimod 5% cream
Herpes gladiatorum	*If >18 years old:*
	• Famciclovir 250 mg 3 times a day for 10 days for initial outbreak; 5 days for recurrence
	• Valacyclovir 1 g twice a day for 10 days for initial outbreak; 5 days for recurrence
	If <18 years of age:
	• Acyclovir 40-80 mg/kg/d, divided, 3-4 times a day for 7-10 days
	• Prophylaxis: 400-800 mg acyclovir daily throughout the sports season
Tinea versicolor	• Topical 2.5% selenium sulfate shampoo (Selsun). Apply from the neck down to thighs for 15-30 minutes before rinsing off for 5-10 days. Alternatively, apply the lotion overnight (for 6-12 hours) from the neck down to thighs, rinsing off the next morning, reapplying weekly to prevent recurrence
	• For extensive disease, ketoconazole 200 mg once a day for 7-10 days or 400 mg once a month; exercising to produce perspiration within 1 hour after taking medication may promote effectiveness
Onychomycosis	• Itraconazole 200 mg once a day for 12 weeks for toenails; 6 weeks for fingernails
	• Itraconazole 400 mg once a day for the first week of 3-4 successive months
	• Terbinafine 250 mg once a day for 12 weeks for toenails; 6 weeks for fingernails
Tinea pedis	• Topical antifungal cream (miconazole, clotrimazole, econazole) twice a day for 6-8 weeks
Tinea corporis	• Fluconazole 200 mg once a week for 4 weeks
	• Terbinafine cream in children for minor cases twice a day for 4 weeks
Tinea cruris	• Topical antifungal cream (miconazole, clotrimazole, econazole) twice a day for 2-4 weeks
Scabies	• 5% permethrin applied from neck down for 8-14 hours, then rinsed off and repeated in 7 days

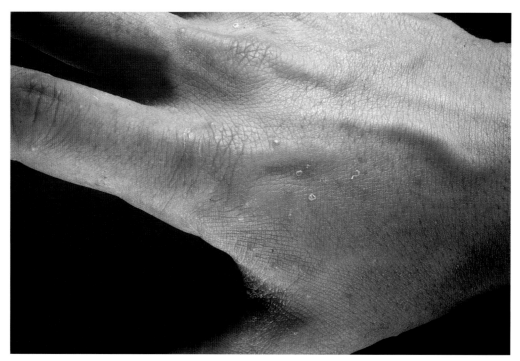

FIGURE 28.15 Scabies on the hand of a wrestler.

TABLE 28.3

NCAA Guidelines for Skin Conditions and Participation in Wrestling

Condition	To Participate, the Wrestler Must:
Abrasions	• Provide occlusive dressing during competition
	• Be removed from competition for active bleeding and universal precautions implemented
Bacterial infections (impetigo)	• Be without new lesions for 48 hours before a meet
	• Have completed 72 hours of antibiotic therapy
	• Have no moist or draining lesions before competition
Tinea corporis	• Have completed 72 hours of topical terbinafine or naftifine
	• Have completed 2 weeks of oral therapy for scalp lesions
	• Adequately cover all lesions with an antifungal cream, gas-permeable dressing, and ProWrap with stretch tape
Herpes gladiatorum	• Be free of systemic symptoms
	• Have not developed lesions in the past 72 hours
	• Have firm, adherent crust on all lesions
	• Have received antiviral therapy for 120 hours
Verruca	• Cover multiple digitate verruca of the face with a mask
	• Have simple coverage of verruca plana or vulgaris
Molluscum contagiosum	• Have lesions curetted or removed before competition; solitary or localized, clustered lesions can be covered with a gas-permeable membrane, followed by ProWrap and stretch tape

NCAA indicates National Collegiate Athletic Association.
Reprinted with permission from Bubb RG. Appendix D: skin infections. In: Halpin T, ed. *NCAA 2007: Wrestling Rules and Interpretations*. Indianapolis, IN: National Collegiate Athletic Association; 2006;WA-14–WA-18.

In these cases, learning that the child is a wrestler while taking the child's history may be the most important diagnostic finding. Questionable cases seen during the competitive season should be immediately referred to a dermatologist.

Treatment of fungal infections in wrestlers has to be rapid and aggressive. Topical cidal-type antifungals such as terbinafine or butenafine, applied 4 times daily, are of some benefit. Minor cases manifest as a single plaque or up to 6 superficial localized plaques. However, when inflamed indurated nodules appear, systemic therapy with terbinafine or itraconazole will usually need to be initiated

and provided for at least 4 weeks, often beyond the point that the infection is clinically evident.

Clearance for return to wrestling competition can be given only when all visible lesions have responded to treatment, which generally represents 10 days of topical treatment in minor cases or at least 2 weeks of systemic therapy in more extensive cases. However, wrestlers with solitary or closely clustered, localized lesions need not be disqualified if involvement is in a body location that can be covered securely with a barrier membrane such as OpSite or Second Skin. Dressings should be changed after each match to allow the area to air-dry.

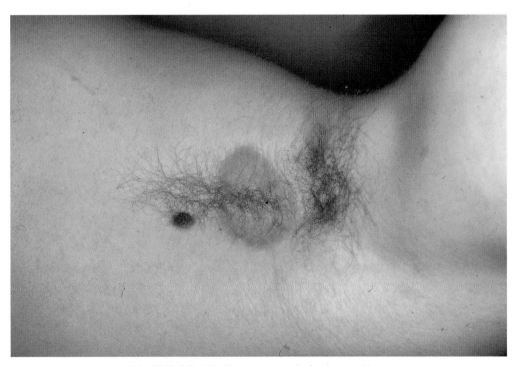

FIGURE 28.16 Tinea corporis in a wrestler.

SUMMARY POINTS

- When identified early and treated properly, most sports-related cutaneous conditions will not cause serious interruption of athletic participation by children or adolescents.

- Athletic injuries to the skin can usually be prevented from recurring in young sports participants by using commonsense methods of intervention.

- The combination of hospitable conditions for invasion, which result from the macerating effect of perspiration, and an abundance of available organisms promotes su-

perficial infections, particularly in skin folds of young athletes.

- Young wrestlers represent a specific subset of athletes at increased risk of various infections because of the skin-to-skin contact and superficial abrasions inherent to the sport.

SUGGESTED READING

Basler RS, Basler DL, Basler GC, Garcia MA. Cutaneous injuries in women athletes. *Dermatol Nurs.* 1998;10:9-18.

Basler RSW. Managing skin problems in athletes. In: Mellion MB, Walsh WM, Shelton GL, eds. *The Team Physician's Handbook.* 3rd ed. Philadelphia, PA: Hanley and Belfus; 2002:311-325.

Basler RSW. Athletic skin injuries: combating pressure and friction. *Physician Sportsmed.* 2004 (May);32, 33-40.

Bubb RG. Appendix D: skin infections. In: Halpin T, ed. *NCAA 2007: Wrestling Rules and Interpretations.* Indianapolis, IN: National Collegiate Athletic Association; 2006;WA-14–WA-18.

Cordoro KM, Ganz JE. Training room management of medical conditions: sports dermatology. *Clin Sports Med.* 2005;24:565-598,viii-ix.

Levine N. Dermatologic aspects of sports medicine. *Dermatol Nurs.* 1994;6:179-186.

Pharis DB, Teller C, Wolf JE Jr. Cutaneous manifestations of sports participation. *J Am Acad Dermatol.* 1997;36(3 pt l):448-459.

SECTION 5

Musculoskeletal Conditions

CHAPTER 29

Introduction to the Musculoskeletal System

Steven J. Anderson, MD

njuries to the musculoskeletal system account for a large proportion of the medical encounters between athletes and their care providers. Accordingly, the field of sports medicine is heavily weighted toward the care of musculoskeletal problems. Greater numbers of young people are participating in organized sports. Regular physical activity is also increasingly being recognized as important for the health of all young people. As a result, the care of active and athletic individuals—including the care of musculoskeletal problems—has become an integral part of general pediatrics.

Primary care providers who work with children are most often the initial contact point for the care of sports injuries and orthopedic problems. Specialized care for every sports injury by an orthopedist or sports medicine expert is neither necessary nor practical. Primary care providers trained to handle orthopedic problems can offer timely access to care for athletic injuries and are more likely to know the patient's medical and family background. Familiarity with the patient's general medical history is useful in understanding an individual's injury risk, the effect of injury on overall health, and a patient's readiness to return to play after injury. Finally, because most musculoskeletal injuries do not require surgical treatment, physicians who focus on nonsurgical care are better oriented to the problems that do tend to occur.

To effectively manage musculoskeletal problems, it is necessary to understand the anatomy and function of the musculoskeletal system, the pathogenesis of common injuries, the tools for efficient clinical evaluation, and strategies for planning effective treatment. This chapter summarizes some of the general principles that can be used when assessing a young athlete's musculoskeletal system. There are predictable patterns to injury and recurring themes in musculoskeletal medicine that connect problems that initially seem unrelated. Appreciating these patterns and themes can make common injuries easier to understand and uncommon injuries easier to evaluate. The efficiency of clinical evaluation can also be enhanced by knowing which diagnostic tools to use in which situations, as well as learning to better interpret the directional signs that the patient provides. Understanding the pathomechanical and clinical characteristics of selected categories of injury can help physicians make a diagnosis from confusing clinical findings or confirm that a suspected diagnosis is correct.

PATHOGENESIS OF INJURY

The primary function of the musculoskeletal system is locomotion. The skeleton gives the muscles and joints a framework for movement. Bony structures also provide protection of internal organs. Musculoskeletal health is critical to all active and athletic individuals. The system that is most responsible for performing sporting activities is also the system most likely to break down from sports participation.

Injury to musculoskeletal structures disrupts musculoskeletal function and affects other systems. For example, the cardiovascular system depends on movement for optimal health and function. Physical inactivity can adversely affect cardiovascular health. Conversely, disease in other organ systems can affect musculoskeletal function. Injury to the central nervous system can compromise muscle contractility, motor control, balance, and coordination. Cardiovascular compromise may affect the development of muscle strength and endurance. Rheumatologic disorders can directly affect muscles, tendons, and joints and can have indirect effects through cardiac, respiratory, and peripheral vascular function. Because musculoskeletal disorders may affect other organ systems, and because disorders in other organ systems may affect the musculoskeletal system, musculoskeletal problems cannot be viewed in isolation. Accordingly, comprehensive assessment and management of musculoskeletal problems may need to extend beyond the musculoskeletal system.

The functional components of the musculoskeletal system include bones, growth plates, cartilage, ligaments, muscles, tendons, and the neurovascular system. Dysfunction of the musculoskeletal system or its component parts may be a result of injury or disease process. Dysfunction of one structural component may lead to disease or dysfunction of related structures or other organ systems. Injury is the most common perturbation of the musculoskeletal system in a sports setting, so this discussion focuses on injury evaluation.

The working components of the musculoskeletal system function as a series of pulleys, levers, and hinges. With movement or activity, there are forces of tension, compression, or torsion on these structures. With sports activities, the movements and forces on these structures are likely to be more forceful and more frequent than the stresses associated with daily activity. Injuries can occur from acute or repetitive stress. With acute injuries, a single, maximal force exceeds a structure's tolerance and can lead to breakdown or failure of that structure. A fracture is an acute injury resulting in failure of bone; a sprain is a failure of ligament; and a strain is a failure of musculotendinous structure.

Repetitive, submaximal forces can also lead to injury. Overuse injuries can occur from the cumulative effect of repetitive forces. A stress fracture is a repetitive stress injury to bone; tendonitis is a repetitive stress injury to a tendon. Bursitis, fasciitis, periostitis, and apophysitis are repetitive stress injuries to the related structures. In cases of overuse injury, the forces causing injury have to be repeated over time to produce clinical evidence of injury.

With each category of injury, there is a particular type of force or mechanism most likely to lead to that injury. For each structure, there is a path of least resistance whereby a predictable combination of circumstances—movement, direction, position, load, tension, or speed—will be most

likely to result in injury. For example, the ankle joint has the least amount of bony stability when it is plantarflexed and inverted. This is the position where ligament support is most crucial for maintaining stability, and accordingly, it is the position where the ankle is most vulnerable to sprains. However, if the ankle is dorsiflexed and everted, there is greater bony stability. Injuries that occur in this position are more likely to be bony in nature. If the distal fibular physis is immature, then the physis may be more susceptible to injury than the associated ligaments or bone.

Virtually all injury categories and anatomic structures have similarly predictable circumstances that lead to injuries. Familiarity with these injury patterns and vulnerabilities can help direct the evaluation of musculoskeletal complaints and can lead to an appreciation of the logic that underlies musculoskeletal injuries. For each of the categories of injuries discussed, the various subtypes of injury are reviewed, as are the most common mechanisms of injury and the positions of greatest vulnerability.

CATEGORIES OF MUSCULOSKELETAL INJURY

Bony Injuries

Although the term *fracture* is a relatively specific reference to bony injury, there are many subtypes and categories of fracture. Long bones have a diaphysis, metaphysis, and epiphysis. *Physis* refers to the cartilaginous growth plate. A growth center that serves as an attachment for a major tendon group is called an apophysis (**Figure 29.1**).

The particular area of the bone that is injured may have different implications for treatment and long-term outcome. The diaphysis or shaft of a long bone can bend through plastic deformation or can bend and fracture through a single cortex in a greenstick fracture. Fracture through both cortices can occur in a transverse, oblique, or spiral pattern.

The metaphysis is the flared portion at the end of a bone. In growing children, the cortex in the metaphysis is thinner than other parts of the bone. Axial loads to the thin metaphyseal cortex can cause a buckling deformity known as a torus or buckle fracture (**Figure 29.2**).

Because the epiphysis contributes to long bone formation, fractures through the epiphysis can lead to disruption of long bone growth. The epiphysis also contributes to the formation of a joint surface. Fractures that displace the epiphyseal portion of the bone or extend into the joint can lead to joint deformity and degenerative arthritis. Fractures through the physeal plate and the epiphysis are categorized according to the Salter-Harris classification (**Figure 29.3**). The risk of growth disruption from an epiphyseal fracture

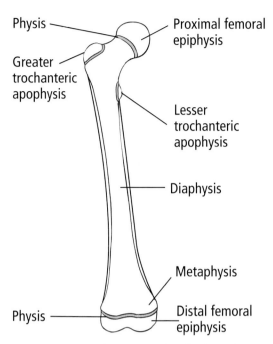

FIGURE 29.1 Components of a long bone.

is generally higher as the Salter-Harris classification number increases. The degree of displacement or deformity of the fracture and the amount of remaining growth in the injured epiphysis also contribute to the risk of long-term growth disruption.

Salter-Harris type I and V fractures may be particularly difficult to diagnose because the injury occurs through the physis. If the typical radiolucent line of a fracture is superimposed on the radiolucent line of the physis, radiographic findings may be subtle or nonexistent. Failure to recognize physeal injuries is a concern because of the risk for long-term disturbances of bone or joint growth. Young athletes with physeal injuries or suspected physeal injuries may benefit from consultation with a pediatric orthopedic specialist. Physeal injuries also warrant long-term monitoring until it is clear that growth has not been altered or until bony maturation has occurred.

The apophysis is a growth center that serves as an attachment point for a major tendon or ligament. Chronic injuries from repetitive stress to the apophysis are common but may not be evident on x-ray. Examples of chronic apophyseal injuries include Osgood-Schlatter disease and Sever's disease. An acute apophyseal avulsion will be evident on x-ray because of visible displacement of the apophysis. Because the apophysis does not contribute to long bone growth or the formation of a joint, apophyseal inju-

ries do not have the same risks for growth disturbance associated with epiphyseal injuries.

A fracture through a bone that has been weakened by prior injury or disease process is a pathologic fracture. Fractures through a bone cyst or a tumor, or fractures in conjunction with osteoporosis, are examples of pathologic fractures. A prior fracture that healed with a fibrous union or nonunion may become painful with activity or become the source of a new fracture.

Fractures that cause more than 2 separate bony fragments are comminuted fractures. Fractures that communicate with an open skin wound are called compound or open fractures.

Fractures should be described by their location, the orientation of the fracture, and the amount of displacement of the fracture fragments. An angulated fracture indicates that the bony fragments are no longer in anatomic alignment. The degree of angulation is measured with the most proximal fragment used as a reference point. The apparent degree of angulation can change with different x-ray views (**Figure 29.4**). In Figure 29.4A, the fracture through the metaphysis is subtle and the alignment of the first metacarpal appears normal. Figure 29.4B was obtained from a slightly different angle. This view revealed significant deformity and indicated a need for closed reduction and percutaneous pinning.

Fracture ends may be separated, or the ends may overlap in bayonet apposition. Compression fractures are most common in vertebral bodies but can occur in the small carpal or tarsal bones of the wrist or foot.

Stress fractures occur from repetitive, submaximal stress to the bone rather than as the result of an acute event. A stress fracture often does not appear on plain radiographs; if it is present, then it may appear as a subtle lucency. A hairline fracture is an acute injury in which the fracture line is thin and the fracture is nondisplaced. Although the radiographic findings may be similar, stress fractures and hairline fractures have different injury mechanisms, require different forms of treatment, and have different recovery times.

Fractures in which a tendon or ligament attachment pulls away a fragment of bone are known as avulsion fractures. Avulsion fractures can be easily confused with a painful accessory ossification center or an apophysis. With avulsion fractures, the avulsed fragment is typically more irregular in appearance than an accessory ossicle, and a donor site or defect from the avulsed fragment can usually be identified. An apophysis or apophyseal avulsion can be distinguished from an avulsion fracture by comparison x-rays of the asymptomatic side. A normal apophysis should

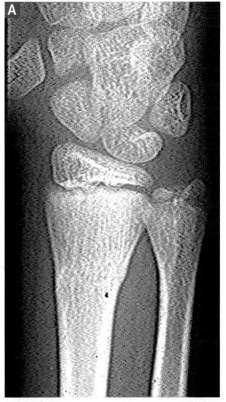

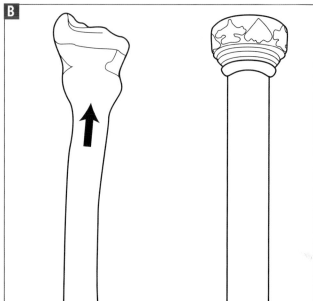

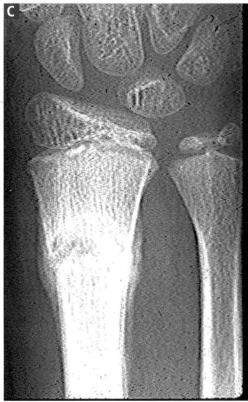

FIGURE 29.2 (A) Metaphyseal fracture of radius. (B) Diagram of torus or buckle fracture. (C) Follow-up x-ray 3 weeks later.

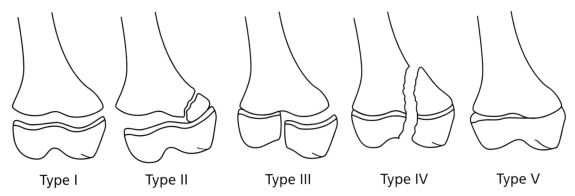

FIGURE 29.3 Illustration of Salter-Harris classification of epiphyseal injuries. Dyment, PG, ed. *Sports Medicine: Health Care for Young Athletes.* 2nd ed. Elk Grove Village, IL: American Academy of Pediatrics; 1991. Based on Salter RB, Harris WR. Injuries involving the epiphyseal plate. *J Bone Joint Surg Am.* 1963;45:587-622.

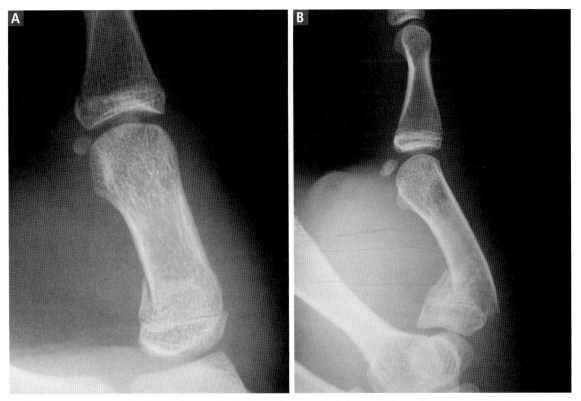

FIGURE 29.4 Salter-Harris II fracture of first metacarpal; lateral (A) and anteroposterior (B) view. Note difference in degree of deformity based on x-ray view. This fracture was treated with closed reduction and percutaneous pinning.

have a similar appearance on both sides. Asymmetric bony abnormalities could be due to an avulsion fracture, an accessory ossification center, an unfused apophysis, or normal variation (**Table 29.1**).

The factors that determine whether a bone will break include the magnitude of the applied force, the direction of force, the rate at which the force is applied, and any inherent weakness of the bone. A bone with an immature physis may be more vulnerable to fracture through the physis. Similarly, if the cortex at the metaphysis is thinner than the diaphysis, it may be the most vulnerable part of the bone to injury. Long bones are more susceptible to translational or

TABLE 29.1

Age of Appearance and Maturation of Apophyses

Apophysis	Related Muscle	Age at Appearance of Apophysis (years)	Age at Fusion of Apophysis (years)	Comments
Anterior superior iliac spine	Sartorius	13-15	16-18	Easily confused with hip pointer.
Anterior inferior iliac spine	Quadriceps	13-15	16-18	Most common acute apophyseal avulsion; often confused with hip flexor strain; can be treated like a quadriceps strain.
Iliac crest	Obliques, iliotibial band	13-15	21-25	Overuse injuries more common than acute injuries; common in sprinters, hurdlers, soccer players.
Ischium	Hamstrings	13-15	20-22	Similar mechanism and findings as hamstring strain except tenderness is proximal (at origin).
Tibial tubercle	Patellar tendon	12-13	15-17	Overuse injuries (ie, Osgood-Schlatter) much more common than acute avulsion.
Calcaneus	Achilles tendon, plantar fascia	7-9	12-14	Sever's disease is common in soccer or sports in which athletes run while wearing cleats.
Fifth metatarsal	Peroneal brevis	7-9	12-14	Apophysitis of Vth metatarsal or Iselin disease is confused with avulsion fracture and Jones fracture; comparison x-rays can help clarify diagnosis.
Medial epicondyle	Common flexor tendon	8-10	13-15	"Little League elbow" is an overuse injury to the apophysis but can lead to acute avulsion of apophysis.

torsional forces, and bones such as the vertebral bodies or carpal bones may be more susceptible to compression forces. When fractures result from forces that appear insufficient to cause a fracture in healthy bone, a pathologic fracture should be suspected.

Repetitive, submaximal stress causes bone to break down with osteoclastic activity and eventually remodel with osteoblastic activity. If the breakdown process exceeds the remodeling process, a weakened area of bone or stress fracture will develop. Muscles that attach along the surface of a long bone have a role in absorbing and dissipating forces applied to the bone. If the muscles fatigue or if the regenerative capabilities of bone are compromised through dietary or hormonal deficiencies, stress fractures are more likely. If there is an area of bone not protected by overlying muscle, such as the junction between the distal third and proximal two thirds of the tibia, stress fractures are more likely to occur at this location.

Simple fractures that are closed and nondisplaced and that do not involve a growth plate may be adequately managed by primary care providers. Fractures that are displaced, angulated, open, intra-articular, involve a growth plate, or are pathologic may require consultation with an orthopedic specialist.

Sprains

Ligaments connect bone to bone and function primarily to provide stability to joints. Ligament injuries are sprains. A grade I or mild sprain indicates microscopic tearing of a ligament without resultant joint instability. A grade II or mild sprain is a partial tear of a ligament whereby some fibers are disrupted and others remain intact. A grade III or severe sprain indicates a complete tear of a ligament.

Ligaments provide joint stability; stability is also afforded by the bony architecture of the joint, joint cartilage, and the surrounding musculotendinous structures. Therefore, the ligaments, bony architecture, cartilage, and musculotendinous structures provide distinct lines of defense that lend stability to a joint. The position of the joint at the time of injury determines which line of defense is going to be most responsible for protecting the joint. When the joint is in a position where there is limited bony stability, ligament sprains are more likely to occur. Examples of positions of low bony stability include a fully extended knee, an inverted ankle, or an externally rotated shoulder. In these positions, ligaments are responsible for stability and are more likely to be injured. Conversely, injuries to a joint in a position of greater bony stability (ie, a flexed knee, a dorsiflexed ankle, or an adducted shoulder) are more likely to be bony in nature. Some joints, such as the hip, have a high degree of bony stability in virtually all positions, making hip sprain a highly improbable diagnosis. By knowing which joint positions have high and low degrees of bony stability and which joints are inherently more or less stable, the risk of sprain can be predicted.

Joint Subluxation and Dislocation

Because bony architecture, ligaments, joint cartilage, and musculotendinous structures maintain joint stability, disruption of any of these structures can be both the cause and an effect of a joint that subluxates or dislocates. A subluxating joint slips partially out of place. The articular surfaces remain in at least partial contact during the subluxation. A subluxated joint usually reduces spontaneously. A dislocated joint slips completely out of place, and the articular surfaces are no longer in contact. A dislocated joint may need external assistance to be reduced. Joints that have a low degree of bony stability, such as the patellofemoral joint or glenohumeral joint, predictably have more frequent subluxations and dislocations than more stable joints like the hip or ankle.

Joint laxity may be acquired or constitutional. Constitutional joint laxity involves all joints, and the laxity is multidirectional. Acquired joint laxity typically involves joints that have been injured; the laxity is usually most pronounced in one direction. When patients have acquired joint instability, they are more likely to have symptoms including pain, weakness, joint clicking, and a sense of joint looseness. Trauma leading to joint instability typically causes damage to one or more of the structures that provide stability. This could be bone, articular cartilage, meniscal cartilage, ligaments, or tendons. Compromise of structures providing joint stability can lead to more instability and progressive injury to joint structures. A subluxating or dislocating joint can be an all-encompassing orthopedic injury with components including fracture, sprain, cartilage injury, strain, and eventually

arthritis. This is also a case in which the effects of the injury may become the cause of further injury.

Strains

Tendons connect muscle to bone. Injuries to musculotendinous structures are strains. Strains are graded in a similar manner to ligament sprains: a grade I or mild strain is a microscopic tear, a grade II or moderate strain is a partial tear, and a grade III or severe strain is a complete tear.

Strains occur from excessive tension to a musculotendinous structure, particularly when the tensile loads are rapidly applied. Eccentric contractions, in which the muscle contracts as it is being stretched, generate the maximal muscle tension and are most likely to cause strains. Eccentric contractions occur with decelerating, landing from a jump, or making a sudden change of direction. The musculotendinous junction is the most vulnerable portion of the musculotendinous unit and the site most likely to have tenderness, swelling, or a palpable defect. Muscles that cross 2 joints are also more likely to be strained. In the calf, the gastrocnemius is at greater risk for strain than the soleus because the gastrocnemius crosses the knee and ankle joint.

With skeletally immature patients, the apophysis or growth center for the tendon attachment is the weak link. Although strains can occur in skeletally immature patients, apophyseal avulsions can occur from the very same mechanisms that would cause a muscle or tendon injury in a skeletally mature patient. With apophyseal avulsions, the pain and tenderness is at the tendon attachment on the apophysis rather than the muscle-tendon junction.

Familiarity with the mechanism and clinical findings of strains is helpful when evaluating any muscle or tendon pain. A diagnosis other than strain should be suspected when muscle or tendon pain occurs without a high-speed, eccentric load; when pain occurs in a musculotendinous structure that crosses only one joint; or when bony pain occurs at a tendon attachment site.

Tendonitis and Tendinosis

Tendonitis occurs from repetitive, submaximal stress to a tendon. The strength of the tendon comes from individual tendon fibers. The tendon sheath or peritenon protects the tendon and facilitates smooth gliding of the tendon. Tendonitis refers to inflammation of the tendon sheath. This inflammation can produce visible swelling; palpable thickening; and symptoms of pain, burning, tightness, and crepitation. Tendinosis is a more advanced form of tendon injury in which microscopic tears of individual tendon fibers can coalesce to form an area where the tendon is swollen and thickened; the tendon fibers may be disrupted and weakened.

The symptoms of tendonitis usually worsen with activity and subside with rest. However, as a result of inflammatory changes in the tendon sheath and adhesions between the tendon and the tendon sheath, patients with tendonitis often report increased pain or stiffness in the morning or after periods of inactivity. The symptoms of tendinosis are similar, but there tends to be more swelling, stiffness, and weakness than occurs with tendonitis. The symptoms of tendinosis tend to be less responsive to basic therapies such as rest, ice, and anti-inflammatory medications.

Although tendons are designed to withstand tensile loads, excessive tension can cause injury. Tendons are less well adapted to withstand torsional forces or compression. Therefore, tendons that are forced to bend, twist, or absorb impact are more likely to be injured. Achilles tendonitis may occur from additional tension on the Achilles in a patient with tight calf muscles or from torsion on the Achilles in a patient with a heel that flares out from a hyperpronated foot.

Symptoms of tendonitis usually subside with rest. However, rest may not correct the stiffness, weakness, or biomechanical abnormalities that caused the injury; nor will it correct the abnormal training patterns or equipment that contributed to the injury. Effective treatment of tendonitis, including prevention of recurrence, requires proper identification and modification of the forces contributing to the injury.

In cases of chronic tendonitis, there may be marked thickening or scar tissue that builds up around a tendon. This may be difficult to distinguish from tendinosis, in which the tendon itself may become swollen and thickened. Tendinosis can weaken the tendon and lead to tendon rupture. Imaging techniques, such as magnetic resonance imaging (MRI), may be helpful in making the important distinction between tendonitis and tendinosis.

In skeletally immature patients, the tendon's attachment on the apophysis is the weak link. With an immature apophysis, the same forces that cause tendonitis in an older patient may cause apophysitis in a younger patient. The causes of apophysitis and the treatment may be the same as for tendonitis. However, with apophysitis, the location of pain is on the bony attachment site for the tendon. Vulnerability to injury at this site will disappear once the apophysis matures.

Apophyseal Injuries

An apophysis is a growth center that serves as an attachment site for a muscle or tendon. Each apophysis appears as a separate center of ossification on x-ray and fuses to the related bone at different ages. When the tensile stress on an apophysis is forceful or rapidly applied, the apophysis may become separated or avulsed. The mechanism of apophyseal avulsion is similar to that of strains.

Chronic or repetitive apophyseal injuries are among the most common problems seen in young athletes. The calcaneal apophysis serves as the attachment point for the Achilles tendon and plantar fascia. The calcaneal apophysis appears on x-ray at approximately age 7 to 8 years and fuses around age 12 to 14 years. If there is excessive tension on the apophysis exerted by the Achilles tendon or the plantar fascia, pain at the junction between the calcaneal apophysis and the calcaneus, or Sever's disease, can develop. Once the apophysis matures, the weak and vulnerable attachment site becomes stronger and more resistant to tension. A similar pathomechanical scenario can occur at other apophyses and produce common and distinct clinical syndromes.

The location of the various apophyses and the patient's age and stage of maturation will determine when and where clinical symptoms of apophysitis will appear.

When pain or tenderness appears on a tendon attachment point of a mature apophysis, or if there is no history of repetitive traction stresses, diagnoses such as enthesitis, stress fracture, or bone tumor should be considered. Enthesitis refers to pain and inflammation at a tendon attachment to bone. The painful attachment site may be an open apophysis or mature bone. Enthesitis should raise concern for a possible systemic inflammatory disorder. A history of trauma is not necessary for an enthesitis to become painful.

Because the apophysis does not contribute to long bone growth, neither acute nor chronic apophyseal injuries are likely to result in long-term growth disruptions. Rarely, however, an apophysis that has been separated or an apophysitis under chronic tension may not fuse properly at the time of maturation. This can result in a permanently weakened tendon attachment site or an unfused bony fragment that becomes a nidus for persistent inflammation and pain.

Bursitis

A bursa is a thin, slippery layer of tissue that functions to reduce friction between moving parts of the musculoskeletal system. Bursae can overlie bony prominences and allow the skin to slide over a convex bony surface like the patella, elbow, or heel. Bursae may function around joints such as the shoulder, where it serves to decrease friction between the rotator cuff and the undersurface of the acromion. Bursitis is an inflammatory reaction in the bursa that can result from acute compressive forces or chronic, repetitive compression or friction. When the bursa is inflamed and swollen, large amounts of fluid can accumulate. If the bursa is superficial, the swelling will be visible and palpable. Bursal swelling near a joint should be distinguished from intra-articular swelling. Bursal swelling near a joint tends to be more superficial and localized to one side of the joint. The swelling from intra-articular effusions is deeper and can be detected on all sides of the joint. An enlarged or swollen bursa can take up additional space between the structures it is designed to protect, thus subjecting it to further compression. This can lead to a vicious cycle in which bursal swelling and pain can escalate with ongoing activity.

Chronic bursitis may produce more subtle swelling or thickening of a bursa. Risk factors for bursitis include internal and external factors that increase pressure or friction on the bursa. An underlying bony prominence from a bone spur, accessory ossification center, or bony deformity can become a pressure point and source of bursitis. External factors contributing to bursitis include poorly fitting shoes or sports equipment, or participation in activities that concentrate pressure over a bursa. For example, tight boots worn by a skier or skater can cause ankle or foot bursitis, and frequent kneeling during wrestling can cause bursitis in the knee.

Both acute and chronic bursitis is generally benign and tends to resolve when the offending forces have been mitigated. However, bursal fluid can become infected. Cellulitis can easily be confused with an infected bursitis. Other conditions in the differential diagnosis of bursitis include hematoma formation, synovial cyst, lipoma, or soft tissue sarcoma.

Arthritis

Arthritis refers to inflammation in a joint. Although the term may raise concern for a rheumatologic or infectious disorder, arthritis can also occur from trauma or through posttraumatic degeneration. Monoarticular joint swelling that persists after a traumatic injury and is not associated with other swollen joints or systemic symptoms may be due to posttraumatic arthritis. Arthritis in sports settings is typically seen in association with cartilage injury. A torn meniscus, a chondral fracture to the articular surface, an osteochondral fracture, an interarticular fracture, an inter-articular loose body, or osteochondritis dissecans can all cause irregularities in the joint or loss of joint cartilage. The injured cartilage leads to reactive changes in the synovium, which results in joint swelling and the clinical finding of arthritis. Over time, these changes can lead to radiographic evidence of joint space narrowing, bone spur formation, subchondral cyst formation, and the changes referred to as osteoarthritis in adults. Because cartilage does not have the regenerative properties of bone, muscle, or tendon, it is critical to recognize the early stages of arthritis, identify and treat the cause of the cartilage breakdown, preserve healthy cartilage, and arrest the progression to irreversible joint degeneration.

Arthritis from trauma needs to be differentiated from arthritis due to systemic inflammatory disorders, gout, pseudogout, and infections. Septic arthritis is rare in sports settings but should treated as a medical emergency. Pigmented villonodular synovitis may cause synovial swelling that mimics arthritis. Bursitis and a joint hemarthrosis may also be confused with arthritis, but injury history, time course for development of findings, and location of fluid accumulation at physical examination should distinguish these diagnoses.

Cartilage Injury

As is the case with other structural elements in the musculoskeletal system, cartilage can be subject to both acute and overuse injury. Acute cartilage injuries include a torn meniscus in the knee, a torn glenoid labrum in the shoulder, or a torn triangular fibrocartilage complex in the wrist. The hyaline cartilage that lines joint surfaces, also known as articular cartilage, can be injured as a result of compression or shearing forces to the joint surface. A chondral fracture can result in fissuring of a joint surface or a section of articular cartilage becoming detached with formation of a loose body.

Injury to any cartilage structure can cause joint pain, swelling, locking, and catching, as well as symptoms of joint instability. Cartilage damage is often seen in association with other injuries, including ligament sprains, joint subluxations, joint dislocations, or intra-articular fractures. If the clinical findings of the associated injury are more prominent, the cartilage injury may be overlooked. Radiographs will not detect cartilage injury; an intra-articular contrast study or an MRI must be performed if there is clinical suspicion of cartilage injury. The presence of marrow edema on MRI or a bone contusion involving a joint surface should raise concern for possible chondral fracture.

Articular cartilage obtains its blood supply and nourishment from underlying subchondral bone. Knee cartilage, such as the meniscus, is relatively hypovascular except for the peripheral rim of the meniscus. Whether a cartilage injury heals depends on the adequacy of the blood supply and the degree of displacement or fragmentation of the injured cartilage. Surgical treatment is often necessary for a cartilage injury that fails to heal. Successful repair from suturing injured cartilage depends on whether the tissue being repaired has an adequate blood supply. Injured cartilage with a good blood supply may heal without surgery. Surgical treatment for an unhealed cartilage injury typically involves resection, without replacement or repair, of damaged cartilage.

Repetitive compression, friction, or shearing stress to articular cartilage can cause softening of the articular cartilage or chondromalacia. The patella is the most familiar location for chondromalacia, but this abnormality can occur in any joint. The softening of the cartilage can progress to cartilage thinning, fibrillation, and ultimately denuding of the protective covering of the articular surface. Patients with chondromalacia initially report activity-related pain in the joint but may develop crepitation, swelling, and joint stiffness, as well as arthritis-like symptoms. Treatment for chondromalacia focuses on minimizing the forces that have contributed to the cartilage breakdown. Surgical treatment for chondromalacia is ineffective at restoring normal cartilage. Arthroscopic shaving of rough or fibrillated cartilage serves only to remove damaged tissue without promoting cartilage growth or healing.

Osteochondritis dissecans is a developmental, or sometimes a traumatic, condition in which blood supply is diminished to a portion of the articular surface of a growing joint. Osteochondritis dissecans tends to manifest during periods of rapid bony growth. In the early stages, the diminished blood supply can result in a focal area of chondromalacia. In later stages, osteochondritis can progress to focal areas of bone demineralization, collapse of the joint surface, or development of a necrotic osteochondral fragment. Osteochondritis dissecans manifests with features of both acute and chronic cartilage injuries. There may be swelling, clicking, and locking consistent with an acute chondral fracture or meniscal injury and insidious pain due to softened or irregular cartilage consistent with an overuse cartilage injury.

When osteochondritis dissecans occurs in the elbow or ankle, there is typically a history of acute or repetitive trauma. Examples include the stress on the radiocapitellar joint associated with pitching in baseball or performing handsprings in gymnastics. In the ankle, a sprain or high-impact injury to the talar dome can precede the appearance of an osteochondral lesion. When osteochondritis dissecans manifests in the knee, antecedent trauma is less frequently observed. If trauma is thought to be a factor, the traumatic forces do not appear to be sufficient to cause the degree of observed joint destruction.

When musculoskeletal findings manifest without a clear history for antecedent injury, there may be an underlying developmental condition, a predisposing risk factor causing increased vulnerability to injury, or a condition such as osteochondritis dissecans. Referral to an orthopedic specialist is appropriate in cases of osteochondritis dissecans or other joint cartilage abnormalities.

Developmental Conditions and Anatomic Variants

Osteochondritis dissecans can be categorized as both an injury and a developmental condition. Other developmental conditions and anatomic variants that may become symptomatic or that may be mistaken for injuries are listed in **Table 29.2**. Developmental conditions and anatomic variants are no more likely to occur in athletes than the general population. However, athletes place more stress on their bones and joints, have more musculoskeletal injuries, and are more likely to be evaluated for musculoskeletal complaints.

A discoid lateral meniscus is a developmental variation that is present in 2% of the population. Of these patients, approximately 2% have symptoms. Symptoms of clicking, locking, or swelling in the knee may occur in conjunction with athletic activity. The clinical evaluation may indicate a possible meniscus tear, but there is no history of the type of injury mechanism that typically leads to a meniscus tear. If clinical findings of a torn meniscus develop in a patient without a history of meniscal injury, a discoid meniscus should be considered as a possible cause.

Similarly, a bipartite patella may be present as an asymptomatic variant or may be confused with a patellar fracture in a patient who falls on a knee and experiences knee pain (**Figure 29.5**).

Other Injury Categories

In addition to the common acute and overuse injuries discussed, musculoskeletal pain in a young athlete could also be due to any number of injury categories or disease processes that affect the musculoskeletal system. Some of the other injury categories and disease processes include periostitis, fasciitis, vasculitis, myositis, myopathy, neuritis, neuropathy, and compartment syndrome, as well as a host of benign and malignant tumors involving soft tissue and bone, infection, rheumatologic disorders, and pain amplification syndromes.

Biomechanical Abnormalities

Repetitive motions such as running, jumping, throwing, and swimming can lead to injury. The techniques that athletes use while performing these activities, as well as alterations in mechanics resulting from anatomic variations, can be factors in injury. *Biomechanics* refers to the dynamic interaction of structures involved with movement.

TABLE 29. 2

Developmental Conditions and Anatomic Variants

Developmental Condition/Anatomic Variant	Comments
Osteochondritis dissecans	Occurs in knee, ankle, and elbow; presents with joint swelling, clicking, catching; mimics torn meniscus or loose body.
Bipartite patella	Involves superolateral patella; may be incidental finding or be confused with fracture; insufficient trauma history to cause fracture.
Bipartite navicular	Easily mistaken for navicular fracture or stress fracture in foot; similar radiographic findings may be present on asymptomatic side.
Bipartite/tripartite sesamoid	A painful sesamoid may appear to be fractures in 2 or 3 pieces when in reality the sesamoid developed as a bipartite or tripartite sesamoid. Prior x-rays, if available; comparison views; a bone scan; or magnetic resonance imaging can help determine whether the findings are due to a fracture.
Accessory navicular	Easily confused with navicular fracture or avulsion fracture; pain pattern similar to tibialis posterior tendonitis; often painful when associated with flat foot.
Os trigonum	Extra bone posterior to talus that causes impingement in posterior ankle; restricts plantarflexion in ballet dancers or athletes who point their toes.
Discoid lateral meniscus	Two percent prevalence in general population; if symptomatic, presents with clicking or popping in lateral knee; worse with active extension; causes swelling or locking if it becomes torn.
Tarsal coalition	Incomplete segmentation of tarsal bones; becomes more painful as bones mature and cartilaginous coalition becomes more rigid; causes painful flat foot, peroneal spasm, and occasional sense of ankle instability.
Scheuermann kyphosis	Causes kyphosis in thoracic spine; x-ray shows 3 consecutive wedged vertebrae; can be confused with vertebral compression fracture.
Spina bifida occulta	Failure of spinous process to fuse; most common at L5-S1; correlates with spondylolysis; not thought to be a direct cause of symptoms.
Transitional lumbar vertebra	The lowest lumbar vertebra may have transverse processes that are enlarged or fused to the sacrum. These changes are not a result of trauma and do not cause pain. However, motion may be restricted at the affected spinal segment.
Osteoid osteoma	Benign bone cyst that appears sclerotic with a central nidus; clinical presentation may be confused with stress fracture.

The biomechanics of a given activity must be understood to appreciate the abnormalities that lead to injury, as well as the requirements for full, functional recovery after injury.

Injury can occur from repetitive motion in patients with optimal movement patterns and optimal mechanical efficiency. Anatomic variation or abnormalities of technique can result in movement patterns that are restricted, uncoordinated, inefficient, or otherwise abnormal. When biomechanical abnormalities are present, the risk of injury increases.

Despite the prominent role of biomechanics in sports injuries, much of the clinical assessment of injuries is based on static evaluation. Detection of swelling, tenderness, crepitation, restricted mobility, or weakness indicates that an injury has occurred, but it does not specify the cause of the injury or how to treat the source. A flat foot or a valgus knee does not constitute an injury. However, when subjected to the repetitive stresses of running, these anatomic variations may contribute to injury of the foot, ankle, leg, knee, or hip. Imaging studies, including MRI, also involve static representations of structures that are subjected to dynamic stress. If there is evidence of injury or structural breakdown, the imaging studies fail to reveal critical information about the cause of injury. Biomechanical abnormalities may explain injuries in which symptoms occur only with activity but do not produce obvious physical or radiographic signs.

It is beyond the scope of this chapter to review biomechanical patterns associated with each sport. However, when evaluating baseball pitchers, tennis players, runners, rowers, swimmers, divers, golfers, dancers, gymnasts, or weight lifters, understanding the underlying biomechanics of the activity can greatly help in evaluating, treating, and preventing injuries.

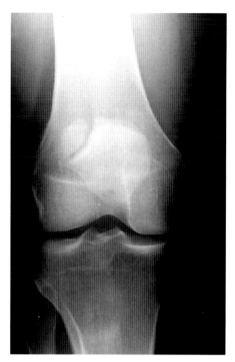

FIGURE 29.5 Bipartite patella.

The axis of rotation of the subtalar joint is 16° from the sagittal plane and 43° from the transverse plane (**Figure 29.6**). Because of the oblique angle of the subtalar joint, lateral movement of the foot is translated to rotation of the leg. Pronation and supination occur at the subtalar joint. Because of the oblique angle of rotation around the subtalar joint, pronation is a combination of eversion of the heel, abduction of the forefoot, dorsiflexion of the ankle, and internal rotation of the tibia. Supination is a combination of inversion of the heel, adduction of the forefoot, plantarflexion of the ankle, and external rotation of the tibia (**Figure 29.7**).

Pronation puts the foot in a flexible, adaptable position. With pronation, the axes of rotation of the transverse tarsal joint are parallel. This unlocks the transverse tarsal joint and consequently makes the foot more flexible and adaptable (**Figure 29.8**). With supination, the axes of rotation of the transverse tarsal joint are at oblique angles that lock the joint and make the foot more rigid.

With normal gait, the foot pronates at the time of heel strike. This allows the foot to adapt to the surface and absorb shock. At midstance, the foot naturally supinates.

Because running is common to many sports, understanding the biomechanics of running can help explain overuse injuries that occur in many sports. The biomechanics of walking and running include a gait cycle with a stance phase and a swing phase. The stance phase is the weight-bearing phase and is composed of heel strike, midstance, and push-off. The swing phase is the non–weight-bearing portion of gait in which the leg swings forward during recovery. Most running injuries are related to the forces and movements associated with the stance or support phase of gait.

Every time the foot hits the ground with running, the equivalent of 2.5 to 3 times the body weight of force needs to be dissipated at the time of impact. For a runner who weighs 150 pounds and takes 1600 steps per mile of running, the musculoskeletal system needs to absorb up to 2 160 000 pounds, or 1080 tons, of force per mile. The foot needs to be able to absorb impact at heel strike, but it also must become sufficiently stable to allow for push-off. Understanding the function of the subtalar joint is the key to understanding how the foot can transition between a flexible shock absorber at heel strike to a rigid lever at push-off. This transition must occur at the speed and frequency of each step that is taken. It must also provide for the level of shock absorption and stability to protect against injury.

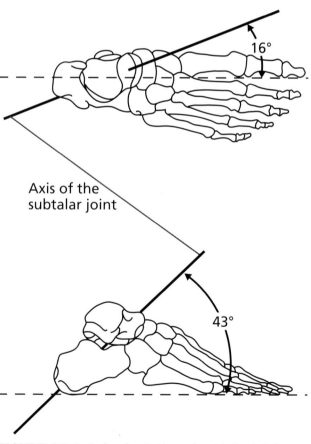

FIGURE 29.6 Axis of rotation of subtalar joint.

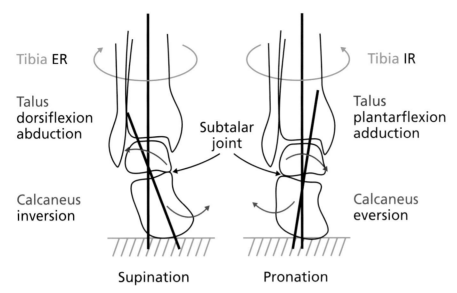

FIGURE 29.7 Linked motions at subtalar joint. Supination: external rotation of tibia; dorsiflexion and abduction of talus; inversion of calcaneus. Pronation: internal rotation of tibia; plantarflexion and adduction of talus; eversion of calcaneus.

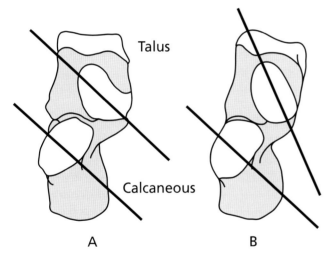

FIGURE 29.8 (A) Transverse tarsal joint during pronation. Parallel axes of rotation allow for increased mobility. (B) Transverse tarsal joint during supination. Oblique or locked axes of rotation allow for increased rigidity of foot.

Supination passively puts the foot in a more stable position and creates a rigid lever to allow for push-off. Pronation and supination are a normal part of gait. However, if patients pronate or supinate excessively, injury may occur.

With excessive or prolonged pronation, the foot stays in a flexible, unstable configuration longer than is optimal. A hyperpronated foot has an arch that flattens with weight bearing. To make the foot rigid for push-off, the muscles of the leg must be recruited to raise the arch and stabilize the subtalar joint. This leads to overload of the muscles along the medial portion of the tibia. Excessive pronation is also linked to increased internal tibial rotation. This can contribute to patellar tracking abnormalities and an increased risk of patellofemoral pain. In general, patients with hyperpronation tend to have more overuse injuries on the medial portion of the leg (ie, shin splints, tibialis posterior tendonitis) and the medial portion of the knee (ie, patellofemoral stress syndrome).

A foot that is excessively supinated appears as a high-arched or cavus foot. This is a foot that is rigid and well adapted for stability and push-off but not designed to absorb shock. This means that more stress is transmitted to the bones in the foot and leg. Patients with a supinated foot are at increased risk for stress fractures and tend to have more overuse injuries to structures on the lateral aspect of the leg, including iliotibial band friction syndrome, trochanteric bursitis, peroneal tendonitis, and fibular stress fracture.

To determine whether patients have excessive pronation or supination, they need to be examined while bearing weight. A foot may appear to have a normal arch while not bearing weight but become flat or remain highly arched while standing. A flexible flat foot implies that there is normal motion in the subtalar joint. Patients with a flexible flat foot will develop a visible arch when they stand on their toes. Because plantarflexion is a component of supination, when patients stand on tiptoe, the heel should invert, the forefoot should adduct, and the combination of these movements should raise the arch of the foot. If plantarflexion does not cause the linked motions of heel inversion and foot adduction, then the subtalar motion is abnormal. A rigid flat foot, or a foot that remains flat during a toe raise, is a pathologic flat foot. This foot type is most likely the result of a subtalar tarsal coalition.

Not every patient with a biomechanical abnormality develops an injury, nor does every biomechanical abnormality need treatment. However, a biomechanical evaluation should be performed on all patients with overuse injuries and on patients who are planning to participate in sports in which specific motions are repeated frequently. For patients being evaluated with overuse injuries, clinicians should consider whether a biomechanical abnormality is present and whether such an abnormality might contribute to the injury. If abnormal biomechanics are indeed a factor in the patient's injury, then the clinician should assess whether the biomechanical abnormality can be corrected.

Clinical Evaluation of Musculoskeletal Problems

The evaluation of a given musculoskeletal problem includes general aspects that are relevant to all musculoskeletal conditions and elements that are specific to the problem at hand. The ultimate goal of evaluation is to reach an accurate diagnosis. Establishing an accurate diagnosis is critical to planning effective treatment, and the tools available for reaching one include the medical history, physical examination, and diagnostic imaging.

This chapter provides a general overview. The individual chapters on specific injuries will emphasize the aspects of the history and physical examination that are relevant to those anatomic areas or conditions.

History

The history of a musculoskeletal problem should allow for proper categorization of the condition and suggest likely diagnoses. Before inquiring about a specific injury, the clinician should obtain a general medical history, asking questions about the patient's general health, presence of acute and chronic medical conditions, medication use, supplement use, tobacco use, and allergies, and perform a medical review of systems. A sports background history should be obtained. This includes which sports the patient plays currently and throughout the year; which position is played; the schedule for practice and competition; and any upcoming changes, deadlines, or events.

The musculoskeletal injury history starts with inquiries about the mechanism of injury. For acute injuries, the patient should be able to explain or demonstrate what happened. For overuse injuries, the patient may be able to identify any recent changes in training or equipment or modifications in technique that preceded the onset of symptoms. Symptoms of pain should be explored, including its location, quality, and severity, as well as what makes it better and what makes it worse. Severity of pain can be judged by how much it interferes with sports activity and whether it affects the activities of daily living. Pain that occurs at rest or that disrupts sleep raises concern for more severe injury or the presence of an underlying medical problem. The patient should also be asked about swelling; stiffness; and joint locking, catching, or instability. A report of weakness needs to be explored to determine whether the weakness is due to muscle injury, pain inhibition, nerve injury, or disuse. Neurologic symptoms—including numbness, tingling, burning, and radiating pain—should be investigated with a focus on determining whether the source is in the spine or a peripheral structure.

The effect of an injury on function can be assessed by asking about restrictions or limitations on sports activity and daily activity. Does the condition affect the ability to stand, walk, climb stairs, kneel, or squat? Does the condition affect the patient's ability to run, jump, or pivot? Does the condition affect bending, arching, twisting, or lifting?

The history should include previous evaluations and consultations, x-ray findings, and test results. The history should include prior and recent treatment, including surgery, and the response to treatment. In addition to a general medical review of systems, the injury history should include descriptions of concurrent injuries and the presence of prior injuries to the affected area, as well as other areas. For symptoms that cannot be explained by an acute or overuse injury, the presence of concurrent illness or constitutional symptoms of fever, sweats, chills, or weight loss should be elicited.

Physical Examination

The physical examination for a musculoskeletal problem begins with an overall inspection of the patient to assess general health, fitness, stature, and maturity. Posture and body habitus can be assessed, and the patient should be evaluated for syndromic features. The skin should also be evaluated for unusual lesions, bruising, hyperelasticity, infection, jaundice, acne, or signs of possible anabolic steroid use. Individual chapters will describe the specific physical examinations for extremity and joint problems, as well as the spine. The common elements of the musculoskeletal examination for each anatomic area include inspection, palpation, assessment of mobility, joint stability, strength, and any specific or provocative tests indicated by the general examination.

For extremity or joint problems, it is helpful to examine the uninjured side first. This establishes a baseline and can reassure an anxious patient about the process of the examination. It is also helpful to examine joints both proximal and distal to the injured site because injuries may affect adjoining or related structures.

Inspection can yield useful information about the presence of swelling, skin discoloration, deformity, postural abnormalities, and malalignment, as well as the quality of movement and pain behavior. For athletes who run and jump or athletes with overuse injuries to the lower extremity, inspection should include an evaluation of foot type and leg alignment. A standing inspection of patients can reveal whether they have a neutral foot, a high-arched (supinated) foot, or a flat (pronated) foot; it can also reveal whether they have external tibial rotation, internal femoral rotation (femoral anteversion), genu varus (bow legs), or genu valgus (knock-knees).

Palpation should be systemically performed, starting with the uninjured side and progressing to the area where pain can be anticipated. Palpation can identify tenderness, swelling, masses, temperature changes, and crepitation. When a patient has pain in an area but no local findings such as tenderness or swelling, the pain may be from another source. The injury or source of pain may not be palpable, and findings that are palpable are not necessarily the cause of the problem. For example, a patient may have a protruding lumbar disk that is not palpable but have muscle spasm in the back that is palpable but that is not the source of the problem.

For joint problems, the joint should be assessed for both swelling and tenderness. The joint examination should check for range of motion and ligamentous stability. Tenderness at or around a joint in a skeletally immature patient should warrant evaluation for possible physeal disruption or metaphyseal fracture. Joint stability may vary according to the position of the joint during the examination and the presence of pain, swelling, and guarding. There is also individual variation in joint stability resulting from age, gender, and genetics. Comparison with the uninjured side is helpful in separating the effects of injury from normal variation.

For extremity injuries, active motion, passive motion, and muscle flexibility should be measured and compared with the uninjured side. Patients with spinal problems can also be assessed for available motion by flexing, extending, bending sideways, and rotating to both sides. Any restriction of motion, asymmetry, or positions that result in pain can be noted, and the pattern of restriction can help identify the injured structure.

Strength testing may not be very helpful in acute extremity injuries. Pain and joint swelling inhibit strength. However, long-term weakness or weakness from chronic injury may manifest as visible atrophy. Detailed strength testing is crucial in both acute and chronic spine injuries. Strength testing is also useful in overuse injuries in which the pattern of weakness can help explain the cause and effects of injury and the need for specific rehabilitation exercises.

When neurologic injury is suspected, strength should be measured, graded, and compared with the asymptomatic side. Grading of muscle strength is shown in **Table 29.3**. With neurologic weakness, it is usually necessary to test several muscle groups to determine whether the weakness follows a pattern for a peripheral nerve or nerve root injury. Manual muscle testing of muscular patients may lack sufficient sensitivity to detect subtle weakness. For the large muscles of the lower extremity, using the patient's own body weight for resistance may be more sensitive than manual muscle testing. Repetitive toe raises can assess calf strength and S1 nerve function, and repetitive single-legged squats can assess quadriceps strength and L4 function.

In addition to strength testing, the neurologic examination should check for paresthesias and deep tendon reflexes. The physical examination, when possible, should also assess

TABLE 29.3

Grading System for Muscle Strength

Strength Grade	Definition
5	Normal strength against maximum resistance through full range of motion.
4	Intact strength against moderate or strong resistance through full range of motion.
3	Patient can move through full range of motion against gravity but cannot tolerate added resistance.
2	Patient can move through full range of motion when gravity is eliminated.
1	Muscle contraction can be palpated in position where gravity is eliminated.
0	No contractile activity can be felt in position where gravity is eliminated.

functional patterns, as well as general characteristics such as balance, coordination, and proprioception. A functional pattern involves the coordinated movement of a series of joints with the pattern representing a movement relevant to the patient's sport. The functional pattern may be running, throwing, a swimming stroke, or performing a plié at the ballet barre. Proprioception can be tested by having patients attempt to balance on one leg with their eyes open and closed.

Finally, many injuries are diagnosed with specific maneuvers or provocative tests. These include maneuvers such as the McMurray test for a torn meniscus or a relocation test for an unstable shoulder. The musculoskeletal physical examination should include any special tests available for the condition being investigated. Such tests are described in the individual chapters on injuries.

The validity and reliability of a given part of the physical examination will vary with the experience of the examiner and the level of cooperation of the patient. Like laboratory tests, each part of the physical examination has a sensitivity, specificity, and predictive value for a given condition. Joint swelling may be a sensitive indicator of intra-articular joint pathology but is nonspecific as to the cause. Crepitation may be a sensitive indication of tendon or joint inflammation but nonspecific as to the cause. A McMurray test may be relatively specific for a torn meniscus but positive in only 60% of patients with a torn meniscus. A 3+ anterior drawer test in the ankle could be due to injury or constitutional laxity, but the test is inadequate to predict who will have problems with instability or may need surgical treatment. Few diagnoses can be reliably made by a single test, and few tests are meaningful in isolation.

In some cases, negative findings can be as helpful as positive findings in reaching a correct diagnosis. A negative Lachman test can confirm that symptoms of knee instability are not due to disruption of the anterior cruciate ligament (ACL). A negative examination for cervical spine pathology can confirm that a patient's hand numbness is not coming from the neck.

An effective physical examination is based more on the quality of information obtained than its volume. Understanding the strengths and limitations of various components of the physical examination will enhance the strength of any conclusions drawn from the physical examination. The physical findings should fit in the clinical context as defined by the medical history and support the presumptive diagnosis. When there are inconsistencies, further information from the history or physical examination should be gathered, and the information should continue to be scrutinized until a conclusion can be drawn.

Laboratory and Imaging Studies

Nonradiologic diagnostic tests may include laboratory studies such as complete blood count, blood chemistry analysis, screening tests for arthritis, joint fluid analysis, cultures, and serology. Electrodiagnostic studies such as electromyography and nerve conduction study can aid in evaluating suspected neurologic injuries. Doppler studies provide a noninvasive means to assess vascular obstruction.

Chapter 30 provides a review of the use of the radiology department in the evaluation of sports injuries. Before ordering an x-ray or other diagnostic test, it is useful to have formulated a differential diagnosis or to have a specific question in mind. It is also useful to know the efficacy of the chosen test in confirming or refuting the suspected diagnosis. Selection of a test can be further challenged by asking whether the results are likely to alter the management of the problem or whether there is another way to get the same information.

Diagnostic Approaches to Musculoskeletal Problems

After performing the initial history and physical examination, clinicians should focus the evaluation of a musculoskeletal problem by asking the questions provided in **Table 29.4**. These questions can help determine which of the various categories of musculoskeletal disorders is likely to yield a diagnosis. If musculoskeletal symptoms occur in a patient who is not active or if there is no history of trauma, medical or nontraumatic causes should be pursued. Nontraumatic conditions include infection, arthritis, neoplastic disorders, and developmental abnormalities.

TABLE 29.4

Evaluation of a Musculoskeletal Problem

- Are the findings due to an injury or an underlying medical condition?
- Which injury or disease process is most likely to explain the clinical findings?
- Is there more than one injury or disease process operating?
- Is the injury acute or overuse in nature?
- Are the predominant symptoms and physical findings the cause of the underlying condition, or are they a secondary effect of the underlying condition?
- Is the location of the symptoms the same as the location of the source of the symptoms?
- Are there contributing nonmedical factors?

The characteristic features of various injury processes were discussed earlier. Identifying the category of musculoskeletal disorder will dictate which additional inquiries, physical examination findings, and diagnostic studies can help confirm the diagnosis. Distinguishing between acute and overuse injuries can further define an effective diagnostic approach.

Acute versus Overuse Injuries

Acute injuries include sprains, strains, fractures, dislocations, contusions, lacerations, and abrasions. Acute injuries result from maximal forces that result in disruption or failure of the injured structure. Acute injuries occur as a result of a single event and usually result in obvious symptoms, physical findings, and/or radiographic changes. Patients with acute injuries know they are injured; they also know when and how they were injured.

Overuse injuries include tendonitis, apophysitis, bursitis, periostitis, fasciitis, shin splints, and stress fractures. Overuse injuries occur from repetitive, submaximal trauma. Symptoms and physical findings develop over time and are often vague and insidious. The patient does not recall a specific time of injury and may not know how or why the injury occurred. There may be a delay seeking medical attention because patients can often continue with their activity and remain free of symptoms with daily activity. The pathologic changes with overuse syndromes are subtle and typically produce minimal findings at physical examination and standard radiographs. The lack of more dramatic symptoms, physical findings, or radiographic changes with overuse syndromes can create an impression that the patient is not actually injured. The differences in the cause and presentation of acute versus overuse injuries call for a difference in the clinical approach (**Table 29.5**).

For acute injuries, the treatment must address the effects of the injury. The effects may be a displaced fracture, a deformity, an unstable joint, or a bleeding wound. The treatment for acute injuries involves reducing the fracture, correcting the deformity, repairing the damaged ligament, stabilizing the joint, or suturing the lacerated skin.

For overuse injuries, the effects of the injury are typically mild and nonspecific. Effects of an overuse injury may include pain, tightness, crepitation, or fatigue. Even if the effects of an overuse injury subside with rest, the condition will recur with activity unless the causes of injury are identified and corrected.

The causes of an overuse injury can be broken down into extrinsic and intrinsic categories (**Table 29.6**). Extrinsic risk factors for overuse injuries are generally related to the risks of the sport, the sports environment, the equipment, and the training regimens. Intrinsic risk factors relate to the age, maturation, gender, health, and fitness of the individual as well as anatomic factors such as flexibility, strength, joint stability, and alignment. There may be several extrinsic and intrinsic factors that cause or contribute to an overuse injury. The degree to which all contributing factors can be identified and corrected will determine the efficacy of treatment.

With acute injuries, the cause of the injury is less critical in planning treatment than the effects. For example, the treatment of an ACL sprain resulting from a ski accident is essentially no different from treating an ACL sprain resulting from football. However, anterior knee pain from chondromalacia in a skeletally immature female gymnast with hypermobile joints may require different treatment than chondromalacia in a skeletally mature basketball player with tight muscles and flat feet.

When the effects of an injury must be understood to administer proper treatment, the history, physical examination, and radiographic evaluation will take on a different character than when identification of the causes of injury is the priority. Effects from acute injuries such as swelling,

TABLE 29.5

Acute Versus Overuse Injuries

Characteristic	Acute Injuries	Overuse Injuries
Examples	Sprains, strains, fractures, dislocations, contusions, lacerations, abrasions	Tendonitis, apophysitis, bursitis, periostitis, fasciitis, shin splints, stress fracture
Timing	Occur as single event	Develop over time
Force	Maximal	Repetitive, submaximal
Importance of cause in planning treatment	Not as important as identifying *effects* of injury	Critical; condition will not resolve until *causes* are identified and addressed

TABLE 29.6

Extrinsic and Intrinsic Risk Factors for Overuse Syndromes

Extrinsic Risk Factors	Intrinsic Risk Factors
Nature/demands of the sport	• Age
Contact/collision	• Maturation
Noncontact	• Gender
Endurance	• Fitness, health
• Rules, supervision	• Flexibility
• Coaching	• Joint stability
• Fields, playing surfaces	• Alignment
• Equipment	• Strength
• Protective equipment (helmets, pads, shin guards)	• Proprioception
	• Psychological
• Equipment for sport (bats, balls, bases, goals, shoes)	
• Equipment for injury treatment or prevention (knee braces, face masks, goggles, neck rolls)	
• Training regimen	
• Level of competition	
• Weather conditions	

deformity, restricted motion, instability, and weakness produce clear positive findings during history, physical examination, and imaging studies.

Eliciting the causes of overuse injuries, such as overtraining, improper footwear, tight muscles, or strength imbalances, requires a different line of inquiry than the evaluation of acute injuries. Evaluating overuse injuries typically requires a more detailed history, whereas acute injuries can largely be diagnosed by physical examination and imaging studies. If the evaluation strategy for an acute injury is applied to an overuse problem, the lack of positive findings may be misconstrued as a lack of real injury. Conversely, dwelling on the causes of injury when the problem is acute will only delay diagnosis and treatment. Therefore, acute injuries warrant an evaluation geared at assessing the effects of injury, and overuse injuries warrant an evaluation geared at assessing the causes of injury.

Separating causes and effects of injury can also be problematic when it comes to interpreting symptoms or physical findings. For example, muscle spasm is the effect of an injury, but its cause may be a direct injury to the muscle, such as a muscle strain, or it could be the result of a pinched nerve or disk herniation. Tingling in the fingers may be due to carpal tunnel syndrome, ulnar neuritis at the elbow, thoracic outlet syndrome, or a cervical radiculopathy. Deltoid pain may be due to a deltoid contusion, rotator cuff tendonitis, or an injury to the proximal humeral epiphysis. In all of these cases, the observed effects of injury all have different causes and will thus require different forms of treatment.

In some cases, several ongoing injury processes, several sources for clinical findings, or a mixture of acute and overuse conditions may simultaneously occur. A shoulder may be unstable after a subluxation that injured the glenoid labrum. There may be associated numbness as a result of an axillary nerve injury, which in turn is most likely a result of instability. There may also be impingement pain as a result of the instability and rotator cuff weakness stemming from the original subluxation. Recognizing the potential for complex interactions among multiple injury processes will minimize the diagnostic shortcomings that occur with oversimplification during the clinical evaluation.

When the history, physical examination, and imaging tests fail to identify objective evidence of injury, nonmedical sources should be considered. Nonorganic musculoskeletal pain should be a consideration when the symptoms vary in location, timing, and quality or when the examination shows pain behavior that is out of proportion to objective findings. If the findings cannot be explained by an underlying systemic illness, referral to a behavioral medicine specialist may be appropriate. If psychological factors are not the sole source of musculoskeletal complaints, there may still be a psychological component that affects the magnitude of symptoms or dysfunction.

A Convergent Approach to Musculoskeletal Diagnosis

Only rarely do patients' actual clinical findings perfectly replicate a textbook description of their condition. When the factors do not match, or when there is question about the level of matching required to make a diagnosis, it becomes increasingly difficult to make a confident diagnosis. The efforts to find a diagnostic match can shift the focus of the evaluation to building a case rather than pursuing the best diagnosis.

Injuries have been diagnosed by using probabilities that are based on likelihood or colloquial terminology. Little League elbow may be a likely cause of elbow pain in a 12-year-old baseball pitcher. However, Little League elbow is a nonspecific term; it can occur in athletes who do not play baseball. It can be the result of different causes, and treatment depends on how the diagnosis is interpreted and applied. Patients who initially seem to have Little League elbow may actually have osteochondritis dissecans. This misdiagnosis and the resulting inappropriate treatment can lead to permanent damage to the elbow. As with Little League elbow, relying on names of disorders such as runner's knee, swimmer's shoulder, tennis elbow, or dancer's fracture should be avoided.

The convergent approach is a way to narrow down sports-related musculoskeletal injuries. This involves starting with a chief complaint and systematically narrowing down the diagnostic possibilities by initially assigning a general injury category and eventually a more specific classification. Knowledge of various injury processes, injury patterns, and evaluation strategies can guide the analysis of incoming clinical information. For musculoskeletal complaints, the list of questions in **Table 29.7** can help systematically arrive at a diagnosis.

The convergent approach to musculoskeletal diagnosis does not require memorizing lists of clinical findings, nor does it require that the clinical findings precisely match a standardized description. By using the history and physical examination to narrow the diagnostic possibilities, diagnos-tic tests, imaging studies, and specialty consultations can be used more selectively.

Implementation of the convergent approach to musculo-skeletal diagnosis starts with an evaluation of the chief complaint, which may take on many forms. It may be a report of a past event, a prominent symptom, a functional limitation, a physical finding, or an area of pain. Patients may complain that their back went out, or that they have a locked knee, a swollen ankle, a numb finger, a sore shoulder, or a muscle spasm. A diagnosis should not be made from the chief complaint alone, but correctly interpreting the manifested findings can help the clinical evaluation. **Table 29.8** reviews common findings at the time the patient seeks care and some of the diagnostic considerations that each finding should raise.

When the complaint is an anatomic area of pain, the *Symptom Locator* illustrations on pages 286-292 may be helpful in identifying diagnostic possibilities. As previously indicated, pain in a given area may be due to an injury to a structure in that area, pain referred to that area, or the result of an injury in another area.

TABLE 29.7

Questions to Ask to Diagnose Musculoskeletal Complaints

- Are the findings due to an injury or an underlying medical problem?
- Are the findings explained by a congenital or developmental abnormality?
- If the findings are due to an injury, is it an acute or overuse injury?
- If it is an acute injury:
    - What are the effects of the injury?
    - Does the injury follow the expected pattern for a fracture, sprain, strain, dislocation, or contusion?
- If it is an overuse injury:
    - What are the intrinsic causes of the injury?
    - What are the extrinsic causes of the injury?
    - Does the injury follow the expected pattern for tendonitis, stress fracture, periostitis, apophysitis, bursitis, or arthritis?
- Are the predominant findings directly related to the cause of the underlying problem?
- Are the predominant findings a direct result of the underlying problem or are they due to compensations that have evolved as a result of the primary problem?
- Is the location of the symptoms and the source of the symptoms the same?
- Is there more than one injury process occurring simultaneously?
- What is the most likely diagnostic category for the problem?
- What is the most likely specific diagnosis within this category?
- What are alternative diagnoses?
- What additional information, including tests or imaging studies, would be most helpful to confirm the diagnosis?

TABLE 29.8

Diagnostic Considerations for Common Presenting Findings

Presenting Complaint or Physical Finding	Diagnostic Considerations	Recommendation for Further Evaluation[a]	Comments
Joint swelling	1. Trauma • Sprains • Subluxation or dislocation • Cartilage tear (torn meniscus, chondral fracture) • Intra-articular fracture	X-ray, MRI, MRI-arthrogram, CT, CT-arthrogram.	The history and physical examination will be sufficient to distinguish various traumatic causes.
	2. Developmental • Osteochondritis dissecans • Discoid meniscus	X-ray, MRI, MRI-arthrogram.	There is typically no history of acute trauma.
	3. Inflammatory • Infection • Rheumatologic • Neoplastic or paraneoplastic	Blood work, joint fluid analysis, synovial biopsy.	Patients have inadequate history of trauma and have nonmusculoskeletal findings.
Joint instability	1. Ligament sprain 2. Constitutional joint hypermobility 3. Intra-articular loose body 4. Torn cartilage (meniscus, labrum, chondral fracture) 5. Subluxation or dislocation 6. Snapping or dislocating tendon 7. Pain inhibition of muscles 8. Proprioceptive deficit	Complete history and physical examination with appropriate imaging studies to confirm suspected diagnosis. With ligament sprain, there should be specific ligament laxity. With cartilage injury, ligaments are stable, but joint is swollen, tender, and/or restricted in motion. With subluxation or dislocation, there is apprehension or instability.	The history, physical examination, and imaging studies can determine whether there is an injury and if the instability is static (ie, due to ligament laxity) or functional (ie, due to pain inhibition).
Weakness	1. Muscle injury • Strain • Contusion 2. Neuropathy or myopathy 3. Pain inhibition 4. Disuse atrophy 5. Joint pain or instability 6. Systemic disease, chronic illness	If history and physical examination do not clarify the source of weakness, MRI can confirm muscle or tendon injury. Electrodiagnostic studies can evaluate neuropathy or myopathy.	Clarify whether weakness is due to direct injury to muscle or whether it is neurologic, the result of a spine problem, the result of disuse or pain, or whether it is part of a systemic or metabolic abnormality.
Muscle spasm	1. Muscle injury • Strain • Contusion 2. Spasm resulting from underlying spinal abnormality • Disk protrusion • Radiculopathy 3. Systemic or rheumatologic disorder • Fibromyalgia • Complex regional pain disorder	Clinical evaluation must include evaluation of spine to look for sources of referred pain, spasm, or guarding; MRI can determine whether there is a local abnormality in the muscle or if there is a source for referred pain.	Clarify whether the findings are the result of a local problem or if they are referred; if spasm is generalized and independent from activity, suspect a systemic disorder.
Numbness	1. Neuritis or neuropathy (peripheral nerve or nerve root injury) 2. Vascular • Vascular obstruction (thoracic outlet) • Raynaud disease • Sympathetic dysfunction 3. Hyperventilation, anxiety	Examination to look for all possible sites of nerve compression or injury (from distal to proximal); EMG-NCV to assess location and severity of nerve injury; ultrasound to screen for thoracic outlet system or vascular obstruction.	Check first for local versus referred sources; see whether distribution of paresthesias follows pattern for nerve root, peripheral nerve root, or spinal cord. Paresthesias due to vascular abnormalities tend to follow stocking-glove distribution with symptoms that are most pronounced distally.

Continued

TABLE 29.8

Diagnostic Considerations for Common Presenting Findings—cont'd

Presenting Complaint or Physical Finding	Diagnostic Considerations	Recommendation for Further Evaluation	Comments
Burning	1. Neuritic, particularly if involving superficial sensory nerves 2. Neuroma 3. Bursitis 4. Cellulitis, fasciitis 5. Myositis ossificans 6. Sympathetic dysfunction	Positive Tinel's sign with neuritis of peripheral nerve. Inflammatory conditions are associated with visible swelling, erythema, and palpable warmth to touch.	With neuritic causes of burning, the patient perceives burning, but the skin looks and feels normal to touch. With inflammatory conditions, the skin is erythematous and feels warm.
Joint locking	1. Torn meniscus 2. Chondral or osteochondral fracture 3. Osteochondritis dissecans 4. Labrum tear 5. Subluxating joint	MRI with or without contrast for suspected cartilage pathology; plain radiographs may show osteochondritis dissecans.	Other than locking resulting from a subluxating joint, most other causes may need surgical treatment.
Joint clicking, popping, or snapping	1. Torn cartilage 2. Loose body 3. Joint hypermobility 4. Subluxating tendons 5. Impingement or snapping or joint capsule, retinaculum	MRI with or without contrast for suspected cartilage pathology.	Many cases of popping or clicking are benign. Pursue workup if there are associated symptoms (pain, swelling, locking, instability).
Bony tenderness	1. Fracture 2. Stress fracture 3. Contusion 4. Subperiosteal hematoma 5. Developmental variant 6. Tumor 7. Osteomyelitis	Plain radiographs; bone scan or MRI if plain films are normal; CT scan to clarify pathology.	Any bony pain or tenderness needs to be explained, even if preliminary plain films are normal.
Soft tissue swelling	1. Contusion 2. Myositis 3. Cellulitis 4. Bursitis 5. Synovial cyst (including ganglion cyst) 6. Lipoma 7. Soft tissue sarcoma 8. Foreign body reaction	MRI is the most useful imaging study if imaging is necessary; some conditions may be evaluated by fluid aspiration, cultures, or biopsy.	Clinical evaluation will be more useful than any specific test.
Extremity deformity	1. Fracture 2. Dislocation 3. Severe muscle strain (complete rupture) 4. Hematoma 5. Congenital or developmental disorder 6. Bone or soft tissue tumor	Plain radiographs indicated for both traumatic and nontraumatic deformity.	For acute deformity due to fracture or dislocation, compromise of neurovascular status may warrant immediate intervention.
Spinal deformity	1. Scoliosis 2. Kyphosis 3. Lordosis 4. Disk herniation with lumbar shift 5. Compression fracture 6. Hemivertebrae	Plain radiographs with anteroposterior and lateral views; MRI can show disk pathology if plain films are normal.	Acute onset of spinal deformity is due to fracture or disk herniation; because of the risk of spinal cord or neurologic compromise, evaluation and treatment are more urgent than spinal deformity due to idiopathic scoliosis or postural deformities.
Flat feet	1. Normal variation 2. Tarsal coalition 3. Joint hypermobility	Evaluate gait and footwear; with a flexible flat foot, the heel inverts and the arch elevates if the patient stands on his or her toes.	Painful flat feet may indicate tarsal coalition; flat feet may contribute to pain in ankles, shins, or knees as a result of associated biomechanical abnormalities.

Continued

TABLE 29.8

Diagnostic Considerations for Common Presenting Findings—cont'd

Presenting Complaint or Physical Finding	Diagnostic Considerations	Recommendation for Further Evaluation	Comments
High-arched feet	1. Normal variation 2. Club feet 3. Spasticity	Evaluate gait, lower extremity muscle tone; x-ray if foot cannot be placed flat on the ground.	No intervention or correction is needed if pain free and if gait and neurologic examinations are normal.
Turned-in toes	1. Internal tibial torsion 2. Femoral anteversion 3. Metatarsus adductus	Torsional examination to evaluate hip rotation, tibial torsion (thigh-foot angle), and foot alignment.	Many problems self-correct with growth; further treatment may be necessary for fixed deformity associated with pain or dysfunction.
Genu valgus (knock-knees)	1. Normal variation 2. Femoral anteversion 3. Hyperpronation	Examination of the hip and subtalar joint is necessary to determine whether the genu valgus is fixed or whether it dynamically changes with weight bearing or gait.	Valgus deformity may further increase if knees hyperextend; rarely does the genu valgus need to be treated, but associated injuries (eg, patellofemoral pain) may need treatment to compensate for associated patellar tracking abnormalities.

MRI indicates magnetic resonance imaging; CT, computed tomography; and EMG-NCV, electromyography-nerve conduction studies.

Diagnostic Pitfalls

Attempts to logically and sequentially converge on a viable diagnosis can be thwarted by stumbling blocks in the diagnostic process. In some situations, the most prominent symptoms or physical findings are not due to the primary underlying diagnosis. Conversely, the primary diagnosis may not always produce the most prominent symptoms or physical findings. For example, with an ACL-MCL-meniscus injury or triad, the medial collateral ligament (MCL) sprain may produce the greatest pain and be the most obvious finding at physical examination. The medial meniscus tear may cause the greatest restriction of function but can be somewhat more difficult to assess during the examination. Ironically, the ACL, which is the most critical component of the triad, is the least likely of the 3 structures to produce pain by itself and can be the most difficult to appreciate at physical examination. In evaluating an anxious and uncomfortable patient, there may be a sense of relief once a plausible explanation for the symptoms has been identified. However, in the case of the ACL-MCL-meniscus triad, terminating the evaluation before the full extent of the injury is recognized will lead to treatment that similarly ends before the full extent of the injury is addressed.

Another area of caution in diagnosing musculoskeletal problems occurs when similar injury mechanisms, similar symptoms, and similar physical findings are associated with distinct injuries. This occurs most frequently in skeletally immature patients in which an unfused epiphysis or apophysis is more vulnerable to injury than the corresponding ligament or tendon. When the distal femoral physis is immature, an apparent MCL sprain could turn out to be a distal femoral epiphyseal fracture. What may appear to be a hamstring strain in a skeletally mature patient could be an avulsion of the ischial apophysis in a skeletally immature patient. Heel pain that appears to be Achilles tendonitis or plantar fasciitis may be calcaneal apophysitis in a skeletally immature patient.

Some of the most common diagnostic pitfalls that can sidetrack a diagnostic evaluation are listed in **Table 29.9**. Knowing where mistakes and diagnostic errors may occur can identify areas in which particular caution is waranted.

TABLE 29.9

Common Pitfalls in the Diagnosis of Sports Injuries in Children

Preliminary Diagnosis	Alternative Diagnosis	Comment
Ankle sprain	Distal fibular epiphyseal fracture	Assess for bony tenderness across physis; x-ray may show widening.
Anterior cruciate ligament sprain	Tibial eminence fracture	Lateral x-ray should be done on skeletally immature patient with positive Lachman test.
Quadriceps strain	Avulsion of anterior inferior iliac spine	Tenderness is over anterior pelvis; x-ray shows open apophysis with or without separation.
Hamstring strain	Avulsion of ischial tuberosity	Tenderness occurs over ischium; x-ray shows immature apophysis with or without separation.
Meniscus tear	(a) Osteochondritis dissecans	(a) Hyperlucency on plain films over lateral portion of medial femoral condyle.
	(b) Discoid lateral meniscus	(b) Presents with meniscal symptoms without history of meniscal injury; widened lateral joint space; confirm with MRI.
MCL sprain	Fracture of distal femoral physis	Tenderness on distal femur extends beyond MCL attachment; x-ray shows widened physis.
Patellar fracture	Bipartite patella	Smooth, curvilinear lucency along superolateral border of patella; appears less irregular than fracture; history of trauma is inadequate to cause fracture.
Lateral epicondylitis (tennis elbow)	Osteochondritis dissecans of radiocapitellar joint	Patient may have swelling, restricted joint motion, clicking/catching, and hyperlucency on x-ray.
Navicular fracture (foot)	(a) Bipartite navicular	(a) Navicular has appearance of old fracture; similar findings may be present on asymptomatic side.
	(b) Accessory navicular	(b) Small, smooth-appearing fragment seen medial to navicular; may be confused with avulsion fracture.
Fifth metatarsal fracture	Iselin disease (apophysitis at base of Vth metatarsal)	X-ray may appear to be avulsion fracture, but the fracture line is parallel to the long axis of bone and may be visible on contralateral side.
Rotator cuff tendonitis	Proximal humeral epiphysitis	X-ray shows open, widened, and possibly displaced proximal humeral physis.
Hip pointer	Iliac crest apophysitis	Tenderness over iliac crest; x-ray shows open apophysis; no history of direct trauma sufficient to cause pain.
Plantar fasciitis and Achilles tendonitis	Sever's disease (calcaneal apophysitis)	Sever's disease occurs at age 8-14 when calcaneal apophysis is immature on x-ray; tenderness is on bone rather than Achilles or plantar fascia.
Patellar tendonitis	(a) Sinding-Larsen Johansson disease	(a) Tender at distal pole of patella. X-ray may show small bony fragment at inferior patellar pole; patients are usually aged 8-12; easily confused with avulsion fracture but there is no history of acute injury.
	(b) Osgood-Schlatter disease	(b) Tender at patellar tendon insertion on tibial tubercle; x-ray shows open apophysis with or without separation; patients are usually aged 12-16.
Peroneal tendonitis	Tarsal coalition	Peroneal spasm and tenderness seen in conjunction with rigid flat foot; may also have symptoms of instability without evidence of ligament laxity.
Lumbar facet syndrome	Spondylolysis	Spondylolysis occurs during rapid bony growth (at age 12-16); defect in pars interarticularis on x-ray, CT, or bone scan.
Vertebral compression fracture	Scheuermann kyphosis	Lateral radiographs of spine show $\geq$3 vertebral bodies with anterior wedging; insufficient trauma to account for fractures.
Acute scoliosis	Disk herniation with lumbar shift	Scoliosis does not develop acutely and does not present with pain; back injury usually precedes restricted mobility and abnormal posture.

MRI indicates magnetic resonance imaging; MCL, medial collateral ligament; and CT, computed tomography.

Symptom Locator — Shoulder

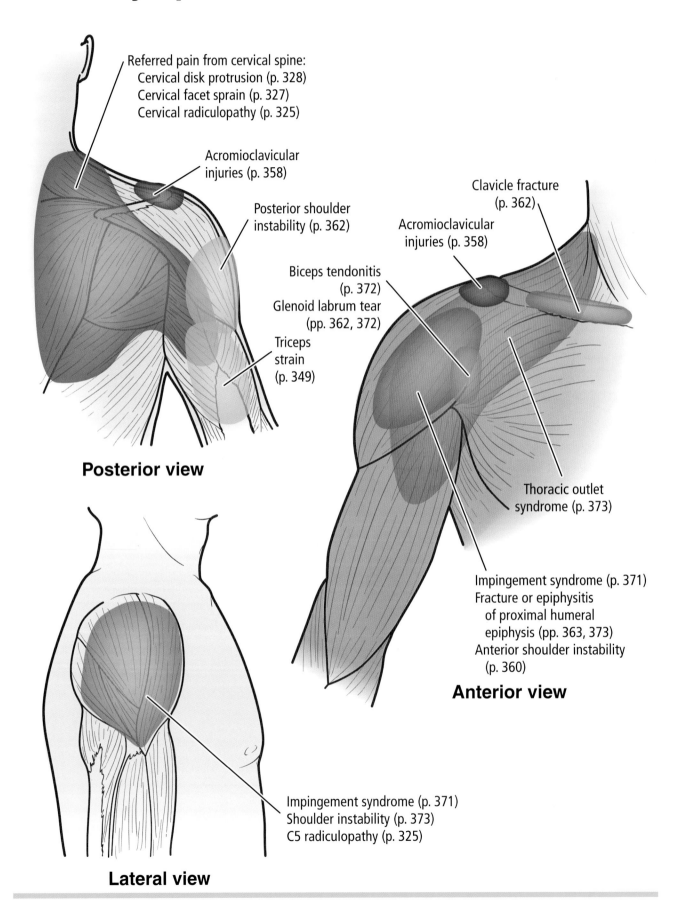

Referred pain from cervical spine:
Cervical disk protrusion (p. 328)
Cervical facet sprain (p. 327)
Cervical radiculopathy (p. 325)

Acromioclavicular
injuries (p. 358)

Posterior shoulder
instability (p. 362)

Biceps tendonitis
(p. 372)
Glenoid labrum tear
(pp. 362, 372)
Triceps
strain
(p. 349)

Posterior view

Clavicle fracture
(p. 362)

Acromioclavicular
injuries (p. 358)

Thoracic outlet
syndrome (p. 373)

Impingement syndrome (p. 371)
Fracture or epiphysitis
of proximal humeral
epiphysis (pp. 363, 373)
Anterior shoulder instability
(p. 360)

Anterior view

Impingement syndrome (p. 371)
Shoulder instability (p. 373)
C5 radiculopathy (p. 325)

Lateral view

Symptom Locator — Elbow and Forearm

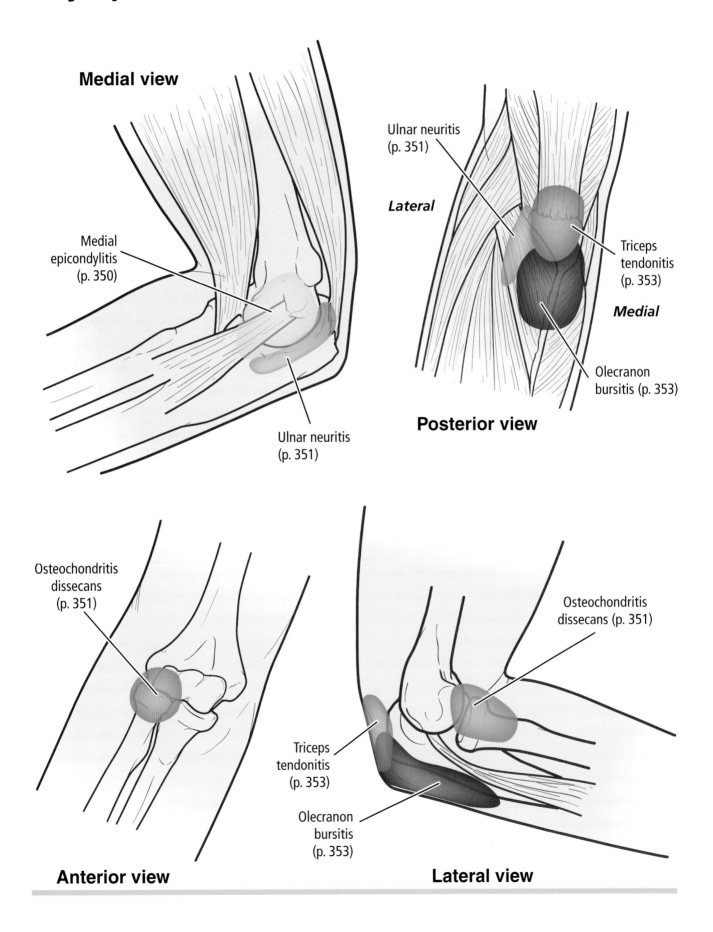

Medial view

Medial
epicondylitis
(p. 350)

Ulnar neuritis
(p. 351)

Ulnar neuritis
(p. 351)

Lateral

Triceps
tendonitis
(p. 353)

Medial

Olecranon
bursitis (p. 353)

Posterior view

Osteochondritis
dissecans
(p. 351)

Osteochondritis
dissecans (p. 351)

Triceps
tendonitis
(p. 353)

Olecranon
bursitis
(p. 353)

Anterior view

Lateral view

Symptom Locator — Hand and Wrist

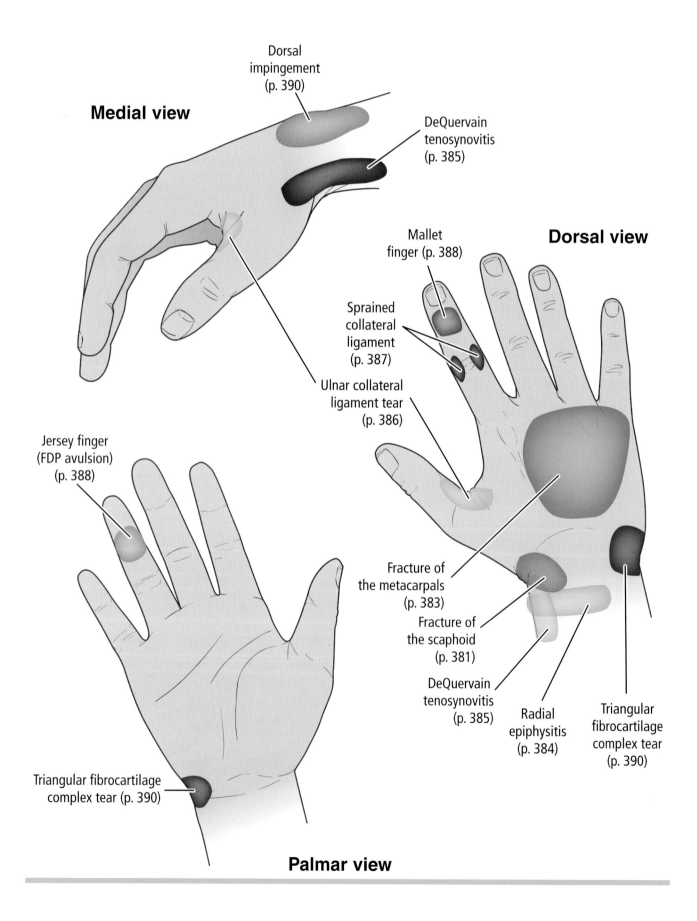

Medial view

Dorsal
impingement
(p. 390)

DeQuervain
tenosynovitis
(p. 385)

Dorsal view

Mallet
finger (p. 388)

Sprained
collateral
ligament
(p. 387)

Ulnar collateral
ligament tear
(p. 386)

Jersey finger
(FDP avulsion)
(p. 388)

Fracture of
the metacarpals
(p. 383)

Fracture of
the scaphoid
(p. 381)

DeQuervain
tenosynovitis
(p. 385)

Radial
epiphysitis
(p. 384)

Triangular
fibrocartilage
complex tear
(p. 390)

Triangular fibrocartilage
complex tear (p. 390)

Palmar view

Symptom Locator — Hip, Thigh, and Lower Leg

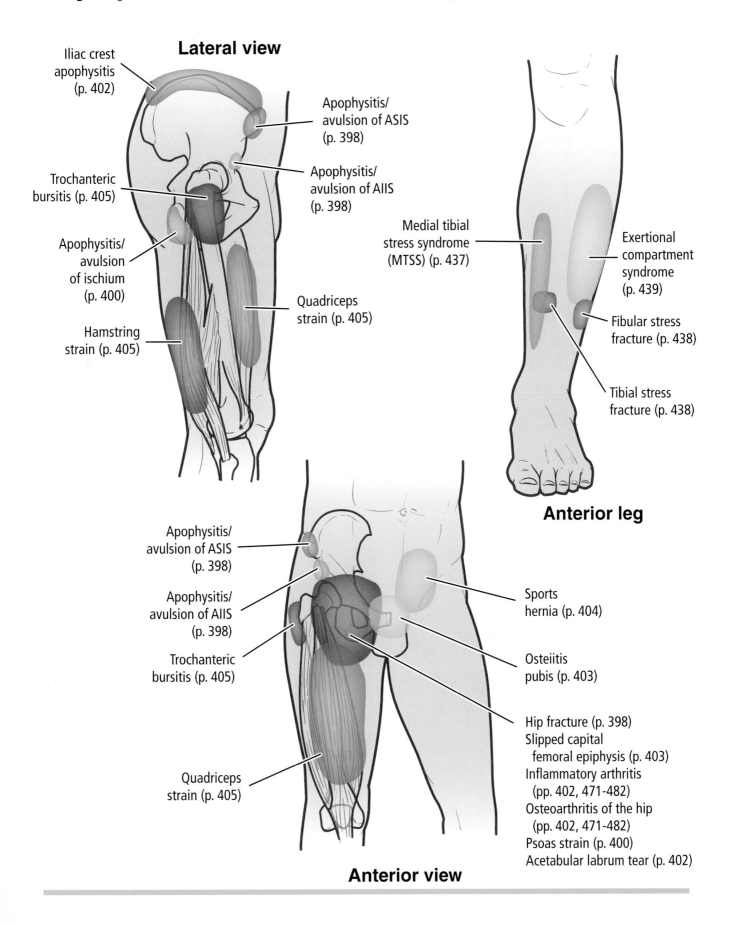

Lateral view

Iliac crest apophysitis (p. 402)

Apophysitis/ avulsion of ASIS (p. 398)

Apophysitis/ avulsion of AIIS (p. 398)

Trochanteric bursitis (p. 405)

Apophysitis/ avulsion of ischium (p. 400)

Quadriceps strain (p. 405)

Hamstring strain (p. 405)

Medial tibial stress syndrome (MTSS) (p. 437)

Exertional compartment syndrome (p. 439)

Fibular stress fracture (p. 438)

Tibial stress fracture (p. 438)

Anterior leg

Apophysitis/ avulsion of ASIS (p. 398)

Apophysitis/ avulsion of AIIS (p. 398)

Trochanteric bursitis (p. 405)

Quadriceps strain (p. 405)

Sports hernia (p. 404)

Osteiitis pubis (p. 403)

Hip fracture (p. 398)
Slipped capital femoral epiphysis (p. 403)
Inflammatory arthritis (pp. 402, 471-482)
Osteoarthritis of the hip (pp. 402, 471-482)
Psoas strain (p. 400)
Acetabular labrum tear (p. 402)

Anterior view

Symptom Locator — Knee and Lower Leg

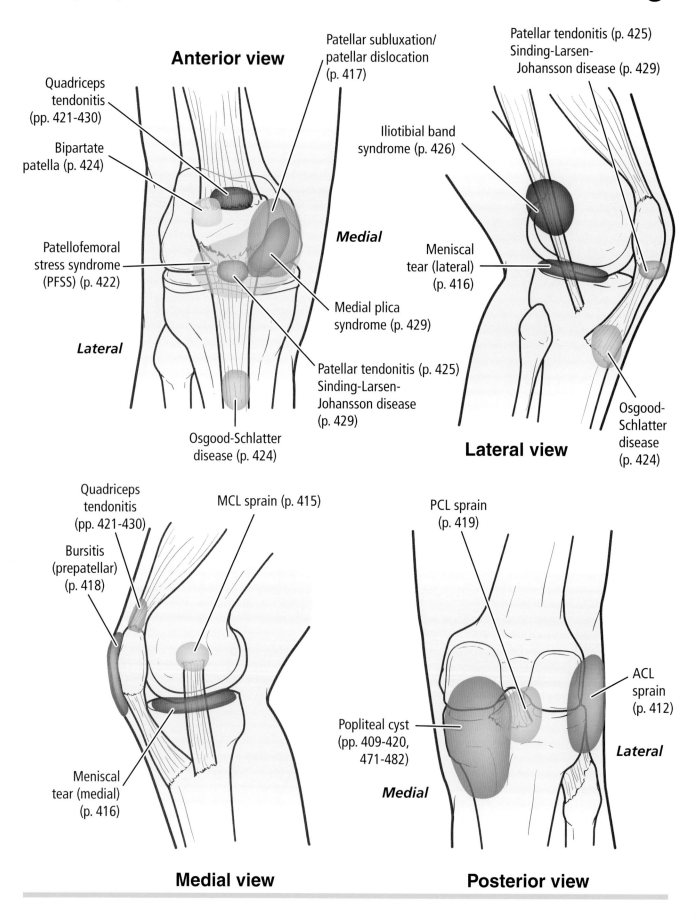

Anterior view

Patellar subluxation/
patellar dislocation
(p. 417)

Quadriceps
tendonitis
(pp. 421-430)

Bipartate
patella (p. 424)

Patellofemoral
stress syndrome
(PFSS) (p. 422)

Medial

Lateral

Medial plica
syndrome (p. 429)

Patellar tendonitis (p. 425)
Sinding-Larsen-
Johansson disease
(p. 429)

Osgood-Schlatter
disease (p. 424)

Patellar tendonitis (p. 425)
Sinding-Larsen-
Johansson disease (p. 429)

Iliotibial band
syndrome (p. 426)

Meniscal
tear (lateral)
(p. 416)

Osgood-
Schlatter
disease
(p. 424)

Lateral view

Quadriceps
tendonitis
(pp. 421-430)

MCL sprain (p. 415)

Bursitis
(prepatellar)
(p. 418)

Meniscal
tear (medial)
(p. 416)

Medial view

PCL sprain
(p. 419)

Popliteal cyst
(pp. 409-420,
471-482)

ACL
sprain
(p. 412)

Lateral

Medial

Posterior view

Symptom Locator — Foot and Ankle

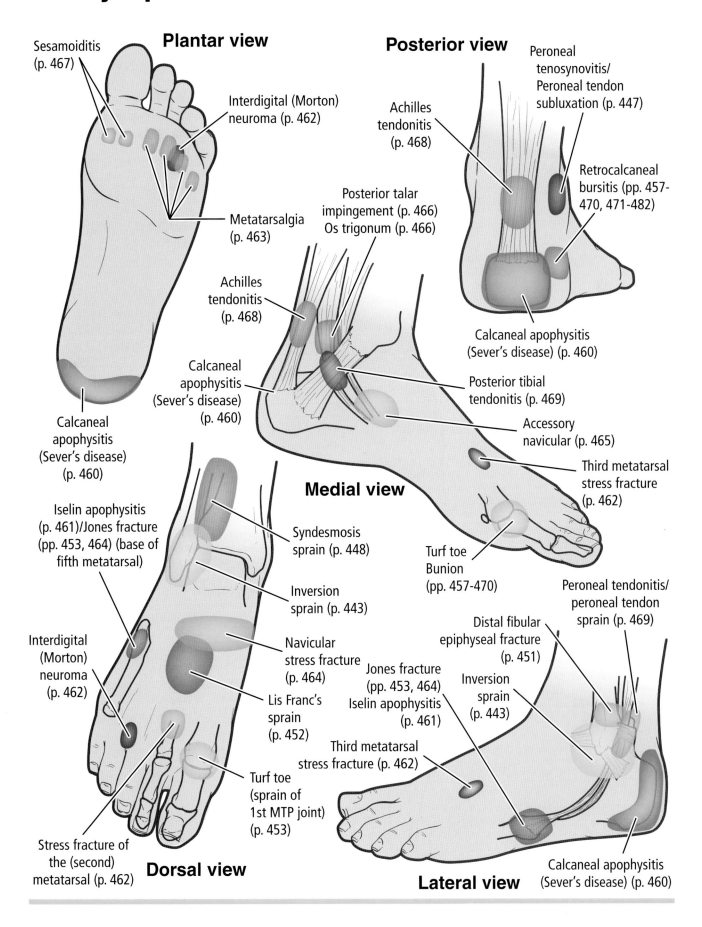

Plantar view

Sesamoiditis (p. 467)

Interdigital (Morton) neuroma (p. 462)

Metatarsalgia (p. 463)

Achilles tendonitis (p. 468)

Calcaneal apophysitis (Sever's disease) (p. 460)

Calcaneal apophysitis (Sever's disease) (p. 460)

Posterior view

Peroneal tenosynovitis/ Peroneal tendon subluxation (p. 447)

Achilles tendonitis (p. 468)

Retrocalcaneal bursitis (pp. 457-470, 471-482)

Posterior talar impingement (p. 466) Os trigonum (p. 466)

Calcaneal apophysitis (Sever's disease) (p. 460)

Posterior tibial tendonitis (p. 469)

Accessory navicular (p. 465)

Third metatarsal stress fracture (p. 462)

Medial view

Iselin apophysitis (p. 461)/Jones fracture (pp. 453, 464) (base of fifth metatarsal)

Syndesmosis sprain (p. 448)

Inversion sprain (p. 443)

Navicular stress fracture (p. 464)

Lis Franc's sprain (p. 452)

Turf toe (sprain of 1st MTP joint) (p. 453)

Turf toe Bunion (pp. 457-470)

Interdigital (Morton) neuroma (p. 462)

Stress fracture of the (second) metatarsal (p. 462)

Dorsal view

Distal fibular epiphyseal fracture (p. 451)

Jones fracture (pp. 453, 464) Iselin apophysitis (p. 461)

Inversion sprain (p. 443)

Third metatarsal stress fracture (p. 462)

Peroneal tendonitis/ peroneal tendon sprain (p. 469)

Calcaneal apophysitis (Sever's disease) (p. 460)

Lateral view

Symptom Locator — General

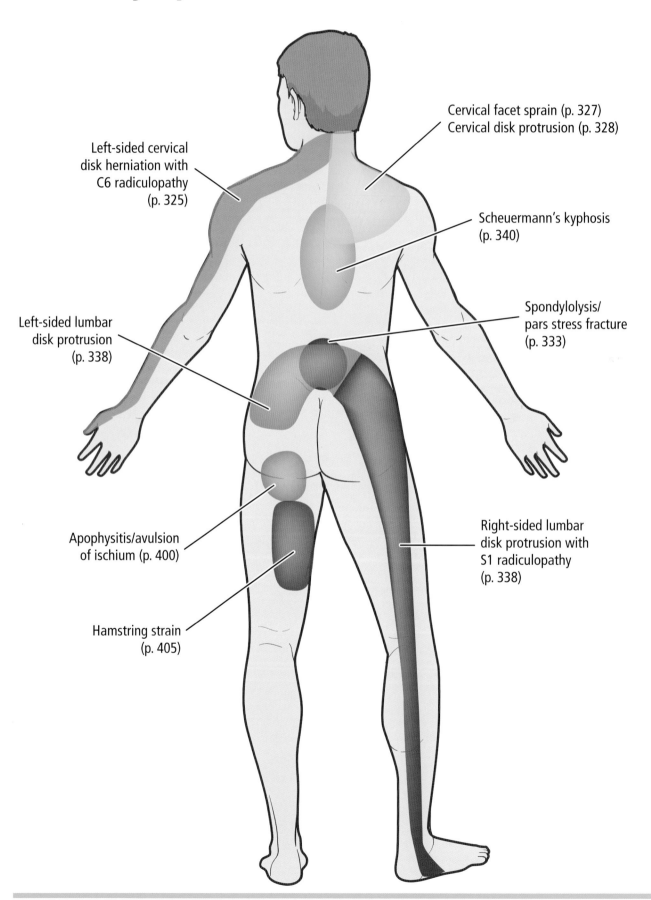

Cervical facet sprain (p. 327)
Cervical disk protrusion (p. 328)

Left-sided cervical disk herniation with C6 radiculopathy (p. 325)

Scheuermann's kyphosis (p. 340)

Spondylolysis/ pars stress fracture (p. 333)

Left-sided lumbar disk protrusion (p. 338)

Apophysitis/avulsion of ischium (p. 400)

Right-sided lumbar disk protrusion with S1 radiculopathy (p. 338)

Hamstring strain (p. 405)

SUMMARY POINTS

- Musculoskeletal symptoms can result from injuries, as well as from underlying medical conditions and developmental abnormalities.

- Because different diagnostic categories call for different diagnostic approaches, appropriate initial categorization of the problem can help ensure that the approach used will be the most efficient and effective in reaching a diagnosis.

- The various subtypes of both acute and overuse injury are associated with predictable antecedents, predictable injury mechanisms, predictable symptoms, predictable physical findings, and predictable x-ray findings.

- Acute injuries demand an accurate assessment of the effects of the injury; overuse injuries require an assessment of the causes of injury.

- Knowledge of known injury patterns can help determine when a diagnosis is plausible and when further evaluation is indicated.

- Establishing an accurate diagnosis is critical for planning effective treatment and determining when it is safe for an athlete to return to play after an injury.

- Some conditions are the result of multiple injury mechanisms or disease processes and require a broad diagnostic approach to properly identify and treat the underlying causes.

- A convergent process for diagnostic evaluation has the advantage of narrowing down the diagnostic possibilities and reducing unnecessary expenditures in the radiology department, with subspecialty consultants, and with ineffective treatment.

- Recognizing common diagnostic pitfalls and making appropriate distinctions between the causes and effects of injury can reduce misdiagnosis and mistreatment.

SUGGESTED READING

Anderson SJ. Sports injuries. *Curr Prob Pediatr Adolesc Health Care.* 2005;35:110-164.

Arrington ED, Miller MD. Skeletal muscle injuries. *Orthop Clin North Am.* 1995;26:411-422.

Best TM. Muscle-tendon injuries in young athletes. *Clin Sports Med.* 1995;14:669-686.

Caine D, Caine C, Maffuli N. Incidence and distribution of pediatric sport-related injuries. *Clin J Sport Med.* 2006;16:500-513.

Garrett WE. Muscle strain injuries. *Am J Sports Med.* 1996;24(6 suppl):S2-S8.

Hawkins D, Metheny J. Overuse injuries in youth sports: biomechanical considerations. *Med Sci Sports Exerc.* 2001;33:1701-1707.

Khan KM, Cook JL, Taunton JE, Bonar F. Overuse tendinosis, not tendonitis. *Phys Sports Med.* 2000;25:38-48.

Kirkendall DT, Garrett WE. Clinical perspectives regarding eccentric muscle injury. *Clin Orthop Relat Res.* 2002;(403 suppl):S81-S89.

Noonan TJ, Garrett WE. Muscle strain injury: diagnosis and treatment. *J Am Acad Orthop Surg.* 1999;7:262-269.

Solomon DH, Simel DL, Bates DW, Katz JN, Schaffer JL. Does this patient have a torn meniscus or ligament of the knee? Value of the physical examination. *JAMA.* 2001;286:1610-1620.

Witvrouw E, Lysens R, Bellemans J, Cambier D, Vanderstraeten G. Intrinsic risk factors for the development of anterior knee pain in an athletic population. A two-year prospective study. *Am J Sports Med.* 2000;28:480-489.

CHAPTER 30

Diagnostic Imaging

Weyton W. Tam, MD

Changes in computer technology over the past decade have produced a number of highly sophisticated imaging modalities, such as computed tomography (CT), magnetic resonance imaging (MRI), ultrasonography, and scintigraphy (bone scans). Given the wide variety of high-quality images available today, physicians must understand the indications for and the appropriate time to order specific images.

GUIDELINES FOR ORDERING IMAGING STUDIES

In the initial communication with the radiologist, physicians must specify the exact areas to be evaluated, the views desired, and the diagnoses under consideration. Poor communication may result in an order for an inadequate or inappropriate study. Providing a clinical history for the radiologist can help in selecting an appropriate imaging study and interpreting it correctly. This is especially true with the more sophisticated imaging modalities. In clinically confusing cases, consultation with the radiologist helps to direct the approach to the study and often improves the final interpretation. Consultation with a specialist may also be helpful in selecting the most appropriate imaging modality, as well as determining if there are alternatives to radiologic studies for making or confirming a suspected diagnosis.

Obtaining previous imaging studies, when available, may better focus the diagnostic possibilities by showing how the patient's condition has changed over time. Whenever possible, all imaging studies should be interpreted in conjunction with a review of all other previously related images. If these previous reports or images originate from another facility, they should be made available to the consulting radiologist.

Comparison views of the contralateral extremity are helpful because children have multiple ossification centers at various stages of maturity. However, in the absence of a comparison view, standard imaging texts can be consulted to identify normal growth patterns and developmental variants. This kind of consultation avoids the additional expense of imaging and the resulting irradiation of the contralateral normal extremity.

COMMON IMAGING TECHNIQUES

Table 30.1 shows the suggested hierarchy for ordering imaging studies for the young athlete.

Radiography

Conventional radiography (x-ray) is the mainstay of imaging. With few exceptions, almost all imaging should begin with radiographs, especially for patients with a history of trauma. Radiographs are almost universally available, inexpensive, and require the least amount of imaging time. Indications for conventional radiography include the evaluation of acute bone trauma, bone pain, joint pain, bone infection, soft tissue masses, and radiopaque foreign bodies.

Follow-up radiographs 14 to 21 days later provide an inexpensive means of confirming a diagnosis of radiographically occult fractures (**Figure 30.1**). Sometimes, however, in circumstances that require a rapid diagnosis (eg, an athlete with an upcoming competition), the more sophisticated and costly imaging techniques such as a CT scan, MRI, or bone scan should be considered.

Anteroposterior and Lateral Views Anteroposterior (AP) and lateral views should be obtained in patients with traumatic injuries whenever clinically possible. Radiographs of the extremities, especially those involving the forearm or leg, should include the joint above and below the involved bone. A minimum of 2 views obtained at 90° from one another should be obtained.

TABLE 30.1

Imaging of the Young Athlete

Consider Consulting a Radiologist

- If unsure of imaging modality of choice
- If complex case
- If unsure of necessity of intravenous or intra-articular contrast

Conventional Radiography

- Acute trauma to bone or soft tissue
- Bone or joint pain
- Epiphyseal or apophyseal injury
- Anatomic variants/developmental abnormalities
- Myositis ossificans

Additional Radiographic Imaging

Follow-up Radiograph (if initial studies are normal)

- Confirm occult fracture
- Evaluation for myositis ossificans

Stress Views[a]

- Ligamentous injury
- Physeal plate injury
- Accessory ossification center

Comparison View of Contralateral Extremity[b]

- Physeal plate injury
- Apophyseal abnormality
- Accessory ossification center

Computed Tomography

- Detailed evaluation of complex or intra-articular fracture
- Assess healing of fracture or stress fracture; evaluate nonunions
- Acute head or visceral trauma
- Further evaluation of potential myositis ossificans

Magnetic Resonance

- Soft tissue trauma (ligament, cartilage, muscle, tendon, bone marrow)
- Combination of soft tissue and bone trauma
- Infection
- Neoplasia

Bone Scan

- Excellent sensitivity, poor specificity
- Confirm occult fracture
- Evaluate generalized bone pain or multifocal trauma
- Reflex sympathetic dystrophy
- Osteomyelitis

Arthrography

- Evaluation of rotator cuff tear, triangular fibrocartilage complex (TFCC) tear, or scapholunate ligament tear
- Increasingly used in combination with magnetic resonance imaging for glenoid and acetabular labral tears in form of magnetic resonance arthrography

Angiography

- Detailed evaluation of vessels, particularly with altered distal pulses, extremity dislocation, or displaced fracture)

Ultrasonography

- Evaluation for presence of soft tissue foreign body
- Gynecologic imaging
- Vascular imaging

[a] Stress views should only be carried out by qualified specialists and only if the suspected instabiltiy cannot be confirmed by other clinical methods or imaging modalities.

[b] Consulation with standard reference texts on radiographic findings and normal variants may obviate the need to obtain comparision views.

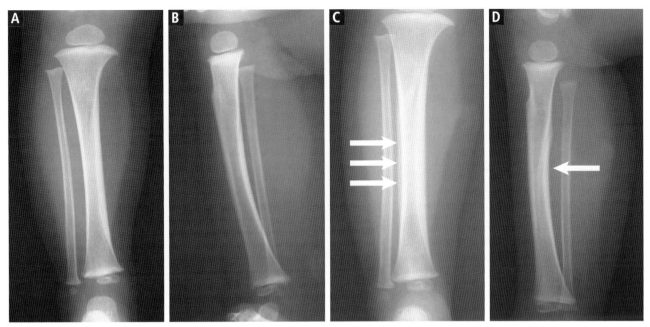

FIGURE 30.1 Follow-up radiographs are useful for identifying some suspected fractures. (A) Normal antero-posterior view. (B) Normal lateral view. (C, D) Repeat radiograph 3 weeks later showing periosteal new bone consistent with an undisplaced fracture.

Stress Views Stress views allow for indirect evaluation of ligamentous injuries. These views include, but are not limited to, weight-bearing views and varus-valgus stress views of peripheral joints. The joint of interest can either be stressed by the physician, the radiology technician, or the patient (weight bearing), or it can be stressed by the use of weights. If the patient has acute trauma, the presence of a physician is often required when obtaining stress views.

In skeletally immature patients, gentle stress views under direct fluoroscopic supervision may reveal an occult physeal plate injury. Weight-bearing views may accentuate joint instability not evident on a typical supine view, and use of weights may demonstrate or accentuate an acromioclavicular joint separation. An AP clenched-fist view of the wrist stresses the scapholunate ligament, accentuating a scapholunate dissociation. Varus-valgus stressing of the thumb can be used to confirm an ulnar collateral ligament injury.

Acute Cervical Injuries In the initial evaluation of acute cervical trauma, radiographs (including AP, lateral, and odontoid views) are indicated. If the problem involves the posterior elements of the cervical spine, base of skull, C1 or C2 vertebrae, or suspected fracture, thin section CT with sagittal and coronal reconstructions should be considered over MRI.

When spinal cord or disk abnormality is of primary concern, MRI is the study of choice. MRI can also demonstrate evidence of cervical spine ligamentous injury by the presence of edema or direct evidence of ligamentous discontinuity. However, soft tissue edema is not specific to ligamentous injury and can be seen with soft tissue contusions or be associated with downward dissection of fluid from an injury cephalad to the cervical spine. In addition, chronic ligamentous injuries do not tend to demonstrate edema and thus are much more difficult to detect on MRI. Lateral flexion-extension radiographs of the cervical spine should be considered in the evaluation of potential spinal instability when other studies are nondiagnostic. Flexion-extension views of the cervical spine are no longer routinely used in the initial evaluation of acute cervical spine trauma. The decision to obtain flexion-extension views should be made and carried out by a qualified specialist in cervical spine trauma. Obtaining these requires that the patient be conscious and able to communicate the presence of neurologic change, such as pain or dysesthesia. Flexion and extension of the cervical spine should be actively performed by the patient while a physician supports the head.

Other Views Radiographs of the chest, abdomen, and pelvis are routinely obtained after traumatic injuries to these areas. Initial imaging should include an AP view of the chest to evaluate for pneumothorax and mediastinal blood. In abdominal radiographs, visceral injury is suggested by the presence of pneumoperitoneum, free fluid, and bony injury. Although radiographs of the skull are commonly obtained, they provide little information about the condition of the brain. Significant, acute head trauma should be evaluated by a CT scan, not plain films.

Computed Tomography

CT results in the reformation of axial images by use of x-rays combined with a sophisticated computer. Because of its versatility in imaging the entire body, it has become widely used. Costs tend to be moderate, and with newer technology, images are obtained relatively quickly.

CT is often the best way to further evaluate cortical bone after radiography. It can diagnose minimally displaced cortical fractures and provide the anatomic detail that may be necessary before definitive reduction. This is especially useful for small bony structures, such as the carpal and tarsal bones, or for clinically sensitive bony sites such as the spine and the articular surfaces (**Figure 30.2**). A CT scan is the image of choice in evaluating severe, acute trauma to the brain (especially in the first 3 days), osseous spinal column, chest, abdomen, and pelvis. It can also be used to identify the presence of nonradiopaque foreign bodies, such as wood or plastic.

With thin-slice (1-3 mm thick) contiguous axial images, the data can be reconstructed into 2-dimensional images in other planes, or into 3-dimensional images. The speed at which 3-dimensional images are reconstructed depends on the sophistication of the scanner. State-of-the-art scanners are now able to reconstruct images almost immediately. In selected circumstances, such as complex facial, spinal, hip,

or foot injuries, 3-dimensional images can provide direct visualization of complex relationships among various bony structures (**Figure 30.3**).

The use of intravenous contrast material with a CT scan varies, depending on the reason for the examination. Because of the potential for a serious life-threatening allergic reaction to the contrast material, which occurs in 1 per 100 000 patients, contrast material should be used only under the supervision of a radiologist and limited to valid clinical indications. Contrast material is not usually required for imaging acute skeletal and head injuries. Rather, it is typically used for imaging of acute abdominal, pelvic, or chest injuries and looking for infection.

Patients with known iodine allergies can be given a non-ionic contrast agent and premedicated with a combination of an antihistamine and corticosteroid at least 12 hours before the study. Coordination between the radiologist and the treating physician should be considered in patients with multiple trauma in which vascular injury is also suspected. These patients may require angiography, and the total contrast agent load administered to the patient's kidneys should be considered.

Magnetic Resonance Imaging

MRI, in its simplest form, represents the use of a magnetic field to excite protons in the body to generate images. MRI is sensitive and specific for a variety of soft tissue and bony abnormalities. Because imaging times are far longer than with CT scans, patient cooperation is critical. Patients with acute trauma, medically unstable patients, or patients who

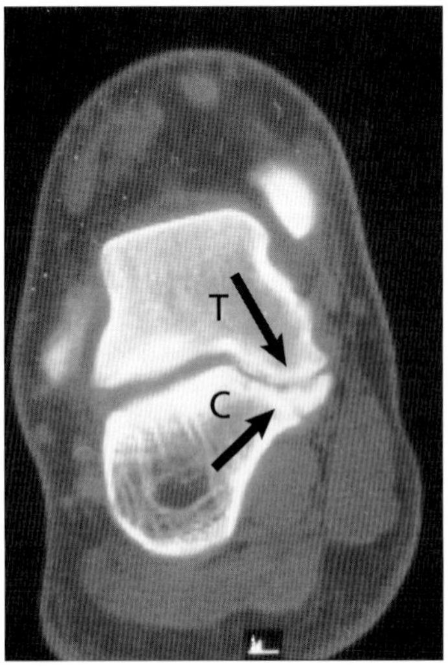

FIGURE 30.2 Computed tomographic scan showing a nonosseous coalition between the talus (T) and calcaneus (C).

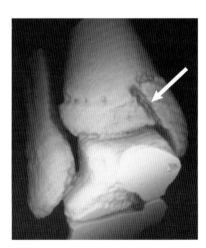

FIGURE 30.3 Three-dimensional reconstruction of an ankle fracture.

are confused, disoriented, uncooperative, or immature may not tolerate the imaging time. Despite the cost and occasional barriers to access, the demand for MRI remains high among athletes who anxiously await confirmation of a diagnosis or initiation of treatment.

The strength of MRI lies in its excellent soft tissue contrast and direct multiplanar capabilities. MRI provides exceptional evaluation of soft tissue injuries to the spinal cord, muscles, ligaments, tendons, menisci, and articular and labral cartilage. It can be used to identify and evaluate underlying abnormalities that may contribute to various impingement syndromes, such as those to the rotator cuff or carpal canal. However, judicious use of MRI is suggested because of its cost. MRI should be limited to clinically valid situations in which the results of imaging will alter treatment. Although MRI can be used to diagnose a lateral collateral ligament injury to the ankle, it is only occasionally required to clarify a clinically confusing picture. The need for rapid diagnosis or exclusion of associated injuries, such as for elite athletes who have an upcoming competition, is becoming a common rationale for MRI.

Increasingly common indications for MRI use in the young athlete include the following: persistent ankle pain despite conservative clinical treatment (due to osteochondral injury to the talar dome, anterolateral gutter syndrome); persistent bone pain (due to slowly healing radiographically occult stress fracture); and lower back pain in young athletes involved in gymnastics, cheerleading, or heavy weight lifting (due to stress fractures to the posterior elements of the lumbar spine). Although the sensitivity of bone scan is excellent, its specificity is poor. Most causes for increased bone turnover result in a focal hot spot on a late-phase bone scan (ie, trauma, tumor, infection, arthritis). Therefore, for many, MRI is the preferred imaging modality for evaluation of stress fracture.

MRI, in conjunction with knowledge of the reasons for increased bone stress or insufficiency fracture, aids in specificity. Imaging studies are similar to laboratory studies and need be interpreted in conjunction with the history. Because MRI has a much greater resolution than bone scan (which has basically no detail), if closely evaluated at a sufficiently high resolution, it often directly demonstrates a fracture line if both fluid-sensitive and T1 images are obtained. Injury will typically demonstrate an area of brightness on fluid-sensitive sequences. MRI sensitivity is generally as good as or better than a whole-body bone scan when the specific body part is imaged appropriately. Determining an exact location is better on MRI than bone

scan, which contributes to determination of the cause: stress fractures and insufficiency fractures tend to occur in certain common locations. MRI specificity can be improved by looking for a microfracture line, confirming the exact site of pain with an externally positioned skin marker, considering the location of MRI lesion, and interpreting the MRI in conjunction with radiographs. When MRI imaging is normal, there is often a level of confidence for return to competition for the coach, trainer, parent, and athlete that a radionuclide bone scan may not provide.

MRI is an excellent technique for evaluating bone marrow edema (**Figure 30.4**). It is extremely sensitive in detecting radiographically occult stress fractures, bone marrow contusions, osteomyelitis, and osteonecrosis. In addition, kinematic studies of the knee can be performed to evaluate dynamic patellofemoral joint subluxation. Recurrent joint effusions can be evaluated for inflammatory synovitis, pigmented villonodular synovitis, or so-called internal derangement. Soft tissue masses can be identified as cystic lesions such as soft tissue ganglion, synovial cyst (eg, Baker's cyst, paralabral cyst, parameniscal cyst), bursitis, hematoma, or solid masses (eg, tumors, ruptured muscle fibers). In certain situations, MRI can be combined with arthrography to better delineate small intra-articular injuries such as those affecting the glenoid and acetabular labrum.

Use of intravenous contrast material in MRI is limited primarily to evaluation of infection, soft tissue masses, and synovitis. As with CT scans, the use of contrast material is best decided by the radiologist.

Bone Scintigraphy

Bone scintigraphy, or bone scan, is a nuclear medicine imaging technique that uses a radioactive-labeled compound such as technetium methylene diphosphonate. Bone scans can evaluate the entire skeleton or can be localized to an extremity. Indications for bone scintigraphy include evaluation of occult fractures, stress fractures, osteomyelitis, and occasionally reflex sympathetic dystrophy (**Figure 30.5**). This imaging modality is sensitive when used to detect bony injury, but it is relatively nonspecific. Abnormalities detected by bone scan may need a more specific imaging modality, such as CT scan, to clarify the cause of the abnormality.

If the lesion is located in a region of complex bony anatomy, such as the spine, hip, or knee, single proton emission computed tomography (SPECT) should be performed.

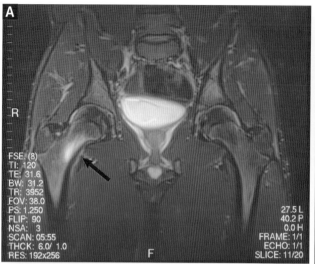

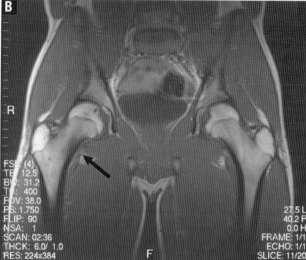

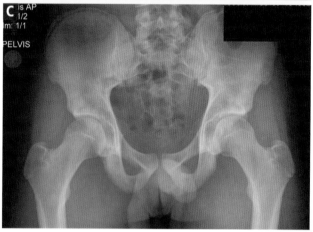

Figure 30.4 (A, B) Magnetic resonance imaging scan of a stress response (early stress fracture) involving the medial cortex of the right femoral neck. Note bone marrow edema. (C) Radiographs taken on the same day were normal. The patient was treated conservatively, and pain completely resolved within 2 months.

SPECT images allow for separation of activity from the lesion from the adjacent or overlying bony structures. This technique improves localization of the lesion to a specific anatomic site and can enhance both the sensitivity and specificity of scintigraphy. Although MRI may supplant scintigraphy as a preferred method for diagnosing stress fractures, bone scans may still be a better screening tool for evaluating a patient with multiple sites of bony pain or for evaluating patients who have experienced multiple traumas or abuse.

Arthrography

Arthrography is a technique in which air and/or contrast medium is injected percutaneously into a joint. Arthrography is used to evaluate the synovium and the structures immediately bordering the joint space. For many years, conventional radiographic arthrography was commonly used to evaluate meniscal injury and tears of the rotator cuff, wrist ligaments, and triangular fibrocartilage. Arthrography is relatively

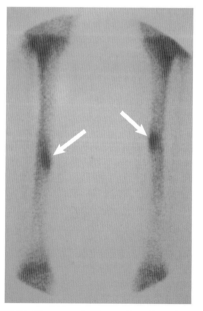

FIGURE 30.5 Bone scintigraphy showing increased uptake in the midshaft of both tibiae.

inexpensive and easily performed, but it is invasive and has largely been replaced by MRI.

Arthrography can also be performed with more sophisticated imaging techniques, such as CT scans and MRI. Magnetic resonance arthrography has replaced CT arthrography in most situations because of its superior contrast and direct multiplanar capability. Magnetic resonance arthrography is most often used to evaluate tears of the glenoid labrum or acetabular labrum. Magnetic resonance arthrography can also be used to evaluate meniscal pathology in patients who have had previous meniscal tears or arthroscopic surgery.

Angiography

Angiography is an invasive procedure used to image the vessels of the body. Iodinated contrast agents are used with conventional angiography. The risk of severe allergic reaction is similar to that associated with a contrast-enhanced CT scan; however, additional potential complications include hemorrhage, infection, and nerve and vascular injury. Conventional angiography is occasionally indicated in the young athlete, particularly for dislocations (especially at the knee—see **Figure 30.6**), displaced fractures with abnormal distal pulses after reduction, and severe deceleration or crush injuries to the chest.

Ultrasonography

Ultrasonography is increasingly being used in musculoskeletal imaging. Ultrasonography is most commonly used to evaluate potential vascular injury and to evaluate for presence of a nonradiopaque (especially wood or plastic) foreign body embedded within the soft tissues. In addition,

ultrasonography of the pelvis is useful for evaluating the incidental soft tissue pelvic mass occasionally seen during MRI of the lumbar spine or during routine physical examination of a female athlete.

EVALUATION OF SOFT TISSUE MASSES

Radiographs are generally the first imaging study ordered when evaluating a soft tissue mass, especially after trauma. A muscle or contusion may ossify in as little as 3 weeks, forming a radiographically characteristic lesion known as myositis ossificans (**Figure 30.7**). Radiographs are the preferred imaging technique because these lesions can mimic a soft tissue sarcoma on MRI; they can also mimic osteosarcoma histologically.

If the diagnosis of myositis ossificans cannot be confirmed by radiography, a noncontrast CT scan can be obtained to identify the typical peripheral zoning phenomenon. Calcified soft tissue masses that do not follow the typical clinical pattern for myositis ossificans may need MR imaging or biopsy.

SUMMARY POINTS

- As with all other diagnostic tests, the value of imaging depends on the initial clinical appropriateness of the test and the proper performance and interpretation of the study.

- A study should not be performed unless there is a specific question that needs to be answered and if that answer will alter the clinical decision and treatment process.

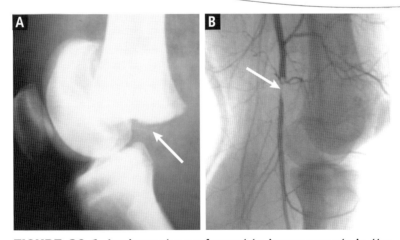

FIGURE 30.6 Angiography performed to image vessels in the body. (A) Radiograph of a distal femoral physeal fracture in a patient without pulses in the foot. (B) Postreduction angiogram showing disruption of the popliteal artery.

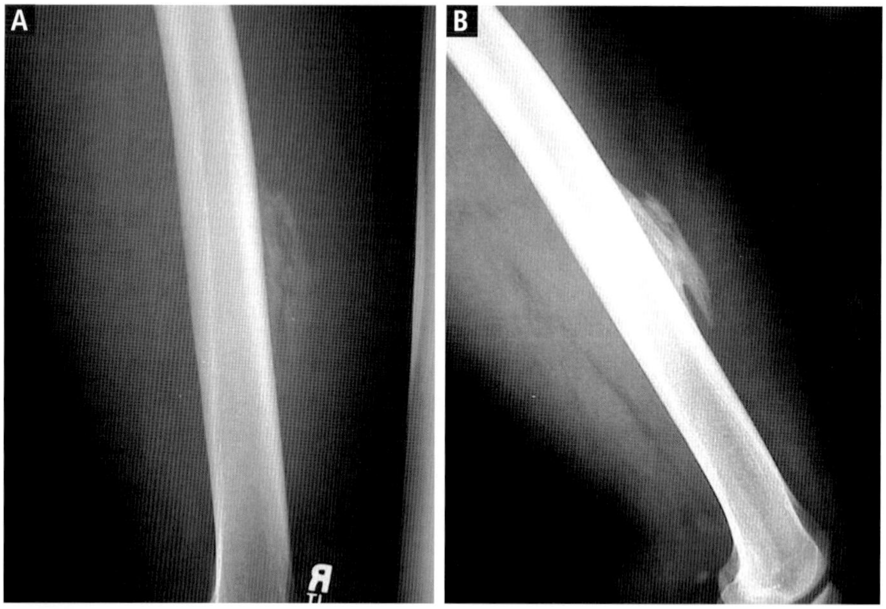

FIGURE 30.7 (A) Faint ossification with early myositis ossificans. (B) Mature myositis ossificans.

- If the problem is complex or if there is a question regarding which imaging technique to order, direct consultation with a radiologist is suggested.

- If the patient is to be sent to a specialist, a phone call to that specialist may prevent unnecessary imaging or inadequate studies. The specialist may have a specific request or question that will alter the imaging approach.

SUGGESTED READING

Collier BD Jr, Fogelman I, Rosenthail L, eds. *Skeletal Nuclear Medicine.* St Louis, MO: Mosby-Year Book; 1996:46, 232, 311-332.

Keats TE, ed. *Atlas of Normal Roentgen Variants That May Simulate Disease.* 5th ed. St Louis, MO: Mosby-Year Book; 1992.

Pavlov H, Dalinka MK, Alazraki N, et al. Acute trauma to the knee. American College of Radiology. ACR Appropriateness Criteria. *Radiology.* 2000:215 Suppl: 365-373.

Rogers LF, ed. *Radiology of Skeletal Trauma.* 2nd ed. New York, NY: Churchill Livingstone; 1992:302.

Stoller DW. *Magnetic Resonance Imaging in Orthopaedics and Sports Medicine.* 2nd ed. Philadelphia, PA: Lippincott-Raven; 1997.

Swischuk LE, ed. *Emergency Radiology of the Acutely Ill or Injured Child.* 2nd ed. Baltimore, MD: Williams & Wilkins; 1986:105-116, 205-279.

CHAPTER 31

Principles of Rehabilitation

Steven J. Anderson, MD

Rehabilitation is a process designed to help athletes restore normal function after injury or illness. Physicians provide a valuable service to athletes by identifying the functional deficits caused by injury, offering options for treatment, organizing a rehabilitation program, supervising the recovery process, and determining when function is restored adequately to permit a safe return to play. The resolution of pain is an important milestone in the recovery process but should not be equated with full recovery. In addition to pain, injuries are associated with losses of flexibility, joint motion, muscle strength, coordination, and general fitness. These losses may persist even after pain or other symptoms have subsided. Before an athlete returns to play, these losses must be addressed with the rehabilitation process to avoid limitations of performance and further injury.

REHABILITATION PLANNING

Planning a rehabilitation program starts with an analysis of the medical needs of the injured athlete (**Table 31.1**). It is essential to establish an accurate diagnosis and to identify the causes and effects of the injury. Without a precise diagnosis and an understanding of the natural history of the condition, it is impossible to measure the efficacy of treatment. With acute injuries, the effects of the injury (ie, swelling, joint instability, deformity, weakness) must be identified and ultimately corrected with treatment. For overuse injuries, the causes of injury (ie, training, equipment, technique, malalignment, strength imbalances, and inadequate flexibility) must be identified and addressed in the course of treatment.

Understanding the demands of the sport is also important in determining the potential effects of an injury on performance, the risk for further injury, the specific goals and end points of rehabilitation, the need to modify the activity or the level of participation, and the requirements for return to play. Factors such as the athlete's general health, motivation, external support systems, access to treatment resources, and time constraints also influence the rehabilitation program and its outcome. Educating athletes about their injuries, the rationale and goals for treatment, and the necessary steps in the rehabilitation program can increase compliance and help the athletes become more invested in their recovery process.

A rehabilitation program is an evolving, sequential process organized to address the specific causes and effects of injury in a given individual. With injury, there is typically pain and swelling, as well as loss of motion, strength, and function. A rehabilitation program uses therapeutic modalities to reduce pain and swelling and therapeutic exercises to restore flexibility, joint motion, strength, and function. The particular rehabilitation tools used depend on what is needed to address the deficits that are present (**Table 31.2**). Each successive step in the rehabilitation process is predicated on completing the previous step. For example, restoring full joint motion may not be possible until joint swelling is resolved. Strengthening exercises will not be fully effective until pain and swelling are controlled and joint motion is restored. Similarly, functional patterns; proprioception; and complex, integrated tasks cannot be performed without first controlling pain and restoring motion and baseline strength.

THERAPEUTIC MODALITIES

The tools available for the various phases of rehabilitation are known as therapeutic modalities and include physical modalities, therapeutic exercises, and orthopedic appliances. These modalities are described next, and some of the common applications are summarized in **Table 31-2**.

TABLE 31.1

Essential Questions for Rehabilitation Planning

- What is the diagnosis?
- Is the injury an acute or overuse problem?
- If acute, what are the effects of the injury? Effects may include:
  - Pain
  - Swelling
  - Loss of motion
  - Weakness
  - Instability
  - Dysfunctional movement patterns
  - Proprioceptive deficits
- If overuse, what are the contributing causes of the injury? Causes may include:
  - Extrinsic factors such as:
    - Training error
    - Surfaces
    - Shoes
    - Equipment
    - Coaching
    - Technique
    - Environmental conditions
  - Intrinsic factors such as:
    - Flexibility
    - Strength
    - Joint stability
    - Alignment
    - Gender
    - Skeletal maturation
    - Overall fitness
- Are there concurrent injuries or other medical conditions that may affect recovery?
- What level of activity modification and injury protection are necessary to permit healing and prevent further injury?
- What are the functional demands of the sport?
- What are the functional limitations due to the injury?
- Are there sport-specific and general conditioning exercises that can be safely continued during the rehabilitation process?
- What are the available tools for reducing pain and inflammation, and what is the plan for using these tools?
- What are the available tools for restoring joint motion and muscle flexibility, and what is the plan for using these tools?
- What are the available tools for restoring strength and endurance, and what is the plan for using these tools?
- What are the available tools for restoring function, and what is the plan for using these tools?
- What are the goals for functional restoration, and how can the level of recovery be objectively measured?
- Have the criteria for determining readiness to return to play been satisfied?

PHYSICAL MODALITIES

Physical modalities facilitate the rehabilitation process by decreasing pain, swelling, spasm, and soft tissue restrictions and by preparing an injured athlete for the therapeutic exercise phase of rehabilitation. Physical modalities include therapies that use cold, heat, and electricity. These modalities are used primarily in the initial phase of treatment to control pain, swelling, and muscle spasm.

Cold Therapy

Cold therapy, or cryotherapy, is the application of cold to the injured area in the form of ice packs, ice massage, and hydrotherapy, including ice baths and ice whirlpools. Cryotherapy is intended to decrease pain, swelling, capillary blood flow, muscle spasm, and local metabolic activity (**Table 31.3**). Cold is the modality of choice for nearly all acute injuries accompanied by pain and swelling. In addition, cold therapy may be used to diminish inflammatory changes associated with overuse injuries such as tendonitis, apophysitis, bursitis, and periostitis. Cold therapy can be used as long as there is inflammation or swelling. However, for most acute injuries, the inflammatory phase tends to subside within 1 to 2 weeks and the indications for icing decrease accordingly.

Ice packs may be applied directly to the skin for 20 minutes at a time and as frequently as once per hour. Chemical ice packs may be colder than frozen water and can cause burns if left in place too long. The use of ice packs is not recommended for athletes with cold-induced urticaria, athletes with Raynaud's disease, or when the injury is in a location that has poor circulation. In addition, ethyl chloride spray can provide rapid, superficial cooling to the skin. This modality is used primarily as a topical anesthetic.

Ice massage is effective for treating injuries that cause localized areas of superficial inflammation, such as tendonitis or bursitis. With this technique, ice is rubbed in a circular pattern over the affected area for approximately 10 minutes per session. Ice baths or ice whirlpools are used if the injured area is relatively diffuse and can be submerged. Contrast baths alternate between cold and heat and may be used to reduce edema.

Heat Therapy

Heat therapy is most commonly administered with hot packs, hydrotherapy, and ultrasound. Hot packs heat the affected body part by conduction, hydrotherapy heats by convection, and ultrasound heats by transduction of mechanical sound waves to heat. Less common heating

TABLE 31.2

Use of Therapeutic Modalities

Symptoms and Physical Findings	Modality	Exercise	Equipment	Comment
Acute swelling	• Ice • EGS	• General exercise permissible as long as the injured area is not affected	• Compression • Braces and splints for immobilization	...
Chronic inflammation	• Ice • Phonophoresis • Iontophoresis • Nonsteroidal anti-inflammatory drugs	• Stretching • Joint mobilization • Isometric and short arc strengthening	• Tape • Soft braces • Neoprene sleeves	...
Restricted joint motion with inflammation	• Ice	• Isometric strengthening • Active exercises in ROM without pain	• Compression wraps • Functional braces	• Assess for intra-articular pathology
Restricted joint motion without inflammation	• Heat • Ultrasound	• Active ROM exercises • Passive ROM exercises • Active-assist ROM exercises	• Progressive splints to maintain motion • Night splints	• Rule out systemic disease and reflex sympathetic dystrophy
Joint instability	• None, unless swelling is present	• Strengthening in pain-free range • Closed kinetic chain exercises • Proprioceptive exercises	• Immobilize acute injury • Functional braces later	• Distinguish between static and functional instability
Muscle atrophy	• EGS	• Progressive resistance exercises	• Weights and tubing for home exercise program	• Distinguish between atrophy due to disuse and neurologic injury
Muscle imbalances	• EGS for retraining weak muscles	• Selective strengthening exercises	• Weights and tubing	• Distinguish between weakness due to disuse and neurologic injury
Loss of flexibility with injury	• Ice • EGS • Ultrasound	• Static stretching • Massage • Progressive resistance exercises	...	...
Loss of flexibility without injury	• Ultrasound	• Active stretching, with and without assistance • Massage • Myofascial release	...	• Address underlying cause of muscle tightness
Proprioceptive deficit	...	• Balance and proprioceptive exercises • Functional exercises	• Neoprene sleeve or wrap for tactile input • Balance board	• Document deficit by modified Romberg test

EGS indicates electrogalvanic stimulation; ROM, range of motion.

modalities use radiant heat, short-wave diathermy, paraffin baths, fluidotherapy, and pulsed infrared laser. Analgesic ointments and sports creams can provide a perception of warmth because they irritate the skin, but they do little to increase the temperature below the skin surface.

Heat therapy can reduce pain and spasm, increase blood flow, increase compliance of soft tissue structures, and increase nerve conduction velocity (Table 31.3). Heat has a limited role in acute injuries or in conditions in which inflammation and swelling are present. The common practice of switching from cold therapy to heat therapy

TABLE 31.3

Physical Effects of Therapeutic Heat and Cold

	Heat	Cold
Pain	Decrease	Decrease
Spasm	Decrease	Decrease
Nerve conduction velocity	Increase	Decrease
Edema	Increase	Decrease
Metabolic activity	Increase	Decrease
Capillary blood flow	Increase	Decrease
Collagen extensibility	Increase	Decrease

48 hours after an acute injury—particularly when swelling and inflammation persist—has no basis in scientific fact. If heat therapy is used, it is best to apply heat before exercise or in the treatment of chronic conditions in which restricted muscle or joint motion hampers recovery. The positive effect of stretching exercises can be enhanced by warming the muscles before stretching, either actively with warm-up exercises or passively with the heating modalities mentioned previously.

Ultrasound heat therapy can penetrate more deeply than other heating modalities and may be the best modality for injuries such as deep thigh bruises. Ultrasound may be used in combination with a corticosteroid cream in a technique known as phonophoresis. The ultrasound increases the permeability of the skin to allow penetration of the corticosteroid into the underlying inflamed structures. Ultrasound should be used with caution over growth plates, and it should not be used over a hollow viscus or over a deep thigh bruise with possible myositis ossificans.

Therapeutic Electricity

Therapeutic electricity can be delivered in the form of electrogalvanic stimulation (EGS), transcutaneous nerve stimulation (TNS), or iontophoresis. EGS causes small muscle contractions to produce a pumping action that mobilizes edema and reduces swelling. In addition, muscle stimulation from EGS may help decrease muscle atrophy that accompanies injury, immobilization, or disuse. TNS uses electric stimulation to block the transmission of pain impulses from musculoskeletal injury, neuritic pain, or postoperative pain. Furthermore, TNS is convenient to use because its units are portable. Iontophoresis establishes an electrical field around an injury that helps to deliver an ionized form of corticosteroid to the injured site. Both iontophoresis and phonophoresis have similar applications,

but iontophoresis uses electricity rather than heat to enhance delivery of the medication.

THERAPEUTIC EXERCISE

Therapeutic exercise improves joint mobility and stretches and strengthens muscles (**Table 31.4**). Therapeutic exercises can begin once swelling and spasm subside and when the athlete can move the injured area without pain.

Joint Mobilization

Deficits of joint mobility may precede an injury and commonly occur as an effect of injury. With acute injuries, a reduction of swelling and inflammation typically allows for restoration of normal joint motion. When restrictions of joint motion persist—even after swelling and mechanical barriers have been removed—active joint mobilization techniques may be needed. Restricted joint motion can impair development of strength, limit performance, and contribute to further injury in the affected area or related structures.

TABLE 31.4

Therapeutic Exercises

Flexibility
- Stretching exercises
  - Static stretching
  - Ballistic stretching
  - Proprioceptive neuromuscular facilitation
- Soft tissue mobilization
- Myofascial release
- Massage therapy

Joint Mobilization
- Active mobilization
- Passive mobilization
- Active-assist mobilization

Strengthening Exercises
- Isometric exercises
- Isotonic exercises
- Isokinetic exercises
- Concentric exercises
- Eccentric exercises
- Closed kinetic chain exercises
- Plyometric exercises
- Functional exercises

The primary responsibility of the treating physician is to assess the source of restrictions of joint motion, including muscle inflexibility, scar formation, and structural abnormalities within the joint, and to prescribe therapy that can restore normal joint motion.

Techniques for improving joint mobility include active mobilization, passive mobilization, and active-assist mobilization. Active joint mobilization requires the athlete to use his or her power to move a joint. It is considered the safest and most readily available technique. Passive joint mobilization requires an assistant, such as a trained therapist, to move a restricted joint. This technique can achieve motion beyond what the athlete is able or willing to perform. However, passive joint mobilization can cause or exacerbate injury, particularly when it is performed by someone who is not qualified. Active-assist mobilization combines techniques of both active and passive mobilization to improve joint mobility. This technique also requires a therapist who is trained and certified in joint mobilization.

Stretching

Stretching restores flexibility after an injury and corrects deficiencies in flexibility that may have contributed to the injury. The primary methods of stretching are static and ballistic stretching. With static stretching, the target muscle is stretched and held for 20 to 30 seconds. Static stretching is safe, effective, and easily performed without any equipment or assistance (**Figure 31.1**). Ballistic stretching involves rapid stretches that are often associated with bouncing motions. Muscle strains can occur with these stretches because they activate the stretch reflex that causes the muscle being stretched to contract. Therefore, ballistic stretching is not recommended for injury rehabilitation.

Flexibility can also be achieved through assisted stretching techniques such as proprioceptive neuromuscular facilitation (PNF). With PNF, the target muscle is contracted against resistance and then passively stretched. By sequentially contracting and stretching the muscle, flexibility gains can be achieved beyond what can be accomplished by other stretching techniques. The use of PNF is limited by the availability of a trained and certified therapist.

In general, warm muscles (achieved by either warm-up exercises or by passive heating modalities) respond better to flexibility exercises. Stretching before activity is commonly recommended; however, stretching after activity may produce greater gains in flexibility because the muscles are already warm.

Manual techniques such as myofascial release and friction massage can improve flexibility and soft tissue mobility. Such techniques again require the assistance of a physical therapist or certified athletic trainer. Massage therapy is another form of manual therapy that can be used to promote gains in flexibility.

Strengthening

Nearly any activity that contracts a muscle also strengthens it. With appropriate training, even pubescent and prepubescent athletes can improve strength. However, muscle weakness and muscle atrophy can occur relatively rapidly with immobilization or disuse, or with the inhibitory effects of pain. As is the case with joint mobility and flexibility, premorbid deficits can lead to injury, and further deficits can occur directly from injury or as a result of the rest and inactivity that follows injury.

Strengthening exercises are categorized according to changes in length of the muscle, the amount of resistance, and the speed of contraction. The gains in strength are specific to the type of strengthening exercise carried out. Multiple repetitions with submaximal resistance are required for muscle endurance. Fewer repetitions with the greatest possible resistance lead to maximal strength. Developing power requires training with greater levels of speed and resistance of muscle contraction. In a rehabilitation program, the strengthening phase may begin with simple isometric exercises or low-resistance, short-arc isotonic exercises. Such exercises can reawaken the muscles and reduce atrophy while minimizing the risk of pain or further injury. Ultimately, the exercises should progress until strength and endurance have been restored throughout the full range of motion of the muscle. If the patient's sport requires endurance, exercises to train for endurance should be included. Similarly, if the sport requires strength or power, the rehabilitation program should train the muscles to meet the demands of the patient's activity.

Isometric Exercises

With isometric exercises, a muscle contracts without changing length. Isometric strengthening is considered a safe way to resume strengthening after an injury because the athlete controls the forces generated during the exercise and performs the exercise without moving the injured joint or muscle. Isometric exercises also allow the athlete to isolate and contract single muscle groups, which aids the process of muscle reeducation. Isometric exercises do not require any special equipment or facilities.

Isotonic Exercises

Isotonic exercises involve contracting a muscle against fixed resistance throughout its arc of motion. Most weight machines, free weights, and pulleys provide isotonic resistance.

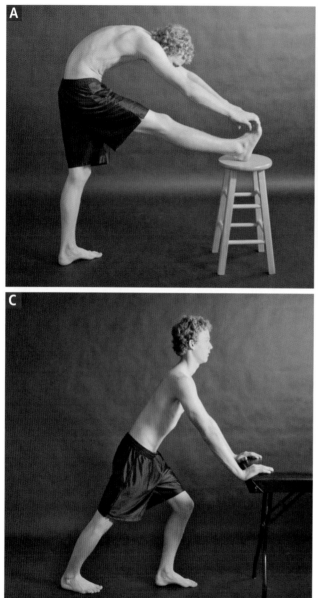

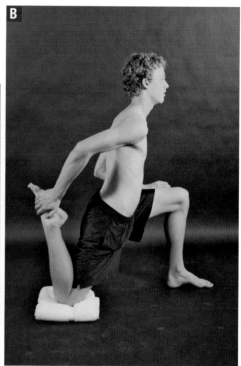

FIGURE 31.1. Static stretching of (A) hamstring, (B) quadriceps, and (C) calf.

If muscle strength is required through the full range of motion, resistance exercises ultimately must be performed throughout the full range of motion. Isotonic strengthening should not be initiated until pain and swelling have been controlled and restrictions ultimately of flexibility and joint motion have been addressed. For an athlete to continue to gain strength, the isotonic resistance must be increased as adaptive changes occur. Progressive resistive

exercises (PREs) refer to a commonly prescribed regimen of incremental strengthening.

Isokinetic Exercises

With isokinetic exercises, the speed of muscle contraction is constant. Typically, isokinetic machines have a lever that sets the machine to move at a predetermined number of degrees of arc per second. The machine then measures the force that the athlete applies against this arm as torque. Conditioning at high speeds on isokinetic machines approximates the speed of muscle contraction during many sports activities. However, isokinetic machines are expensive to own and operate. In addition, some iso-kinetic exercises cause nonphysiologic loading or place abnormal shear forces on joints that may contribute to injury.

Strengthening exercises may be further characterized as concentric, eccentric, closed kinetic chain, and functional. Clinically, these distinctions are important because each type of exercise is designed to meet the specific functional demands of different athletes and sports.

Concentric and Eccentric Exercises

Concentric exercises contract or shorten muscles during exercise. Many traditional exercises for strength training such as biceps curls, bench press, and leg press are con-centric exercises. With eccentric exercises, the muscles elongate during contraction. Eccentric exercises, some-times called "negative contraction exercises," oppose the forces of gravity. The quadriceps contract eccentrically when an athlete lands from a jump, decelerates, or walks down stairs. With a biceps curl, lifting the weight involves a concentric contraction of the biceps, while a controlled lowering of the weight involves an eccentric contraction of the biceps.

With eccentric contractions, the combination of simul-taneous stretch and contraction of muscle generates high levels of tension in the muscle-tendon unit. Because the development of strength is related to the level of tension in the muscle, significant improvements in strength are possible with eccentric exercises. Eccentric strengthening can be useful during rehabilitation to prepare an athlete to withstand the eccentric loads that often lead to muscle injury. However, given the high levels of tension generated with eccentric exercises, they can also cause muscle strain injury.

Closed and Open Kinetic Chain Exercises

A closed kinetic chain exercise involves a concentric-eccentric loop whereby the muscle is strengthened in both a shortening phase and a lengthening phase. With closed kinetic chain exercises, the foot or hand is fixed to the floor, as with a squat lunge or push-up. The exercise starts and ends at the same position. With open kinetic chain exercises, the distal portion of the extremity is not fixed. A biceps curl or knee extension is an example of an open chain exercise. Closed chain exercises are thought to more closely mimic functional patterns used in sports

and to improve strength in both the concentric and eccentric phase of contraction.

Plyometric Training

Plyometric exercises are useful for training for power and explosiveness and are commonly used as condition-ing drills for athletes in running or jumping sports such as basketball, volleyball, gymnastics, diving, and track. A plyometric exercise may involve jumping off a plat-form, landing, and immediately jumping back on. With landing, there is a rapid stretch of the quadriceps while it is simultaneously contracting to decelerate knee flexion and preparing to jump again. During this high-speed eccentric contraction, the elastic properties of the muscle generate tension, as well as the contractile properties of the muscle. The combination of these forces generates considerable forces that stimulate the development of greater muscle strength and power, but it may also cause injury. Plyometric training may be recommended to prepare athletes for the particular demands of a given sport, but because of the risk of muscle-tendon injury, caution and skilled supervision are encouraged.

Functional Exercises

Functional exercises strengthen muscles in their position of normal use or function. Usually, functional exercises repli-cate movements or patterns of movement required by a sport. Unlike exercises that isolate a single muscle in a single plane of motion, functional exercises involve the integrated action of multiple muscle groups working in multiple planes of motion. Functional exercises are the most advanced strengthening exercises because they require mastery and in-tegration of all the earlier types of strengthening, including concentric, eccentric, closed kinetic chain, and isokinetic ex-ercises. Before functional exercises can begin, strength must be restored in individual muscle groups and in simpler pat-terns or planes of motion.

Functional exercises require intact proprioception to maintain proper balance and control. Proprioception can be restored with balancing exercises, such as those done using a balance board or standing on one foot while play-ing catch with a ball or performing a distracting activity. Adequacy of proprioception can be tested with a modified Romberg test. With this test, the athlete stands on one foot with his or her eyes closed. When proprioception is restored, the athlete will be able to maintain balance on the affected extremity, as well as the uninjured extremity.

Functional testing provides an objective means to document effective restoration and integration of strength before continuing with the rehabilitation program.

Strength Testing

Objective measures of strength provide evidence of the athlete's improvement and readiness to proceed in the rehabilitation process. Manual muscle testing is convenient and easy to perform but is limited by interobserver variability and relative strength differences between the examiner and the patient. When testing strong muscles such as the quadriceps or calf, it may be helpful to use gravity as resistance and have the patient perform multiple repetitions of a given exercise. For example, in testing the quadriceps, the patient can do a series of 10 one-legged squats. The athlete's speed and ease in performing the exercise can easily be observed and compared with the performance using the uninjured extremity. Similarly, for testing calf strength, repetitive toe raises can be performed, with the speed of contraction and height of heel elevation observed and compared with that of the opposite side. Strength can also be tested by having the athlete lift a weight repeatedly. Isometric strength can be tested by observing how long a patient can maintain a given posture. A wall-sit measures isometric quadriceps strength, and a side plank exercise measures the ability to use trunk muscles to stabilize the spine.

Isokinetic machines assess muscle power at various speeds of contraction and at various points in the movement arc. Isokinetic machines may provide the best measurements of strength imbalances between paired muscle groups.

Functional Testing

Functional testing can examine proficiency at specific functional patterns of movement, as well as sport-specific skills. Functional tests can be created simply by identifying a movement performed in the sport that is likely to be affected by the injury, and then devising an exercise that tests the athlete's ability to perform that movement. For example, if a sport requires running and cutting movements, athletes should be tested to determine whether they can perform these movements before returning to play. Running grapevines or karaoke are examples of functional training and can be used for functional testing. Functional tests can help with return-to-play decisions because the decisions about readiness are based on the functional ability of the athlete rather than arbitrary lengths of time.

Orthopedic Appliances

Orthopedic appliances protect an injured area and minimize the negative impact on uninjured structures. A wide range of orthopedic appliances are used for rehabilitation, and recommendations for their use are detailed elsewhere, including Chapter 46 on injury prevention.

Usually, acute injuries that cause pain, swelling, joint instability, or weakness will need some level of protection and immobilization. Orthopedic devices that provide such protection include splints, casts, braces, tape, crutches, and slings. For injuries associated with significant swelling, a splint is preferable to a cast. Splints may be prefabricated or made with casting material. Wrist splints, finger splints, knee immobilizers, and cast boots can be adjusted to allow for swelling and removed to apply ice or to repeat an examination. A splint can be converted to a cast once any swelling is controlled or if there is reason to believe that an athlete may not comply with wearing a removable splint. Also, crutches and slings may be used in conjunction with splints or casts to further protect and immobilize the injury. In addition, elastic bandages provide compression, hold ice packs in place, and remind an athlete to protect the injury during the initial phases of recovery.

When the athlete is ready to start exercising, the injured area may still require some protection but not complete immobilization. A functional brace allows exercise and motion within a controlled range while still protecting the injured site.

Orthotic devices may facilitate recovery from overuse injuries caused by biomechanical abnormalities. Orthotics are designed to offer stability, support, and control, or they may be designed to offer cushion or shock absorption. An orthotic prescription, whether it is for a custom or off-the-shelf product, should be based on the foot type and specific needs of the patient. In general, a patient with a hyperpronated flat foot *and* an injury in which the instability of the foot structure is a contributing factor will benefit from a rigid or semirigid orthotic. A patient with a high-arched, cavus foot rarely needs additional stability and control in footwear but may benefit from additional cushioning. An orthotic is rarely sufficient by itself to treat an injury, and an improper orthotic can actually cause injury.

Protective equipment such as custom pads, flak jackets, face shields, goggles, and playing casts may protect the injured area and allow the athlete to return to limited play before the injury has completely healed. Such protective equipment should be used only if the injury and the protective equipment do not significantly impair function and if the protective equipment effectively reduces the risk of further injury. An example of appropriate use of protective equipment may be a playing cast for a soccer player with a stable wrist fracture or goggles for a basketball player with a corneal abrasion. Officials for the sport must approve the protective equipment. Often when an athlete requires equipment beyond what is normally used in the sport, the physician must submit a letter of explanation, and the parents must sign a liability waiver.

If the equipment used for the sport contributed to the injury because of faulty design, poor fit, or improper maintenance, it may have to be modified or corrected before the athlete can return to the sport.

PHASES OF A REHABILITATION PROGRAM

The rehabilitation program may be divided into 3 phases: (1) initial care, which addresses the immediate effects of injury; (2) intermediate care, which restores normal motion and strength through therapeutic exercises; and (3) functional rehabilitation, which involves more complex movement patterns, sport-specific skills, and transition back to play (**Table 31.5**). Each of these phases of rehabilitation occurs sequentially and lasts approximately one-third of the total time required for rehabilitation. For example, if pain and swelling resolve after 2 weeks of initial care, restoration of motion and strength during intermediate care will require approximately 2 weeks, and fitness and function will require another 2 weeks in later care. This formula can help to estimate recovery times and serves as a reminder that return to play depends more on measurable restoration of function than it depends on time.

The specific goals for each phase of rehabilitation are addressed by selecting and implementing the appropriate treatment options available in each phase. In general, pain and swelling need to be controlled before motion and strength can be restored. It is also necessary to restore motion and strength before proprioception and more complex functional exercises can be carried out. For overuse injuries, intrinsic and extrinsic factors contributing to the injury must be identified and corrected during the rehabilitation process.

The progress through the course of rehabilitation should be monitored with a follow-up visit ideally occurring at the transition point between each of the 3 phases of rehabilitation. If it is not possible to have the patient return for an office visit, progress can be monitored through reports from a physical therapist or certified athletic trainer who may be helping with the rehabilitation. If progress is slow or if unexpected complications arise, follow-up with the physician may be necessary to determine whether the treatment will simply take more time, whether additional diagnostic information is necessary, or whether other forms of treatment should be considered.

INITIAL CARE

Usually initial care for an acute or overuse injury includes rest and protection from the injury-producing activity. The amount and duration of rest depend on the nature and seriousness of the injury.

With relative rest, the injured area is protected while the athlete continues a modified training regimen or carries out conditioning exercises that will not interfere with recovery. When patients are given viable options for maintaining their fitness, the recovery process may not be as long in perception or in reality.

In addition to prescribing an appropriate level of rest as well as options for cross training, initial care must also address pain and inflammation. For acute injuries, applying ice; elevating the injured area; and applying compressive wraps, splints, or braces are most helpful during this phase of treatment. For conditions with persistent inflammation, modalities such as electric stimulation can be an adjunct to treatment with ice. Anti-inflammatory medication for acute injuries can help reduce pain and swelling but does not promote tissue healing. For conditions such as tendonitis, bursitis, periostitis, and arthritis, the presence of inflammation has a less obvious role in helping the injury heal. Therefore, use of anti-inflammatory medications for overuse or nonacute injuries has a more logical basis of support.

Analgesics play a limited role in the treatment of injured athletes. Athletes who need medication for pain should not play. Most pain from musculoskeletal injury can be controlled adequately with rest, immobilization, and therapeutic modalities. A similar caution is warranted for muscle relaxants. These medications have no direct effect on the

---

TABLE 31.5

Phases of Rehabilitation

Initial Care
- Relative rest
- Protection and support
- Control of pain and inflammation

Intermediate Care
- Resolution of residual pain and inflammation
- Restoration of joint motion
- Restoration of flexibility
- Restoration of strength
- Address biomechanical abnormalities
- Restoration and maintenance of fitness

Functional Rehabilitation
- Progressive strengthening exercises
- Proprioceptive training
- Functional exercises
- Sport-specific skills
- Determine readiness to return to play

Follow-up Care
- Protective equipment
- Maintenance therapy
- Recheck visit if symptoms persist or recur

muscle or the cause of the muscle spasm. The side effects and addictive potential of narcotic analgesics and muscle relaxants make them undesirable for use in young athletes.

Modalities such as EGS and TNS can be used for swelling and pain during initial care, but they require referral to a physical therapist or athletic trainer. Similarly, acupuncture has been shown to help both acute and chronic pain.

INTERMEDIATE CARE

The goals of intermediate care are to resolve residual pain and swelling and to restore flexibility, joint motion, and strength. Biomechanical abnormalities and deficits in flexibility and strength that contributed to the injury should also be addressed during this phase.

Athletes may begin intermediate care when pain and swelling subside and the injury has had sufficient time to begin healing. By this time, athletes should not require any splints, casts, slings, crutches, or other devices that can limit joint motion or muscle contraction. However, tape, elastic or neoprene sleeves, functional braces, pads, and orthotic devices may offer some protection as athletes begin this more active phase of rehabilitation.

Physical therapists or certified athletic trainers can teach athletes exercises to restore flexibility, joint motion, and strength, both by demonstration and by printed handouts. In addition to giving proper instruction, trained personnel can supervise the exercises to increase compliance and the likelihood of a successful outcome. Prescribing and demonstrating rehabilitation exercises after the effects of acute injury have subsided will increase the chances of the patient performing the exercises at the correct time and in the correct manner. When exercises for intermediate care are prescribed at the initial visit for an acute injury, the patient may be unable to physically perform the exercises or grasp the important details of the information. Usually, injured athletes will be more receptive to learning rehabilitation exercises once they have had time to recover from the initial effect of the injury and are feeling well enough to participate actively in the rehabilitation process.

Strengthening exercises should be performed only within the range of motion that does not cause pain. Initially, isometric or short-arc isotonic exercises may be the only exercises that do not cause pain. If pain or swelling develops, the exercise should be modified or curtailed. An athlete who responds favorably to strengthening exercises will be able to perform the exercises through wider ranges of motion with increasing resistance and/or more repetitions.

The end points for therapeutic exercise are restoration of symmetry and balance of motion and strength. The injured extremity should be equal to the uninjured extremity in motion and strength. Because muscles work in agonist and antagonistic pairs, strengthening exercises should be designed for both pairs to restore balances that are normal for the joint. Visible deficits or asymmetries warrant further attention before the athlete progresses to the later phase of rehabilitation.

During the intermediate phase of rehabilitation, the athlete can begin general conditioning exercises to maintain fitness as long as the general conditioning exercises do not overload the injured area. For example, an athlete with a knee or ankle injury may be able to tolerate swimming, whereas an athlete with a shoulder or elbow injury may be able to tolerate running, bicycling, stair climbing, elliptical trainers, or skating. By maintaining fitness, the athlete will be better prepared to return to play once the injury has healed. In addition, cross training can provide a safe outlet for the athlete's desire to be active while allowing the necessary time to progress through the rehabilitation process.

FUNCTIONAL REHABILITATION

When the athlete regains normal joint motion, muscle flexibility, and strength, he or she is ready to advance to the last phase of rehabilitation, known as functional rehabilitation. During this phase, exercises are designed to develop more complicated, demanding, and sport-specific skills.

By the time the athlete is ready for functional exercises, there should be little need for physical modalities or medications. However, functional braces, taping, orthotics, and protective equipment may still be used. Flexibility and joint motion should be normal, but ongoing maintenance exercises can help preserve the gains made earlier.

The most significant changes during the later phase of rehabilitation occur with strengthening. The athlete should be pain free while performing any of the exercises in this phase. Strengthening exercises can be expanded to include work at higher speeds of contraction, as well as exercises designed to enhance power and endurance. Closed kinetic chain exercises and functional exercises can be introduced during this later phase. Also, exercises that restore proprioception or position sense are an important element of functional rehabilitation. Balance boards or balancing exercises can be used to identify proprioceptive deficits and to restore proprioceptive function. Training in functional exercises requires integration and coordination of multiple muscle groups and helps restore neuromuscular mechanisms that will be used in the athlete's sport.

Specific requirements for muscle speed, power, endurance, and coordination will vary among the different sports. The physician can help ensure adequate functional rehabilitation by identifying the demands of a sport, assessing the deficits of the athlete, prescribing appropriate exercises, monitoring recovery, and testing functional ability before allowing the athlete to return to play.

FOLLOW-UP CARE

Usually, once athletes successfully complete a functional rehabilitation program, they can return to play. Depending on the injury and the sport, modifications or restrictions of activity may initially be warranted. The longer the athlete has been away from the sport during rehabilitation, the longer the time required to build up to full activity.

By the time an athlete returns to practice, the rehabilitation program can usually be simplified to include a few essential maintenance exercises. Integrating these maintenance exercises into the training routine for the sport is an easy way to continue rehabilitation. Maintenance exercises may be continued for the duration of the season or until the athlete has fully participated in the activity for a month without recurrent symptoms or injury.

Athletes who participate in seasonal sports may develop seasonal injuries. A common example is elbow or shoulder pain that coincides with the beginning of baseball season. For athletes with these injuries, year-round maintenance exercises are impractical. Instead, selected rehabilitation exercises may be started 4 to 6 weeks before the next season begins. Continuing a limited set of exercises, combined with a gradual buildup to full activity, may help prevent recurrent injury.

After discussion of the type and duration of maintenance exercises, the final step of follow-up care is instructing athletes about the early warning signs of further injury or the criteria for scheduling a follow-up evaluation. Selected conditions, such as physeal injuries or osteochondritis, may require scheduled follow-up. If the athlete changes sports or the level of participation, a follow-up visit may also be helpful to confirm that the original recommendations for treatment and participation still apply.

INFORMED CONSENT

A successful rehabilitation program will help an injured athlete regain full function and return to play while minimizing the risk of further injury. However, even with the best-conceived rehabilitation program, athletes and their parents should understand that risks of further injury cannot be eliminated entirely. The physician should help identify injury risks and recommend options for reducing the risks related to the injury and the sport. Athletes can be medically cleared to return to play when the risks of further injury return to baseline. In some cases, recognition of baseline risks may discourage athletes from returning to play. When the risks for further injury are disproportionately high, medical clearance to return to full activity may be denied, regardless of the athlete's or family's willingness to accept those risks. Documenting the rationale for return-to-play decisions, as well as patients' and families' understanding and acceptance of the risks, may prove useful, if a return-to-play decision is ever questioned.

SUMMARY POINTS

- Injuries are typically associated with pain, inflammation, restricted motion, weakness, deconditioning, and diminished function.

- Rehabilitation of sports injuries uses a sequential implementation of physical modalities, orthopedic appliances, and therapeutic exercise to reduce pain and inflammation; restore flexibility and joint motion; restore strength, endurance, and fitness; and correct functional deficits.

- Rehabilitation of acute injuries focuses primarily on correcting the effects of an injury.

- Rehabilitation of overuse injuries focuses on identifying and correcting the intrinsic and extrinsic causes of injury.

- Objective measurements of functional restoration can help ensure that rehabilitation goals have been met and that the athlete is ready to return to play.

SUGGESTED READING

Allen RJ. Physical agents used in the management of chronic pain by physical therapists. *Phys Med Rehabil Clin North Am.* 2006;17:315-345.

Anderson SJ. Sports injuries. *Curr Probl Pediatr Adolesc Health Care.* 2005;35:110-164.

Elder CL, Dahner LE, Weinhold PS. A cyclooxygenase-2 inhibitor impairs ligament healing in the rat. *Am J Sports Med.* 2001;29:801-805.

Fuller CW, Walker J. Quantifying the functional rehabilitation of injured football players. *Br J Sports Med.* 2006;40:151-157.

Fyfe I, Stanish WD. The use of eccentric training and stretching in the treatment and prevention of tendon injuries. *Clin Sports Med.* 1992;11:601-624.

Geffen SJ. Rehabilitation principles for treating chronic musculoskeletal injuries. *Med J Aust.* 2003;178:238-242.

Harris GR, Susman JL. Managing musculoskeletal complaints with rehabilitation therapy: summary of the Philadelphia Panel evidence-based clinical practice guidelines on musculoskeletal rehabilitation interventions. *J Fam Pract.* 2002;51:1042-1046.

Hubbard TJ, Denegar CR. Does cryotherapy improve outcomes with soft tissue injury? *J Athl Train.* 2004;39:278-279.

Jette AM, Haley SM. Contemporary measurement techniques for rehabilitation outcomes assessment. *J Rehabil Med.* 2005;37:339-345.

Khalsa PS, Eberhart A, Cotler A, Nahin R. The 2005 Conference on the Biology of Manual Therapies. *J Manipulative Physiol Ther.* 2006;29:341-346.

Kibler WB. Closed kinetic chain rehabilitation for sports injuries. *Phys Med Rehabil Clin North Am.* 2000;11:369-384.

Kibler WB, Chandler TJ, Pace BK. Principles of rehabilitation after chronic tendon injuries. *Clin Sports Med.* 1992;11:661-671.

Kibler WB, Lee PA, Herring SA, Press JM, eds. *Functional Rehabilitation of Sports and Musculoskeletal Injuries.* Gaithersburg, MD: Aspen Publishers; 1998.

Mair SD, Seaber AV, Glisson RR, Garrett WE. The role of fatigue in susceptibility to acute muscle strain injury. *Am J Sports Med.* 1996;24:137-143.

Nyland J, Nolan MF. Therapeutic modality: rehabilitation of the injured athlete. *Clin Sports Med.* 2004;23:299-313.

Prentice WE, ed. *Rehabilitation Techniques in Sports Medicine.* 2nd ed. St Louis, MO: Mosby-Year Book;1994:94.

Simpson CA. Complementary medicine in chronic pain treatment. *Phys Med Rehabil Clin North Am.* 2006;17:451-472.

Young JL, Press JM. The physiologic basis of sports rehabilitation. *Phys Med Rehabil Clin North Am.* 1994;5:9-36.

CHAPTER 32

Stress Fractures

Andrew J. M. Gregory, MD

A stress fracture or fatigue fracture is a weakening of bone that occurs from repetitive compressive or tensile stresses on the bone. Stress fractures are overuse injuries as distinct from acute fractures in which the bony injury occurs after a single traumatic event. Stress fractures are common injuries in young athletes and must be considered in any active young person who seeks care for bone pain or a limp. Stress fractures are usually treatable by rest alone. Once the bone has healed and the contributing training errors and biomechanical risk factors have been addressed, the athlete may fully return to the activity. However, if left unrecognized or untreated, stress fractures can progress to complete fracture or malunion. With careful attention to training, biomechanics, diet, and menstrual function, many stress fractures can be prevented. This chapter reviews the epidemiology, pathogenesis, evaluation, diagnosis, treatment, and prevention of stress fractures in young athletes.

CAUSE AND EPIDEMIOLOGY

Bones are in a constant state of turnover, with new bone being laid down and old bone being resorbed. This complex process is controlled by regulatory factors that are affected by hormones, dietary factors, and mechanical forces. Stress fractures develop when the damage caused by stress occurs too fast for the healing to keep up. Under these conditions, bone resorption by osteoclasts exceeds bone formation by osteoblasts.

The process leading to a stress fracture follows a continuum from simple edema in the marrow with no visible fracture line (termed *stress reaction*) all the way to a complete fracture. Stress reactions can be seen only on magnetic resonance imaging (MRI) or bone scans (**Figure 32.1**),

whereas a fracture or fracture callus can be seen on plain films (**Figure 32.2** and **Figure 32.3**). If the diagnosis of a stress injury to the bone is made before changes are visible on plain films, recovery time may be decreased.

Risk Factors

Stress fractures can occur from normal stress to abnormal bone or abnormal stress to normal bone. Risk factors for stress fracture include genetically determined bone abnormalities, female gender, white ethnicity, low body weight, lack of weight-bearing exercise, oligomenorrhea, inadequate calcium and caloric intake, and disordered eating. Children with a history of 2 or more acute fractures have a greater risk of lower bone density and thus are at a higher risk for further fractures, including stress fractures. Children receiving chronic corticosteroid therapy, children with severe osteopenia, or children with osteogenesis imperfecta may get stress fractures from ordinary daily activity.

A number of risk factors, including low bone mineral density, menstrual irregularities, dietary factors, and history of prior stress fractures, have been associated with an increased risk for stress fractures in female athletes (see Chapter 16, Female Athletes) The female athlete seems to be at particular risk for stress fracture if the menstrual cycle is disrupted. If caloric intake does not match energy expenditure, then the body protects itself by stopping menses. The female athlete triad comprises 3 criteria that together are associated with an increased risk of stress fractures: disordered eating, amenorrhea, and osteopenia.

Biomechanical factors may contribute to development of a stress fracture. Flat feet or high arches, anterior bowing of the tibia, excessive lordosis of the lumbar spine, and leg

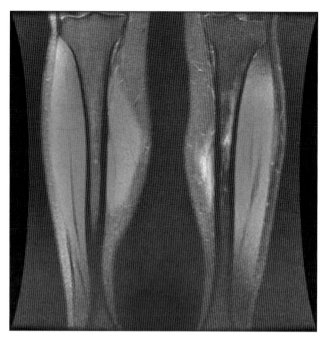

FIGURE 32.1 Stress reaction of left tibia with periosteal hemorrhage; coronal proton density fat saturation.

length discrepancies have all been implicated. Inflexibility and strength imbalances may also be risk factors.

Errors in training (extrinsic factors) are usually important contributors to stress fractures. When stress fractures develop, there typically has been some change in the training regimen, such as starting a season without preconditioning or abruptly increasing the intensity, duration, and frequency of workouts.

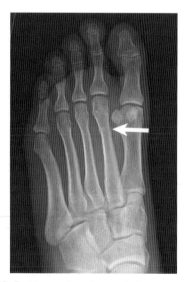

FIGURE 32.2 Stress fracture of the second metatarsal neck.

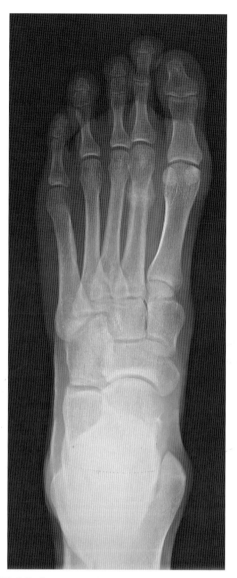

FIGURE 32.3 Stress fracture shown in Figure 32.2 after 5 weeks of healing.

Athletes should be asked how much they are exercising and training because they will frequently work out in addition to what is expected of their sport.

Poor footwear can also contribute to the development of stress fractures. Shoes lose their cushioning ability; they need to be replaced not according to time but according to the amount of wear and use. A person with a flat foot should have a stable, supportive shoe, and a person with a high-arched, rigid, cavus foot should have a well-cushioned shoe with shock absorption. If an appropriate shoe is not available for the foot type and training regimen, then orthotics may be helpful. Orthotics can provide added cushioning for a rigid foot or stability for a flexible foot. Orthotics are available off the shelf, or they can be custom-made.

Training on an inappropriate surface may result in stress fractures. Hard surfaces such as concrete, asphalt, or hardwood gym floors are particularly implicated in stress fractures. Modifying training by substituting softer surfaces such as grass, a cushioned track, trails, or a treadmill may reduce this risk.

There may be several causes for a stress fracture in a given individual; both intrinsic and extrinsic. The more contributing factors that can be identified, the better the chances of eliminating the causes and preventing recurrences.

Prevention

Prevention of stress fractures involves identifying and addressing risk factors during the athlete's preparticipation examination and annual physicals. The approach should be multidisciplinary, including nutritional, exercise, and psychological therapy for patients with disordered eating. Supplements, such as vitamin D and calcium, may be recommended, and there may be medical indication to prescribe hormonal therapy for patients with amenorrhea. Patient education, including instruction on the early warning signs of impending stress fracture, may also reduce injuries.

Sites of Fractures

Stress fractures occur most commonly in the long bones of the lower extremities, particularly the tibia, metatarsals, and fibula, but fractures of the femur, tarsal navicular (**Figure 32.4** and **Figure 32.5**), and sesamoids may also occur. Stress fractures of an upper extremity may occur in special circumstances—for example, in the humerus or ulna in baseball pitchers or in the forearm in volleyball players and rodeo riders. Stress fractures of the axial skeleton have also been described with pars or pedicle stress fractures of the spine. Rib stress fractures may occur in rowers and pelvic stress fractures in long-distance runners. **Table 32.1** lists the sites of stress fractures.

CLINICAL EVALUATION

History

If a young athlete experiences bone pain in association with physical activity, then a stress fracture must be considered. Location, severity, quality, and aggravating and alleviating factors must be elicited. Typically stress fractures are associated with pain that is insidious in onset, worsens with activity, and improves with rest. The pain usually begins as a diffuse ache or soreness and becomes much more focal and sharp as the

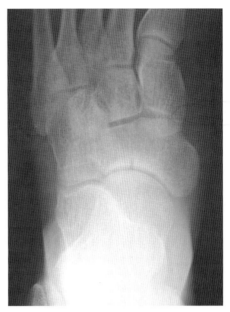

FIGURE 32.4 Stress fracture of the tarsal navicular of the left foot; anteroposterior view.

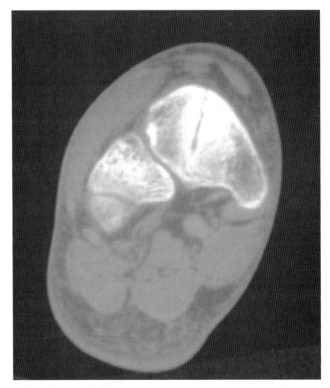

FIGURE 32.5 Computed tomography of the foot in Figure 32.4 with tarsal navicular stress fracture on axial cut.

TABLE 32.1

Sites of Stress Fractures

Tibia
• Posteromedial, midshaft
• Anterior cortex*
• Medial malleolus*

Fibula
• Midshaft
• Lateral malleolus*
• Fibular head*

Metatarsals
• Midshaft of 2nd-4th
• Base of 5th (Jones fracture)*

Tarsals
• Navicular*
• Calcaneus
• Cuneiform
• Cuboid

Sesamoids*

Femur
• Midshaft
• Femoral neck*

Pelvis

Pars interarticularis of spine*

* Indicates high-risk stress fractures

stress fracture develops. Initially, the pain may be noticeable only after activity. However, with continued activity, the pain occurs during activity and at rest, and eventually the pain becomes so severe that the athlete can no longer continue the activity. The number and location of previous stress fractures can be a risk factor for development of subsequent stress fractures.

The athlete's activity history should include the days per week, hours per day, and intensity for each activity. Errors in training are typically made when training intensity or volume is precipitously increased or when an additional sport is added. Use of orthotics can point to a previously identified biomechanical abnormality.

Nutritional history must be part of routine questioning. Questions should be specifically asked about intake of meat, fat, dairy, and fruits and vegetables, as well as calcium and vitamin D supplementation. Menstrual history is important to obtain for female athletes, including age of menarche, regularity (menses per year), and use of oral contraception.

Physical Examination

The physical examination should start with an inspection to assess general health, leanness, and lower extremity alignment. In addition to evaluating the athlete's foot type, the physician should examine his or her shoes, orthotics, and wear pattern. Tenderness to palpation is the primary method of physical diagnosis of a stress fracture. Stress fracture tenderness tends to be localized. The tenderness for conditions such as shin splints tends to be diffuse and corresponds to the areas of increased activity that are shown on a bone scan (**Figure 32.6**). Occasionally, fracture callus can be palpated even before changes are visible on x-ray. Palpation is more difficult when there is overlying muscle or soft tissue, as is the case with femoral stress fractures. When there is question about the significance of a given degree of tenderness, palpation of the opposite extremity can be used for comparison.

A complete examination of the surrounding joints and muscles must be performed to exclude other diagnoses. Additional tests to support the diagnosis of stress fracture include the hop test, the fulcrum test, the squeeze test, and the stork test. The hop test can be used for any stress

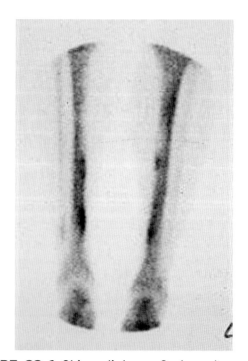

FIGURE 32.6 Shin splints on 3-phase bone scan. Note diffuse, patchy areas of increased uptake.

fracture of the lower extremity and is considered positive if pain is elicited with hopping on the affected side and not on the unaffected side, or if the athlete is unable to hop. The fulcrum test is used only on the long bones and is performed by bending the bone over the examiner's leg or the edge of the examination table. The test is considered positive if pain is elicited at the site of tenderness. The squeeze test can be used when multiple bones are in close proximity, such as metatarsals or the tibia and fibula. The bones are squeezed together, away from the site of pain. The test is considered positive if pain is elicited not where the bones are being squeezed but over the area of tenderness to palpation. The squeeze test is sensitive but not specific and can be positive in other conditions, such as Morton's neuroma of the foot. The stork test can reproduce the pain that occurs from a pars fractures of the spine. The test involves standing on a single leg while extending the spine (bending backwards). The test is repeated after switching the stance leg. A positive test results in back pain that is not caused when the spine is in a neutral or flexed position. (see Chapter 34, Lumbar and Thoracic Spine). A vibrating tuning fork may produce pain over a stress fracture, as may therapeutic ultrasound. These provocative tests must be used in conjunction with other examination findings and history and are not meant to stand alone for diagnosis.

Imaging Studies

Plain films are still the cheapest and easiest way to diagnose a stress fracture. However, they are not particularly sensitive. If a stress fracture is detectable on plain films, it may not appear until 2 to 4 weeks after the injury. This is because fracture lines and callus formation do not appear until later in the evolution of a stress fracture. Medullary edema is an earlier stage in the evolution of a stress fracture but does not appear on plain films.

Bone scan has been used for early diagnosis of stress fractures because it reveals increased osteoblastic activity before regular x-rays will show abnormalities. A bone scan can detect stress fractures 3 to 5 days after the onset of symptoms. Bone scans can remain positive well after healing has occurred. Accordingly, use of a follow-up bone scan to document healing is not clinically useful.

A positive bone scan is not specific as to the cause of bony abnormality. Stress fractures, acute fractures, bony tumors, or bony infections can all produce a positive bone scan. Active individuals may have multiple areas of increased activity on bone scan that are not tender or are

not clinically significant. This accounts for a number of false positive findings on bone scan.

With MRI, marrow edema can be detected much sooner (within 24 hours of the onset of pain), abnormalities can be more precisely localized, and staging stress fractures for prognosis is more accurate. Marrow edema in the presence of tenderness to palpation confirms the diagnosis. As is the case with bone scans, marrow edema may be an incidental finding in MR imaging and false positive may appear on MR images. Again, clinical correlation is necessary to confirm the diagnosis. MRI has advantages over bone scan or serial plain films for the diagnosis of stress fractures in terms of sensitivity and specificity. **Figure** 32.7 and **Figure** 32.8 demonstrate stress fractures in the proximal femur and the distal tibia, respectively. MRI staging is based on the presence of edema on T2 sequences and a fracture line (hypodense signal) on T1 sequences.

Computed tomography (CT) can be useful for providing additional information about staging or healing of a stress fracture, but this modality lacks the sensitivity for early diagnosis. CT can also help distinguish stress fractures from other pathologic sources of bone pain.

Other conditions that also cause bone pain and must be excluded are periostitis (eg, shin splints), bone cysts, osteoid osteoma, tumor, infection, and anatomic variation

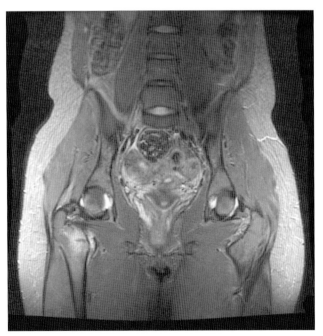

FIGURE 32.7 Right hip stress fracture with surrounding marrow edema on coronal STIR (short T1 inversion recovery) magnetic resonance imaging.

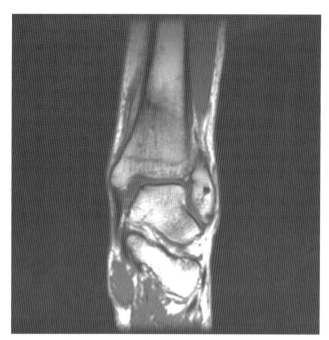

FIGURE 32.8 Left distal tibia stress fracture on coronal T1 magnetic resonance imaging.

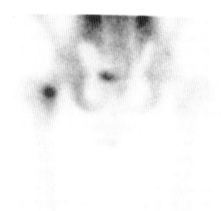

FIGURE 32.9 Bone scan of a compression-sided stress fracture of the femoral neck.

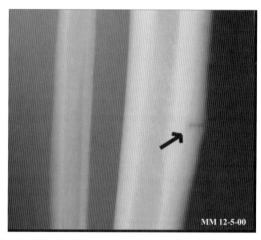

FIGURE 32.10 Stress fracture of anterior cortex of the tibia.

(eg, bipartite navicular). Shin splints are covered in depth in Chapter 42, Lower Leg. Pain at night or with rest is more suggestive of a diagnosis of neoplasm or osteoid osteoma than a diagnosis of stress fracture. Acute osteomyelitis occurs with fever, but subacute osteomyelitis can occur without fever and must be considered in a child with unexplained bone pain. A working knowledge of anatomic variations in the pediatric skeleton is necessary because some of these conditions are fairly common (eg, bipartite sesamoid or patella, apophysitis at the base of the fifth metatarsal) and can be confused with stress or acute fractures (see Chapter 30, Diagnostic Imaging). Plain films are still appropriate for the initial evaluation of suspected bony pathology but additional studies are often necessary to confirm the diagnosis.

TREATMENT

Most stress fractures heal with removal of the offending stress. However, certain stress fractures have a lower capacity to heal; these are called high-risk stress fractures (**Table 32.1**). These include stress fractures to the femoral neck (**Figure 32.9**), anterior tibia (**Figure 32.10**), medial malleolus of the tibia, tarsal navicular, base of fifth metatarsal (Jones fracture) (**Figure 32.11**), and sesamoids. These fractures may require a non-weight-bearing period of up

to 2-3 months and up to 4-6 months to heal. Occasionally, bone grafting or internal fixation is required to heal a high-risk stress fracture.

Conventional stress fractures typically require 6 to 8 weeks of rest from impact activities and another 4 to 6 weeks to gradually transition to full activity. Common sites of conventional stress fractures include the posteriomedial tibia, fibula, and metatarsals (**Table 32.1**). **Table 32.2** lists the steps for treating stress fractures.

Healing of a stress fracture can commence once the stressor is removed. The time required to heal the stress fracture depends on the duration of symptoms, the site of injury, and the individual body's underlying healing ability. Ice, acetaminophen, and rest are the main treatment modalities for pain. In general, anti-inflammatory medications

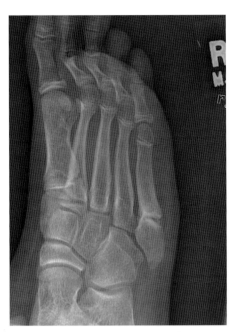

FIGURE 32.11 Nonunion of stress fracture of right fifth metatarsal on oblique view.

should be avoided because they can potentially delay fracture healing. Crutches, cast boots, and/or casts may be used until walking is free of pain. Prolonged immobilization causes joint stiffness, muscle wasting, and osteopenia, so immobilization should be limited to the amount of time necessary to become pain free. It is also important for athletes to keep physically fit while they are recovering from their injury. During treatment, running or impact activity may not be tolerated but lifting weights, swimming, riding a bike, or using an elliptical trainer may be done without

TABLE 32.2

Treatment of Conventional Stress Fractures

- Relative rest (avoid the offending activity).
- Engage in nonimpact activities, such as swimming, bicycling, or lifting weights.
- Ice or take analgesics such as acetaminophen as needed for pain.
- Wear a walking boot or use crutches for high-risk stress fractures.
- Address risk factors related to training regimens, footwear, biomechanics, nutrition, and general health.
- Allow time to gradually transition back to preinjury level of activity after bone healing has occurred.

pain or risk of compromising healing. Biomechanical, nutritional, and menstrual problems must be addressed during the treatment to optimize healing and to set the stage for prevention of recurrent or future stress fractures.

Objective assessment of healing is necessary before the athlete returns to play. Absent or decreased tenderness to palpation, after a suitable period of rest, is the primary indicator for clinical healing at examination. Mature callus and complete bridging of the fracture is the indicator of healing on x-ray. If the stress fracture never appeared on plain films, follow-up plain films will not be useful to document healing. Low-risk fractures that are deemed clinically healed do not necessarily warrant further imaging. High-risk stress fractures deserve follow-up imaging such as CT or MRI to confirm the healing.

If the stress fracture goes untreated and develops into a complete fracture, it can still be treated conservatively. However, if the fracture does not heal, then open reduction with internal fixation and bone grafting should be considered. Bone growth stimulators may be considered for nonunions or delayed unions, but surgery may still be necessary. Bone growth stimulators work by providing a low-dose electric current to fractures to stimulate healing, and although they have been shown to facilitate healing in some fracture nonunions, they are expensive and work slowly (3-6 months).

Once healing has been confirmed clinically or radiographically and after underlying biomechanical, nutritional, and/or hormonal abnormalities have been addressed, the athlete may gradually resume activities specific to their sport. This may include sport-specific drills, transitioning back to practice sessions, and finally, returning to competition.

SUMMARY POINTS

- Stress fractures are common in young athletes who train intensely or participate in endurance sports.
- Most stress fractures are caused by an error in training—doing too much too fast. However, intrinsic factors, including dietary and hormonal abnormalities, can also contribute to stress fractures.
- Stress fractures manifest as an insidious onset of bone pain.
- The hallmark during physical examination is tenderness to palpation of the affected bone.
- X-rays are helpful if evidence of fracture or callus is present, but they may not show a stress fracture until 3 to 4 weeks after the onset of pain.

- Bone scan or MRI provides options for diagnosis of stress fracture when plain films are normal.

- Relative rest (avoiding only the offending activity) and correcting underlying abnormalities of training, equipment, and biomechanics is the preferred treatment for low-risk stress fractures.

- High-risk stress fractures require the same basic treatment as low-risk stress fractures but, in some instances, may require longer treatment durations, consultation with a specialist, or additional interventions such as bone stimulators or surgical intervention.

- The female athlete triad should be considered in girls with stress fractures.

SUGGESTED READING

Arendt E, Agel J, Heikes C, et al. Stress injuries to bone in college athletes: a retrospective review of experience at a single institution. *Am J Sports Med.* 2003;31:959-968.

Coady CM, Micheli LJ. Stress fractures in the pediatric athlete. *Clin Sports Med.* 1997;16:225-238.

Nattiv A. Stress fractures and bone health in track and field athletes. *J Sci Med Sport.* 2000;3:268-279.

Nattiv A, Armsey TD Jr. Stress injury to bone in the female athlete. *Clin Sports Med.* 1997;16:197-224.

Snyder RA, Koester MC, Dunn WR. Epidemiology of stress fractures. *Clin Sports Med.* 2006:25(1);37-52.

CHAPTER 33

Cervical Spine

Gregory L. Landry, MD

njuries to the neck are common in collision sports and are estimated to occur in 10% to 15% of players of American football. They are nearly as common as head injuries and are outnumbered only by injuries to the ankles, knees, and shoulders. Other sports associated with an increased risk of neck injury are ice hockey, gymnastics, rugby, snowboarding, cheerleading, and equestrian sports. Serious injuries are rare, but the examining physician must carefully look for any symptoms or signs of injuries to the spine, intervertebral disks, nerve roots, or spinal cord in athletes with neck pain.

The cervical spine is designed for a high degree of mobility, which makes it more vulnerable to injury than the thoracic or lumbar spine. It is also important to know what symptoms and findings at physical examination occur with more severe injuries, when to perform imaging studies on injured athletes, and when to refer athletes to a specialist.

ANATOMY

The cervical spine comprises 7 vertebrae between the head and thorax. The cervical spine has the smallest bodies of all the vertebrae. The vertebral canal is larger at the cervical level than at all the lower levels. The third through the sixth vertebrae are similar to each other and are called typical cervical vertebrae; the first, second, and seventh are specialized and are considered atypical. The typical vertebrae have small ovoid bodies that are curved superiorly like a bucket seat. These partially interlock with the adjacent vertebrae with their uncovertebral joints; they provide additional stability. These are important clinically because the posterior part forms the margin of the intervertebral foramen, which is where the spinal nerve emerges. The right and left transverse processes have grooves on their superior aspect to support

the spinal nerve. Right and left superior and inferior articular processes sit at the junction of the root (pedicle) with the lamina of the neural arch (**Figure 33.1**). These articular processes form 2 columns of joints posteriorly. Each typical vertebra has a bifid spinous process. These form a straight line posteriorly and are easily palpated. Any deviation of a spinous process from this line is abnormal.

The first, second, and seventh vertebrae are atypical because of their specialization. The first cervical vertebra, known as the atlas, is the most superior. It has 2 superior articular facets to support the condyles of the occiput, but it lacks a vertebral body. The inferior facets are rounded to match the superior facets of the second vertebra. The plane between the C1 and C2 joints is more horizontal and is designed for rotatory motion. The body of the axis, or the second vertebra, supports the odontoid process, which serves as a pivot about which the atlas rotates. The seventh cervical vertebra is called the vertebra prominens because of the prominence of the spinous process, which is longer than that of the other cervical vertebrae. Occasionally the transverse process develops excessively and becomes a cervical rib.

The articulation between the first cervical vertebra and the occiput, known as the atlanto-occipital joint, allows for about one-third of the flexion and extension and about one-half of the lateral bending of the neck. The articulation between the first and second vertebrae is called the atlanto-axial joint, and it produces approximately 50% of the rotation of the neck. The articulations from the second through the seventh cervical vertebrae account for two-thirds of the flexion and extension, 50% of the rotation, and 50% of the lateral bending.

Below the axis, intervertebral disks fill each interval between the vertebral bodies. Each disk is composed of a peripheral annulus fibrosus and a central nucleus pulposus.

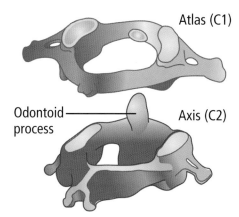

Atlas (C1)

Odontoid process

Axis (C2)

FIGURE 33.1 Anatomy of first and second cervical vertebrae.

In flexion of the cervical spine, the anterior part of the disk is compressed and the posterior part is extended. In addition to the bony architecture and disks, ligaments are a critical component of the stability of the spine.

There are 8 pairs of cervical spinal nerves. The first is unusual in that it emerges through the atlanto-occipital membrane just above the posterior arch of the atlas instead of an intervertebral foramen. The eighth nerve emerges through the foramen between the seventh cervical vertebra and the first thoracic vertebra.

The cervical and trapezius muscles support and permit movement for the head and neck; they also protect the spinal cord. The normal cervical spine has a slight lordosis, which is maintained by the neck muscles. This curvature allows the spine to withstand more force without injury. When the cervical spine is flexed or when lordosis is lost, the spine is more rigid and less able to withstand axial loads.

EVALUATION

History

Any blow to the head or neck can produce a serious cervical spine injury. The mechanism of injury can help the clinician form an initial diagnosis. Axial loading and hyperflexion are associated with cervical disk injury as well as vertebral body and spinal cord injury. Hyperextension is associated with facet joint, ligament, and brachial plexus injury.

When performing an initial evaluation of an athlete on the playing field, it is imperative to obtain a good history before moving the athlete. If there is evidence of a concussion or if the athlete is unconscious, a cervical spine injury should be suspected until proved otherwise. If the athlete is responsive, the athlete should not be permitted to move until an assessment can be made. The first questions that

should be asked are "Does your neck hurt?" "Is there any numbness or tingling in your arms or legs?" "Can you move your fingers?" and "Can you move your toes?" Any symptoms in the extremities that are bilateral or that involve an arm and leg imply a spinal cord injury. In these cases, the athlete's spine should be immobilized, and he or she should be sent to an emergency facility. Numbness, tingling, or pain in one arm may be the result of a nerve root injury, a brachial plexus injury, or a peripheral nerve injury. On the playing field, it should be assumed that any neurologic symptoms are related to the cervical spine until a thorough physical examination can be performed. Even if the athlete is ambulatory and neurologic involvement is not evident, a spine injury should still be suspected if neck pain is present.

If the athlete seeks care in an office environment, and if the injury is subacute or chronic, the clinician should ask the athlete about any previous injuries, as well as the mechanism of the current injury, the symptoms at the time of injury, and the duration of the symptoms. The clinician should elicit reports of stiffness, muscle spasm, numbness, tingling, burning, weakness, and radiating pain. Pain at rest, night pain, and pain with daily activities are also of concern. Finally, the results of any previous tests and the response to previous treatment should be elicited.

Physical Examination

In the acutely injured athlete, the clinician should determine whether the cervical spine is tender; any tenderness of the spine in the acute setting implies a bony injury or a disk injury. Tenderness limited to soft tissue and muscle is less worrisome, but it does not preclude serious injury.

If the athlete is down on the field and there is no midline cervical spine tenderness and no symptoms in the extremities, the athlete may sit and then stand when comfortable doing so. The athlete should be asked to carefully try to move the neck in different directions. The examiner should demonstrate the motions as they are described in words, asking the athlete to do as the examiner does. The athlete should be asked to perform neck extension (average 75°) and flexion (average 60°), lateral flexion to both sides (average 45°), and rotation in both directions (average 90°). Any asymmetry in range of motion is important. Upper cervical spine abnormalities (C1-C3) will be more likely to affect rotation, whereas lateral flexion impairment is more prominent with lower cervical spine injuries (C4-C7).

In the presence of normal range of motion, applying downward pressure on the head and axial loading the cervical spine may produce pain consistent with a spine injury.

A more sensitive test is the Spurling maneuver, (**Table 33.1**). The Spurling maneuver is performed with the head extended, ipsilaterally rotated, and ipsilaterally tilted (**Figure 33.2**). Reproduction of the symptoms extending beyond the shoulder is a positive test. The Spurling maneuver is specific for cervical nerve root compression, but its sensitivity is low. Reproduction of neck pain alone is nonspecific but is consistent with spine injury. Strength of the neck muscles should be tested isometrically with the spine at neutral.

Any athlete with radicular symptoms needs a thorough neurologic examination that checks sensation, muscle strength, reflexes, and gait. Sensation to light touch or pinprick should be assessed for dermatomes from C5 to T1 (**Figure 33.3**). Muscle strength should be tested in shoulder abduction, elbow flexion, elbow extension, wrist extension, wrist flexion, and grip. Strength should be recorded according to the Medical Research Council manual muscle

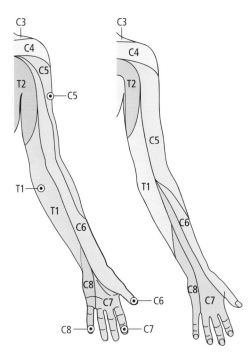

FIGURE 33.3 Dermatomes for sensory testing.

TABLE 33.1
Spurling Maneuver for Examination of Cervical Spine
• Mechanical stress, such as excessive vertebral motion, may exacerbate symptoms.
• Pain is provoked in the patient's arm by inducing narrowing of the neuroforamen.
• Gentle neck hyperextension with the head tilted toward the affected side will narrow the size of the neuroforamen and may exacerbate the symptoms or produce radiculopathy.
• Downward head compression increases the patient's radicular pain and paresthesias, especially if the neck is rotated to the side of involvement.

testing scale, as follows: 0, no muscle contraction; 1, visible muscle twitch but no movement of the joint; 2, weak contraction insufficient to overcome gravity; 3, weak contraction that can overcome gravity but no additional resistance; 4, weak contraction able to overcome some but not full resistance; and 5, normal ability to overcome full resistance. The cervical root and corresponding functions are listed in **Table 33.2**. Muscle stretch reflexes should be checked at the biceps, brachioradialis, and triceps. Knee and ankle reflexes should be assessed for evidence of myelopathy (hyperreflexia).

Imaging Studies

Any athlete with midline cervical spine tenderness or marked loss of range of motion after an injury needs cervical spine radiographs. Additional indications for cervical radiographs are severe cervical pain at rest, pain with active range-of-motion testing, neurologic deficit, or severe cervical rigidity. The minimum radiographic views are the anteroposterior (AP) view, the lateral view, and the open-mouth view to image the first and second cervical vertebrae. The AP view should be examined for any asymmetry of the superior and inferior end plates of the vertebrae, the pedicles, and the spinous processes. The open-mouth view is the AP view for C1 and C2, and it should be checked to ensure that the odontoid process is equidistant from the lateral masses of C1 and that the lateral

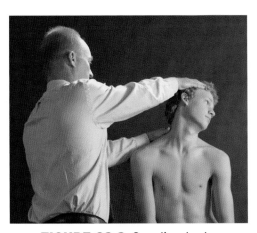

FIGURE 33.2 Spurling test.

TABLE 33.2

Neurologic Examination for Cervical Spine Injuries

Disk	Nerve Root	Reflex	Sensation	Muscle	Test Movement
C4-5	C5	Biceps	Lateral deltoid	Deltoid	Shoulder abduction
C5-6	C6	Brachioradialis	Thumb	Biceps, wrist extensors	Elbow flexion or wrist extension
C6-7	C7	Triceps	Middle finger	Triceps	Elbow extension
C7-T1	C8		Small finger	Flexor digitorum superficialis	Finger flexion
T1-T2	T1		Medial forearm	Hand intrinsics	Abduction/adduction of fingers

masses of C1 and C2 are aligned. The lateral view is the most important. The soft tissues should be examined. At the level of C3, the soft tissues are normally less than one-half of the AP width of the C3 vertebral body. At the C6 level, the soft tissues are approximately equal to the width of the C6 vertebral body.

Computed tomography (CT) scanning is helpful in the acute setting when a significant injury is suspected and plain radiographs are normal. CT scanning is fast and readily available at most emergency facilities. It is good at identifying bony problems such as occult fractures. It is not as good as magnetic resonance imaging (MRI) for diagnosing intervertebral disk pathology. Magnetic resonance imaging is a sensitive test and is useful when a significant injury is suspected, especially of the disks. It will show edema of the bone or in the soft tissues.

CERVICAL EMERGENCIES

When an injury is witnessed by the physician, the most worrisome mechanism of injury is axial loading with the neck flexed. The cervical spine is weaker in this position because the physiologic lordosis is lost and the space for the spinal cord is narrowed. This injury can occur with so-called spear tackling in American football—that is, when the player uses the helmet at the point of impact when tackling. The physician should always ask about neck pain and should suspect a cervical spine injury in the event of a concussion. It is not unusual to have an injury to both the brain and neck.

If the athlete is injured in a remote area or in a location where there is limited medical assistance, emergency services should be summoned, and the athlete should be kept still. If the athlete is unconscious, an airway must be maintained, and the cervical spine should be stabilized until emergency personnel can take over. For the helmeted athlete in American football, the helmet can help with stabilization because of its tight fit. The helmet and chin strap should be kept in place. Removal of a football helmet

is difficult without moving the cervical spine. The mask can usually be removed with a screwdriver or the snaps can be cut if the airway must be accessed. In other sports with helmets that fit more loosely, it may be more prudent to remove the helmet to stabilize the cervical spine, but the cervical spine must be kept immobile during this process.

Physicians who regularly cover athletic events should have a plan to handle a possible spine injury. Medical personnel should have the proper equipment and practice a possible transport. A spine board with proper straps to immobilize various parts of the body should be available.

When a spine injury is suspected, prevention of further injury is the main objective. The first step is to immobilize the head and neck in a neutral position. It is also important to check for breathing, pulse, and level of consciousness. If there is a mouth guard in place, it should be removed. Athletes who are lying facedown or on one side will need to be moved to a supine position so that they can be attached to the spine board. If there are enough medical personnel available (usually 4 people in addition to the person controlling the head and neck), the athlete can be "logrolled" onto the spine board. The person controlling the head and neck acts as the leader and provides instructions for the others to move the shoulders, hips, and legs in unison with the head to prevent any movement of the spine. If there are not enough trained people to properly move the athlete onto the spine board, the athlete should stay completely still until emergency personnel arrive.

DIAGNOSIS AND TREATMENT OF COMMON ACUTE AND CHRONIC CERVICAL SPINE INJURIES

Stinger (Burner) Syndrome

The stinger or burner syndrome is so named because an athlete may acutely experience shooting pain and/or a burning sensation down the arm with associated numbness of the hand and arm. It has long been thought to be the result of a stretch of the brachial plexus from a blow to the head that pulls the head laterally, in the opposite direction from the affected arm. This is not the only mechanism of injury to account for these symptoms. The brachial plexus can be compressed acutely from a direct blow to the anterior shoulder. A blow to the head may also cause a stinger with axial loading, resulting in compression of the dorsal root nerve root ipsilateral to the affected arm. Axial loading can also cause a cervical disk injury and produce a clinical presentation similar to a stinger. Stingers are most common in football but can occur in wrestling, diving, or any contact/collision sport.

The typical stinger affects the upper brachial plexus and results in weakness of the deltoid, supraspinatus, infraspinatus, biceps, brachioradialis, pronator teres, or the wrist extensors. Symptoms last from seconds to several days. Permanent nerve damage is possible but uncommon. If the athlete experiences midline cervical tenderness, further evaluation is imperative, and the athlete should not play until further evaluation has been completed. It is common to have trapezius muscle tenderness in the typical stinger; by itself, it does not indicate a more serious injury.

Nerve injuries can be classified as grade I, which includes neuropraxia and transient loss of motor and sensory function without axonal injury. All grade I injuries should resolve in 2 weeks; most resolve in minutes. A grade II injury is an axonotmesis that results in marked motor and occasional sensory deficits that last at least 2 weeks and may take months to resolve. A grade III injury, which consists of neurotmesis, lasts a year or more and is associated with permanent deficits. This is a rare injury. Most brachial plexus injuries are mild grade I injuries.

For most stingers, the symptoms are transient. The athlete can return to play as soon as the symptoms resolve, provided there is no residual weakness at physical examination. If the symptoms persist or if weakness is present at the examination, the athlete must rest and must not participate in sport. Anti-inflammatory medication can be used for pain control, although its efficacy has not been demonstrated in terms of neurologic recovery. Athletes with trapezius muscle pain may be more comfortable if they wear a soft collar. Ice should be applied for the first 48 to 72 hours. Once the initial symptoms have subsided, the athlete may apply moist heat and work on range of motion with gentle stretching and light isometric strengthening exercises. Once range of motion is normal and pain is gone or minimal, a more aggressive neck muscle strengthening program should be initiated.

An athlete who has weakness from a stinger that persists more than 2 weeks should be referred to a neurologist or spine specialist. Electromyography and nerve conduction studies should be considered in patients with prolonged symptoms or when profound weakness is present. Rarely, the injury occurs at the cervical nerve root and can involve a nerve root avulsion. A sports medicine specialist or a spine specialist should be consulted if the athlete has recurrent stingers, especially if the symptoms worsen or last longer with each subsequent injury.

Athletes may return to play after a stinger once they have regained full, pain-free cervical motion; normal sensation and strength in the upper extremities; and normal strength of cervical musculature. If the stinger occurred from football, a neck roll or "cowboy collar" (**Figure 33.4**) may provide additional protection against further injury.

Cervical Strain/Sprain

An acute cervical sprain is a ligamentous injury that may occur from a head-on collision with another athlete, a lateral blow, or neck hyperextension. It may be difficult to distinguish from a muscle strain. In the neck, muscle injuries and ligamentous injuries often occur simultaneously. Athletes will often say they jammed or stretched their neck. A common mechanism is whiplash, or acceleration-deceleration force on the neck. Sprains result in tenderness to palpation over the cervical spine and limited motion. If only a muscular injury is present, tenderness primarily occurs over the muscles.

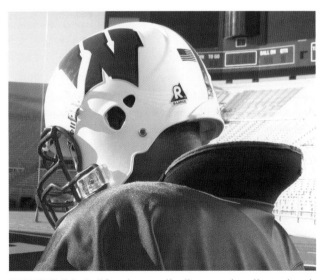

FIGURE 33.4 "Cowboy collar" or neck roll on shoulder pads on a football player.

Assessing range of motion should be done only when athletes can move under their own power. Neck strength can be tested with gentle resistance with the neck in a neutral position. Examiners should never push the athlete's head out of neutral position. The neurologic examination should be completely normal if there is a simple sprain. When tenderness is present directly over the cervical spine, radiographs should be obtained to rule out a fracture or significant ligamentous laxity. While awaiting radiographs, athletes with possible fracture or ligamentous laxity should be immobilized in a Philadelphia collar or a similar device that allows virtually no neck motion. If range of motion is diminished, CT or MRI imaging should be done to identify any significant fracture or disc injury. Flexion and extension radiographs should be considered to rule out any segmental instability only when range of motion has been restored and a CT or MRI has excluded any significant injury. Decisions about MRI, CT scan, or flexion-extension view of a suspected cervical spine injury are best made by a specialist in cervical spine trauma.

For initial treatment of sprains or strains, the athlete may be more comfortable wearing a soft collar for the first 48 to 72 hours. Analgesic medication may be used, especially at night to help with sleep. Ice can be applied for acute pain and spasm. For more chronic stiffness, moist heat is helpful before carrying out mobilization exercises. Manual therapy by a qualified spine physical therapist may also provide pain relief and facilitate recovery. The goal of rehabilitation is to restore normal range of motion and normal strength. Once normal range of motion is restored, the athlete can begin a strengthening program. If the athlete is not improving or has persistent pain, consultation with a spine specialist should be considered.

Intervertebral Disk Injury

Cervical disk injuries are rare in adolescents but occur more often in adults. Most patients with an acute cervical disk herniation complain of a sudden onset of severe posterior neck pain. Neck pain may be the only symptom, or it may be associated with referred pain to the shoulder, arm, and/or hand. Coughing or sneezing may exacerbate the pain. There is often a family history of cervical or lumbar disk disease. Young athletes are more likely to have herniation of the gelatinous nucleus pulposus into or through the annulus of the cervical disk compared with adults, who are more likely to have a progressive degeneration of the disk. The referred extremity pain may be associated with paresthesias and sense of muscular weakness due to nerve root compression and edema. A dermatomal pattern may allow for a presumptive diagnosis of the involved root level (**Table 33.2**). The athlete

will likely have an extremely limited range of motion and may experience tenderness over the spinal process at the level of injury. If the disk herniates centrally, it can compress the cord and produce symptoms and signs of myelopathy. Electric shock sensations with forward flexion of the neck, or Lhermitte's sign, indicate cord compromise. Disturbances in balance or gait, leg weakness, or alterations in bladder or bowel function also imply cord compression and myelopathy.

Initial treatment for a patient with a disk injury may include ice, analgesic and anti-inflammatory medication, and use of a soft cervical collar. Physical therapy can help relieve pain, reduce spasm, and restore cervical motion. Cervical traction reduces stress of the spine and intervertebral disk spaces. If traction is of benefit in a session with a rehabilitation professional, a home traction unit may be rented or purchased to achieve the same relief. In rare cases, pain and radicular symptoms persist, and an epidural corticosteroid injection is performed under fluoroscopic guidance in an effort to reduce swelling and avoid surgical intervention. Surgery is rarely necessary in the young athlete. Referral to a spine specialist is warranted if instability or fracture of the cervical spine is suspected. Similarly, associated congenital abnormalities, myelopathy, or any condition that may cause cervical stenosis should be evaluated by a spine specialist.

Return to play after a cervical disk injury is possible once cervical motion is restored, neurologic changes have resolved, strength is normal, and risk factors for further injury have been addressed.

Cervical Cord Neuropraxia

Cervical cord neuropraxia is a transient numbness and/or weakness that can affect both arms, both legs, all extremities, or an ipsilateral arm and leg. When all 4 extremities are affected, it is called transient quadriparesis. Transient neuropraxia can develop after an axial load or hyperextension of the spine. Athletes will often report bilateral burning pain, tingling, and loss of sensation in the arms and/or legs. They may have weakness that ranges from mild to complete paralysis. Symptoms usually last from 10 to 15 minutes but can take up to 48 hours to resolve completely. Radiographs are usually normal. MRI may be normal or may reveal spinal cord edema. Appropriate imaging studies should be used to look for any bone, disk, or ligamentous abnormality that may narrow the spinal canal and compromise the spinal cord. Radiographs should be examined carefully for evidence of fracture, instability, congenital or acquired stenosis, spondylolysis, or congenital abnormalities such as Klippel-Feil syndrome (fusion of some or all of the vertebrae in the neck) (**Figure 33.5**).

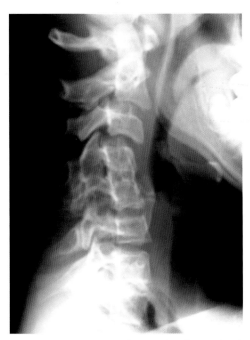

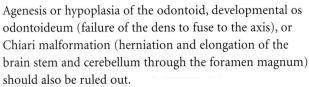

FIGURE 33.5 Lateral radiograph of cervical spine showing C4-C5 fusion.

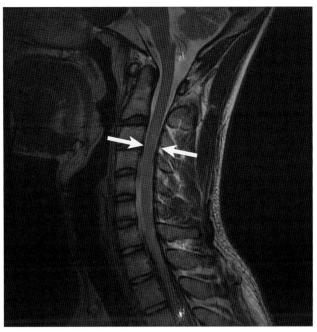

FIGURE 33.6 MRI of functional stenosis with loss of CSF on T2 sagittal image.

Agenesis or hypoplasia of the odontoid, developmental os odontoideum (failure of the dens to fuse to the axis), or Chiari malformation (herniation and elongation of the brain stem and cerebellum through the foramen magnum) should also be ruled out.

The criteria for diagnosis of cervical stenosis are controversial. In the 1950s, stenosis was defined as a cervical canal measuring less than 13 mm from the posterior aspect of the vertebral body to the most anterior point of the spinolaminar line on plain radiographs. In the 1980s, the Torg ratio was defined as spinal canal width divided by the width of the vertebral body. A ratio of less than 0.8 was considered to indicate the presence of spinal stenosis. This ratio was found to be unreliable as a result of a large number of false-positive findings attributed to the disproportionately large vertebral bodies in football players. However, because the Torg ratio can be measured on plain radiographs, it is still considered a good initial screen for stenosis. MRI has become the study of choice for diagnosing stenosis. The term *functional cervical stenosis* refers to a spinal canal that is so narrow that the protective cerebrospinal fluid (CSF) is obliterated. In more extreme cases, the stenosis may cause deformation of the spinal cord itself (**Figure 33.6**). Any canal measuring less than 13 mm on MRI is also considered stenotic, including those that are narrow from an injured disk.

Athletes with cervical cord neuropraxia need prompt emergency care in the event there is a bony, disk, or ligamentous injury causing injury to the cord. Because of the controversy over management of the athlete with cervical cord neuropraxia, an athlete with this history should be referred to a spine specialist. Any injury that results in signs of myelopathy, such as hyperreflexia, poor balance, or change in control of bladder or bowels, requires an urgent referral to a spine specialist. Once instability, stenosis, and significant injury have been ruled out, pain can guide the activity level of the patient. Rehabilitation and return-to-play decisions should also involve a spine specialist. If the source of stenosis is not reversible, the athlete's return to contact and collision sports may be inadvisable.

PROTECTIVE EQUIPMENT

Few sports permit protective equipment for the neck. The exception is American football because of the structure of the shoulder pads and helmet. A variety of collars and neck rolls are available that attach to the shoulder pads to prevent excessive lateral bending of the neck and hyperextension (**Figure 33.4**). Care should be taken to choose a collar that still allows for extension of the neck when the athlete is blocking or tackling. The inability to make contact with the neck slightly extended makes the athlete more vulnerable to a catastrophic injury. Use of these neck collars is controversial, but they may help prevent stingers, strain/sprain, and disk injuries.

RETURN-TO-PLAY CRITERIA

Athletes with a neck injury should not return to play until their symptoms have resolved and their physical examination is normal. Athletes should not be allowed to participate if there is decreased neck motion, pain with neck motion, or torticollis. In addition, there should be no tenderness of the spine to palpation and no pain with axial loading or Spurling testing. There should be symmetric strength of the neck muscles in all planes. The neurologic examination must be completely normal, including sensation and strength in the muscles of the upper extremity. The treating physician must be certain there is no bone, disk, or ligament injury before returning the athlete to play and that cervical stenosis and instability have been ruled out. In some cases, a safe return to preinjury activities may not be possible. Sports with a lower risk of cervical injury may have to be suggested as alternatives.

SUMMARY POINTS

- Neck injuries occur at approximately the same rate as head injuries in collision sports. Catastrophic injury to the spinal cord is rare but should be considered during the evaluation of all cervical spine injuries.

- Compared to the thoracic or lumbar spine, the cervical spine has more mobility and less support from bony and muscular structures. This vulnerability may increase the risk of injury to cervical disks, facet joints, and the spinal cord.

- Athletes with a neck injury and midline cervical spine tenderness or loss of cervical motion should have radiographs to rule out fractures or instability of the cervical vertebrae.

- A stinger or burner is an injury that causes pain, burning, numbness, and occasional weakness of the affected arm. These neurologic findings typically occur from forced extension or side bending of the cervical spine that stretches the brachial plexus or compresses a cervical nerve root.

- The presence of radicular symptoms warrants a careful evaluation for the source of neurologic compromise.

The source may be the brachial plexus or a cervical nerve root being compressed by a herniated disk.

- Physicians attending athletic events should make sure an emergency plan is in place to stabilize and transport athletes with a possible cervical spine injury.

- Rehabilitation of most cervical spine injuries involves restoring a pain-free normal range of motion and normal strength of the neck and upper extremity musculature.

- Athletes should not be allowed to return to play until they have regained full range of motion, normal cervical muscle strength, and normal neurologic function.

- Athletes with cervical cord neuropraxia should be referred to a spine specialist.

SUGGESTED READING

Dorshimer GW, Kelley M. Cervical pain in the athlete: common conditions and treatment. *Prim Care Clin Office Pract.* 2005;32:231-243.

Fagan K. Transient quadriplegia and return-to-play criteria. *Clin Sports Med* 2004;23:409-419.

Kleiner DM, Almquist JL, Bailes J, et al, for the Inter-Association Task Force for Appropriate Care of the Spine-Injured Athlete. *Prehospital Care of the Spine-Injured Athlete.* Dallas, TX: National Athletic Trainers' Association; March 2001. http://www.nata.org/statements/consensus/NATAPreHospital.pdf. Accessed November 8, 2007.

McAlindon RJ. On field evaluation and management of head and neck injured athletes. *Clin Sports Med.* 2002;21:1-14.

Morganti C. Recommendations for return to sports following cervical spine injuries. *Sports Med* 2003;33:563-573.

Sanchez AR, Sugalski MT, LaPrade RF. Field-side and prehospital management of the spine-injured athlete. *Curr Sports Med Rep.* 2005;4:50-55.

Torg JS. *Athletic Injuries to the Head, Neck and Face.* 2nd ed. St Louis, MO: Mosby Year-Book; 1991.

Wilson JB, Zarzour R, Moorman CT. Spinal injuries in contact sports. *Curr Sports Med Rep.* 2006;5:50-55.

CHAPTER 34

Lumbar and Thoracic Spine

Daniel E. Kraft, MD

Lower back pain is a common problem that will cause young athletes to seek care. These athletes have often been told to work through their pain by coaches and other adults who may themselves have been treated for lower back pain. When these young athletes are treated using an adult model for lower back pain, the diagnosis and management may not be appropriate. The differential diagnosis and treatment plans for young athletes with lower back pain differ greatly from adults. This chapter will examine the common causes of lower back pain in young athletes and practical approaches to care.

ANATOMY

The anatomic features of the spine allow it to provide stability and support, as well as flexibility and motion. The spine is made up of a series of vertebrae with related facet joints, spinous processes, and transverse processes (**Figure 34.1**). By the time a child is age 10 years, each vertebra has assumed a normal adult shape consisting of an anterior body and a posterior arch, which surrounds the spinal canal (**Figure 34.2**). The disks form the joints between the individual vertebral bodies, and the facets are the joints between the posterior arches of the vertebrae. The pedicle is the vertebrae portion that connects the anterior body to the posterior arch in each vertebra. The pars interarticularis is part of the posterior arch between the upper and lower facet joints.

The vertebral bodies and intervertebral disks help keep the body upright and are responsible for most of the load-bearing function of the spine. The facet joints control the amount of extension and rotation of the spine. The central bony canal provides for protection of the spinal cord and nerve roots.

In general, injury to the spine occurs when the load-bearing structures are exposed to excessive loads and when motion-controlling structures are subjected to excessive motion. In addition, when load-bearing structures are exposed to excessive motion or motion-controlling structures are exposed to excessive loads, injury may result.

One of the differences in injury patterns in young athletes versus adults is due to the proportionally higher levels of cartilage in preadolescent and adolescent vertebrae and the secondary centers of ossification in skeletally immature vertebral end plates. This may make the vertebrae more vulnerable to injury with compressive loads. The pars interarticularis also appears to be susceptible to repetitive extension stresses in skeletally immature individuals.

EVALUATION

History

Obtaining a complete history from the athlete will help lead the physician toward the correct diagnosis when evaluating lower back pain. The physician should know all the sports in which the athlete participates and the level of the athlete's involvement. Specific sports activities that cause pain can help direct the physician to the source of the symptoms. The physician should know whether the athlete's pain developed as a result of an injury or was gradual in onset. Has the athlete missed any games or practices? This answer helps a physician understand the effect and severity of the athlete's pain. Many athletes will not seek medical attention for back pain until it affects their ability to participate in practices and games. An adolescent athlete with persistent pain for 2 weeks or longer should be evaluated by a physician. Pain at night

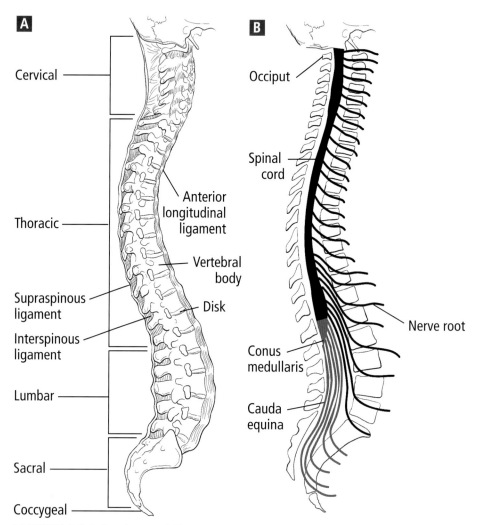

FIGURE 34.1 Anatomy of the spine. (A) Bony and ligamentous components of the spine. (B) Neural elements of the spine.

or pain without activity could signal a significant non–sports-related problem, such as a tumor.

Physical Examination

The physical examination of the athlete with lower back pain should evaluate the spine, sacroiliac (SI) joints, and hips and should include a neurologic examination. Many athletes with lower back problems will not experience any palpable tenderness over the spine at examination, but they may have lumbar paraspinous muscle spasm. Range of motion in forward flexion, side bending, and extension should be noted, along with any pain that coincides with these movements (**Figure 34.3**). The single leg standing extension test can indicate pathology in the pars interarticularis or facet joints (**Figure 34.4**). This test is positive if it produces pain when the patient stands and has his or her back extended by the examiner.

Problems in the lumbar disk, vertebral body, or vertebral end plate should be suspected if the patient has painful or restricted trunk flexion. The slump test is also useful when evaluating the young athlete for pathology in the disk or vertebral body. The test is performed with the patient sitting on the side of the bed, slumping the head down and straightening a leg away from the table. The maneuver is repeated a second time, but without the patient slumping the head. The test is positive when the slumping head causes radicular pain that is relieved or made better with the patient sitting up straight.

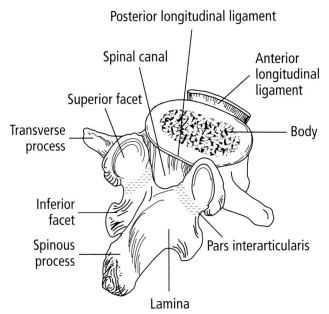

Posterior longitudinal ligament

Spinal canal

Superior facet

Anterior
longitudinal
ligament

Transverse
process

Body

Inferior
facet

Spinous
process

Pars interarticularis

Lamina

FIGURE 34.2 Anatomy of vertebral body, facet joints, and pars interarticularis.

A positive straight leg raising test is also an indicator of lumbar nerve root compression, which most commonly occurs from a lumbar disk protrusion.

SI joints can be evaluated by palpation and the FABER (flexion, abduction, and external rotation of the hip) test. The athlete's hip examination should document range of motion in internal and external rotation, document any palpable areas of pain, and describe the patient's gait pattern. All patients with lower back pain should undergo a neurologic examination that checks for reflexes, sensation, and strength in the lower extremities. Similarly, patients with pain, paresthesias, or weakness in the lower extremities should undergo a thorough evaluation of the lumbar spine.

Imaging Studies

Structural problems are a common cause of lower back pain in adolescent athletes. Therefore, radiologic testing is an important component in the athlete's medical evaluation. Plain films that include anteroposterior, lateral, and oblique views are the initial radiologic step. If the plain films are normal and the athlete has a positive single leg standing extension test, further evaluation can then be done with a bone/single photon emission computed tomography (SPECT) scan to look for a pars stress fracture. The SPECT scan is more sensitive than planar bone scans in detecting pars stress fractures and better shows the localization of

radioisotope uptake in the posterior vertebral elements. Magnetic resonance imaging (MRI) is an alternative to the bone/SPECT scan for detecting pars stress fractures.

Computed tomography (CT) scans can be used to evaluate the pars and help determine the amount of healing of pars stress fractures. Either reverse-angle CT scans or 3-dimensional reformatted CT scans provide excellent images that can help the clinician determine the degree of bony healing at the pars interarticularis. To decrease the patient's radiation exposure, these scans should be limited to viewing the spine from the vertebral level above the stress fracture site to the one below it. Use of CT scanning permits stress lesions to be categorized as full bony healing, partial healing, or cartilage nonunions.

MRI is also an important component in imaging the spine in young athletes. In some areas of the country, MRI is used as a detection test for pars interarticularis problems. More commonly, MRI is the test of choice when looking for soft pathology in the disk, nerve root, or spinal cord.

PARS INTERARTICULARIS PROBLEMS

Problems involving the pars interarticularis comprise a large percentage of the structural problems in young athletes. The terms *pars stress fracture*, *spondylolysis*, and *spondylolisthesis* have been used interchangeably to describe various clinical abnormalities in the pars interarticularis. All of these conditions can cause lower back pain that is typically worse with extension. These conditions are distinguished by their radiographic features. A pars stress fracture connotes a stress-related injury to the pars that typically has normal plain radiographs of the spine but a positive bone/SPECT scan. Spondylolysis refers to a radiographic lucency in the pars interarticularis that may be an asymptomatic developmental variant or an acquired and sometimes painful result of chronic stress to the pars. Bone/SPECT scans may be positive (hot) or negative (cold) with spondylolysis. Spondylolisthesis refers to an anterior slippage of a vertebra that occurs secondary to a bilateral spondylolysis. Spondylolisthesis can be visualized and graded based on the amount of anterior slippage demonstrated on a standing lateral radiograph of the lumbar spine

Pars Stress Fracture

Pars interarticularis problems are common in adolescent athletes with lower back pain. The pars stress fracture is the most acute of the pars interarticularis problems, and it is the most common of the 3 problems seen in sports medicine clinics. Athletes with pars stress fractures typically seek

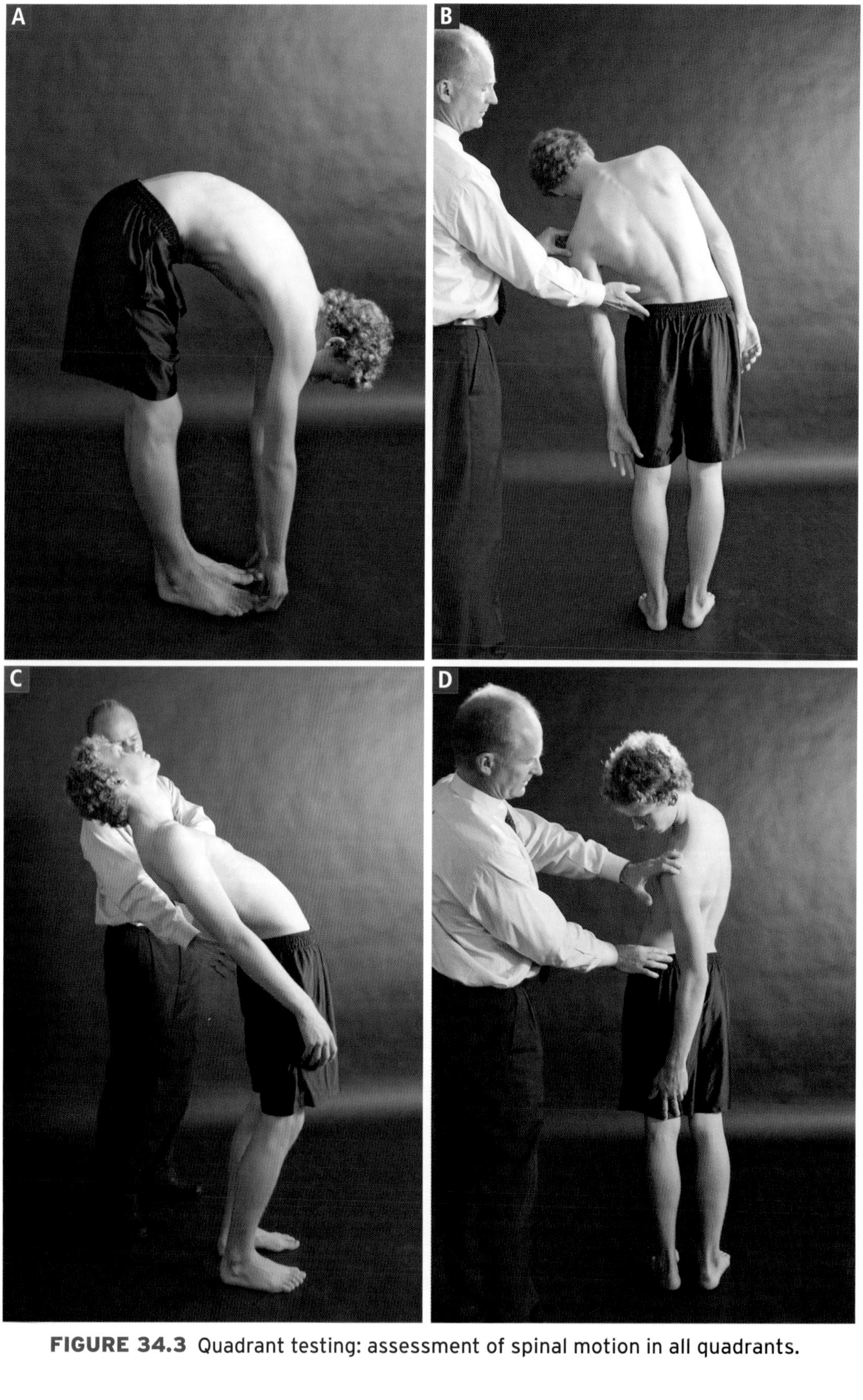

FIGURE 34.3 Quadrant testing: assessment of spinal motion in all quadrants.

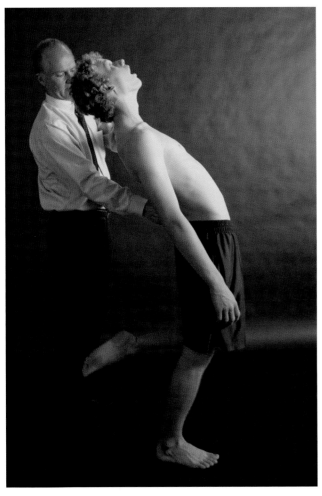

FIGURE 34.4 Single leg standing extension test.

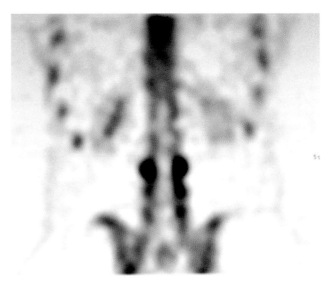

FIGURE 34.5 SPECT scan showing bilateral increased activity in pars interarticularis.

care after weeks to months of lower back pain that increasingly affects their sports activities. The diagnosis can be seen across the full spectrum of sports but seems to be more common in sports associated with jumping or repetitive back arching, such as gymnastics, soccer, and ballet.

At physical examination, the athlete may or may not have any bony point tenderness, but he or she may exhibit paraspinal muscle spasm along the lumbar spine. The hallmark findings at examination include pain with extension and a positive single leg standing extension test. The hip, SI joint, straight leg raising and slump tests, and neurologic examinations will be normal. Radiographic evaluation should begin with plain films. If a bony abnormality is not noted, a bone/SPECT scan or MRI should be considered. Athletes with positive bone/SPECT scan or MRI findings and normal plain films can be diagnosed as having a pars stress fracture (**Figure 34.5**). A baseline CT performed at diagnosis can help confirm the diagnosis because occasionally other

entities, such as an osteoid osteoma, can have similar-appearing bone scans as the pars stress fracture.

Currently, no gold standard exists for the treatment of a pars stress fracture. Patients with pars stress fractures have an active bony healing process occurring because their bone scans are positive. Therefore, treatment should be aimed at bony healing if possible. The most common treatments for pars stress fractures include wearing a Boston overlap brace (**Figure 34.6**), a Warm-N-Form orthosis, or a lumbar corset or modifying activity without bracing.

Athletes who choose the Boston brace or other brace options are most commonly treated with the brace for

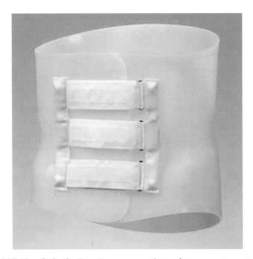

FIGURE 34.6 Boston overlap brace. Reproduced with permission from bostonbrace.com

3 to 6 months, wearing their brace 12 to 23 hours a day. The time frame for return to play varies with the treatment protocol and ranges from 1 to 6 months. Typically, the most important factor determining return to play is the patient's pain. Most physicians require athletes to be asymptomatic before they return to play and to remain asymptomatic to continue competing. Athletes should also have normal, pain-free lumbar motion with normal trunk strength and overall fitness before returning to practice and play. Exercises intended to increase trunk strength or improve overall fitness need to be done cautiously during the rehabilitation process. Strengthening exercises may require supervision from a physical therapist and should be modified or curtailed if there is any associated pain. Some athletes who have been treated with braces may be able to wear the brace when they return to practices and games.

Athletes who are treated without braces are typically kept out of all sports activities for 6-12 weeks until they are asymptomatic. They are not able to participate in any practices, games, or physical education classes during the healing phase. As is the case for athletes treated in a brace, athletes treated without a brace need to be pain free and have normal lumbar motion and trunk strength before resuming activity.

The goal of treatment for a pars stress fracture, as with other fractures, is to obtain complete bony healing. Currently, the CT scan is thought to be the best tool to assess healing at the completion of treatment. Athletes who achieve complete bony healing will have more normal-appearing CT scans 10 years after treatment than those with partial or no healing. If treatment of a pars stress fracture results in partial healing or a nonunion, there will be more degenerative changes on the CT scan 10 years later. It should be noted that complete bony healing is not necessary for a good clinical outcome. Patients who have regained full motion, strength, and function do not need CT scans or other imaging prior to returning to sports.

Rehabilitation is also an important component in the treatment of these athletes. Rehabilitation emphasizes a rigorous core strengthening/trunk stabilization program and stretching of hamstrings and hip flexors. Initially, the athlete is taught a posterior pelvic tilt and then progresses through various levels of a trunk stabilization program. The higher levels of the program will typically use a foam roller or exercise ball to improve functional use of core strength. Stabilization exercises can be initiated while the patient is in a brace and should be continued as the patient is weaned from wearing the brace and transitions to full activity. As patients progress with rehabilitation exercises and return to activity, they should remain free of pain.

Spondylolysis

Athletes who are diagnosed with spondylolysis, a more chronic pars interarticularis problem, typically have a similar clinical history and physical examination findings as previously described for the pars stress fracture. In fact, these 2 groups of athletes are often identical until the radiologic evaluation. With spondylolysis, the plain films will show a pars defect. The athlete with a pars stress fracture will have normal plain films. Even if plain films are noted to show a pars defect, a bone/SPECT scan can be useful to rule out a new pars stress fracture at another vertebral level. It is possible for plain films to show a spondylolysis at one level and a bone scan/SPECT scan to show a pars stress fracture at a different level.

Treatment of patients with spondylolysis may not result in visible healing of the bony defect. However, a fibrous union of the pars can become asymptomatic with conservative therapy and can permit a return to sports activity.

The Boston brace, a Warm-N-Form orthosis, or a lumbar corset can be effective brace treatments for these athletes. These braces work equally well for control of symptoms, although the Warm-N-Form orthosis and lumbar corset are less expensive than the Boston brace. Brace treatment starts at 23.5 hours per day. Once the patient has become pain free with daily activity, he or she may start an active rehabilitation program that includes general conditioning exercises as well as flexibility exercises for the lower extremity and core strengthening. The total length of brace treatment depends on the athlete's symptoms and the demands of the sport. Return to sports can occur when the patient is pain free and when he or she has optimized lower extremity and core strength. Many practitioners recommend that the patient successfully wean from the brace prior to returning to sports. With the flexible corset-type braces, it may be possible to wear the brace during the transition back to sports activities. Follow-up x-rays to document healing are generally not useful with spondylolysis, because visible bony defects may persist even in patients who are clinically doing well. Flexibility and core strengthening exercises should be continued for at least 2 additional months after athletes have successfully returned to full activity.

Spondylolisthesis

Spondylolisthesis is the forward slippage of one vertebra in relation to the vertebra below. Spondylolisthesis is a sequela of bilateral spondylolysis. In athletes, spondylolisthesis is far less common than the pars stress fracture or spondylolysis. As with other pars interarticularis problems, athletes will experience activity-related pain. The clinical examination will reveal pain with lower back extension and a positive single leg standing extension test. A standing lateral x-ray is typically used to diagnose spondylolisthesis and to monitor for progression of the slippage (**Figure 34.7**). **Table 34.1** provides the grading system used when assessing the severity of spondylolisthesis (**Figure 34.8**).

Athletes with grade I spondylolisthesis (L5 slips ≤25% forward on S1) can be treated with a Warm-N-Form orthosis, a lumbar corset, or the Boston brace for symptoms of pain. Treatment for a symptomatic spondylolisthesis requires an initial period of rest from running, jumping, and impact activities along with protection from arching of the spine. With use of a lumbar brace or corset, most patients will be pain free within 2 to 3 weeks. At this point, it is usually safe to commence general conditioning exercises that can be performed in the brace. This includes stationary bikes, stairsteppers, and elliptical trainers as well as general flexibility exercises. If this level of exercise is tolerated, patients can begin a trunk stabilization program. Trunk strengthening exercises are initially done in a neutral spine position but progress through a wider range of motion that requires removal of the back brace during the exercises. When trunk strength has been restored, patients may gradually transition back to sports activity. Some experts recommend weaning from the brace before resuming sports activities. Others recommend continuing to use a softer, more flexible brace such as the Warm-N-Form or lumbar corset for added protection during the transition back to sports.

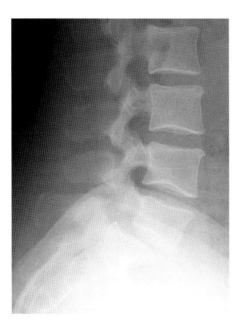

FIGURE 34.7 Lateral radiograph of grade II spondylolisthesis.

For patients with spondylolisthesis, follow-up yearly plain films are necessary until age 19 to check for any progression of vertebral slippage. With persistent or increasing pain, follow-up radiographs to rule out progressive slippage may need to be taken sooner. Athletes with higher-grade spondylolisthesis (L5 slips 50% or more forward on S1), athletes who show evidence of progressive slippage, or athletes who remain symptomatic with treatment should be referred to a pediatric orthopedist specialist.

SACROILIAC (SI) JOINT PAIN

Another possible diagnosis for young athletes who experience lower back pain is SI joint pain. Clinically, athletes with SI joint pain will manifest activity-related pain in the lower back or posterior hip. The clinical examination reveals pain with lumbar extension and/or with the single leg standing extension test. The SI joint or ilium may be observed to be elevated or move asymmetrically as the patient flexes the trunk or bends sideways. Typically patients with SI dysfunction will experience pain at palpation over the SI joint, and the FABER test will reproduce their symptoms. The straight leg raising test and the slump test are both negative, and the hip examination is normal.

Radiologic evaluation should begin with 4-view plain films of the lumbar spine. Unless the clinician suspects that the patient has an underlying rheumatologic disorder, SI joint films are typically not very helpful. Because athletes with SI joint pain often have a positive single leg standing extension test, further evaluation with the bone/SPECT scan to rule out pars stress fracture may be necessary. The diagnosis of SI joint pain must be considered in athletes with a positive single leg standing extension test who have normal lumbosacral spine films and a normal bone/SPECT scan.

Rehabilitation is the mainstay of treatment for SI joint pain. As they are with other lower back problems in young athletes, physical therapists experienced in treating SI joint pain are valuable to the physician. The mainstays of rehabilitation are to restore normal motion in the SI joint and to stabilize the muscles of the hip, spine, and pelvis. A lumbar corset or an SI belt may augment the role of stabilizing muscles. Gross instability of the SI joint stemming from major trauma such as a motor vehicle collision may require operative fixation. Athletes may return to play once their symptoms have resolved and they are able to pass a sport-specific functional progression test. SI joint corticosteroid injection under fluoroscopy is a further treatment option if the athlete's injury does not respond to conservative treatment.

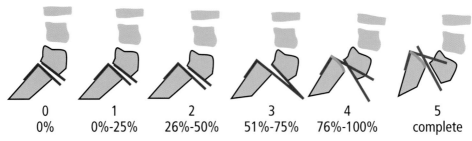

| 0 | 1 | 2 | 3 | 4 | 5 |
| 0% | 0%-25% | 26%-50% | 51%-75% | 76%-100% | complete |

FIGURE 34.8 Measuring percentage slip of L5 on S1.

TABLE 34.1

Grading System for Spondylolisthesis

Grade	Percentage Anterior Slip of L5 on S1
I	0% to 25%
II	26% to 50%
III	51% to 75%
IV	76% to 100+%

Source: Meyerding HW. Spondylolisthesis. *Surg Gynecol Obstet* 1932; S4:371-377.

LUMBAR DISK DISEASE

Another cause of lower back pain in young athletes is lumbar disk pain. This diagnosis is less common in young athletes than pars interarticularis problems. Athletes with disk injuries typically have lower back, buttock, or hamstring pain that is more pronounced with trunk flexion, lifting, sitting, and lying supine. Activities that would aggravate a pars defect, such as arching, may be asymptomatic in a patient with a disk injury. Radiating pain or symptoms of sciatic nerve irritation may be present only if the disk is compressing a lumbar nerve root. Occasionally, patients will seek care for hamstring or calf pain that is due to a disk protrusion or herniation, even if they do not report back pain.

At physical examination, patients with disk problems may have painful or restricted trunk flexion or a lumbar shift. With a bulging disk, patients tend to shift their posture or bend away from the protruding portion of the disk. This lumbar shift can give the appearance of an acutely painful scoliosis. Dural tension signs, such as a positive straight leg raising test, are less common in young athletes than in adults with a diagnosis of lumbar disk pain. The slump test may be positive in adolescent athletes with lumbar disk injuries.

Plain radiographs in young patients with disk injuries are usually normal. With long-standing disk problems, the intervertebral disk space may narrow. Vertebral end-plate irregularities or vertebral wedging may also be seen in patients with disk-related symptoms. MRI is the best imaging modality to confirm the diagnosis of disk pathology and to assess compression on lumbar nerve roots (**Figure 34.9**). A lumbar disk does not have to be herniated or compressing a nerve root to be a source of back pain. Furthermore, smaller disk protrusions or degenerative changes that may be considered normal in an adult may not be normal in an adolescent with back pain.

Adolescent athletes with lumbar disk disease are usually treated with a rehabilitation program and anti-inflammatory medication. Initially, activities need to be modified or restricted to whatever level is necessary

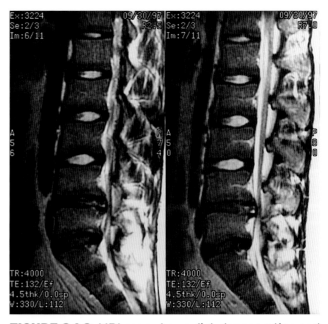

FIGURE 34.9 MRI scan shows disk degeneration and protrusion at L4-L5 and L5-S1. Reproduced with permission from Richards BS, McCarthy RE, Akbarnia BA. Back pain in childhood and adolescence. In: Zuckerman JD, ed. *Instructional Course Lectures 48*. Rosemont, IL: American Academy of Orthopaedic Surgeons; 1999:525-542.

to avoid further disk injury or pain. Lifting, bending, twisting, and high-impact activities create stresses to the spine that are most likely to cause pain or disrupt healing. Therapeutic exercises focus on improving lower extremity flexibility, restoring normal lumbar motion, and establishing adequate trunk stability.

As symptoms improve, the athlete can begin general conditioning with elliptical or stair-stepper machines and advance to running and then sport-specific drills. Neutral spine exercises, in which excessive flexion, rotation, and extension of the spine are avoided, tend to be better tolerated in patients with disk injuries. Lifting free weights or any lifting associated with trunk flexion may need to be limited until the athlete has fully recovered.

Epidural corticosteroid injections can be a helpful adjunct to reduce inflammation around a disk for athletes who experience continued pain that prevents them from carrying out rehabilitation exercises or returning to full activity. Surgery is generally reserved for patients whose injuries do not respond to nonsurgical measures or for patients who have a herniated disk associated with persistent or progressive neurologic deficits. Performing repeat MRIs to document disk healing is not a prerequisite for return to play because visible disk abnormalities tend to persist even after the patient has become symptom free and has successfully resumed full activity.

MUSCULAR LOWER BACK PAIN

Most patients with back pain experience muscular tightness, spasm, or pain. These symptoms may be a result of multiple underlying problems but are rarely a result of a primary muscle injury. If the evaluation for structural sources of muscle pain, spasm, or guarding is negative, mechanical or muscular lower back pain may be considered as a possible diagnosis.

Athletes who are diagnosed with muscular lower back pain have clinical histories and examination results similar to those described for the other causes of lower back pain discussed earlier. Their physical examination may show various signs such as generalized paraspinal muscle spasm or pain with lumbar extension. However, patients with muscular lower back pain rarely have localizing signs such as a lumbar shift, positive slump test, positive single leg standing extension test, or dural tension signs.

If symptoms persist and clinical evaluation has ruled out more specific diagnoses of back pain, the athlete may benefit from a rehabilitation program. In addition to use of ice or heat and antiinflammatory medications, the athlete may respond to

stretching exercises, massage, low- to moderate-intensity aerobic exercise, or core strengthening exercises, as well as instruction in proper posture and spine mechanics. Return to sports may occur once the patient is asymptomatic and has regained normal spinal motion, core strength, and function.

DIFFERENTIAL DIAGNOSIS OF LOWER BACK PAIN

Although most young athletes with lower back pain have structural problems or mechanical pain, other conditions should always be considered in the differential diagnosis. As with other musculoskeletal problems, both infection (such as diskitis) and tumors can manifest as back pain in active, athletic individuals. Diskitis presents with unrelenting pain that does not diminish with rest or simple treatment measures such as ice, anti-inflammatory medications, or stretching. Patients with diskitis may not develop fever or other constitutional symptoms during the diagnosis period.

Night pain that awakens the athlete can be a hallmark symptom of tumors, including osteoid osteomas. Patients with tumors may have pain that does not correspond with activity. Both infection and tumors can produce abnormalities on bone scans and may need further diagnostic evaluation with either CT or MRI. Both diagnoses should always be considered in athletes whose back pain is not clearly associated with injury or activity, or in athletes whose injuries are not improving with standard treatment.

Young athletes with symptoms of lower back pain and stiffness may be suffering from an inflammatory disease such as ankylosing spondylitis or Reiter syndrome. Boys are more likely than girls to fall into this diagnostic group. Chronic Achilles insertion pain or enthesopathy in the athlete with lower back pain may be a tip-off to an underlying inflammatory disorder. Back pain may also be the result of an intra-abdominal or retroperitoneal abnormality such as kidney stones, an ovarian cyst, an infection, or a tumor.

Normal lumbar spine variants can be seen on plain films and are often mentioned in the radiology report. Spina bifida occulta and transitional vertebrae are the most commonly mentioned. Neither of these variants will typically cause pain by themselves. However, these 2 variants may be correlated with pars interarticularis problems.

THORACIC BACK PAIN

Although thoracic or midback pain is less common than lower back pain, it can also be seen in adolescent athletes. The differential diagnosis list for thoracic pain includes thoracic disk disease, vertebral end-plate injuries, Scheuermann kyphosis, myofascial pain syndromes, and postural/mechanical pain.

Disk Pain

Thoracic disk problems are less common than cervical and lumbar disk problems because the rib cage restricts thoracic motion and provides bony support and stability to the thoracic spine. Disk protrusions or herniations in the thoracic spine cause back pain that is worse with trunk flexion or compression of the spine, or paraspinal muscle spasm, but rarely any signs or symptoms or neurologic compromise.

End-Plate Irregularities

Radiographs of the thoracic spine may reveal end-plate irregularities such as Schmorl's nodes or vertebral wedging (**Figure 34.10**). These findings are commonly observed in asymptomatic patients. However, if there is associated pain,

further imaging such as a bone scan/SPECT scan, CT scan, or MRI may help clarify the diagnosis.

Scheuermann Kyphosis

Scheuermann kyphosis, a structural deformity that affects the thoracic spine, can manifest with midback pain. Patients with Scheuermann kyphosis may have a rounded back and the appearance of poor posture but are unable to correct their posture by trying to sit up. Lateral radiographs of the thoracic spine will show anterior wedging of at least 3 consecutive thoracic vertebrae. Abnormal growth and development of thoracic vertebral end plates is one possible explanation for this condition. The classic form of Scheuermann kyphosis tends to involve the upper portion of the thoracic spine. This condition can lead to progressive pain and deformity during growth and may require bracing and follow-up care with a pediatric spine specialist.

If the kyphosis involves the lower thoracic spine or upper lumbar spine, repetitive impact and compressive forces may

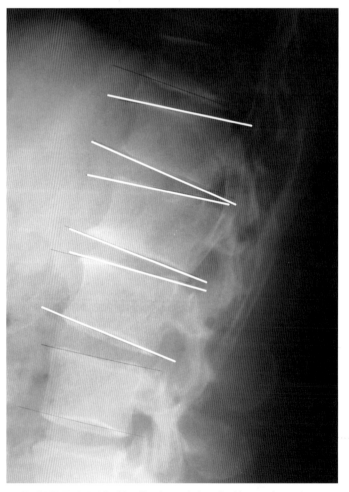

FIGURE 34.10 Vertical wedging in thoracic spine.

be the cause. Gymnasts, rowers, football players, and weight lifters are among the athletes who may have the acquired or traumatic form of Scheuermann kyphosis. Physical therapy can help diminish pain-related symptoms but will usually have little effect on the structural kyphosis. Therapeutic exercises aim to extend kyphotic segments, correct posture, and strengthen extensor musculature of the back. Patients with significant kyphosis, progressive kyphosis, or kyphosis associated with persistent pain may need bracing, as well as consultation with a pediatric spine specialist.

Myofascial Pain

Thoracic muscular/myofascial pain can be diagnosed if disk injuries, vertebral end-plate injuries, and vertebral wedging have been excluded as causes of back pain. Patients with myofascial pain typically have no specific injury history. Their symptoms of muscular pain and spasm are not associated with specific activities and are not relieved by rest. The physical examination may reveal a kyphotic posture, rounded shoulders, forward head position, abducted scapulae, and generalized joint hypermobility. Trigger points are typically found along the medial and superior border of the scapula and the paraspinal muscles in the cervical, thoracic, and lumbar regions. The thoracic spine is not typically tender to direct palpation, and there are no obvious structural deformities or neurologic abnormalities. Patients with thoracic or scapulothoracic myofascial pain will also have normal pulmonary and cardiac examinations. Radiologic evaluation with plain films of the thoracic spine will be normal. Treatment can include massage therapy, as well as physical therapy with emphasis on postural correction and scapular stabilization exercises. Athletes can typically return to play as symptoms allow.

Scoliosis

Scoliosis is the most common bony anomaly affecting the thoracic spine but is rarely a cause of back pain. The incidence of scoliosis in some sports may be slightly higher than in the general population, indicating there is a possibility that sports participation may have a small effect on the development of scoliosis. Athletes with scoliosis are usually detected by scoliosis screening. When athletes have x-rays to evaluate back pain, scoliosis may be present but should not be assumed to be the source of the patient's symptoms. A scoliosis curve that appears rapidly and is associated with pain may be caused by a tumor or an infection. Another cause of acute-onset, painful scoliosis may be a disk herniation with a compensatory lumbar shift. Athletes with less than 20° curves can be followed with periodic plain films. Athletes with curves over 20° should be

referred to a pediatric spine specialist. Athletes with mild scoliosis who have had other, more specific sources of back pain excluded can be treated with physical therapy. Athletes with scoliosis and no back pain should be able to participate in sports. However, for those with scoliosis curves more than 30°, unstable curves, or scoliosis-associated back pain, sports participation may have to be restricted.

SUMMARY POINTS

- Lower and midback pain is common in active and athletic individuals. Although a variety of underlying structural and mechanical abnormalities may be found, non–activity-related sources of back pain, including tumor and infection, should also be considered in the differential diagnosis.

- Any individual with persistent back pain should be evaluated; a thorough medical and orthopedic history should be taken; and a physical examination should be performed that includes the spine, extremities, and relevant organ systems.

- Plain radiographs are commonly indicated in the evaluation of back pain, but more sophisticated imaging, such as bone scan/SPECT scan, CT, and MRI, may be necessary to confirm the diagnosis and to plan proper treatment.

- Back pain associated with lumbar extension should raise concern for abnormalities in the pars interarticularis. Pars interarticularis lesions associated with abnormal bony activity on bone scan/SPECT scan or MRI warrant sufficient rest or protection in a brace to permit bony healing.

- Lumbar disk injuries can also cause back pain in young athletes. Disk problems in young patients are less likely than in adults to produce abnormalities on plain radiographs and are less likely to produce radiculopathy. The abnormalities of a symptomatic disk on MRI may be more subtle than for adults, but early diagnosis and treatment of a disk injury is associated with a better response to conservative therapy.

- Thoracic pain is less common than lumbar pain in young athletes. Thoracic disk disease, vertebral end-plate irregularities, and vertebral wedging with Scheuermann kyphosis may be sources of thoracic pain.

- Scoliosis may be the most commonly observed radiographic abnormality in the thoracic spine but is unlikely to be the source of back pain.

- Muscular and myofascial pain syndromes should be diagnosed only after ruling out more specific structural, mechanical, or medical sources for back pain.

- Most young athletes with back pain can benefit from a rehabilitation program that identifies and corrects the abnormalities in posture, flexibility, strength, and spinal mechanics that contributed to the pain or resulted from the pain. For the majority of conditions that do not warrant surgical intervention, physical therapy can be a beneficial part of most rehabilitation programs.

SUGGESTED READING

Congeni J, McCulloch J, Swanson K. Lumbar spondylolysis: a study of natural progression in athletes. *Am J Sports Med.* 1997; 25:248-253.

Kraft D. Low back pain in the adolescent athlete. *Ped Clin North Am.* 2002; 643-653.

Papanicolaou N, Wilkinson RH, Emans JB, et al. Bone scintigraphy and radiology in young athletes with low back pain. *Am J Roentgenol.* 1985; 145:1039-1044.

D'Hemecourt PA, Gerbino PG 2nd, Micheli LJ. Back injuries in the young athlete. *Clin Sports Med.* 2000;19(4):663-79.

Sassmannshausen G, Smith B. Back pain in the young athlete. *Clin Sports Med.* 2002; 21(1):121-132.

Stanitski CL, Delee JC, Drez D Jr. *Pediatric and Adolescent Sports Medicine.* Philadelphia, PA: WB Saunders; 1994.

Watkins RG, Dillin WH. Lumbar spine injury in the athlete. *Clin Sports Med.* 1990; 9:419-448.

Wood K. Spinal deformity in the adolescent athlete. *Clin Sports Med.* 2002;1:77-92.

CHAPTER 35

Elbow

Joseph A. Congeni, MD

The elbow joint is unlike any other joint in the human body. The unique architecture of the elbow allows the joint to pivot and rotate, as well as function like a hinge. The variety of available joint movements contributes to the functionality of the upper extremity as a whole. The ability of the radius and ulna to rotate about one another at the elbow allows for remarkable precision and dexterity in handling objects. The ability of the elbow to flex and extend allows for objects to be lifted, moved, and propelled. This combination of movements is especially useful with tasks such as throwing a ball or hitting a ball with a racquet, bat, or golf club. Despite the wide range of available motions, the elbow can be sufficiently stable to support considerable weight and impact, as is the case with a gymnast doing a back handspring.

The demands placed on the elbow subject it to a variety of acute and chronic injuries. Many of the traumatic injuries to the elbow are caused by falling onto an outstretched hand. In the growing child, many of the bony structures have not ossified, diminishing their ability to withstand impact and contribute to elbow stability. Thus, children are more likely than adults to experience elbow fracture dislocations. In addition, the elbow is often subjected to sub-maximal repetitive stresses with certain sporting activities, especially overhead throwing. The presence of open growth centers about the elbow predisposes the skeletally immature athlete to unique overuse injuries not seen in adults.

ANATOMY AND BIOMECHANICS

The elbow functions as a hinge joint, allowing flexion and extension. The bony articulation involves the distal humerus with the proximal radius and ulna (**Figure 35.1**). At its distal end, the humerus broadens, forming the capitellum and trochlea on the articular surface. The trochlea, on the medial aspect of the distal humerus, is spool shaped. It articulates with the trochlear notch of the olecranon of the proximal ulna, which surrounds nearly 180° of the trochlea. This expansive contact area provides much of the inherent stability to the elbow. Adding to this stability is the presence of the coronoid process, a bony projection of the ulna that lies anterior to the trochlea when the elbow is flexed. This structure further surrounds the trochlea, making the joint far more stable. On the lateral side, the capitellum of the humerus articulates with the radial head. The bony congruence between the radial head and the capitellum is much less than the medial portion of the joint, which allows for great mobility of the proximal radius as it rotates about the ulna. The radiocapitellar joint is important in transmitting force from the hand to the humerus over a wide range of elbow positions and in load bearing through an extended elbow. The third bony articulation at the elbow is the association between the proximal ends of the radius and ulna. This is classified as a gliding joint, with the radius rotating about the ulna. This joint does not contribute to elbow stability per se, but it is crucial in allowing forearm rotation.

The soft tissue stability of the elbow is provided by the joint capsule as well the medial and lateral collateral ligaments. The medial ligament complex includes the 2-part ulnar collateral ligament, which is a key resistor to valgus stress applied to the elbow. Injury to this structure is a common source of elbow pain and weakness in throwing athletes. On the lateral side, the lateral ulnar collateral ligament serves to stabilize the elbow joint. Tears of this ligament complex often result in recurrent posterolateral dislocations of the elbow.

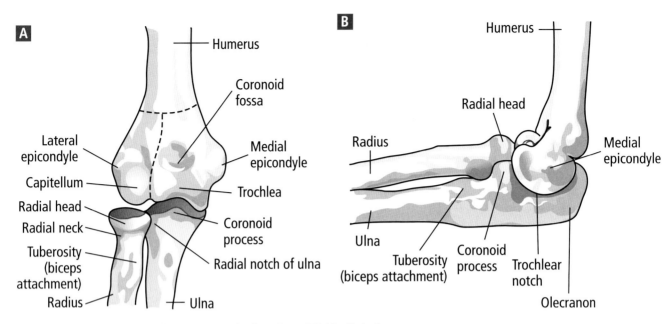

FIGURE 35.1 Elbow anatomy. (A) Anterior view. (B) Medial view.

The muscles that cross the elbow serve as the final contribution to joint stability. In particular, the anconeus, brachialis, and triceps muscles stabilize the elbow by exerting compressive forces on it. In addition, the flexor-pronator group of the forearm, which originates on the medial epicondyle, contributes to medial stability.

Normal motion of the elbow includes flexion-extension as well as supination-pronation. Younger children typically have more joint mobility than adolescents and adults, and it is not unusual for them to be able to hyperextend 10° to 15°. When the elbow is fully extended, there may be a slight valgus orientation called the carrying angle. The degree of this valgus alignment is typically greater in women than men. With the elbow fully flexed, the angle between the arm and forearm changes to a varus alignment.

When evaluating a young athlete with elbow pain, it is important to consider the skeletal maturity of the patient and to understand the normal ossification of the elbow. There are 6 secondary ossification centers of the elbow that appear at predictable times during development. The mnemonic CRITOE is used to remember the order of appearance of each of these centers: C (capitellum) at age 1 to 2 years, R (radial head) at age 3, I (internal/medial epicondyle) at age 5, T (trochlea) at age 7, O (olecranon) at age 9, and E (external/lateral epicondyle) at age 11

(see **Figure 35.4**). Knowing when these ossification centers appear may be important in differentiating them from fracture fragments on radiographs. The fusion of the ossification centers shows more variation but typically occurs in the following manner: capitellum, trochlea, and olecranon at age 14; medial epicondyle at age 15; and radial head and lateral epicondyle at age 16. Familiarity with normal ossification patterns can help minimize confusion among ligament injuries, apophyseal injuries, and fractures.

CLINICAL EVALUATION

A thorough and complete history and physical examination are the most important diagnostic tools for the clinician. They are often sufficient to make a diagnosis, or at least raise the most likely diagnostic possibilities. They also help the clinician make decisions on diagnostic imaging.

History

The first objective in obtaining the history is to inquire about the onset of symptoms and to classify the injury as acute or overuse. For acute injuries, information should be gathered on the activity or sport the athlete was engaged in, the mechanism of injury, the position of the elbow at the time of injury (ie, flexed, extended, or rotated), the location of pain, the presence of swelling, restricted mobility, instability, weakness, and radiating symptoms such as numbness or tingling. For symptoms with an insidious onset, the clinician should note the sport and position played, volume of play (number of games per week), any recent changes in volume of play, and any other factors that may have chronically increased the stress to the elbow. Again, the location of pain; the presence of swelling or joint restrictions; and numbness, tingling, and/or radiating pain should be evaluated. The presence of concurrent symptoms or injury in other areas, such as the shoulder, neck, hips, or lower extremity, should also be explored.

Other important information to obtain during the history is the patient's handedness; the presence of symptoms with activities of daily living; and any previous injury, evaluation, and treatment.

Physical Examination

The clinician should begin the physical examination by evaluating the uninjured elbow, paying particular attention to the patient's baseline range of motion, alignment, and stability. These results can then be compared with the injured side, taking note of swelling, bruising, deformity, and station (how the patient is holding his or her arm and elbow). Next, the clinician should palpate for areas of tenderness or swelling. Point tenderness may suggest fracture. An elbow joint effusion suggests intra-articular injury, such as a fracture or articular cartilage injury. Range of motion is assessed by having the patient actively flex and extend the elbow, as well as pronate and supinate the forearm. Pronation/supination should be tested both with the elbow fully extended and flexed at 90°. All movements should be full and pain free and compared with the unaffected side. Pain with these movements could indicate fracture, and mechanical obstruction to movement could suggest loose bodies within the joint, such as fracture or cartilaginous loose bodies.

The integrity of the ulnar collateral ligament can be assessed by performing a valgus stress test, in which a valgus stress is applied with the elbow flexed 20° to 30° (**Figure 35.2**). If there is a suspicion of fracture, this test should be deferred until after radiographs are obtained.

A complete neurovascular examination should be performed, especially in the setting of traumatic injuries. Any abnormalities require prompt evaluation to prevent further damage. The extremity distal to the injury should be examined for color, temperature, and pulses to rule out vascular compromise. The clinician should be alert to signs of compartment syndrome, including swelling and increasing pressure in the forearm as well as pain and decreasing sensation in the hand. Traumatic injuries to the elbow may

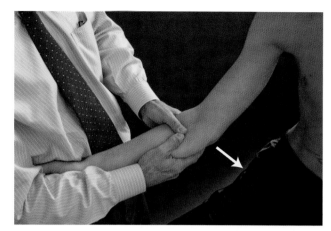

FIGURE 35.2 Valgus stress test of the elbow.

also affect nearby nerves, including the ulnar, radial, and median nerves. Sensation to light touch, pinprick, or 2-point discrimination can be assessed for each peripheral nerve. Some simple tests of motor function for these nerves include ability to flex the thumb and index finger (median), extend the thumb (radial), and move the index finger (ulnar) medially/laterally. The proximal and distal joints should be examined for the presence of associated injuries. The shoulder and wrist should be carefully assessed because the mechanisms leading to injury in the elbow often lead to injuries in these areas, too. In the case of overuse injuries to the elbow, the examiner may find an abnormality that contributes to poor throwing mechanics, such as shoulder weakness or instability.

Imaging Studies

Plain radiographs may be indicated for many patients with elbow pain, both acute and chronic. Anteroposterior and lateral views of the affected side are usually sufficient, but if there is uncertainty in differentiating injury from anatomic variants or normal growth, views of the contralateral elbow may be obtained for comparison. This is commonly needed to assess for widening or subtle avulsion of an epiphysis.

When interpreting radiographs of the elbow in children, it is helpful to confirm normal alignment of structures. On lateral views, a line drawn along the anterior aspect of the humerus should bisect the capitellum. If this does not occur, a supracondylar fracture should be suspected. Also, in all views, the radius should point to the capitellum. Failure to do so could indicate fracture or dislocation. The presence of an anterior or posterior fat pad indicates an intra-articular effusion (**Figure 35.3**). While a fat pad sign can be seen with septic arthritis, a fat pad that is visible following trauma suggests an intra-articular fracture.

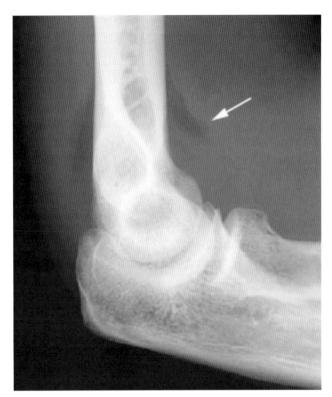

FIGURE 35.3 Radiograph indicating intra-articular effusion with an anterior fat pad or "sail sign."

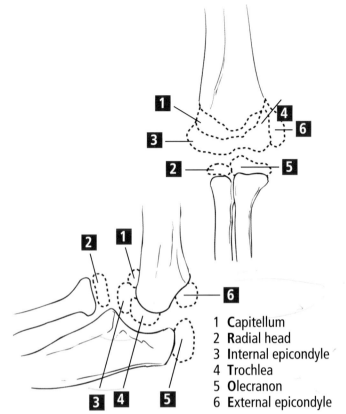

1 Capitellum
2 Radial head
3 Internal epicondyle
4 Trochlea
5 Olecranon
6 External epicondyle

FIGURE 35.4 The ossification centers of the elbow in order of their appearance.

Skeletally immature patients often experience fractures through unossified cartilage. This can make interpretation of radiographs difficult because fracture fragments are often much larger than they appear on films. It is also important to remember the sequence and timing of the structure's ossification (CRITOE mnemonic) to differentiate ossification centers from fracture fragments (**Figure 35.4**).

When visualization of soft tissue structures is needed, magnetic resonance imaging (MRI) is the study of choice. It is most commonly used to identify tears to the ulnar collateral ligament, but it can also show articular cartilage abnormalities, tendonitis, and muscle or tendon strains. MRI may also permit more detailed visualization of fracture lines and osteochondral defects.

ACUTE INJURIES

Fractures and Dislocations

Fractures and dislocations are common results of trauma to the elbow. Approximately 10% of all fractures in children occur in the elbow. The most common mechanism of injury is a fall onto an outstretched hand.

If a fracture or dislocation is suspected, great care should be taken to prevent further damage to neurovascular structures. Thus, after thorough physical and neurovascular examinations, the arm should be carefully splinted to allow for safe transport for radiographic evaluation. Most fractures and dislocations should be referred to orthopedic surgeons because of the high complication rate and the frequent need for surgical fixation.

Supracondylar Fracture Supracondylar fractures are the most common elbow fractures in children. The average age of patients with this injury is 5 to 8 years. Ninety-five percent of supracondylar fractures are the extension type and occur when falling on an outstretched hand results in hyperextension of the elbow. The relatively lax ligaments in the pediatric elbow allow for hyperextension, driving the olecranon into the supracondylar area and producing the fracture (**Figure 35.5**).

If a supracondylar fracture is suspected, the clinician should try to splint the arm with the elbow flexed 20° to 30°, and the patient should be referred for x-rays and orthopedic consultation. Urgent surgical intervention is indicated if

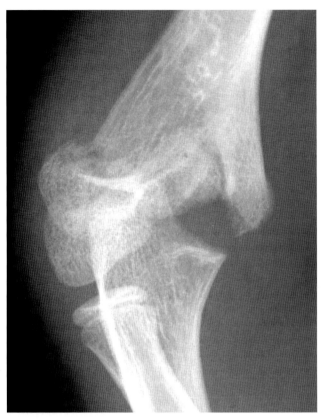

FIGURE 35.5 Radiograph showing supracondylar fracture of the elbow.

distal pulses are absent or if the hand is poorly perfused. Vascular ischemia is suggested if paresthesias follow the distribution of more than one peripheral nerve. Nondisplaced fractures are casted for 3 to 4 weeks. Displaced fractures require reduction and possible surgical fixation. Because the fracture usually occurs proximally to growth centers, there is rarely growth arrest. The most common deformity resulting from a supracondylar fracture is a cubitus varus angulation, in which the normal carrying angle is lost.

Neurovascular injuries are relatively common with this fracture. Those with nerve injuries, which occur in 10% to 18% of cases, usually recover within several weeks. Vascular injuries occur in 3% to 12% of cases, but they rarely require vascular surgical intervention.

Lateral Condyle Fracture Fractures to the lateral condyle of the humerus are the second most common fracture in the elbow of children. As with supracondylar fractures, they are more common in younger children (especially children younger than 7 years), but they may also occur in older children and adolescents. The mechanism of injury is typically a fall onto an outstretched hand combined with a varus force. At examination, pain and swelling will be pres-

ent on the lateral side of the elbow. Radiographic findings are often subtle as a result of the nonossified lateral condyle in young children. Lateral condyle fractures often appear as a small avulsion fragment, but occasionally will extend from the humeral metaphysis to the elbow joint surface. These injuries, which are often classified as Salter-Harris type IV injuries, place the bone at high risk for growth arrest or nonunion. Fragments that are displaced and/or rotated may require surgical intervention.

Radial Neck Fracture Falls onto an outstretched hand may also result in fractures to the proximal radius, most commonly in the radial neck region (**Figure 35.6**). These are often compression fractures induced by axial loading. They should be suspected in a patient who has lateral elbow pain and swelling that is distal to the lateral condyle. Pain is exacerbated by pronation/supination more than flexion/extension of the elbow. Radiographs often show a posterior fat pad, but this sign may be absent if the fracture occurs distal to the attachment of the joint capsule. The presence of a radial neck fracture should alert the examiner to look for associated injuries, especially olecranon and medial epicondyle fractures as well as elbow dislocations. If angulation is greater than 30°, closed reduction under anesthesia is suggested. Otherwise, brief immobilization with splinting or a sling followed by early range-of-motion exercises is sufficient.

Proximal Ulna Fracture Olecranon fractures are relatively uncommon, but they are often associated with other injuries. An extreme valgus stress may result in an olecranon fracture in conjunction with a compression fracture of the radial neck and a medial epicondyle fracture. Other fractures involving the proximal ulna include those of the

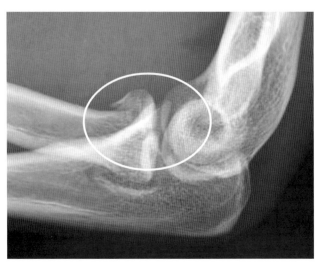

FIGURE 35.6 Radiograph of radial neck fracture.

coronoid process, which are commonly associated with elbow dislocations. A proximal ulna fracture in conjunction with dislocation of the proximal radioulnar joint is called a Monteggia fracture. A Monteggia fracture can also occur in the midshaft of the ulna (**Figure 35.7**) or with a plastic deformation of the ulna. Whenever the ulna is fractured and the radius is not, a Monteggia fracture should be suspected and dedicated x-rays of the elbow should be part of the evaluation.

Elbow Dislocations Dislocation of the elbow is relatively common in young athletes, especially those between the ages of 11 and 15 years. Simple dislocations are those without an associated fracture. They are almost always posteriorly directed (**Figure 35.8**). A dislocation of this type usually implies complete disruption of the ligamentous structures about the elbow. Radiographs should be done to rule out associated fracture or growth plate injury. Closed reduction is performed under anesthesia, and the stability provided by the osseous and muscular elements is usually sufficient to prevent further dislocation. The clinician should treat simple dislocations with a sling for comfort for 5 to 7 days, followed by range-of-motion exercises. Immobilization for more than 2 weeks may lead to a poor long-term prognosis with persistent stiffness. The ligamentous structures heal and regain function in most cases.

A fracture in conjunction with an elbow dislocation defines a complex dislocation. Most common are fractures to the radial neck and avulsion of the medial epicondyle.

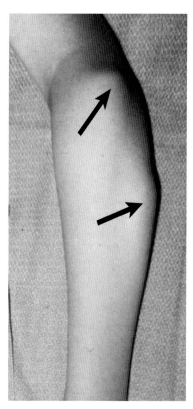

FIGURE 35.7 Clinical presentation of Monteggia fracture/dislocation in the midshaft of the ulna. Adapted with permission from Letts M, ed. *The Management of Pediatric Fractures*. Philadelphia, PA: Churchill Livingstone; 1994:302. Copyright Elsevier.

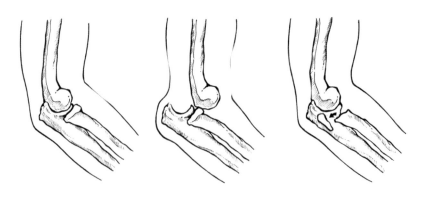

Normal anatomic position

Elbow dislocation

With reduction humerus impinges on radius, shearing off radial head

FIGURE 35.8 Elbow dislocation. Adapted with permission from Letts M. Dislocation of the child's elbow. In: Morrey B, ed. *The Elbow and Its Disorders*. Philadelphia, PA: WB Saunders; 1993:309-310. Copyright Elsevier.

In some cases, the medial epicondylar fragment may be displaced into the elbow joint, requiring surgery.

The Monteggia fracture, as described earlier, is an alternative pattern of injury that occurs when the osseous, rather than ligamentous, structures fail, leading to posterior dislocation.

Anterior dislocations of the elbow are rare. To occur, they typically require a fracture of the olecranon and/or coronoid process. The most common mechanism of injury is a direct blow to the dorsal forearm with the elbow in midflexion. This injury differs from the Monteggia fracture in that the radioulnar joint remains intact. This type of dislocation also usually spares the ligamentous structures of the elbow. Treatment involves surgical fixation of the fracture and reduction of the elbow.

Elbow dislocation in association with radial head and coronoid process fractures is known as the terrible triad because of the high rate of complications, including chronic instability with recurrent dislocations and arthrosis.

Traction Injuries

Injuries often occur as a result of a sudden, forceful tensile stress on a tendon or ligament that attaches to the elbow. A common mechanism is a single, forceful, overhead throw such as a pitched baseball. Patients often describe feeling a pop or a sensation of the elbow giving out. After the injury, athletes cannot continue with their sport because of pain and weakness.

Medial Epicondyle Avulsion Fracture Avulsions to the medial epicondyle can occur from a fall or from a sudden valgus stress applied to the elbow from hard throwing, such as pitching. Because of the relative strength of the ulnar collateral ligament compared with the medial epicondyle epiphysis, it is the physis that fails in this injury. This injury can also occur from a fall onto an outstretched hand. Radiographs may reveal that the avulsed fragment from the medial epicondyle has become displaced into the joint.

Treatment of nondisplaced avulsion (<2 mm) involves immobilization for 2 to 3 weeks, followed by application of a hinged brace, allowing for range-of-motion exercises. Strengthening may begin when there is no tenderness to palpation. Once joint motion and strength have been restored, the athlete may transition back to normal activites. For throwing athletes, the final step in the rehabilitation process is a throwing program with a gradual increase in number of throws, distance, and velocity. These rehabilitative measures should be carefully monitored by therapists trained to care for these types of injuries.

Surgical intervention may be necessary for fragments that are rotated, intra-articular, or displaced more than 2 mm. Valgus instability or ulnar nerve dysfunction may also require surgical treatment. Postoperative rehabilitation follows a similar pattern to the program just outlined.

Ulnar Collateral Ligament Tear In a skeletally mature athlete, a sudden valgus stress, hyperextension, or elbow dislocation may injure the ulnar collateral ligament. The mechanism of injury and history are identical to those of medial epicondyle avulsion, but examination reveals the tenderness to be distal to the medial epicondyle (**Figure 35.9**). There is instability with valgus stress testing, but radiographs are necessary to distinguish an ulnar collateral ligament sprain from an avulsion fracture.

Treatment involves a 4- to 6-week period of conservative management, including rest, ice, and physical therapy directed at range of motion and strength. Splinting with a hinged brace may be used in some cases; this treatment should be individualized on the basis of the severity of injury. If pain and valgus instability persist, surgery to reconstruct the medial collateral ligament may be suggested for those who wish to continue playing sports that involve overhead throwing.

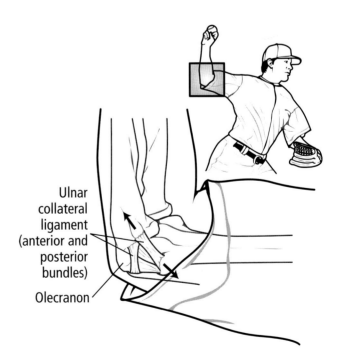

Ulnar collateral ligament (anterior and posterior bundles)

Olecranon

FIGURE 35.9 Ulnar collateral ligament anatomy and the mechanism of injury.

CHRONIC INJURIES

Overuse injuries are characterized by an insidious onset of pain and gradual worsening of symptoms with continued activity. They are a result of repetitive microtrauma and may be the result of abnormalities of training, technique, or anatomic factors such as skeletal immaturity, joint instability, or weakness. Classic examples of overuse injuries to the elbow are seen in baseball pitchers and gymnasts. Because they are not the result of a single, identifiable traumatic event, many athletes, parents, and coaches dismiss the pain as growing pains or tendonitis.

Little League Elbow (Medial Epicondyle Apophysitis)

The term *Little League elbow* may be used to refer to a variety of causes of elbow pain in young throwing athletes (**Figure 35.10**). However, Little League elbow is intended to refer to an apophysitis resulting from repetitive valgus stress on the elbow from overhead throwing. Medial elbow pain is usually felt as the arm accelerates forward during the throwing motion, when maximal valgus stress is exerted on the medial elbow. Although pitchers are the most frequently affected, any position that requires frequent, hard throws can lead to the injury.

The age range for Little League elbow is 8 to 15 years, which corresponds to the age of maturation of the medial epicondylar physis. Once the medial epicondylar physis has matured, forces are transmitted to the ulnar collateral ligament and flexor-pronator muscle mass, leading to ulnar collateral ligament sprain or flexor-pronator tendonitis. The clinician should ask what position the athlete plays and should also ask about the exposure to throwing, including the number of practices and games, the pitch counts, and the duration of season. Athletes should also be asked whether they play on more than one team. In baseball, the position associated with greatest risk for overuse injury to the elbow is pitcher, followed by catcher, third base, shortstop, and outfield.

Patients with Little League elbow often experience pain in the medial elbow as well as weak or ineffective throws. There is usually no history of specific injury or trauma. Pain occurs with throwing, but in more severe cases, it may persist after throwing or nonthrowing activities such as lifting or grasping.

Physical examination often reveals tenderness over the medial epicondyle and pain with valgus stress. The athlete may also experience pain with resisted wrist flexion and forearm pronation. Ulnar nerve pathology should be ruled out, as should pain or dysfunction in the cervical spine or shoulder. Radiographs commonly show a normal medial epicondylar physis in Little

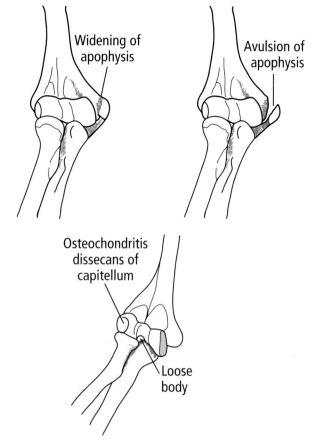

FIGURE 35.10 The spectrum of anatomic injuries associated with Little League elbow.

League elbow; however, subtle widening of the physis or a frank avulsion fracture (pull-off fracture) is not uncommon (**Figure 35.11**). Comparison views should be obtained to determine whether physeal widening is normal or pathologic.

Treatment consists of complete rest from throwing activities. Ice and NSAIDs are effective in the first few weeks for relief of symptoms. Brief immobilization may be required in advanced cases. Physical therapy may help maintain range of motion and strength. Rehabilitation should focus on shoulder, trunk, and lower extremity strengthening as well as the elbow. Abnormalities of training and technique must also be addressed in order to prevent further injury. Throwing may resume only after a repeat clinical evaluation reveals that the symptoms and tenderness have resolved. Demonstration of healing on radiographs is not required. A carefully supervised throwing progression must be undertaken to ensure safe return to play.

Suggestions for prevention of Little League elbow include a preseason strengthening program and a graded return to throwing program that starts 6 to 8 weeks before the first

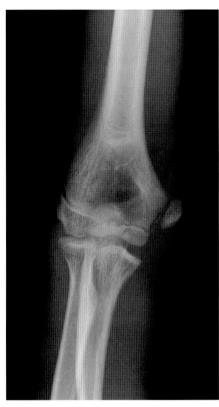

FIGURE 35.11 Radiograph showing avulsion fracture of medial epicondyle apophysis.

practice of the new season. Strengthening exercises should address the rotator cuff as well as the muscles of the hip, trunk, and lower extremity. Any abnormality of technique or mechanics would ideallly be addressed during this time. Athletes should also use the off season to fully rehabilitate any deficits from prior injury.

During the season, baseball pitchers should follow guidelines regarding pitch counts and innings pitched per game and per week. When not pitching, they should be cautious about playing other positions requiring frequent or hard throws, such as catcher, shortstop, or center field. Time spent in both formal practice and backyard play should be closely monitored because these activities can add to the cumulative stress on the elbow. The types of pitches thrown and the mechanics used for throwing can be factors in injury risk. Sidearm deliveries can place extra strain on the elbow and shoulder, so they should be discouraged. Young pitchers should first concentrate on getting the ball in the strike zone (control). This is followed by learning to place pitches in certain parts of the strike zone (command). Next, they can work on increasing speed. While some note that pitch counts are most important, it is generally agreed that pitches with movement (eg, curve balls, sliders) should be reserved for older adolescents and young adults.

Pain or discomfort should be taken seriously. Early diagnosis can lead to more rapid return to play. Persistent symptoms with throwing could indicate serious injury and should be evaluated by a physician.

Ulnar Neuritis

Pathology of the ulnar nerve should be considered in the differential diagnosis of medial elbow pain, especially if there is associated hand weakness or numbness in the ring and small finger. The ulnar nerve can be injured from repetitive traction due to valgus stress on the medial elbow or from the nerve subluxating in the ulnar groove. Medial instability is a risk factor for ulnar neuritis.

Patients with ulnar neuritis may first notice hand clumsiness or cramping. At physical examination, full wrist and elbow flexion reproduces symptoms. Other findings are a weak adductor pollicis muscle, a positive Tinel's sign (reproduction of tingling with percussion in the ulnar groove), and tenderness in the ulnar groove (**Figure 35.12**). Electrodiagnostic studies, including an electromyograph and nerve conduction studies, may be helpful to evaluate more severe or persistent cases of ulnar neuritis.

Conservative treatment consisting of avoiding full elbow flexion, using elbow splints at night, and wearing elastic or neoprene elbow sleeves during activity is usually sufficient. If conservative treatment fails, the athlete may require surgical decompression or anterior transposition of the nerve.

Osteochondritis Dissecans of the Capitellum

Osteochondritis dissecans (OCD) is an injury to subchondral bone and its overlying articular cartilage. It has been described in several characteristic locations, including the distal femur, talar dome of the ankle, and the capitellum of the distal humerus. Capitellar OCD is most common in athletes aged 11 to 16 years who participate in baseball, gymnastics, and football (particularly quarterbacks); these athletes experience chronic valgus stresses to their elbows. The valgus forces exert a compressive force on the lateral elbow, compromising the already tenuous blood supply in that region. The combination of poor blood supply and microtrauma from chronic compression leads to degeneration of subchondral bone. As the injury progresses, the overlying cartilage may become softened, fragmented, or displaced to form loose bodies in the joint.

Clinically, patients manifest an insidious onset of lateral elbow pain with activity that gradually worsens. They may lack full extension of the elbow, and if a loose body has formed, they may experience mechanical symptoms such as locking. Examination will reveal tenderness in the anterolateral aspect

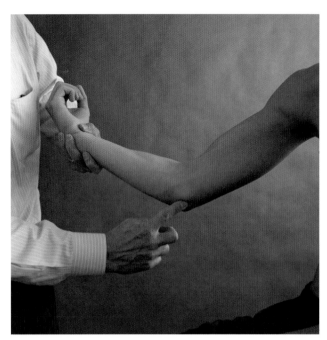

FIGURE 35.12 Eliciting tenderness in the ulnar groove associated with diagnosis of ulnar neuritis.

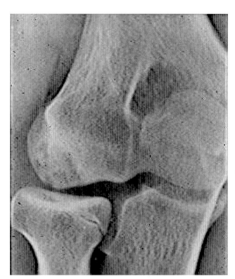

FIGURE 35.13 Radiograph of osteochondritis dissecans (OCD) of the capitellum.

of the elbow as well as mild swelling and restricted joint motion. The radiocapitellar compression test is used to reproduce symptoms and is done by having the patient pronate and supinate the forearm with the elbow in full extension. Radiographs often show lucency or rarefaction of the capitellum, and they may reveal sclerotic bone surrounding the involved area. Early lesions may have no obvious radiographic abnormalities or subtle changes such as radiolucency of the capitellum (**Figure 35.13**). More advanced lesions are associated with joint collapse, joint deformity, or loose bodies. MRI may be used to evaluate the extent of the lesion, the degree of articular surface deformity, and the integrity of overlying structures. Outcomes of OCD lesions are difficult to predict, even with advanced imaging techniques. It is thus difficult to know ahead of time which lesions will progress to collapse, loose body formation, or both. In general, OCD lesions detected before joint collapse or deformity has occurred and lesions diagnosed at earlier stages of skeletal maturation have a better chance of healing with conservative treatment.

Patients with OCD should be referred to an orthopedist or sports medicine specialist early in the clinical course because of variations in outcome and risk of complications. Treatment of early or stable OCD lesions, especially in the skeletally immature athlete, consists of conservative management. This includes strict restriction of throwing or impact activity and early range-of-motion exercises. Ice

and NSAIDs may help relieve symptoms. Serial radiographs or magnetic resonance imaging may be performed to ensure that healing is occurring. Return to play is guided by improvement of symptoms and radiographic evidence of the lesion stabilizing or healing. If symptoms or radiographic findings persist, or if lesions continue to progress during conservative treatment, surgical intervention may be required. Surgical treatment may involve debridement or drilling of the lesion to promote blood supply and healing. Larger osteochondral fragments may be fixed with a pin or compression screw. Smaller loose bodies are removed. For athletes who have permanent joint irregularities after treatment of OCD, activities that place lower demand on the elbow may have to be considered. For baseball pitchers and gymnasts, the compressive stresses on a compromised joint surface will not only limit performance but hasten the development of permanent arthritic changes.

Other Causes of Chronic Lateral Elbow Pain

Lateral epicondylitis (also known as tennis elbow) is an extremely common cause of lateral elbow pain in adults, but it is exceedingly rare in children. Thus, in the child or adolescent with lateral elbow pain, the clinician must rule out the more common diagnoses, such as OCD and Panner disease. Lateral epicondylitis is a tendinopathy of the wrist extensors, especially the extensor carpi radialis brevis, which inserts onto the lateral epicondyle (**Figure 35.14**). It may be encountered in an adolescent athlete who has reached skeletal maturity. Treatment is usually conservative, with only a small percentage requiring surgery.

Nerve entrapments of branches of the radial nerve may occasionally be encountered. They have symptoms similar to those of lateral epicondylitis and are often identified after 6 months of failed conservative treatment for tennis elbow. The posterior interosseus branch of the radial nerve may be entrapped 4-5 cm distal to the lateral epicondyle as it passes through the radial tunnel. Nerve entrapments generally respond to conservative treatment. Surgical exploration and release of the entrapped nerve are rarely necessary.

Olecranon Apophysitis

Athletes who perform repetitive, forceful elbow extensions are at risk for developing an overuse injury to the apophysis of the olecranon. The injury is a result of microtrauma induced by traction applied by the triceps over time, and it is commonly seen in throwing athletes and football linemen. Patients may manifest pain, swelling, and loss of active elbow extension. Examination reveals pain with palpation over the olecranon and with resisted elbow extension. Radiographs may be normal or may show varying degrees of widening at the olecranon physis. Conservative treatment consists of activity modification, ice, NSAIDs, and physical therapy to regain range of motion. Those who do not respond to conservative therapy or who have a physis that does not fuse normally with skeletal maturation may benefit from surgical fixation.

Triceps tendonitis occurs in the skeletally mature athlete. Symptoms are similar to those of olecranon apophysitis. Weight lifters, gymnasts, and divers are at risk for triceps tendonitis as a result of bearing high tensile loads or of absorbing impact with the upper extremity.

Olecranon bursitis can develop with friction or impact over the olecranon process. This may be seen in wrestling or football, or from friction on an armrest in wheelchair athletes. It results in pain and varying degrees of swelling or fluid accumulation superficial to the elbow joint (**Figure 35.15**). Avoiding repeated trauma and using elbow pads hasten recovery, and athletes may continue to play as pain allows. Aspiration of the bursal sac may be advantageous, with tight wrapping of the elbow to minimize the risk of reaccumulation of fluid. Infection of a swollen bursa is a concern, both with and without attempted aspiration.

SUMMARY POINTS

- Evaluating acute and overuse injuries to the elbow requires understanding the anatomic features of the elbow that allow for motion and stability as well as the effects of deficits or related injuries in the shoulder, trunk, hips, or lower extremities.

- The process of skeletal maturation accounts for a complex and evolving pattern of unique injuries and vulnerability to injury in the young athlete.

- Overuse injuries to the elbow are typically the result of poor training or technique. Identifying and correcting these are essential to effective treatment and prevention of reinjury.

- Rehabilitation of elbow injuries requires correcting the deficits of motion, strength, and stability that result from injury as well as the deficits that may have contributed to the injury.

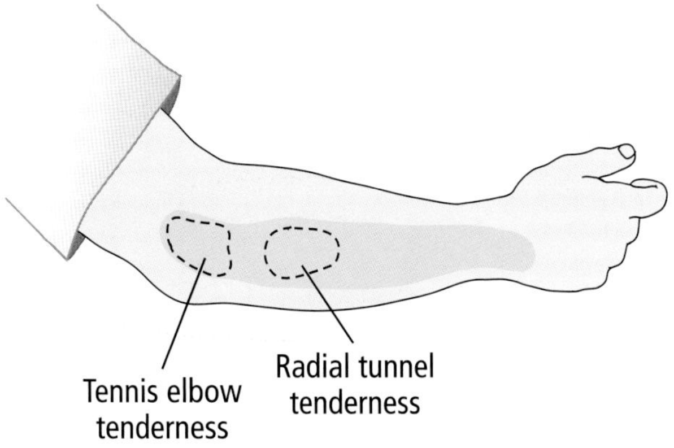

FIGURE 35.14 Location of pain and tenderness with lateral epicondylitis and radial tunnel syndrome.

Tennis elbow tenderness

Radial tunnel tenderness

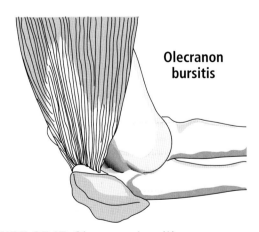

Olecranon bursitis

FIGURE 35.15 Olecranon bursitis.

SUGGESTED READING

Cain EL, Dugas JR, Wolf RS, Andrews JR. Elbow injuries in throwing athletes: a current concepts review. *Am J Sports Med.* 2003;31:621-635.

Congeni JA. Treating—and preventing—Little League elbow. *Phys Sports Med.* 1994;22:54-64.

Mehta JA, Bain GI. Elbow dislocations in adults and children. *Clin Sports Med.* 2004;23:609-627.

Pring ME, Rang M, Wenger DR. Elbow—distal humerus. In: Wenger DR, Pring ME, eds. *Rang's Children's Fractures.* 3rd ed. Philadelphia, PA: Lippincott Williams & Wilkins; 2006: chap 8, p 95.

Pring ME, Wenger DR, Rang M. Elbow—proximal radius and ulna. In: Wenger DR, Pring ME, eds. *Rang's Children's Fractures.* 3rd ed. Philadelphia, PA: Lippincott Williams & Wilkins; 2006: chap 9.

Protecting young pitching arms: the Little League pitch count regulation guide for parents, coaches, and league officials. January 2007. http://www.littleleague.org/media/Pitch_Count_Resource_Page.asp. Accessed July 20, 2008.

Rudzki JR, Paletta GA. Juvenile and adolescent elbow injuries in sports. *Clin Sports Med.* 2004;23:581-608.

Safran MR. Ulnar collateral ligament injury in the overhead athlete: diagnosis and treatment. *Clin Sports Med.* 2004;23:643-663.

Skaggs D, Pershaud J. Pediatric elbow trauma. *Pediatr Emerg Care.* 1997;13:425-434.

Townsend DJ, Bassett GS. Common elbow fractures in children. *Am Fam Physician.* 1996;53:2031-2041.

Walter KD, Congeni JA. Don't let Little League shoulder or elbow sideline your patient permanently. *Contemp Pediatr.* 2004;21:69-88.

CHAPTER 36

Acute Shoulder Injuries in the Young Athlete

Paul R. Stricker, MD

valuating and treating shoulder injuries requires a good understanding of shoulder anatomy and biomechanics. Due to the shallow bony socket of the glenohumeral joint and the flexible, accommodating soft tissue support structures, the shoulder maximizes mobility at the cost of joint stability. Balancing mobility with stability is an ongoing challenge for athletes attempting to balance performance requirements with injury risk.

ANATOMY

The shoulder joint is a complex of 4 joints: the glenohumeral (GH), the acromioclavicular (AC), the sternoclavicular (SC), and the scapulothoracic joints. The GH joint is the articulation of the humeral head onto the glenoid, which is part of the scapula.

The architecture of the GH joint offers little bony stability. The articular surface of the glenoid maintains contact with about a third of the surface area of the humeral head. The glenoid sits at about 20° to 35° of anteversion from the sagittal plane, allowing the humeral head freedom to move anteriorly without bony resistance. This anterior migration is common in athletes with extra laxity or instability.

The shoulder includes both static and dynamic stabilizers. Static stabilizers include the glenohumeral ligaments, glenoid labrum, and concavity of the glenoid fossa. Dynamic stabilizers involve primarily the rotator cuff but include contributions from the biceps, deltoid, and scapular stabilizing musculature. Because of the low degree of bony stability in the GH joint, the dynamic stabilizers play an

important role in maintaining joint congruity of the shoulder.

Bony Anatomy

The humerus, clavicle, and scapula—including the glenoid fossa—comprise the key bony structures of the shoulder. The humerus articulates with the glenoid. Rotator cuff tendons attach to the humeral head in an inverted horseshoe fashion, with the supraspinatus tendon attaching to the greater tuberosity. The proximal humerus growth plate (physis) is distal to the rotator cuff attachment and is vulnerable to injury in skeletally immature patients. The scapula contains the glenoid fossa, which articulates with thehumeral head. The coracoid process is the site for the attachment of the pectoralis minor and the short headof the biceps, and the acromion articulates with the distal clavicle to form the AC joint. The clavicle articulates with the sternum at the SC joint and the acromion at the AC joint.

Muscles and Tendons

Musculotendinous structures of the shoulder include the deltoid and trapezius, which function to elevate and abduct the upper extremity. There are 4 rotator cuff muscles of which the supraspinatus assists in abduction with the arm in slight forward flexion. The infraspinatus and teres minor aid in external rotation of the humerus. The subscapularis functions in internal rotation of the humerus along with the pectoralis major. The rhomboids and serratus anterior help stabilize the scapula against the thoracic wall and control scapular rotation. The long head of the biceps lies in the anterior groove of the humeral head and fuses intra-articularly with the superior portion of the glenoid labrum. The short head of

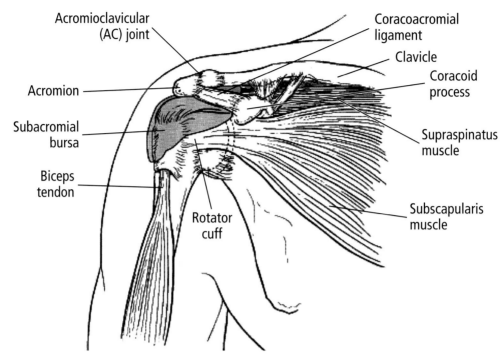

FIGURE 36.1 Anatomic features of the shoulder (anterior view).

the biceps attaches to the coracoid process of the scapula. The biceps acts to flex the elbow and supinate the forearm and aids with forward flexion of the arm. Anatomic features of the shoulder are shown in **Figure 36.1.**

Ligaments

Static stabilizers include the fibrous capsular ligaments and the glenoid labrum. The slinglike inferior GH ligament provides an important source of static stability. The labrum is a fibrocartilage ring that sits on the periphery of the glenoid. The labrum increases the contact surface with the humeral head and provides joint stability. Coracoclavicular ligaments and coracoacromial ligaments help anchor the clavicle to the scapula.

HISTORY

Understanding the mechanism of injury is crucial in evaluating acute problems in the shoulder. When the shoulder is in an adducted position, the joint is relatively stable. Injuries in this position most commonly result in fractures of the clavicle, sprains of the AC joint, or sprains of the SC joint. The shoulder is least stable when it is abducted and externally rotated. Injuries that occur in this position are more likely to result in subluxation or dislocation of the glenohumeral joint or injuries to the soft tissue structures that afford stability to the shoulder.

Pain, swelling, or deformity over the AC joint, SC joint, or clavicle suggests injury to one of those structures. With subluxations or dislocations, the pain tends to be less well localized. Shoulder pain that is posterior or pain that radiates proximally or distally from the shoulder should raise concern about a referred problem from the cervical spine.

In addition to the mechanism of injury and location of pain, the patient should be asked about mobility, strength, and stability in the joint. A history of prior injuries and problems in the cervical spine should also be elicited. The patient's activities, training regimen, and handedness are also important in assessing disability and planning treatment.

PHYSICAL EXAMINATION

The physical examination should commence with an inspection of the injured shoulder, including a comparison with the uninjured shoulder. The SC and AC joints should be visualized as well as the clavicle, position of the humeral head, and scapula. Evaluation should include an assessment for swelling, deformity, and muscle development. Key anatomic structures should be palpated, including the SC joint, clavicle, AC joint, humeral head, anterior joint line, posterior joint line, and biceps tendon.

Active and passive range of motion should be tested while observing for restricted or asymmetric motion, pain inhibition, and substitution patterns. Patients who have had recent subluxations or dislocations may exhibit pain or apprehension with abduction and external rotation. Stability of the glenohumeral joint can be assessed by grasping the humeral head and translating the joint anteriorly, posteriorly, and inferiorly (**Figure 36.2**). Traumatic instability typically results in instability that is most pronounced in one direction—usually anteriorly. With multidirectional instability or constitutional laxity, there is instability in all directions and usually a similar degree of laxity on the asymptomatic shoulder. Patients with multidirectional instability may also have a positive sulcus sign whereby the joint can be readily subluxed inferiorly as well as anteriorly and posteriorly (**Figure 36.3**). Tenderness and range of motion in the cervical spine should be evaluated as well as the presence of referred pain to the shoulder or upper extremity associated with cervical motion.

The neurovascular examination of acute shoulder injuries should include pulses and skin temperature in the upper extremity as well as sensation and strength in the upper extremity. Pain or restricted joint motion may limit the ability to properly evaluate strength in all muscle groups of the shoulder. The examination may need to be modified or repeated to test muscles in a less painful position or test muscles once pain has subsided. When a cervical nerve root or brachial plexus injury is suspected, it is usually possible to

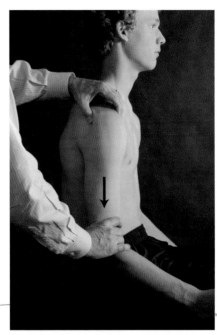

FIGURE 36.3 Eliciting sulcus sign to test for inferior laxity.

test representative muscles for each neurologic level by evaluating muscles of the forearm, wrist, and hand.

Selected provocative tests are also available for assessing acute shoulder injuries. However, pain and guarding may require deferment of these tests in the acute setting. The apprehension test and relocation test both assess symptomatic anterior instability. When the arm is abducted and externally rotated (**Figure 36.4**), patients with instability may demonstrate pain, guarding, or apprehension and resist further motion. The relocation test involves having patients lie supine and positioning their arm in an abducted and externally rotated position. If there is pain or apprehension secondary to anterior instability, the symptoms can be reduced by the examiner pushing the humeral head posteriorly to "relocate" it in its normal position (**Figure 36.5**).

A click or pop associated with a glenoid labrum tear may be detected by circumducting the arm through an adducted and internally rotated position. The O'Brien maneuver, as described in Chapter 37, can also be used to detect labral injuries.

DIAGNOSTIC IMAGING

Plain radiographs are indicated for acute shoulder injuries associated with bony tenderness, deformity, and restricted joint motion. Radiographs should also be considered for suspected subluxations, dislocations, and suspected physeal

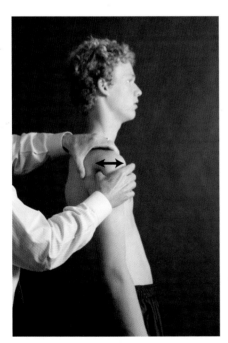

FIGURE 36.2 Load and shift test to evaluate glenohumeral laxity.

injuries. A shoulder series should include an AP view with the shoulder internally rotated and an AP view with the shoulder externally rotated. Additional views, such as a "swimmer's view" or an axillary view, can be added with indication. MR-arthrography is the standard imaging modality for evaluating soft tissue pathology such as the glenoid labrum and rotator cuff.

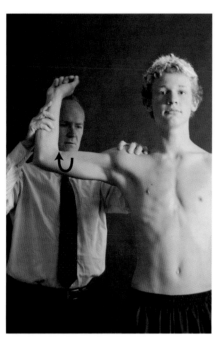

FIGURE 36.4 Apprehension sign. Positive in patients with symptomatic anterior instability.

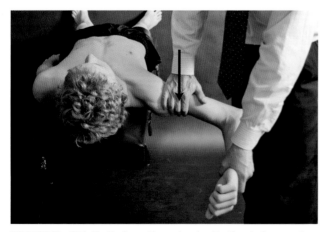

FIGURE 36.5 Relocation test. Patient is supine with arm in abducted, externally rotated position. Posterior reduction relieves pain.

COMMON INJURIES

Sprain of the AC Joint

The AC joint is the junction of the clavicle and the acromion and is stabilized by the AC ligament as well as coracoclavicular (CC) and coracoacromial (CA) ligaments. It is vulnerable to direct trauma, and it is most commonly injured by falling on an adducted shoulder during activities such as biking, snowboarding, and skateboarding, or by a direct blow to the shoulder in sports such as football or ice hockey. If the AC ligament is disrupted, the clavicle will tend to elevate as a result of the pull of the sterno-cleidomastoid muscle. Six different levels of injury to the AC joint have been described; the 3 most common are type I, II, and III AC sprains.

In a type I AC sprain, the AC ligament is partially torn. However, because the coracoclavicular ligament is intact, the clavicle is not elevated. A type II injury disrupts the AC liga-ment and is associated with a partial tear of the coracoclavic-ular ligament. This results in a visible and palpable step off the AC joint and evidence of elevation of the distal clavicle on radiographs. Type III injuries involve complete separation of the acromion and clavicle with complete tearing of the AC and coracoclavicular ligaments. Radiographs show the clavicle elevated above the top of the acromion (**Figure 36.6**). A type IV injury involves a posterior dislocation of the clavicle; a type V injury involves the clavicle being detached from the trapezius and deltoid; and a type VI injury finds the clavicle dislocated inferiorly below the coracoid. **Figure 36.7** illustrates the spectrum of AC injuries.

Examination of the AC sprain reveals pain and swelling at the AC joint. Pain may be reproduced or worsened by having the patient move into positions that load the AC joint, including full abduction overhead, reaching behind the back in internal rotation, and cross-chest adduction. Clavicle fractures need to be considered in the differential diagnosis of AC sprains. Clavicle fractures and AC sprains

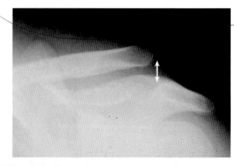

FIGURE 36.6 Radiograph showing the clavicle elevated above the top of the acromion.

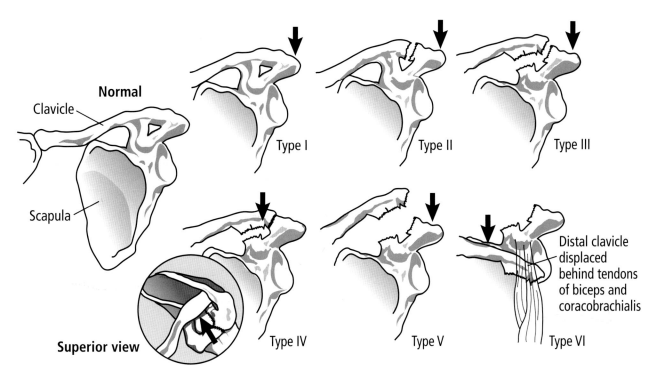

FIGURE 36.7 Spectrum of acromioclavicular injuries. Adapted from Rockwood CA Jr, Williams GR Jr, Young, DC. Disorders of the acromio-clavicular joint. In: Rockwood CA Jr, Matsen FA III. *The Shoulder.* 2nd ed. Philadelphia, PA: WB Saunders; 1998.

have similar mechanisms of injury. With clavicle fractures, the bony tenderness and deformity is over the clavicle. Radiographs may be necessary to differentiate between the 2 injuries. An os acromialis, or accessory ossification center on the lateral portion of the acromial process, may clinically and radiographically be confused with a fracture or AC sprain.

AC joint injuries may be treated conservatively with ice, analgesic medications, and a sling as needed for comfort. Range-of-motion exercises should be commenced as symptoms allow. Strengthening of the surrounding musculature can be carried out in the pain-free range. Overhead lifting or adduction may have to be limited as a result of stress on the AC joint. Length of time for recovery varies according to the severity of injury and the nature and demands of sport activity. Recovery can be as short as a few weeks or as long as a few months. Restoration of full motion and strength in the shoulder should ideally occur before return to play. If the sport is a noncontact one, or if it places minimal demands on the shoulder, it may be possible for the patient to return to play earlier. A protective donut pad can be worn over the AC joint for activities that involve contact or collisions.

Type III injuries are also treated conservatively but may require surgical correction if there is tenting of the skin or neurologic compromise. Type IV, V, and VI injuries typically require surgical intervention with open reduction and internal fixation. If AC arthritis develops as a result of frequent or severe AC sprains, corticosteroid injections or surgical resection of the AC joint may be indicated.

SC Joint Sprains

Injuries to the SC joint are less common than AC sprains. SC sprains can occur when athletes land on an adducted shoulder or other players land on top of them. As the shoulder is compressed, disruption of the SC ligament can occur (**Figures 36.8 and 36.9**). Pain will be located at the proximal end of the clavicle. Injury to the SC ligament may produce swelling, tenderness, and instability at the SC joint. Anteriorly displaced injuries to the SC joint will heal over time with fibrous remodeling. The physis for the proximal clavicle is the last growth plate to fuse. Injuries in this area may actually be Salter-Harris fractures rather than ligament sprains. Fortunately, these fractures do tend to heal and remodel over time.

Posterior displacement of the clavicle can cause compromise of the airway or neurovascular structures. A posteriorly dislocated clavicle becomes wedged behind the sternum. If airway compromise occurs, urgent reduction is necessary. If the clavicle cannot be grasped and reduced manually, a surgically clamp, such as a towel clamp, may be used.

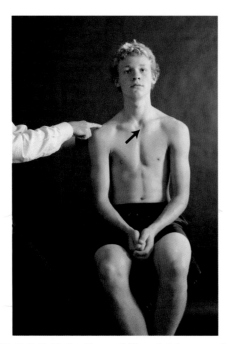

FIGURE 36.8 Palpation of the right acromioclavicular (AC) joint indicating location of tenderness in a patient with a right-sided AC sprain. The arrow indicates where tenderness would be found in a patient who sustained a left sternoclavicular (SC) sprain.

Imaging the SC joint with plain radiography may fail to reveal subtle fractures or displacement. Computed tomography may be necessary to adequately assess the integrity of the joint and rule out fracture. Most SC sprains can be treated nonsurgically. Return to activity is based on resolution of pain and restoration of strength and motion. If the SC joint remains unstable, surgical stabilization may need to be considered before clearance to play can be

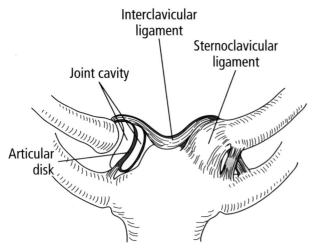

FIGURE 36.9 Sternoclavicular (SC) joint.

granted. If it is not possible to clearly delineate anterior from posterior dislocation based on clinical examination, a CI Scan should be obtained. Patients with a posterior dislocation should be referred to a sugical specialist. If there are signs of respiratory distress after an AC sprain, immediate transfer to an emergency department should take place.

Anterior Dislocation of the Shoulder

Anterior shoulder dislocations occur when the arm is forcefully abducted and externally rotated. Ninety-five percent of all shoulder dislocations are anterior in nature, with the humeral head becoming displaced anterior to the glenoid. The large, slinglike inferior GH ligament is disrupted in anterior dislocations. In most cases, the attachment of the labrum is also torn or separated from the surface of the anterior glenoid, causing what is known as a Bankart lesion (**Figure 36.10**). The presence

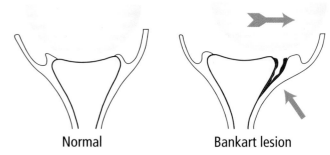

Normal   Bankart lesion

FIGURE 36.10 Bankart lesion secondary to anterior glenohumeral dislocation.

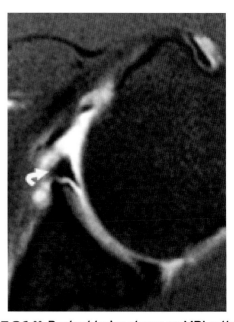

FIGURE 36.11 Bankart lesion shown on MRI-arthrogram of shoulder.

of a Bankart lesion, in association with a glenohumeral subluxation or dislocation, can be confirmed with an MRI-arthrogram of the shoulder (**Figure 36.11**). The disruption of the anterior glenoid labrum contributes to further instability of the GH joint. When the humerus is dislocated anteriorly, the posterior humeral head lies compressed on the anterior rim of the glenoid. This results in a compression fracture that occurs on the posterior-lateral humeral head known as a Hill-Sachs lesion (**Figure 36.12**).

Athletes with glenohumeral dislocations will usually be aware that their shoulder is out of place. At examination, the shoulder is visibly flattened at the deltoid area, with a fullness in the anterior axilla from the dislocated humeral head. Neurovascular status should be checked for wrist pulses, and function of axillary, musculocutaneous, median, ulnar, and radial nerves should be assessed. The axillary nerve provides sensation to the shoulder and motor function to the deltoid muscle. Intact sensation and strength of the deltoid suggests an intact axillary nerve.

Experienced clinicians may be able to reduce a dislocated shoulder on the field unless signs of fracture exist, such as bony tenderness, crepitus, or bony deformity. In skeletally immature patients, a proximal humeral epiphyseal fracture needs to be considered. If reduction attempts are unsuccessful, or if fracture is suspected, the patient should be transported to an emergency facility. Prereduction radiographs should be performed to determine the direction of the dislocation and the presence or absence of fracture (**Figure 36.13**).

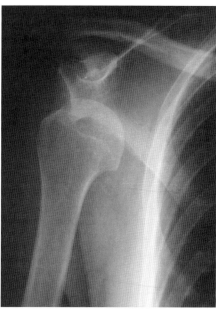

FIGURE 36.13 Radiograph demonstrating anterior-inferior glenohumeral dislocation.

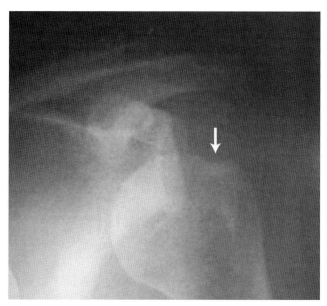

FIGURE 36.12 Hill-Sachs lesion on posterior humeral head secondary to anterior glenohumeral dislocation.

TABLE 36.1	
Methods for Relocating an Anterior Glenohumeral Dislocation	
METHOD	**DESCRIPTION**
Traction-countertraction maneuver (requires 2 people)	One person stabilizes patient's torso with a sheet or towel. The other person applies anterior traction to the arm.
Stimson maneuver	The patient lies prone on an examining table with weights attached to the wrist. The affected arm hangs off the edge of examining table; the weight causes gentle, sustained anterior traction to the arm.
Milch technique	The patient attempts to forward flex the arm while the examiner applies longitudinal traction and external rotation to the humerus.
Hennipen technique	The arm is held at the side with elbow flexed to 90°. The examiner slowly rotates the arm externally.
Scapula manipulation maneuver	The examiner pushes the scapula medially while the arm is longitudinally distracted with slight abduction and forward flexion.

True anteroposterior, axillary, and trans-scapular Y views should be obtained if possible. Multiple relocation techniques have been described, and various methods for relocation of an anterior GH dislocation are listed in **Table 36.1**.

All of the methods for reduction of anterior dislocation involve pulling the arm in the direction of instability. Combining the anterior distraction with forward flexion and internal rotation allows the humerus to slide back over the anterior edge of the glenoid.

Posterior dislocations occur when a person attemps to break a fall by reaching forward with an extended arm and internally rotated humerus. Posterior dislocations are reduced by abducting and externally rotating the arm. Therefore, an anterior dislocation can be treated by moving the shoulder in the position that causes it to move posteriorly, and posterior dislocations can be treated by moving the shoulder in the position that causes it to move anteriorly.

Follow-up radiographs can establish evidence of successful reduction and identify any fractures that were not initially apparent on the prereduction films.

A sling is used for comfort and protection against excessive or painful movement. Strict immobilization with a sling and swath does not decrease the rate of recurrent dislocations. After a period of rest and pain control, treatment involves progressively increasing the range of motion and performing strengthening exercises of the rotator cuff and scapular stabilizing muscles. Because abduction and external rotation are the most vulnerable positions of an unstable shoulder, exercises in these positions are the last to be done. A shoulder harness that restricts abduction and external rotation may provide protection to athletes in sports such as football.

Controversy exists about the surgical versus nonsurgical treatment of a first-time dislocation. Studies show that athletes younger than 20 have a high recurrence rate of dislocation (55%-100%), and these high rates of recurrent dislocations occur even after conservative management. Predictors of recurrence include younger age at the time of the first dislocation and presence of a Bankart lesion. Arthrogram–magnetic resonance imaging is the diagnostic study of choice for identifying a Bankart lesion.

If surgery needs to be performed, controversy exists regarding the optimal procedure. Arthroscopic repair has the advantage of being less invasive, but an open procedure may be more widely available and may be better for achieving long-term stability. Because of the high rate of recurrent dislocations and the limited success of nonsurgical treatment, surgical consultation should be considered for first-time or recurrent anterior shoulder dislocations.

Acute Labral Tear

The fibrocartilage labrum is at risk for tearing during an anterior dislocation of the shoulder. Because this markedly affects the stability of the GH joint, surgical treatment of anterior dislocations involves reattachment of the labrum to the glenoid. In children and adolescents, shoulder dislocation is the most common reason for an acute tear of the labrum. Acute biceps contractions can also tear the labrum at the biceps attachment, causing a SLAP (superior labrum, anterior-to-posterior) lesion (**Figure 36.14**). Labral injuries can also occur in young athletes who perform repetitive or forceful overhead motions, such as baseball pitchers and swimmers. This is discussed in more detail in Chapter 37, Chronic Shoulder Problems in the Young Athlete.

Clavicle Fractures

Clavicle fractures are common in athletic and nonathletic young people. Fractures of the clavicle can occur from either direct or indirect trauma to the shoulder. At examination, a clavicle fracture will often produce a visible bump or deformity. There is tenderness to palpation and pain with active or passive shoulder motion. Neurovascular injury in conjunction with clavicle fracture is rare, but distal pulses and sensation should nonetheless be evaluated.

Fractures occur in the distal, middle, or proximal one-third of the clavicle, with 80% to 85% occurring in the middle one-third. Distal one-third fractures are the

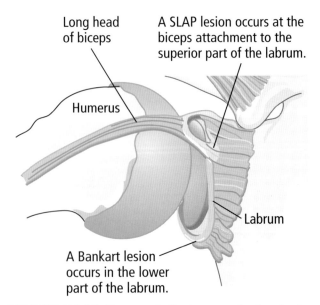

Long head of biceps

A SLAP lesion occurs at the biceps attachment to the superior part of the labrum.

Humerus

Labrum

A Bankart lesion occurs in the lower part of the labrum.

FIGURE 36.14 Tear and displacement of anterior-inferior glenoid labrum (SLAP lession) and anterior inferior glenoid labrum (Bankart lesion).

next most common, at 12% to 15%. An anteroposterior x-ray is usually sufficient to visualize most clavicle fractures (**Figure 36.15**). The fracture fragments can be overlapping, angulated, or comminuted. The medial portion of the clavicle is more tubular in its architecture, whereas the distal portion is more flat. The transition between the 2 zones is relatively weak and is the most vulnerable to fracture.

Middle one-third fractures are the most common; in younger children, this usually manifests as a greenstick fracture. Most of these fractures heal well with conservative management. Overlapping fragments have a higher rate of nonunion and may require orthopedic referral if skin tenting is present or separation of fracture fragments jeopardizes healing. Once the fracture has stabilized, aerobic exercises may be commenced as well as strengthening for the lower extremities and trunk. In general, return to play can take about 5 to 6 weeks for noncontact sports and about 3 to 4 months for contact sports. Noncontact activities that require the use of the upper extremity, such as throwing or swimming, may fall somewhere in between.

Distal one-third fractures are located distal to the coracoclavicular ligaments. These less common fractures can be subdivided into 3 categories: types I, II, and III. A type I fracture of the distal one-third of the clavicle is nondisplaced with intact coracoclavicular ligaments. Such fractures usually require sling immobilization for up to 3 to 6 weeks. Displacement with ruptured coracoclavicular ligaments characterizes a type II fracture. A type III fracture involves the articular surface of the AC joint and may be confused with an AC separation. These latter 2 fractures require treatment with a sling and orthopedic referral because they may need surgical correction.

Nondisplaced or greenstick middle clavicle fractures do not require radiographs at each visit. However, when the

patient has regained full motion and strength, a radiograph can confirm bony healing. With displaced or comminuted fractures, delayed bony healing may be evident on radiographs. With fibrous union, the bone may be sufficiently strong to resume low-demand activities. Full bony union is optimal before contact or collision sports can be resumed.

Other Fractures

Scapula High-velocity, direct trauma to the scapula can cause a scapular fracture. If a suspected fracture is not clearly defined by plain radiographs, computed tomography may be indicated. Scapular fractures are rarely displaced. Treatment with rest or in a sling is usually sufficient to allow healing. Restriction from vigorous upper extremity movement and contact sports may be necessary for up to 3 months.

Fracture involving the acromion is also uncommon. In many cases in children, an unfused apophysis of the acromion (os acromiale) is mistaken for a fracture. Glenoid fractures occur with dislocation of the humeral head as it moves off the glenoid. Surgical treatment is usually necessary because of the disruption of the joint articular surface.

Proximal Humerus Abrupt, forceful contraction of the supraspinatus, such as landing with the arm extended, can cause an avulsion fracture of the greater tuberosity of the humeral head. Displacement of more than 1 cm may require reduction and surgical fixation of the displaced fragment. If there is persistent rotator cuff weakness after the fracture has healed, a magnetic resonance imaging arthrogram should be obtained to identify a tear of the supraspinatus tendon. Overall, isolated tears of the rotator cuff are extremely rare in children. Nondisplaced avulsion fractures require sling immobilization for 3 to 4 weeks, followed by range-of-motion and rotator cuff strengthening exercises.

In skeletally immature patients, fracture through the physis can occur and can be mistaken for a dislocation. Nonphyseal fractures of the proximal humerus are uncommon in children. Fractures of the metaphyseal region usually occur between ages 5 and 10 years and usually heal unless there is significant angulation or gross displacement.

Nerve Injuries

Neurologic symptoms in the upper extremity can come from an injury to the cervical spine, brachial plexus, or peripheral nerve. Numbness or tingling in the shoulder girdle after a cervical injury or in association with cervical pain may be due to a cervical disk herniation. A burner or stinger is a brachial plexus injury due to either stretch or compression of the plexus or cervical nerve root. Immediately after a

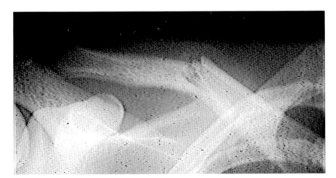

FIGURE 36.15 Fracture of central third of right clavicle.

stinger, athletes may hold their affected arm motionless at their side as they come off the field; this is a characteristic posture for this injury. Examination of the upper extremity reveals paresthesias and weakness that commonly affects nerves in the upper trunk of the brachial plexus. Long-standing nerve injuries may produce visible atrophy. The severity of deficit varies with the injury, but return to play is allowed only after strength and range of motion have been fully restored.

Shoulder dislocations are the most common source of axillary nerve injuries. Examination may reveal loss of sensation to the lateral deltoid as well as deltoid weakness. Suprascapular nerve injuries can occur from blunt trauma, fractures, or a synovial cyst in the suprascapular notch. If the injury or cyst is at the suprascapular notch, both the supraspinatus and infraspinatus muscles will be affected. An injury at the spinoglenoid notch can cause weakness and atrophy of the infraspinatus. Magnetic resonance imaging can help locate the cyst, and electromyography can be helpful for assessing the extent of and prognosis for nerve function.

Winging of the scapula can indicate injury to the long thoracic nerve. Injury to the long thoracic nerve can occur with direct trauma, but such injury has also been seen with heavy strength training. Weakness of the serratus anterior accounts for the scapular winging whereby the abducted scapula fails to lie flat against the thorax. Electromyography can be helpful in assessing the severity of nerve injury and prognosis. Physical therapy can help patients regain strength of the serratus anterior, but shoulder exercises may be ineffective or even harmful until the nerve has shown signs of recovery.

SUMMARY POINTS

- The bony architecture of the shoulder allows for a wide range of joint motion but makes the shoulder inherently unstable and vulnerable to subluxations and dislocations.

- When the arm is adducted, the shoulder is more stable. In this position, injuries are more likely to affect the clavicle or AC and SC joints and are less likely to cause subluxation or dislocation.

- Clavicle fractures are most commonly located in the middle third of the clavicle and typically heal well with nonsurgical treatment.

- AC separations occur most frequently from a fall directly onto the shoulder with the arm in an adducted position. Nonsurgical treatment is usually effective in restoring full motion, strength, and function even though there may be a residual bump at the site of injury.

- When the arm is abducted and externally rotated, there is a greater risk of subluxation or dislocation. Most dislocations occur anteriorly and cause injury to the glenoid labrum and GH ligaments. Injury to these structures contributes to further problems with instability.

- There is a high rate of recurrent dislocations in athletes younger than 20 involved in contact, collision, or overhead sports. Surgical stabilization may need to be considered earlier in athletes who participate in high-risk activities, or who have failed to improve with nonsurgical care.

- Traction or compression injuries to the brachial plexus occur with contact trauma, causing burners and stingers. Any neurologic findings in the shoulder or arm should also prompt an evaluation of the cervical spine and an examination of the peripheral nerves that supply the symptomatic area.

SUGGESTED READING

Andrews J, Carson W Jr, McLeod W. Glenoid labral tears related to the long head of the biceps. *Am J Sports Med.* 1985;13:337-341.

Bottoni C, Wilckens J, DeBerardino T, et al. A prospective randomized evaluation of arthroscopic stabilization versus nonoperative treatment in patients with acute traumatic first-time shoulder dislocation. *Am J Sports Med.* 2002;30:576-580.

DeBerardino T, Arciero R, Taylor D, et al. Prospective evaluation of arthroscopic stabilization of acute, initial anterior shoulder dislocations in young athletes: two to five year follow-up. *Am J Sports Med.* 2001;29:586-592.

Good C, MacGillivray J. Traumatic shoulder dislocation in the adolescent athlete: advances in surgical treatment. *Curr Opin Pediatr.* 2005;17:25-29.

Housner J, Kuhn J. Clavicle fractures. *Physician Sportsmed.* 2003;31:30-36.

Hovelius L, Augustini B, Fredin H, et al. Primary anterior dislocation of the shoulder in young patients: a ten-year prospective study. *J Bone Joint Surg Am.* 1996;78:1677-1684. O'Connell P, Nuber G, Mileski R, et al. The contribution of the glenohumeral ligaments to anterior stability of the shoulder joint. *Am J Sports Med.* 1990;18:579-584.

Paterson P, Waters P. Shoulder injuries in the childhood athlete. *Clin Sports Med.* 2000;19:681-692.

Post M. Current concepts in the treatment of fractures of the clavicle. *Clin Orthop.* 1989;245:89-101.

Saha A. Dynamic stability of the glenohumeral joint. *Acta Orthop Scand.* 1971;42:491-505.

Stetson W, Templin K. The crank test, the O'Brien test, and routine magnetic resonance imaging scans in the diagnosis of labral tears. *Am J Sports Med.* 2002;30:806-809.

CHAPTER 37

Chronic Shoulder Problems in the Young Athlete

Paul R. Stricker, MD

Understanding the functional anatomy of the shoulder, including the balance between mobility and stability, is critical when evaluating the young athlete with an overuse shoulder problem. A high degree of shoulder joint mobility is required to perform many sports activities. Shoulder motion is controlled by ligaments, joint cartilage, and the function of the rotator cuff and scapular stabilizers. If control of shoulder motion or stability is compromised, abnormal mechanics combined with repetitive overhead activity can lead to shoulder injury. The symptoms of overuse often occur over time, which can make awareness of the injury and recognition of the causes of injury more difficult. Common scenarios leading to overuse injuries include commencing a new or unfamiliar exercise program that involves the upper extremity; adding additional weight or resistance to exercises involving the shoulder; increasing intensity, duration, or frequency of an activity that uses the upper extremity such as throwing, swimming, racquet sports, or volleyball; changing or modifying the technique for a repetitive activity that uses the shoulder; using equipment, such as hand paddles in swimming, that places additional stress on the shoulder; or sustaining an injury to the lower extremity, hip, or spine, producing weakness or restrictions that result in additional stress to the shoulder.

The motion and stability of the shoulder are influenced by a balance of bony architecture, glenohumeral (GH) ligaments, the glenoid labrum, and muscles of the rotator cuff and scapular stabilizers. The GH joint is extremely mobile, with the larger humeral head resting on the smaller glenoid. The fibrocartilage ring of the glenoid labrum increases the surface area of contact with the humeral head in order to enhance the static stability afforded by the large surrounding ligaments that make up the shoulder capsule. Because these static stabilizers cannot keep the shoulder completely stable, additional stability is provided by the dynamic stabilizers of the rotator cuff and muscles that control the scapula. The muscles of the rotator cuff attach to the scapula (**Figure 37.1**). The muscles that stabilize the scapula are essential to the function of the rotator cuff. The scapular stabilizers also control rotation of the scapula and are necessary to retract the acromion to allow humeral head clearance with overhead activity. If the scapular movement is dysfunctional, GH motion may be impaired. If the GH ligaments are too tight or too loose, GH motion is also affected. Imbalance or weakness of the rotator cuff muscles and scapular stabilizers also affects GH motion and may contribute to narrowing or impingement in the subacromial space. Some of the anatomic factors contributing to overuse injuries of the shoulder are shown in **Table 37.1**.

Arm strength and the power generated from the shoulder greatly rely on trunk strength as well as the strength of the muscles of the hip and lower extremity. The pelvis is the foundation from which the torso can move. The lower extremity and hips generate forces that travel through the trunk to the shoulder. If these forces are not properly harnessed, the power output through the upper extremity will be diminished. The scapular stabilizing muscles and rotator cuff work in a coordinated manner to

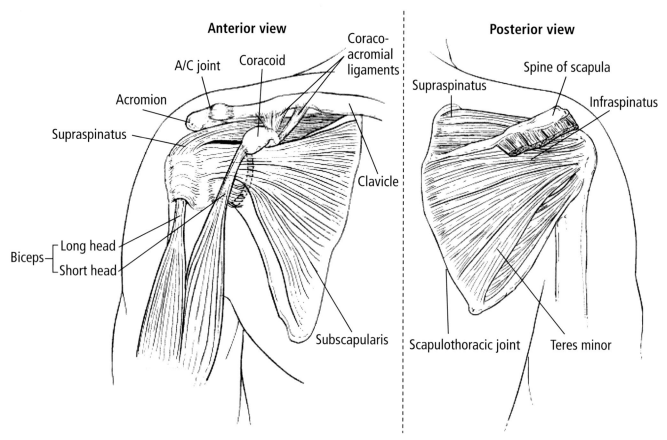

FIGURE 37.1 Anterior and posterior views of shoulder demonstrating rotator cuff muscles.

TABLE 37.1

**Anatomic and Biomechanical Factors
Contributing to Overuse Injuries of the Shoulder**

• Glenohumeral instability

• Dysfunctional scapular motion

• Weakness of scapular stabilizers

• Weakness/imbalance of rotator cuff musculature

• Glenoid labrum abnormalities

• Forward positioned acromial process

• Forward shoulder posture

• Weakness/dysfunction in leg, hips, and/or trunk

• Abnormalities in technique with overhead activity

maintain the humeral head on the glenoid fossa during movement of the upper extremity. When these smaller and weaker muscles are called on to generate greater forces, the additional stresses can cause shoulder injury.

A slumped or forward shoulder posture can contribute to injury. Overdevelopment of anterior chest wall musculature or underdevelopment of posterior musculature contributes to slumped posture. The associated weakness of the scapular stabilizers and the anterior positioning of the acromial process cause subacromial impingement. Impingement causes inflammation and swelling of the subacromial bursa and compression on the supraspinatus tendon. The resulting pain and weakness cause further muscle imbalance, further disruption of shoulder mechanics, and further impingement.

The technique used to perform repetitive overhead activities, such as throwing or swimming, can also play a significant role in overuse injuries to the shoulder. Common technique flaws that place improper forces on the shoulder include overhead throwing without rotating the trunk, breathing on only one side in swimming, and inadequate follow-through in tennis. Proper identification and correction of abnormalities in technique are crucial for effective treatment of shoulder injuries.

CHRONIC SHOULDER PROBLEMS IN THE YOUNG ATHLETE

EVALUATION

History

The history provides information that helps formulate the diagnosis of an overuse injury or chronic shoulder pain. It is necessary to find out what hurts, where and when it hurts, and what the main symptoms are. For any shoulder pain, it is critical to determine whether there are any radicular symptoms coming from a possible disk problem in the neck, such as pain with numbness and tingling down to the hand. Pain caused by an underlying cervical spine problem often manifests as posterior shoulder pain early on, especially with referred trigger point pain in the trapezius. In general, problems originating in the shoulder usually manifest with anterior or lateral shoulder pain. With occasional exceptions, when pain presents in the posterior aspect of the shoulder—especially around the scapula or trapezius— a source in the cervical spine should be considered.

The questions listed in **Table 37.2** can help sort out the cause of shoulder pain and identify factors that need to be addressed in the treatment.

TABLE 37.2

Questions to Ask While Taking a History for Overuse Injury or Chronic Shoulder Pain

- How would you describe the pain and its location?
- Does the pain involve the dominant arm, the nondominant arm, or both?
- How much does the pain interfere with your sport?
- Does it hurt just after the activity, during activity, or all the time?
- What is your current exercise regimen?
- Have you recently changed your exercise program?
- Have you changed your technique for your sport?
- Are you engaging in multiple sports using the shoulder?
- Are you participating on several teams for the same sport?
- What activities exacerbate the pain? What things make it better?
- Does the pain interfere with daily activities or sleep?
- Have you had previous shoulder pain, fractures, dislocations, or surgery?
- Have you had previous medical consultations or diagnostic tests on your shoulder pain? If so, what were the results?
- Have you had this problem before?
- What previous treatments have been tried, and which ones helped?
- Have you used medication to treat your shoulder?
- Have you tried physical therapy for your shoulder?

Physical Examination

The examination of the shoulder should include an assessment for pain, weakness, restricted mobility, or dysfunction in the lower extremities and spine. Limitations in any of these areas can affect shoulder motion or strength. With cervical spine disorders, there may be pain, paresthesias, or weakness directly referred to the shoulder.

Inspection of the shoulder and trunk may reveal postural abnormalities, including thoracic kyphosis, as well as muscle asymmetry or atrophy (see Figure 37.7 later in this chapter). Many of the structures involved with injury may not be directly palpable. However, it is possible to palpate the acromioclavicular (AC) joint, the sternoclavicular joint, the greater tuberosity of the humerus, the biceps tendon, and the anterior joint line.

Active and passive range of motion should be assessed and compared between the symptomatic and asymptomatic shoulders. Forward flexion as well as internal and external rotation are particularly important motions functionally. During the evaluation of passive motion, impingement signs may be elicited. The Neer impingement sign involves the athlete passively flexing the shoulder while the clinician observes for restricted motion or reproduction of pain (**Figure 37.2**). The Hawkins maneuver involves flexing the elbow to 90°, forward

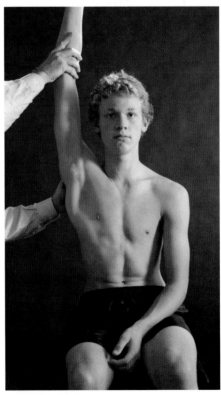

FIGURE 37.2 Neer impingement test.

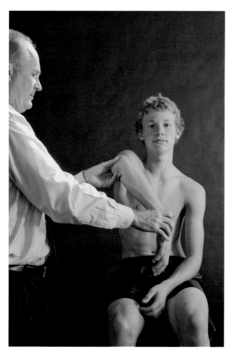

FIGURE 37.3 Hawkins maneuver for evaluation of subacromial impingement.

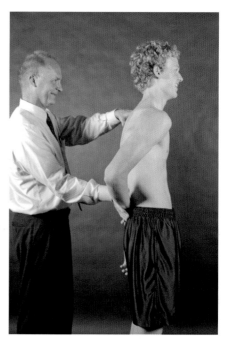

FIGURE 37.5 Strength testing of internal rotators with push-back test.

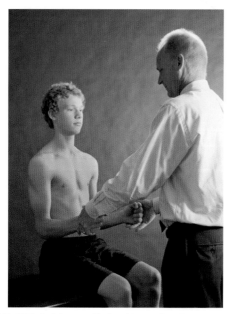

FIGURE 37.4 Strength testing of external rotators.

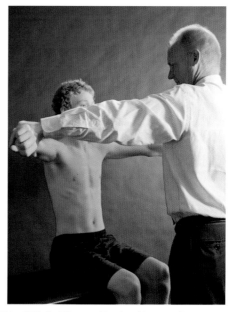

FIGURE 37.6 Strength testing of supraspinatus with hands in "empty-can" position.

flexing the arm to 90°, and internally rotating the arm (**Figure 37.3**). This test may reproduce shoulder pain if there is inflammation in the subacromial space.

Strength testing includes the rotator cuff, biceps, deltoid, and trapezius. Rotator cuff testing includes resistance to internal and external rotation and elevation in the scapular plane for asssessing the suspraspinatus

(**Figures 37.4, 37.5, and 37.6**). The optimal position for testing the supraspinatus requires the straightened arm to be at 90° of abduction and approximately 30° of forward flexion. The forearm is pronated and the thumb points downward as if emptying an imaginary can. Neurologic testing checks for deep tendon reflexes, sensation, and strength of the upper extremity, including testing the strength of muscles that represent each cervical nerve root level.

Shoulder joint instability can be assessed by passively translating the humerus anteriorly and posteriorly. Increased anterior laxity in the symptomatic shoulder may indicate prior subluxation or dislocation. However, some patients have multidirectional instability (MDI) in which both shoulders have increased laxity in all planes of motion. This can be evaluated with a sulcus test, in which the arm is pulled inferiorly. If a dimple appears below the acromion, MDI is present. Symptomatic anterior instability may produce a positive apprehension sign. With this test, a patient's arm is abducted and externally rotated. If the arm is further rotated externally, the patient may guard or express apprehension with a positive test. The relocation test may also be positive in patients with anterior instability. With this test, the patient lies supine while the arm is abducted and externally rotated. During external rotation, the arm and humeral head are gently pulled forward toward the examiner. If this causes apprehension or pain, then the maneuver is repeated with a posterior force on the humeral head. If this relieves the pain and apprehension, then it is positive for anterior instability (symptomatic laxity).

SECONDARY IMPINGEMENT SYNDROME

Older athletes may get primary bony impingement from bone spurs or degenerative changes of the AC joint that narrow the subacromial space and impinge the rotator cuff. In contrast, young athletes are less likely to have bone spurs or degenerative changes. However, subacromial impingement can occur from the upward migration of the humeral head that occurs from relative instability of the joint and inadequate strength of the rotator cuff muscles responsible for preventing this upward migration. The repetitive compression of structures in the subacromial space eventually results in pain and inflammation in the subacromial bursa and supraspinatus tendon.

The muscle imbalances and asymmetries that contribute to injury may be acquired from uneven use of muscles during sports activity. Many activities such as swimming, throwing, racquet sports, wrestling, and weight lifting disproportionately use the anterior muscles (pectoralis, biceps, anterior deltoid, and subscapularis). The increased use of muscles that internally rotate and adduct the shoulder makes these muscles stronger than the muscles that externally rotate and abduct the shoulder or stabilize the scapula. The imbalance of strength alters the ability of the muscles to center the humeral head on the glenoid fossa during overhead activity. This causes secondary subacromial impingement syndrome and results in

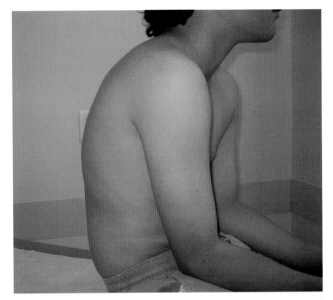

FIGURE 37.7 Lateral view of patient with forward shoulder posture.

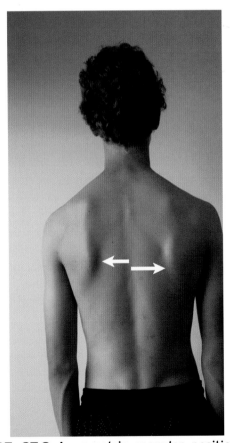

FIGURE 37.8 Asymmetric scapular position with abduction and inferior displacement of the right scapula. Note that the medial border of the right scapula is further from the midline than the left scapula.

inflammation of soft tissues between the humeral head and the coracoacromial arch.

Pain from impingement syndrome usually occurs during the overhead motion and resolves shortly thereafter. With progressive inflammation and tendinopathy, patients may experience pain at rest. Positive findings on physical examination include tenderness at the insertion of the supraspinatus tendon on the greater tubercle. Patients with impingement syndrome may have a slumped shoulder posture (**Figure 37.7**), scapula winging (**Figure 37.8**) or abducted scapula, and pain with impingement maneuvers. Strength testing typically reveals weakness in the external rotators and supraspinatus. The external rotators (infraspinatus and teres minor) function as downward stabilizers of the humerus and counteract the upward pull of the deltoid muscle. Their weakness contributes to the upward migration of the humerus with overhead activity. The supraspinatus may be weak or painful because it is the portion of the rotator cuff that is impinged. Shoulder instability may be seen in association with secondary subacromial impingement syndrome, as can areas of additional inflammation such as the biceps tendon.

Because true bony impingement is unusual in young athletes, radiographs are not routinely necessary. For cases refractory to therapy, or if patients have constant, disabling pain, further evaluation by arthrogram–magnetic resonance imaging (MRI) may be indicated.

Initial treatment involves reducing inflammatory changes in the subacromial space with ice, anti-inflammatory medication, and relative rest. Relative rest involves allowing the athlete to perform nonpainful aspects of their sport to continue to improve skills and maintain strength and aerobic conditioning in a manner that does not cause pain or further injury to the area being treated. Rehabilitation must address not only the training and technique errors that lead to injury but also the underlying muscle imbalances that are present. Typically, this involves strengthening of the external rotators, supraspinatus, and scapular stabilizers, as well as the core muscles (abdomen, lower back, and gluteals). Once the pain and inflammation have subsided, posture and strength deficiencies have been corrected, and the technique and training errors have been addressed, the athlete can gradually resume full activity.

GLENOID LABRUM INJURIES

Instability of the GH joint, coupled with inadequate muscle control, can permit increased anterior migration of the shoulder and encroachment on the anterior portion of the glenoid labrum. In addition, repetitive traction of the long head of

the biceps on the superior portion of the labrum can result in tearing or detachment of the labrum. Symptoms of possible labral pathology include painful popping in the shoulder, a catching sensation, or a sense of the shoulder being out of place. Examination findings include symptomatic laxity of the shoulder along with positive labral entrapment tests. Passive adduction or internal rotation of the shoulder may produce a painful clunk in patients with a torn labrum. Other techniques that may increase suspicion for a labral tear include pain during resistance of straight-arm forward flexion with the forearm supinated. Passively rotating the humerus and compressing the humeral head against the glenoid can elicit pain from patients with a labral tear, much like the grind test for a meniscus tear in the knee. The O'Brien maneuver involves applying resistance to the arm in the empty-can position with the arm slightly adducted (**Figure 37.9**). The test is first performed with the thumb pointing down and is repeated with the thumb pointing up. Pain during the thumb-down position that resolves with the thumb up is a positive test. The resisted supination external rotation test correlates better with a SLAP lesion, which is a superior labral tear that runs anterior to posterior. Suspicion for a labrum tear can be confirmed with an MRI-arthrogram.

Treatment for labrum tears should primarily be aimed at correcting underlying muscle imbalances, using exercises to enhance stability, and addressing any training or technique issues that exist. Often if humeral head motion is well controlled, then labral symptoms may decrease. If conservative management is not successful, surgical correction of an isolated labral tear can be performed

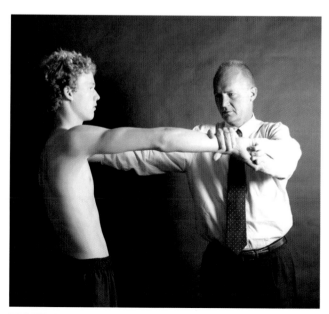

FIGURE 37.9 O'Brien test for glenoid labrum tear.

through the arthroscope. Postoperative rehabilitation is still necessary to address associated muscle and soft tissue abnormalities.

NONTRAUMATIC INSTABILITY

Patients with MDI may be asymptomatic, may have symptoms of instability in the shoulder, or may have pain from related conditions such as impingement or labral pathology. Patients with MDI will have a positive sulcus sign. Treatment of symptomatic MDI focuses on strengthening the dynamic stabilizers. Surgical correction is rarely necessary or effective for MDI.

HUMERAL EPIPHYSITIS

Humeral epiphysitis, also known as Little League shoulder, manifests with shoulder pain that is most often associated with throwing. Patients with humeral epiphysitis are typically boys between 11 and 16 years of age. They are usually among the more accomplished and harder throwers. Repetitive torsional stress to the immature proximal humeral physis can cause widening or separation of the epiphysis. The repetitive microtrauma to the physis causes tenderness over the physis and pain or weakness with resisted internal and external rotation.

Anteroposterior radiographs of both shoulders are necessary to compare the proximal humeral physis. The diagnosis is confirmed with widening of the painful physis compared with the uninjured physis (**Figure 37.10**). Widening is most commonly seen toward the lateral portion of the physis.

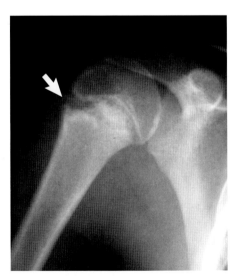

FIGURE 37.10 X-ray showing widening of physis in patient with proximal humeral epiphysitis.

Treatment consists of rest with restriction of throwing. The time frame for rest varies but can be 3 months or longer. Once the bony tenderness has subsided and the patient has regained full motion and strength in the shoulder girdle, he or she may be able to slowly resume full activity. A rehabilitation program for athletes who perform throwing actions must address the shoulder, elbow, trunk, and hip, with progressive return to throwing and attention to proper technique and accumulation of throws.

AC JOINT ARTHRITIS

Repetitive or acute trauma to the AC joint can lead to degenerative arthritis. Repetitive stress from weight lifting, particularly bench press, military press, and even push-ups, can overload the joint and initiate the onset of joint degeneration. Posttraumatic changes from AC sprains can also cause articular surface disruption, instability, and degeneration of the AC joint.

Patients with AC arthritis have AC joint pain that is worse with overhead, behind the back, or across-the-chest movements. Radiographic findings that are the most helpful include narrowing of the AC joint, joint surface irregularity, bone spurs and cystic degenerative changes, or osteolysis of the distal clavicle. Treatment includes modifying activity to reduce painful loading of the AC joint and anti-inflammatory measures. Refractory cases may benefit from corticosteroid injection or even surgical resection of the distal clavicle.

THORACIC OUTLET SYNDROME

Thoracic outlet syndrome generally manifests as nontraumatic shoulder girdle pain that can be associated with radiating pain, numbness or temperature change into the arm or hand. Symptoms are present from the compression of the brachial plexus, subclavian artery, or subclavian vein as they exit the space between the clavicle and the ribs. The thoracic outlet is also bordered by the scalene muscles of the neck. Causes of thoracic outlet narrowing include hypertrophy of the neck muscles, an anatomic cervical rib, or external compression from carrying a backpack. Examination includes the Adson and Wright maneuvers, in which the arm is abducted to horizontal from the side of the body and the examiner's fingers are placed on the wrist pulse. In the Adson maneuver, the head is turned to the affected shoulder while the patient takes a deep breath. This maneuver is then repeated while turning the head away from the affected shoulder (Wright maneuver) (**Figure 37.11**). During these maneuvers, symptoms of pain or numbness may be reproduced, and the examiner may detect a diminished or absent pulse. Conservative management includes stretching the scalene and pectoralis

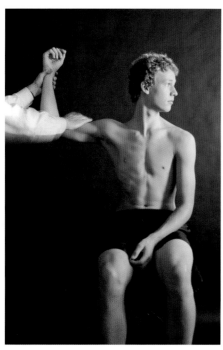

FIGURE 37.11 Wright maneuver for thoracic outlet syndrome. Adson maneurer has patient turn head toward affected shoulder.

muscles and strengthening the inner scapular muscles. Surgical treatment to release the scalenes or resect the first rib is rarely necessary.

SUMMARY POINTS

- The shoulder operates with a delicate balance between mobility and stability. Dysfunction of any of the determinants of shoulder motion or stability can lead to injury. Clinical evaluation must identify the relevant deficits, and rehabilitation must correct the deficits and restore normal integrated function.

- Secondary subacromial impingement syndrome is a common problem in athletes who perform repetitive overhead activities. Imbalances of strength and inadequately controlled motion can lead to impingement of and injury to soft tissues in the subacromial space.

- The lower extremities and trunk are important in generating forces that are transmitted to the shoulder and arm. Injury or weaknesses in these areas can alter shoulder mechanics or place added demands on the shoulder for force production. Therefore, evaluation and treatment of shoulder injuries should address any associated dysfunction in the lower extremity or trunk.

- Shoulder pain can originate from nonshoulder sources such as the cervical spine or thoracic outlet. When shoulder pain is more posterior than anterior, when the pain radiates down the arm, or when there are neurologic symptoms, these other sources should be evaluated.

- Familiarity with common injury mechanisms can serve as the basis for injury prevention programs. If specific patterns of weakness, instability, technique abnormalities, or equipment use predictably lead to injury, correcting these problems in advance may reduce injuries.

SUGGESTED READING

Council on Sports Medicine and Fitness. Overuse injuries, overtraining, and burnout in child and adolescent athletes. *Pediatrics.* 2007;119(6):1242-1245.

Andrews J, Kupferman S, Dillman C. Labral tears in throwing and racquet sports. *Clin Sports Med.* 1991;10:901-911.

Barden J, Balyk R, Raso V, et al. Atypical shoulder muscle activation in multidirectional instability. *Clin Neurophysiol.* 2005;116:1846-1857.

Burkhart S, Morgan C, Kibler W. Shoulder injuries in overhead athletes: the "dead arm" revisited. *Clin Sports Med.* 2000;19:125-158.

Carson W Jr, Gasser S. Little Leaguer's shoulder: a report on 23 cases. *Am J Sports Med.* 1998;26:575-580.

Hawkins R, Kennedy J. Impingement syndrome in athletes. *Am J Sports Med.* 1980;8:151-158.

Kelly B, Kadramas W, Speer K. The manual muscle examination for rotator cuff strength. *Am J Sports Med.* 1996;24:581-588.

Kibler W, McMullen J, Uhl T. Shoulder rehabilitation strategies, guidelines, and practice. *Orthop Clin North Am.* 2001;32:527-538.

Kocher M, Waters P, Micheli L. Upper extremity injuries in the pediatric athlete. *Sports Med.* 2000;30:117-135.

Lyons P, Orwin J. Rotator cuff tendinopathy and subacromial impingement syndrome. *Med Sci Sports Exerc.* 1998;30(suppl):12-17.

Myers T, Zemanovic J, Andrews J. The resisted supination external rotation test: a new test for the diagnosis of superior labral anterior posterior lesions. *Am J Sports Med.* 2005;33:1315-1320.

Nadler S, Sherman A, Malanga G. Sport-specific shoulder injuries. *Phys Med Rehabil Clin N Am.* 2004;15:607-626.

Olsen S, Fleisig G, Dunn S, et al. Risk factors for shoulder and elbow injuries in adolescent baseball pitchers. *Am J Sports Med.* 2006;34:905-912.

Sabick M, Kim Y, Torry M, et al. Biomechanics of the shoulder in youth baseball pitchers: implications for the development of proximal humeral epiphysiolysis and humeral retrotorsion. *Am J Sports Med.* 2005;33:1716-1722.

Stricker P. Swimming: a case-based approach to exercise-induced asthma and rotator cuff tendonitis. *Pediatr Ann.* 1999:29:166-171.

CHAPTER 38

Wrist and Hand Injuries

Amanda Kay Weiss Kelly, MD

Pediatric athletes are at risk for both chronic and acute injuries to the wrist and hand. Acute injures are especially common in contact or collision sports like football, soccer, and skateboarding. Chronic injuries, on the other hand, are seen in sports such as gymnastics, rowing, and racquet sports, where repetitive motion of the wrist and hand are required. An understanding of the anatomy of the wrist and hand and of the elements of a complete history and physical are essential to the accurate diagnosis and proper treatment of these injuries. This chapter reviews the diagnosis, workup, and management of common wrist and hand injuries in the young athlete.

ANATOMY

Bony Anatomy

The bony anatomy of the wrist includes the articulations of the distal radius and ulna with the 8 carpal bones and the carpal bones with the proximal metacarpals (**Figure 38.1**). The radius is, on average, 9 mm longer than the ulna, which is referred to as negative ulnar variance. A positive ulnar variance indicates that the ulna is longer than the radius.

The radius articulates with the scaphoid and lunate, and about 80% of axial load forces to the wrist are absorbed by the radiocarpal joint. The ulna does not articulate directly with the triquetrum and pisiform because the TFCC is interposed between the distal ulna and the carpal bones. The TFCC is composed of a fibrocartilaginous disk (the triangular fibrocartilage), the dorsal and volar radioulnar ligaments, the ulnolunate and ulnotriquetral ligaments, the extensor carpi ulnaris sheath, and the ulnar capsule (**Figure 38.2**). These structures bear 20% of the axial load

forces applied to the wrist. The TFCC also contributes to the stability of the distal radioulnar joint, as do the pronator quadratus and interosseous ligament.

The carpal bones are divided into a proximal row and a distal row. The proximal row consists of the scaphoid, lunate, triquetrum, and pisiform bones. The distal row contains the trapezium, trapezoid capitate, and hamate. The scaphoid bridges the proximal and distal carpal rows (**Figure 38.1**).

The distal row of carpal bones articulates with the metacarpal bases of the hand. The metacarpals articulate with the proximal phalanx of each finger via the metacarpal phalangeal (MCP) joints. Each of the fingers has 3 phalanges with proximal and distal interphalangeal (DIP) joints between them. The thumb has only 2 phalanges with a single interphalangeal joint.

Ligamentous Anatomy

The ligaments of the wrist can be classified as either intrinsic or extrinsic. Intrinsic ligaments originate and insert on the carpals. Extrinsic ligaments join the carpals to the distal radius or metacarpals. The ligaments on the volar aspect of the wrist are thicker than the dorsal ligaments. Each carpal bone is joined to the carpal bones adjacent to it by intrinsic ligaments, except that there is no longitudinal ligament found between the lunate and capitate. Each of the interphalangeal joints of the hand has radial and ulnar collateral ligaments. The collateral ligaments of the proximal interphalangeal (PIP) joint are the most commonly injured hand ligaments.

Muscular Anatomy

The muscles that flex, extend, and radially and ulnarly deviate the wrist originate proximal to the wrist and insert on the metacarpal bases, rather than the carpals, except for the

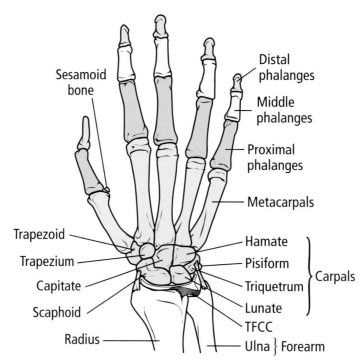

FIGURE 38.1 Bony anatomy of the hand and wrist.

flexor carpi ulnaris (FCU), which inserts on the pisiform. The flexors and extensors of the fingers also originate proximally and insert on the phalanges. The wrist and hand flexors originate from the medial epicondyle as a common tendon. The flexor tendons of the wrist insert on the volar aspect of the metacarpals, and the finger flexors insert on the volar aspect of the phalanges. The flexor digitorum profundus (FDP) tendons, which act to flex the DIP joints, insert on the base of the distal phalanges, and the flexor digitorum superficialis (FDS) tendons, which flex the PIP joints, insert on the bases of the middle phalanges. The FDP and FDS are commonly involved in finger injuries.

The wrist and hand extensor muscles originate as a common tendon from the lateral epicondyle. The extensor tendons of the wrist insert on the dorsal aspect of the metacarpals, and the extensor tendons of the fingers insert on the dorsal aspect of the phalanges. The primary wrist extensors are the extensor carpi radialis longus (ECRL), the extensor carpi radialis brevis (ECRB), and the extensor carpi ulnaris (ECU). The finger extensor muscles include the extensor pollicis longus (EPL) and extensor pollicis brevis (EPB), extensor indicis, extensor digitorum (ED), and extensor digiti minimi (EDM). Each of the wrist extensor tendons attaches at the metacarpal bases, and the finger extensors attach at the bases of the middle and distal phalanges. There are 6 dorsal synovial compartments that divide

the extensor tendons of the wrist and hand (**Figure 38.2**). The extensor tendon groups that most commonly cause problems in athletes are the abductor pollicis longus (APL) and EPB tendons, found in the first compartment, and the ECU, found in the sixth dorsal compartment.

The FCU and ECU act to ulnarly deviate the wrist, and the ECRL and flexor carpi radialis (FCR) radially deviate the wrist.

INNERVATION

Several important nerves cross the wrist to innervate the hand and wrist. The median nerve travels along the volar aspect of the wrist within the carpal tunnel and supplies sensory innervation to the palmar aspect of the thumb, index finger, middle finger, and radial portion of the ring finger, and motor innervation to the thenar muscles and radial 2 lumbricals. The carpal tunnel also contains the FDS, FDP, and flexor pollicis longus (FPL) tendons, which flex the interphalangeal joints of the fingers. The Guyon canal is found ulnar to the carpal tunnel and contains the ulnar artery and ulnar nerve, which supplies sensory innervation to the small finger and ulnar portion of the ring finger and motor innervation to the deep head of the flexor pollicis brevis (FPB) and all of the intrinsic muscles of the hand except the thenar muscles and radial 2 lumbricals. Finally, the superficial radial nerve travels on the dorsal aspect of

Cross section at proximal wrist

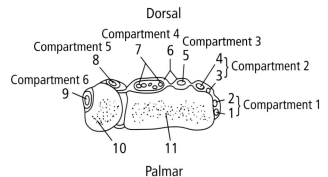

1. Abductor pollicis longus
2. Extensor pollicis brevis
3. Extensor carpi radialis longus
4. Extensor carpi radialis brevis
5. Extensor pollicis longus
6. Extensor retinaculum
7. Extensor digitorum and extensor indicis
8. Extensor digiti minimi
9. Extensor carpi ulnaris
10. Ulna
11. Radius

FIGURE 38.2 Axial view of dorsal compartments of the wrist.

the wrist just superficial to the first dorsal compartment and supplies sensory innervation to the dorsoradial hand and thumb. Motor branches of the radial nerve supply the wrist and finger extensors.

EVALUATION

History

A detailed history of injury can be helpful in making an accurate diagnosis in hand and wrist injuries. A complete history of an acute injury should include a detailed account of the mechanism of injury, including the level and type of impact and the position of the hand and wrist at the time of injury. For overuse injuries, the clinician should identify the sport or activity that resulted in the pain and whether or not any changes in participation occurred before the onset of symptoms. Certain sports, such as rowing and gymnastics, are associated with an increased risk for overuse injury of the hand and wrist. Thus, rowers or gymnasts who have recently increased their level of competitiveness or amount of practice time may be at increased risk for wrist pain. It is also important to ascertain whether the patient can identify a specific site of pain or specific activities or hand motions that exacerbate the pain. In both acute and chronic injuries, the pres-

ence of symptoms such as clicking, popping, or instability should be elicited. Finally, a history of symptoms that might indicate neurologic or vascular disease, including numbness, tingling, weakness, and paresthesias, should be obtained.

Clinical Evaluation

The examination of the hand and wrist should start with inspection for deformity, swelling, bruising, or abrasions. An evaluation of the range of motion of all joints of the wrist and hand in comparison with the unaffected hand and wrist should be performed. A thorough neurovascular examination, including an assessment of motor and sensory capabilities, should be performed in all patients.

Imaging Studies

Most injuries are adequately assessed with posteroanterior, lateral, and oblique radiographs. However, certain injuries warrant other views or special testing, such as magnetic resonance imaging (MRI) or computed tomographic (CT) scan. Consultation with a specialist may be appropriate prior to ordering more detailed imaging studies. A consultation may obviate additional studies, or, when additional studies are indicated, it may ensure that the proper studies are requested.

FRACTURES

Fractures of the hand and wrist are common in young athletes because the hand and wrist are relatively unprotected in most sports. Most wrist and hand fractures cause swelling and pain of the affected area. Neurovascular status should be evaluated in all wrist and hand fractures. Also, evaluation of the elbow is important in all wrist fractures because elbow injuries may accompany distal radius and ulna injuries.

Distal Radius Fracture

Distal radius fractures are among the most common long bone fractures in children. The most common mechanism of injury is the fall onto an outstretched hand (FOOSH).

Physeal fractures are unique to the growing pediatric athlete. The typical patient has a swollen wrist, decreased range of motion, and pain with palpation of the distal radial physis. The Salter-Harris (SH) classification system is most commonly used to define physeal injuries (see Figure 29.3 on page 267). SH I fractures are through the physis without metaphyseal or epiphyseal involvement. Nondisplaced or minimally displaced SH I fractures are often difficult to diagnose, and comparison views of the uninjured wrist may be needed to make the diagnosis. Nondisplaced and minimally displaced SH I fractures can be treated in a short arm cast or splint for 3 or 4 weeks. Significantly displaced SH I fractures (**Figure 38.3**) require reduction and should be referred to a physician who can reduce fractures. If radiographs appear normal but the athlete has a history and physical examination consistent with an SH I fracture, the injury should be treated as a fracture, and repeat radiographs can be obtained in 2 or 3 weeks to look for callus formation, which is increasingly evident as the fracture heals. Growth disturbance due to physeal arrest is more common in displaced than nondisplaced SH I fractures, and long-term follow-up is suggested for displaced SH I fractures.

SH II fractures are through the growth plate and metaphysis. The metaphyseal fragment is often referred to as the *Thurston-Holland fragment.* Nondisplaced SH II fractures can be treated with a short arm cast for 4 to 6 weeks. Displaced SH II fractures may require either closed or open reduction, and patients may require extended follow-up to monitor for physeal arrest. Thus, such patients may warrant referral to a pediatric specialist.

SH III and IV fractures have a much greater risk for growth arrest and should be referred to an orthopedic specialist for management. SH III fractures are through the physis and exit out the epiphysis into the joint space. SH IV fractures are through the metaphysis, physis, and epiphysis. Because SH III and IV fractures are intraarticular, it is important to achieve reduction without significant step-off of the articular surface in order to preserve optimal joint function and avoid long-term arthritis.

SH V fractures are a crush injury to the physis. Like the SH I fracture, there is no metaphyseal or epiphyseal involvement, and diagnosis may be difficult. Comparison views of the uninjured extremity may be useful in aiding diagnosis. SH V fractures should also be referred to a orthopedist for management.

The torus, or buckle, fractures of the distal radius or ulna are also unique to the pediatric athlete. This fracture is a compressive plastic deformation of the bony cortex (**Figure 38.4**). Injury may be caused by a FOOSH or by a direct blow. Athletes typically experience pain and swelling of the affected bone. Torus fractures are usually stable and

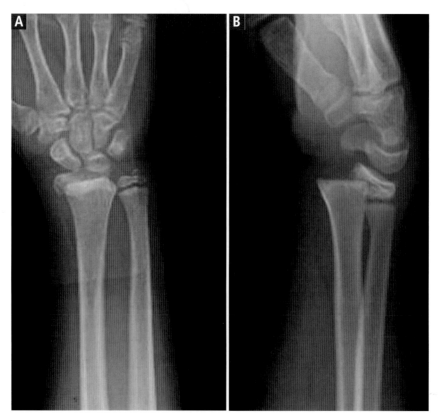

FIGURE 38.3 Dorsally displaced Salter-Harris I distal radius fracture as shown on AP (A) and lateral (B) views.

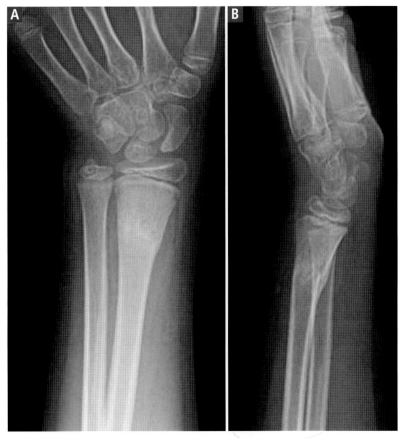

FIGURE 38.4 Metaphyseal buckle fracture of radius as shown on AP (A) and lateral (B) views.

rarely require reduction or open fixation. Primary care physicians can manage these injuries by use of a splint or short-arm cast for 3 or 4 weeks.

Scaphoid Fracture

The scaphoid is the most commonly fractured carpal bone. Scaphoid fractures are also typically caused by FOOSH. Generally, patients experience pain and swelling on the radial side of the wrist, although swelling may be more diffuse. Tenderness with palpation of the snuffbox (**Figure 38.5**) is typically present. The dorsal and volar aspects of the scaphoid may also be tender. A standard wrist radiographic series with dedicated scaphoid views may provide the diagnosis. However, scaphoid fractures are often subtle, and athletes with suspected scaphoid fracture should be treated as though they have a scaphoid fracture until the diagnosis has been ruled out. Repeat radiographs should be performed in 2 to 3 weeks if initial radiographs appear normal. If fracture is still suspected but not visible on plain radiographs at that time, CT or MRI may be used to diagnose occult fracture.

Scaphoid waist fractures, or midbody fractures, are the most common type of scaphoid fracture, followed by proximal third, distal third, and distal tubercle. Nondisplaced scaphoid fractures of the distal pole or waist can be treated conservatively in a short arm thumb spica cast for 6 to 10 weeks, although some physicians advocate use of a long arm cast for the first 2 to 4 weeks of immobilization. Proximal pole or displaced waist fractures, those with more than 1 mm of displacement, or visible step-off on radiograph require surgical consultation for internal fixation. Early surgical intervention for nondisplaced waist fractures may be considered for athletes who do not want to risk additional time off if the fracture fails to heal with conservative treatment.

Nonunion and avascular necrosis of the proximal pole of the scaphoid are both concerns in scaphoid fractures, especially those of the waist and proximal third. The proximal pole of the scaphoid is perfused by retrograde interosseous blood flow from the distal pole that can be disrupted in these types of fracture. Scaphoid fractures may also be associated with injury to the scapholunate ligament. Scapholunate ligament injuries are suspected when widening of

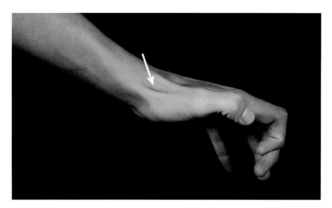

FIGURE 38.5 Snuffbox. The extensor pollicis longus on one side and the abductor pollicis longus and extensor pollicis longus on the other.

the space between scaphoid and lunate (called the *scapholunate interval*) is noted on anteroposterior radiographs. MRI arthrogram can be used to definitively diagnose scapholunate ligament injuries. Suspected ligamentous instability warrants surgical referral.

Hand Fractures

Metacarpal Neck Fracture Metacarpal neck fractures usually occur as a result of direct contact injuries, such as when an athlete falls on or strikes an object with a closed fist (**Figure 38.6**). The athlete will experience swelling and tenderness of the involved metacarpal. Angulation may be palpable during the examination, and the knuckle of the involved metacarpal may be depressed as a result of volar angulation of the fracture. Assessment of rotational deformity can made by assessing the direction of the fingers with the MCP and PIP joints in flexion. All fingers should point in the direction of the scaphoid. If the affected finger deviates, rotational angulation is present (**Figure 38.7**). Also, looking at the fingers on end can be useful in identifying rotational deformity. Posteroanterior, lateral, and oblique radiographs of the hand are used for diagnosis and for further evaluation of rotational and angular deformity.

Rotational deformity of the metacarpal is poorly tolerated. Fractures with rotational deformity require reduction. If closed reduction is unsuccessful, open reduction and internal fixation will be required. The amount of angular deformity that can be tolerated depends on which metacarpal is injured. Usually 10° of angular deformity can be allowed in the second metacarpal, 20° in the third metacarpal, 30° in the fourth metacarpal, and 40° in the fifth metacarpal. Metacarpal neck fractures with an acceptable amount of angular deformity and no rotational deformity can be managed in a cast with the radius slightly extended and the MCP joint in 60° to 70° of flexion for 4 to 6 weeks. If a metacarpal neck fracture involves a physis, there may be greater potential to correct an angular deformity.

Bennett Fracture The Bennett fracture is an intraarticular fracture involving the base of the first metacarpal

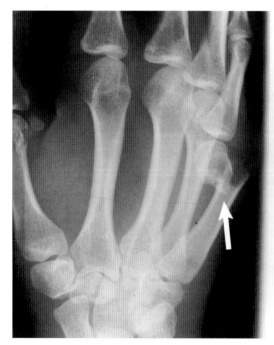
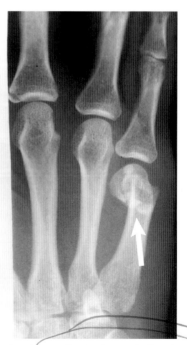

FIGURE 38.6 Fracture of the fifth metacarpal neck, also called a boxer's fracture.

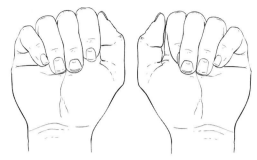

FIGURE 38.7 Diagram showing effects of a left 2nd metacarpal fracture with rotation.

(**Figure 38.8**). The usual mechanism is an axial load to the flexed, adducted thumb, such as when the thumb of a quarterback strikes an opposing player's helmet during the follow-through of a throw. In this fracture, a small fragment of the metacarpal base, held by a volar ulnar ligament, remains in articulation with the trapezium, while the rest of the metacarpal is pulled radially by the APL tendon. All Bennett fractures should be referred to a hand surgeon for management because they often require open reduction and internal fixation. Rolando fractures are similar except that there is comminution of the fracture.

Metacarpal and Phalangeal Shaft Fractures Shaft fractures of the phalanx and metacarpal are similar. They can be

caused by a direct blow or a twisting-type mechanism. The athlete usually experiences swelling, pain, and limited range of motion of the affected bone and surrounding joints.

As in metacarpal neck fractures, reduction should be performed if there is rotational deformity. Rotational deformity can be assessed in the same manner as for metacarpal neck fracture (**Figure 38.9**). Nondisplaced metacarpal shaft fractures should be managed in a short arm cast with the radius slightly extended and the MCP joint in 60° to 70° of flexion for 3 to 4 weeks. Nondisplaced phalangeal shaft fractures should be splinted in an aluminum finger splint that immobilizes the joints proximal and distal to the injured phalanx for 2 to 4 weeks and then taped to the adjoining finger ("buddy taped") until pain free.

Phalanx Fractures SH fractures are also common in the phalanges. SH II fractures are the most common SH injury in the phalanx (**Figure 38.10**), followed by SH III fractures. SH I and IV fractures are rare in the phalanx. Displaced SH fractures of the phalanx should be reduced, especially if the fracture extends to the joint surface. Closed reduction may be possible, but if not, open reduction with internal fixation may be performed. Nondisplaced SH fractures of the phalanx can be managed in an aluminum splint by buddy taping.

Tuft Fractures Tuft fractures of the distal phalanx are common in sports, especially football, and are usually the result

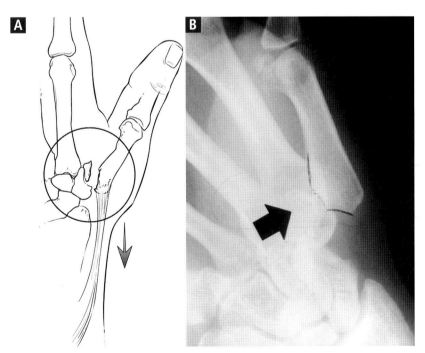

FIGURE 38.8 (A) Fracture-dislocation of the base of the thumb metacarpal (Bennett fracture). (B) Radiograph showing the same.

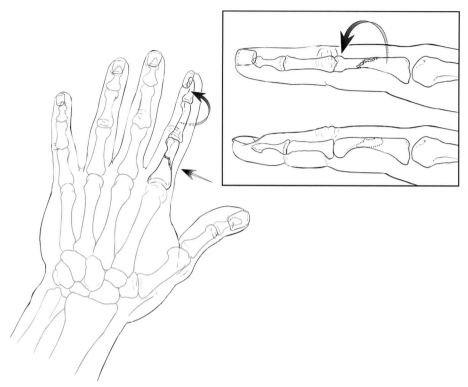

FIGURE 38.9 Rotation of the left index finger with full extension.

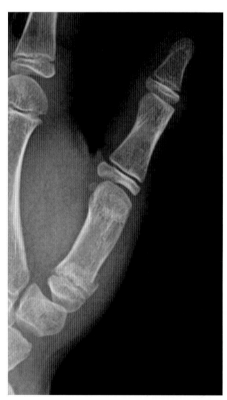

FIGURE 38.10 Salter-Harris II fracture involving the proximal aspect of the first metacarpal.

of the athlete's finger being crushed by another player's cleat. The injured athlete will complain of pain, bruising, and swelling of the affected distal phalanx. It is important to evaluate these fractures carefully because open fractures may be missed if careful examination of the nail bed is not performed. Closed tuft fractures with minimal or no displacement can be managed with an aluminum splint to protect the injured digit for 2 to 3 weeks. Tuft fractures can be associated with injuries to the nail. Subungual hematomas can be aspirated with an 18-gauge needle. Injuries to the nail bed should be repaired with sutures.

Distal Radial Physeal Stress Injury Stress injury of the distal radial physis can occur in gymnasts who perform upper-extremity weight-bearing activities. The gymnast will notice dorsal wrist pain during activities such as handstands and handsprings. At examination, the clinician will find tenderness upon palpation of the dorsal portion of the distal radial physis. Asking the athlete to place his or her palms on the examining table and push off, lifting the body and axially loading the wrist, may reproduce pain (push-off testing). A bilateral wrist series should be obtained; results may show widening and irregularity of the physis and beaking of or cystic changes (**Figure 38.11**). Treatment should include restriction of upper extremity weight-bearing activities for 4 to 12

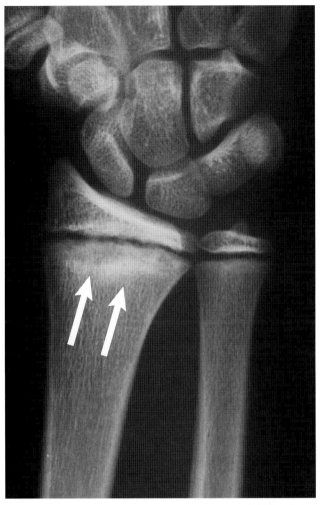

FIGURE 38.11 Metaphyseal sclerosis of the distal radius consistent with radial epiphysitis.

weeks due to the potential for long-term growth inhibition of the radius. Casting or splinting can also be used but is not always necessary. The athlete may gradually resume weight-bearing activities when he or she is pain free with palpation and at push-off.

Keinböck Disease Keinböck disease, or avascular necrosis of the lunate, is most common in upper extremity weight-bearing athletes, such as gymnasts. The cause is unknown, but repetitive trauma and negative ulnar variance have been identified as risk factors. Athletes will complain of dorsal wrist pain and swelling. They may also report pain with wrist extension or gripping and decreased grip strength. Plain radiographs may demonstrate sclerosis, collapse, or fragmentation of the lunate. In early Keinböck disease, bone scan or MRI may demonstrate changes in the lunate, even when plain radiographs are normal.

A classification system for Keinböck disease has been established. In the mildest form of disease, an MRI or bone scan is positive but plain radiographs are normal. In the latest and most severe form, there is collapse, fragmentation, and sclerosis of the lunate with surrounding arthritic changes. Progression of disease is inconsistent, and not all affected athletes will have progressive disease. There is no way to determine which athletes will have progressive disease, and no treatment protocol is universally accepted.

Conservative treatment with rest, ice, nonsteroidal antiinflammatory drugs (NSAIDs), and immobilization in a splint may be helpful in stage 1 disease. However, surgical referral should be made if symptoms persist or in athletes with more advanced disease. Joint leveling, joint unloading, or revascularization procedures may be considered by the surgeon in treating stage 2 disease. In more advanced disease, salvage procedures such as proximal row carpectomy or arthrodesis may be required to alleviate symptoms.

CHRONIC TENDON INJURIES

DeQuervain Tenosynovitis

DeQuervain tenosynovitis is a tenosynovitis of the APL and EPB, the tendons found in the first dorsal compartment of the wrist (see **Figure 38.2**) most commonly seen in golfers, rowers, and racquet sport athletes. It is caused by repetitive stretch of the APL and EPB when the hand is gripped tightly in ulnar deviation or with activities involving active radial deviation of the thumb. Athletes typically complain of pain along the radial aspect of the wrist and thumb. At examination, pain is noted with palpation of the first dorsal compartment, and the Finkelstein test is positive. The Finkelstein test is performed by first having patients lightly grasp their thumb in a fist, followed by passive ulnar deviation of the wrist by the examiner. Reproduction of pain along the first dorsal compartment is considered a positive test (**Figure 38.12**). Resisted extension and abduction of the thumb will also typically reproduce the athlete's pain. Rest from the offending activity and a 7- to 10-day course of NSAIDs will usually relieve pain. However, immobilization in a thumb spica splint and/or injection of the tendon sheath with corticosteroid and local anesthetic may be used in resistant cases. Corticosteroid injections should be done with caution because of the risk of attrition and weakening of the tendon. Once the inflammatory changes have subsided, the athlete should work with a coach to identify any technique errors that may have contributed to symptoms.

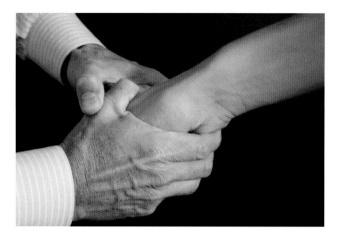

FIGURE 38.12 Finkelstein test.

ECU Tendonitis

ECU tendonitis is commonly seen in athletes participating in racquet sports or rowing and is the second most common overuse injury of the wrist and hand. Athletes usually experience pain along the dorsal-ulnar side of the wrist. At examination, palpation reveals tenderness and swelling of the ECU tendon sheath just dorsal to the ulnar styloid. Resisted extension of the wrist in ulnar deviation should reproduce the athlete's pain. Rest, splinting, and a 7- to 10-day course of NSAIDs will usually be successful in treating ECU tendonitis. When conservative management is unsuccessful, injection with corticosteroid and local anesthetic can be performed. Again, athletes should have a coach carefully evaluate their technique upon return to play to correct errors that may have led to this injury.

Intersection Syndrome

Intersection syndrome is an inflammation at the site where the first dorsal compartment crosses over the second dorsal compartment, about 4 to 6 cm proximal to the radiocarpal joint. It is likely due to friction at this crossover site. Intersection syndrome is commonly seen in rowers, weight lifters, gymnasts, and racquet sport athletes as a result of the repetitive flexion and extension of the wrist required in these activities. Pain at the intersection site can be noted on palpation. This injury is sometimes referred to as a "squeaker" by athletes because of the crepitus noted with active wrist flexion and extension, which can be palpated during the examination. Conservative therapy with rest, ice, and NSAIDs and a short period of splinting in a thumb spica splint is usually successful. However, injection with corticosteroid and local anesthetic may be used in resistant cases.

LIGAMENTOUS INJURY

Ulnar Collateral Ligament Injury

Ulnar collateral ligament (UCL) injury of the thumb is commonly referred to as skier's or gamekeeper's thumb because the most common mechanism of injury is forced abduction and extension of the thumb while falling with a ski pole in the hand. Athletes with a UCL injury experience pain and swelling over the ulnar aspect of the first MCP joint. Stability of the UCL should be assessed by radially deviating the proximal phalanx, which applies an ulnarly directed stress to the UCL with the MCP joint in 0° and 30° of flexion. Firmness of end point and laxity compared with the uninjured thumb are ascertained. When there is significant swelling or bony tenderness, radiographs should be obtained prior to stress testing to rule out physeal fractures. More than 15° of laxity compared with the uninjured side is considered abnormal. Stress radiographs comparing the injured and uninjured thumbs may also be helpful. More than 30° difference between sides is diagnostic for a complete tear of the UCL (**Figure 38.13**). Plain radiographs may also reveal a small bony avulsion fragment.

An attempt at conservative therapy with thumb spica splinting and close follow-up can be made if a partial tear is suspected. If significant laxity persists, referral to a surgical specialist is suggested. A complication of the UCL injury is the Stener lesion, which occurs when the abductor aponeurosis becomes interposed between the 2 ends of the completely torn ligament, preventing healing of the ligament. Confirmation of a Stener lesion may not be possible until the time of surgery, so it is important to consider this complication and refer the patient to a hand surgeon if significant laxity persists after 2 weeks of splinting.

Distal Radioulnar Joint Instability

Distal radioulnar joint (DRUJ) injuries are usually the result of a FOOSH. Other injuries such as distal radius fracture and TFCC injury are commonly associated with DRUJ injuries, but isolated injuries of the DRUJ also occur. Isolated DRUJ injury causes ulnar-sided wrist pain with pronation and supination. With dorsal dislocations, the ulna will appear prominent dorsally when the wrist is flexed. In palmar dislocations, the ulna will appear less prominent. The piano key sign can typically be found during examination when DRUJ instability is present; significant displacement of the ulna is noted when the examiner stabilizes the volar aspect of the pisiform and

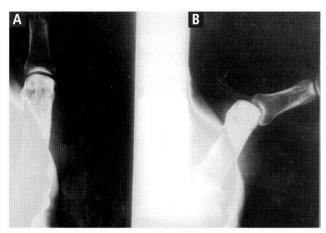

FIGURE 38.13 Metacarpal phalangeal joint of the thumb. (A) Relaxed view. (B) Stress view showing complete rupture of the ulnar collateral ligament.

applies a palmarly directed force to the dorsal aspect of the distal ulna.

Posteroanterior radiographs are useful for demonstrating associated radius fracture and widening of the DRUJ. Displacement of the ulna with respect to the radius may be noted on lateral radiograph. Comparison with the uninjured side may be helpful in demonstrating radiographic abnormality. MRI or CT may be needed to make the diagnosis.

Dorsal DRUJ instability should be treated in a long arm cast with the forearm in supination for 6 weeks, and volar dislocations should be placed in a position between neutral and full pronation. If the ulna does not reduce easily or remains unstable after casting, the patient should be referred to a surgeon.

Scapholunate Ligament Instability

Scapholunate ligament injuries are the most common of the ligamentous injuries of the wrist. A FOOSH is the usual cause of scapholunate ligament injury. The athlete will experience pain and swelling of the affected wrist. The Watson test should be performed by the examiner placing the thumb and index finger over the scaphoid and passively moving the wrist from ulnar to radial deviation. When the scaphoid can be felt to shift and clunk as the wrist is moved into radial deviation, the Watson sign is positive. In the normal wrist, the scaphoid flexes smoothly with radial deviation.

Plain radiographs can be helpful in diagnosing scapholunate ligament injury. Widening of the scapholunate interval more than 3 mm on a standard posteroanterior view or on a clenched-fist view may be noted on the radiograph.

Comparison of the scapholunate interval to the uninjured side should be made. The signet ring sign may also be seen on the posteroanterior view as a result of the flexing of the scaphoid. The lateral wrist film should be evaluated for increased scapholunate angle. The scapholunate angle is the angle created by the intersection of a line through the long axis of the scaphoid and a line through the center of the lunate that parallels the long axis of the forearm (**Figure 38.14**). The scapholunate angle should measure 30° to 60° in the normal wrist. Angles that exceed 60° strongly suggest scapholunate ligament disruption. A magnetic resonance arthrogram may be helpful when the plain radiographs do not permit a clear diagnosis.

Partial scapholunate ligament injuries, without evidence of instability at examination, can be treated with splinting, ice, and NSAIDs. Splinting for durations as long as 3 months may be required to allow for healing. Large tears with obvious scaphoid instability at examination and radiographic studies require surgical referral with open reduction and internal fixation. Left untreated, scapholunate ligament injury can lead to scapholunate advanced collapse (or SLAC wrist), where the scapholunate interval progressively widens, allowing the capitate to shift proximally and the carpal rows to collapse.

PIP Collateral Ligament Sprain

The collateral ligaments of the PIP joints are injured as a result of axial loading with lateral bending force, such as when a ball strikes the end of the finger. Athletes will often say that the finger was "jammed." There will be swelling and tenderness with palpation of the PIP joint. Pain with or without laxity will be noted when the ligaments are stressed. Radial- and ulnar-directed stress should be performed with the joint in 20° of flexion and

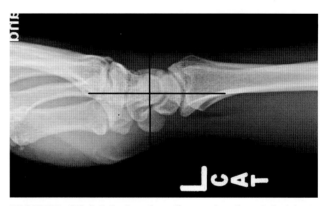

FIGURE 38.14 Lateral radiograph of wrist. Lines indicate scapholunate angle of 90° indicative of scaphulonate dissociation.

full extension, with the examiner looking for laxity. The clinician should compare firmness of end point and laxity to the uninjured hand. Collateral ligament injuries are treated with buddy taping to the adjacent finger. Depending on the amount of laxity, buddy taping will be needed for 2 to 4 weeks. Complete collateral ligament injuries only rarely require surgical intervention. Concurrent volar plate injuries may be present, and if so, splinting in flexion will be required.

ACUTE TENDON INJURIES

Jersey Finger

Jersey finger is an injury of the FDP tendon. Avulsion of the FDP occurs as a result of forced extension of an actively flexed DIP joint, such as when a finger is stuck in an opposing player's jersey as the player pulls away. The athlete will experience pain and swelling of the affected distal phalanx and DIP joint and an inability to actively flex the DIP joint. To test FDP function, the clinician should hold the PIP in extension and ask the patient to actively flex the DIP joint (**Figure 38.15**). Jersey finger requires surgical repair, and referral should be made as quickly as possible because the tendon can recess into the palm, making repair difficult.

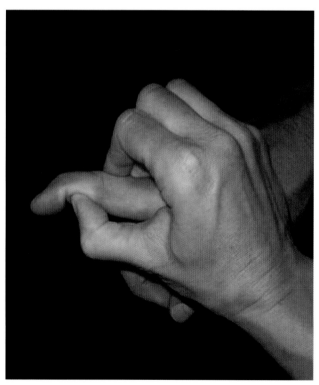

FIGURE 38.15 Active DIP flexion testing the integrity of the flexor digitorum profundis tendon.

Mallet Finger

Mallet finger is an avulsion injury of the distal extensor tendon and occurs as an actively extended DIP joint is forced into flexion. The athlete typically reports that the tip of the finger was struck during an attempt to catch a ball. The athlete presents with pain and swelling on the dorsal aspect of the joint with the DIP in a flexed position. The athlete is unable to actively extend the DIP joint (**Figure 38.16**). Radiographs will help rule out bony involvement. If there is no bony injury or only a small bone fragment is present, conservative treatment is typically successful, but compliance with treatment is sometimes difficult. A splint holding the DIP joint in extension must be worn at all times for 8 weeks and then for 4 to 6 more weeks with activity and while sleeping. Participation in sports can be permitted during treatment as long as the finger is appropriately splinted. If the DIP joint is allowed to fall into flexion during this time, the treatment period must be restarted from the beginning. If there is bony injury that involves more than 30% of the joint surface, surgical repair may be needed, so an appropriate referral should be made.

Central Tendon Slip Rupture

Rupture of the central slip of the extensor tendon at the PIP joint occurs as a result of forced flexion of the PIP joint

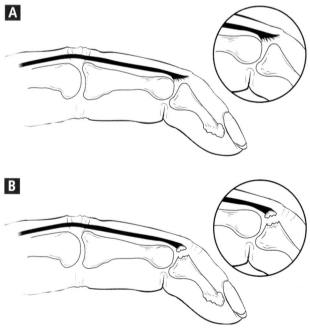

FIGURE 38.16 Mallet finger deformity. (A) Deformity from tendon rupture. (B) Deformity from bony avulsion.

while it is being actively extended, as when a ball directly hits the end of an extended finger. Acutely, the athlete experiences pain on the dorsal aspect of the PIP joint and an inability to actively extend the PIP joint. The DIP joint will be in a position of hyperextension at rest. However, passive extension of the PIP joint is possible. In the chronic form, boutonnière deformity develops, the PIP joint has a flexion contracture, and the DIP joint is hyperextended (**Figure 38.17**). The athlete can be treated with a splint holding the PIP joint in extension for 6 to 8 weeks. As with mallet finger, continuous splinting is essential for healing. Radiographs will permit evaluation of bony avulsion.

Small avulsion fractures can be treated as described earlier. Larger fragments—those involving more than 30% of the joint surface—require surgical referral. Serial splinting, dynamic splinting, or surgery may be needed once a fixed boutonnière deformity develops.

Volar Plate Injury

The volar plate is usually ruptured when the PIP is forced into hyperextension, as when a ball strikes the tip of the finger. The athlete experiences pain and swelling along the volar aspect of the PIP joint. Radiographs may show a bony avulsion fragment off the volar aspect of the middle phalanx. Volar plate injuries should be treated with a splint

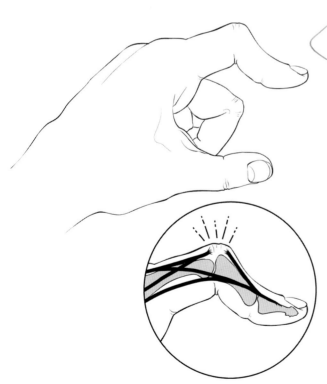

FIGURE 38.17 Boutonnière deformity of the index finger with rupture of the central slip.

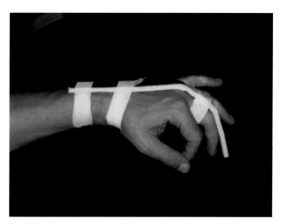

FIGURE 38.18 Extension block splint: The aluminum splint prevents PIP extension but allows flexion.

that blocks the last 30° of extension; flexion may be permitted (**Figure 38.18**). A splint that holds the PIP joint in 30° of flexion can also be used. Splinting will be needed for 2 to 4 weeks, and buddy taping can be used for 2 to 4 more weeks. Left untreated, a flexion contracture of the PIP joint with extension of the DIP joint will occur, creating a pseudo-boutonnière deformity. Injuries with large bony fragments should be referred to a surgeon.

PIP Dislocations

Dorsal dislocation of the PIP joint is the most common dislocation of the hand. Axial loading with dorsal hyperextension causes dorsal dislocation of the middle phalanx on the proximal phalanx and usually rupture of the volar plate and collateral ligaments. Reduction is performed by applying gentle hyperextension of the PIP joint to unlock the middle phalanx from its position on the proximal phalanx, followed by longitudinal traction and flexion of the middle phalanx. Splinting in 30° of flexion for 2 to 4 weeks followed by buddy taping should be undertaken after reduction to allow for healing of the volar plate and collateral ligaments. If reduction cannot be accomplished easily, surgical referral is necessary. As in other finger injuries, radiographs to evaluate for accompanying fracture should be performed, and fractures involving more than 30% of the joint space should be referred for possible surgical fixation.

Volar dislocations are rare and are associated with central tendon and collateral ligament rupture. Reduction is often difficult because the distal aspect of the proximal phalanx can become trapped in the lateral bands of the extensor tendon, and open reduction may be needed. After reduction, splinting in full extension for 6 to 8 weeks will allow the central tendon and collateral ligaments to heal.

TFCC Injury

The TFCC is an important stabilizer of the DRUJ and bears about 20% of the compressive load across the wrist. The TFCC can be injured during a FOOSH or as a result of repetitive wrist loading, such as in gymnastics, weight training, racquet sports, or playing baseballl catcher. Patients will have ulnar-sided wrist pain that is worse with weight bearing on the hands or with activities such as opening jars. At examination, pain can be found with palpation of the TFCC in the space between the pisiform, FCU, and ulnar styloid. The examiner can reproduce pain by placing the wrist in ulnar deviation, applying an axial load, and then flexing and extending the wrist. The patient may also have ulnar-sided wrist pain with push-off testing. Radiographs are typically normal, but they can rule out additional injuries and may show positive ulnar variance, a risk factor for TFCC injury. Magnetic resonance arthrogram of the wrist can be used for diagnosis of TFCC injuries. The primary care physician can order this study, or referral to a specialist can be made. Most patients will respond to conservative therapy with rest and splinting or a short arm cast for 4 to 6 weeks. However, if pain persists, surgical debridement may be needed.

Dorsal Impingement Syndrome

Capsulitis of the dorsal wrist is noted in gymnasts and divers as a result of repetitive wrist extension and axial loading activities. Athletes will experience dorsal wrist pain during extension activities. Pain can be reproduced with push-off testing. Pain with palpation of the dorsal wrist is typically present. Treatment involves relative rest with ice and NSAIDs. Splinting may be needed. Gradual resumption of wrist extension and loading activities is suggested.

Dorsal wrist ganglion cysts can arise from an injured scapholunate joint. Ganglion cysts may be asymptomatic or painful. Conservative therapy with 10 to 14 days of NSAID treatment often resolves the cysts, especially in young athletes. If rest and NSAID treatment are unsuccessful, painful ganglia can be aspirated or injected with corticosteroid, although they often recur. If a painful cyst recurs after multiple aspirations, referral to a hand surgeon for excision may be necessary.

NERVE ENTRAPMENT SYNDROMES

Carpal tunnel syndrome is uncommon in young athletes. However, it may occasionally occur in athletes who participate in activities that require repetitive flexion, such as racquet sports, rowing, and gymnastics, and in wheelchair athletes. Athletes with carpal tunnel syndrome notice pain and paresthesias in the distribution of the median nerve. Associated motor deficits may cause decreased grip strength or difficulty with grasping. Findings at physical examination include reproduction of symptoms with the Phalen maneuver and Tinel testing. Direct compression of the carpal tunnel with the examiner's thumbs may also reproduce numbness, tingling, or pain. In long-standing cases, wasting of the thenar eminence and weakness with thumb adduction may also be noted. In addition to the clinical exam, electromyographic nerve conduction testing may help clarify the diagnosis. MRI can be helpful in identifying mass lesions, such as ganglions, which can cause carpal tunnel compression. However, if the diagnosis is clear at examination, further testing may not be necessary, especially if the patient responds to conservative therapy. Initial therapy should include abstinence from the offending activity and wrist splinting (day and night) for 4 to 6 weeks, along with a course of NSAIDs. Some physicians inject local corticosteroids. If conservative therapy is unsuccessful, additional testing to confirm the diagnosis should be undertaken, and surgical referral for decompression should be made.

The ulnar nerve can be compressed in the wrist at the Guyon canal. As a result of the frequency of this problem in cyclists, ulnar neuropathy is often referred to as *cyclist's palsy*. Afflicted athletes complain of pain and paresthesias in the IVth and Vth fingers. Findings at physical examination may include positive Tinel test over the Guyon canal, decreased sensation of the ulnar digits, and weakness of the interosseus muscle of the fourth and fifth fingers. Plain radiographs of the wrist, including a carpal tunnel view, may permit exclusion of bony pathology. Conservative treatment is usually successful. Rest and wrist splinting for 2 to 6 weeks with a short course of NSAIDs should be performed. Because poor bike fit or worn handlebar padding may contribute to ulnar neuropathy, these issues should be remedied before the athlete returns to the sport. Use of cycling gloves with palmar wrist padding may help prevent return of symptoms. As in carpal tunnel syndrome, if conservative therapy is unsuccessful, electromyography and MRI may be helpful, and surgical referral may be required.

SUMMARY POINTS

- A good working knowledge of the anatomy of the wrist and hand is important in understanding injury mechanisms, performing a detailed physical examination, and making an accurate diagnosis of injury.

- Acute injuries of the wrist are most commonly caused by a fall on an outstretched hand. This mechanism can lead to sprains as well as fractures of the distal radius and scaphoid. Because of the vulnerable nature of the physis in the distal radius and ulna, physeal injury is an important consideration in the differential diagnosis of acute trauma to the wrist. Fractures and physeal injuries are also common occurrences in the metacarpals and phalanges.

- Many wrist and hand injuries require plain radiographs as part of the initial work-up and some may require advanced imaging. Comparison views may be useful in evaluating physeal injuries or variations in bony alignment following injury.

- Blunt trauma to the end of the finger may cause a fracture, ligament sprain, or tendon strain. Tendon injuries that disrupt flexor or extensor function may require surgical treatment.

- Tendonitis and other overuse injuries of the hand and wrist are typically found in athletes who participate in sports requiring repetitive wrist motions such as throwing, racquet sports, or rowing. Weight-bearing or repetitive impact sports, such as gymnastics, can produce stress fractures and other overuse injuries.

- Chronic hand and wrist injuries are more likely to respond to conservative treatment measures such as rest, bracing, and rehabilitation exercises. Surgical treatment may still be necessary for stress fractures, synovial cysts, nerve entrapments, or conditions that fail to improve with conservative measures.

SUGGESTED READING

Cohen P, Aish B. The acutely injured wrist. In: Puffer JC, ed. *20 Common Problems in Sports Medicine.* New York, NY: McGraw-Hill; 2002:69-106.

Eathorne S. The wrist: clinical anatomy and physical examination—an update. *Prim Care Clin Office Prac* 2005;32:17-33.

Hecht S, Luftman J. Fractures in pediatric athletes. In: Puffer JC, ed. *20 Common Problems in Sports Medicine.* New York, NY: McGraw-Hill; 2002:367-408.

Hong E. Hand injuries in sports medicine. *Prim Care Clin Office Pract.* 2005;32:91-103.

McCue F, Bruce J, Koman J. The wrist in the adult. In: *DeLee and Drez's Orthopaedic Sports Medicine.* 2nd ed. Philadelphia, PA: WB Saunders; 2003:1337-1364.

Parmelee-Peters K, Eathorne SW. The wrist: common injuries and management. *Prim Care Clin Office Pract.* 2005;32:35-70.

Peterson J, Bancroft L. Injuries of the fingers and thumb in the athlete. *Clin Sports Med.* 2006;25:527-542.

Rettig AC. Athletic injuries of the wrist and hand. Part 2: overuse injuries of the wrist and traumatic injuries to the hand. *Am J Sports Med.* 2004;32:262-273.

Wen D. The injured finger. In: Puffer JC, ed. *20 Common Problems in Sports Medicine.* New York, NY: McGraw-Hill; 2002:107-130.

Wyzykowski R, Lovallo J, Simmons B. Wrist injuries in the child. In: *DeLee and Drez's Orthopaedic Sports Medicine.* 2nd ed. Philadelphia, PA: WB Saunders; 2003:1365-1377.

CHAPTER 39

Hip, Pelvis, and Thigh

Jorge E. Gómez, MS, MD

Hip, pelvis, and thigh problems occur commonly among young athletes, particularly in adolescent athletes. Physical diagnosis of these problems is challenging as a result of the large muscle mass located around the hip joint, even in lean athletes. The proximity of the pelvic and genital organs to the hip expands the differential diagnosis of hip, pelvis, and thigh pain beyond purely musculoskeletal causes.

ANATOMY AND BIOMECHANICS

The pelvis includes the ilium, ischium, and pubis. The sacrum completes the pelvic ring. The hip joint is composed of the head of the femur articulating in the acetabulum. During the process of skeletal maturation, the secondary ossification centers appear radiographically in the ilium, pubis, ischium, and femur (**Figure 39.1**). These ossification centers serve as origins and insertions of hip and pelvic muscles.

The major muscles of the hip and pelvis are shown in **Figure 39.2**. Flexion of the hip is produced by the iliopsoas, the rectus femoris, and the sartorius. The iliac portion of the iliopsoas originates on the anterior aspect of the iliac crest, and the psoas portion originates on the L2, L3, and L4 vertebrae. The iliopsoas inserts on the lesser trochanter of the femur, which is buried under the quadriceps and adductors. Because the rectus femoris crosses both the hip joint and the knee joint, injury to the rectus femoris often results in weakness of both hip flexion and knee extension. Hip extension is produced primarily by the gluteus maximus, which originates from the sacroiliac joint and inserts on the posterior aspect of the femur. The hamstrings, which originate on the ischial ramus, secondarily assist with hip extension. Hip abduction is effected by the gluteus medius and minimus, which originate on the posterior iliac

crest and insert on the greater trochanter. The tensor fascia lata makes a small contribution to hip abduction. The gluteus medius and minimus, as well as the pyriformis, are responsible for external rotation of the femur. Hip adduction is produced by the adductor minimus, magnus, and longus and by the pectineus and gracilis, all of which originate at the pubic ramus. The adductors and the pectineus are the main internal rotators of the femur.

The hip abductors act to keep the pelvis level during walking and running. Weakness of the hip abductors, or shortening of the femoral neck, such as happens in Legg-Calvé-Perthes disease (LCPD), will cause the pelvis to drop on the opposite side when standing on the affected leg.

The spiral-oriented fibers of the hip capsule allow for increased volume of the hip joint with external rotation and decreased volume of the hip joint with internal rotation. When excessive joint fluid is present in the hip, the patient may be observed to hold the joint in an abducted, externally rotated position to accommodate the excessive fluid. Similarly, internal rotation is restricted and painful as a result of narrowing of the joint capsule and compression of the joint fluid. This anatomic feature of the hip joint makes it possible to detect joint effusions that would otherwise be difficult to detect by inspection or palpation.

EVALUATION

History

The location of pain provides the first clue as to diagnosis. The differential diagnosis of hip and pelvis pain by location is listed in **Table 39.1**. Patients should be evaluated for associated pain in the low back as well as pain that radiates

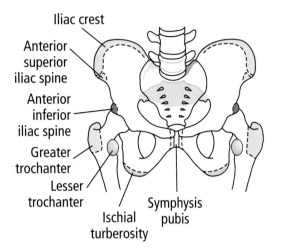

FIGURE 39.1 Bony hip and pelvis; secondary centers of ossification.

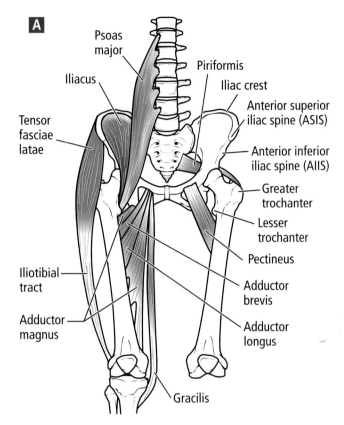

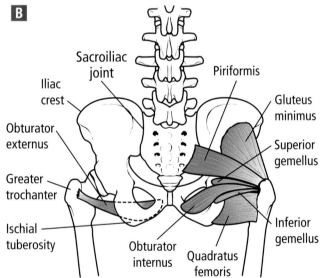

FIGURE 39.2 (A) Anatomy of the anterior hip. (B) Anatomy of the posterior hip.

distally to the thigh or knee. It is also helpful to note whether the pain developed as a result of an acute, traumatic event, or whether it developed gradually. For acute problems, the injury mechanism and resultant limitations should be determined. Common acute problems include hip pointers (iliac crest contusions), apophyseal avulsion fractures, and muscle strains. Chronic or overuse problems in the hip and pelvis include tendonitis, apophysitis, stress fractures, LCPD, and slipped capital femoral epiphysis (SCFE). For repetitive stress or overuse problems, the patient's activities and training regimen should be evaluated.

Pain quality is important, especially in distinguishing visceral from musculoskeletal pain. Pain severity can be gauged by asking patients to rate pain on a scale of 1 to 10 using a visual analog scale such as the Wong-Baker FACES scale, or alternatively by asking them to describe the level of disability being caused by the pain. Popping or snapping sensations in the hip may be associated with tendonitis, bursitis, or pathology in the acetabular labrum. Symptoms of stiffness, restricted joint motion, or a limp suggest intra-articular hip pathology.

A review of systems is helpful, particularly in the patient with hip pain who appears ill or in the patient with gradual onset of pain. The review of systems should address constitutional symptoms (malaise, fever, loss of appetite, weight loss, easy fatigability), head and neck symptoms (sore throat, photophobia, eye redness or pain), abdominal symptoms (pain, diarrhea, dark stools), other musculoskeletal pain, and the skin (rashes).

Medical history may reveal a history of toxic synovitis, which is believed to be a factor predisposing patients to

TABLE 39.1

Differential Diagnosis of Hip and Pelvis Pain by Location

Anterior/Medial	Lateral	Posterior
• Hip flexor strain	• Iliac apophysitis	• Lumbar strain
• Hip flexor tendonitis	• Iliac crest avulsion	• Gluteus medius tendonitis or strain
• Abdominal strain	• Hip pointer	• Sacroiliac sprain
• Anterior superior iliac spine, anterior inferior iliac spine, or lesser trochanter avulsion	• Tensor fascia lata strain	• Pyriformis syndrome
• Hernias; inguinal, femoral	• Trochanteric bursitis	• Lumbar disk herniation
• "Sports hernia"	• Hip joint problems (ie, Legg-Calvé-Perthes disease, slipped capital femoral epiphysis)	
• Osteitis pubis	• Femoral neck stress fracture	
• Hip joint problems (ie, Legg-Calvé-Perthes disease, slipped capital femoral epiphysis)	• Gluteus medius tendonitis or strain	
• Acetabular labrum tear		
• Hip arthritis		
• Toxic synovitis		
• Femoral neck stress fracture		
• Nerve entrapment		
• Pelvic problems		
• Testicular problems		

SCFE. A history of prior stress fracture or oligomenorrhea is common in young women athletes who develop stress fractures.

Physical Examination

Inspection should start with an evaluation of the patient's hip and pelvic alignment, including the presence of anterior tilting of the pelvis or pelvic obliquity from a leg length discrepancy or abductor weakness. Gait should also be evaluated, with particular attention directed toward stride length, limp, or the presence of a Trendelenburg sign whereby the contralateral hip drops during stance phase. Palpation is useful for identifying problems of the pelvic brim (apophysitis, avulsion fractures), muscle injuries, diseases of the pelvic organs (salpingitis, ovarian cyst), or scrotal contents (torsion). Palpation should begin with the bony prominences. With the patient supine, the examiner can readily palpate the iliac crest, anterior superior iliac spine, anterior inferior iliac spine (**Figure 39.3**), greater trochanter, and pubic symphysis. Next, the examiner should examine the inguinal area, the hip flexor and adductor musculature, the femoral triangle, the tensor fascia lata, the lower abdominal musculature, and the pelvic organs. In boys with hip or groin pain of uncertain cause, the scrotal contents should be palpated. Palpation should continue while the patient lies on the unaffected side with the affected hip flexed about 45° so that the examiner may palpate the posterior iliac crest, sacroiliac joints, and the ischial ramus approximately at the inferior gluteal cleft. Then the examiner should palpate the gluteal muscles and the insertion of the gluteus medius and minimus at the greater trochanter. The low lumbar region may also be palpated in this position.

Hip range of motion should be assessed in flexion, extension, abduction, and adduction as well as in internal and external rotation (**Figure 39.4**). Restricted, painful, or asymmetric motion in the hip joint raises concern for intra-articular hip pathology. Motion should first be assessed actively, while the patient performs the motion, and then passively. Hip flexion, abduction, and adduction are assessed with the patient supine. As the examiner flexes the hip, he or she can look for 2 helpful diagnostic signs.

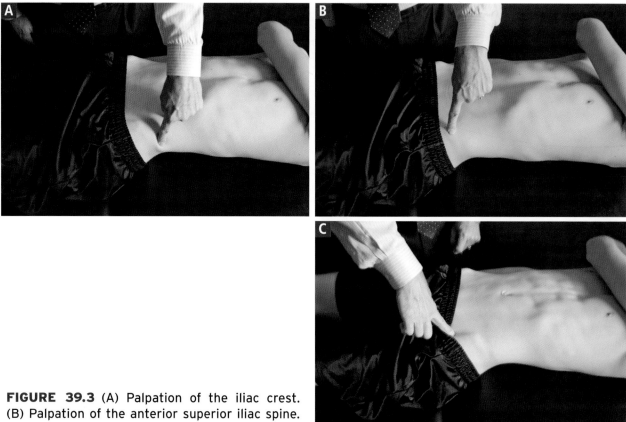

FIGURE 39.3 (A) Palpation of the iliac crest. (B) Palpation of the anterior superior iliac spine. (C) Palpation of the anterior inferior iliac spine.

The first is the Thomas sign, in which flexion of the contralateral hip causes the affected leg to flex at the hip and rise off the table. The Thomas sign indicates a hip flexion contracture that might be present with a hip flexor strain or a hip joint problem (**Figure 39.5**). The second useful sign is the Perthes sign, in which maximum passive flexion of the hip is limited. When intra-articular effusions are present, hip flexion decreases the volume of the joint capsule and compresses the joint fluid. As a result, further attempts to flex the hip result in abduction and external rotation of the hip to accommodate the extra fluid volume.

With the patient lying on the unaffected side, hip extension can be assessed. With the patient prone, internal and external rotation of the hip may be assessed by first stabilizing the pelvis, flexing the knee to 90°, and then internally or externally rotating the leg (**Figure 39.4B and 39.4C**). At least 45° of internal and external hip motion should be present. Affectations of the hip joint, especially LCPD, SCFE, toxic synovitis or septic arthritis, and femoral neck stress fractures all result in a hip joint effusion. Because joint fluid is relatively incompressible, the presence of an

effusion within the hip joint capsule causes pressure pain; therefore, the patient prefers a position in which the volume of the hip joint is maximized, namely flexion, abduction, and external rotation. The presence of a hip joint effusion also limits full motion of the hip, particularly flexion and internal and external rotation. A joint effusion from any cause can result in a positive Perthes sign as well as limited hip flexion and rotation.

Strength testing of the hip muscles should begin with the patient sitting at the edge of the examination table. Hip flexion and adduction can be tested by manually resisting flexion and adduction in this position. With the patient lying on one side, hip abduction can be tested. With the patient lying prone, hip extension can be tested.

Tightness of the iliotibial band can be evaluated with the Ober test (**Figure 39.6**). The patient is asked to lie on one side, with the affected side facing up. The hip is passively extended while the leg is supported, and the pelvis is maintained in vertical alignment. With a tight iliotibial band (or positive Ober test), the knee and leg of the

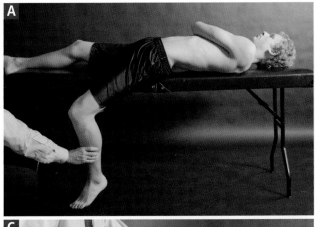

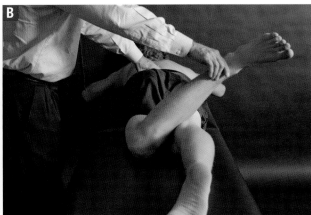

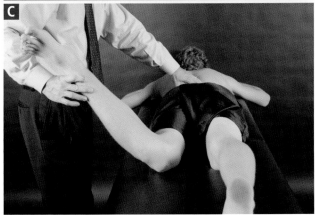

FIGURE 39.4 (A) Physical examination for hip range of motion. Hip extension. (B) Hip external rotation. (C) Hip internal rotation.

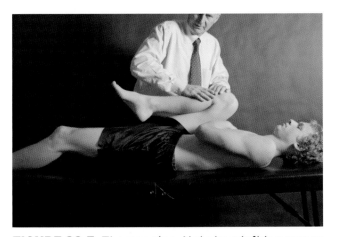

FIGURE 39.5 Thomas sign. Note how left leg comes of table when right hip is maximally flexed.

lever arm over which they exert force, namely the femoral neck, has become shortened. Shortening of the femoral neck occurs with LCPD and SCFE.

Imaging Studies

Initial radiographic evaluation should consist of an antero-posterior (AP) view of the pelvis to include both hips, and an AP view of the pelvis with the legs in a frog's-leg

affected leg remain suspended even after the leg is no longer supported.

The Trendelenburg test is used to identify hip abductor weakness. The Trendelenburg test is done by simply having the patient stand on each leg separately and looking for sagging of the pelvis to the opposite side. The pelvis will sag if the hip abductor muscles themselves are weak or the

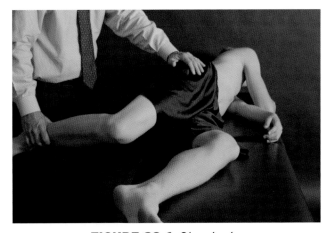

FIGURE 39.6 Ober test.

position. The frog's-leg view essentially provides a lateral view of the femoral neck. In general, evaluation of a long bone for suspected fractures and stress fractures should ideally include 3 views. Problems of the femoral neck that require at least 2 views for evaluation include the SCFE and femoral neck stress fractures.

Laboratory Evaluation

When the possibility of inflammatory processes involving the hip joint exists, screening labs including a complete blood count, erythrocyte sedimentation rate, and C-reactive protein are appropriate. Joint fluid may be analyzed for crystals or bacterial infection.

ACUTE INJURIES OF THE HIP AND PELVIS

Avulsion Fractures

During puberty, 6 secondary centers of ossification are visible radiographically and eventually fuse with the parent bones (**Figure 39.1**). These growth centers or apophyses serve as attachment points for related muscles and do not contribute to long bone growth or stature. Some of these ossification centers may not fuse until long bone growth is complete. Unfused apophyses in the pelvis may be present

in patients who are in their early 20s. Complete maturation may not occur until the patient reaches his or her early or mid-20s. Until these ossification centers mature and fuse with the parent bones, the ultimate tensile strength of the immature physes is less than that of the attached muscle-tendon unit. Under these conditions, powerful contraction of the associated muscle often results in avulsion of the secondary center through the physis (**Figure 39.7A-C**).

Pelvic avulsion fractures are common during puberty. When the apophyses are unfused, apophyseal injuries are more likely than a strain to the related muscle. Pelvic avulsion fractures usually present with sudden onset of intense pain during a sudden, explosive movement. There may be an associated pop or snap as well as pain and weakness associated with contraction of the involved muscle. Despite muscle weakness, the patient may be able to localize the pain to the site of the avulsion rather than in the muscle.

Examination of the athlete with a pelvic avulsion fracture often reveals an antalgic gait. Active range of motion of the hip and associated muscle strength is limited, depending on which muscle attachment is involved. However, passive range of motion may be normal. Hip flexion is limited and weak with avulsions of the anterior superior

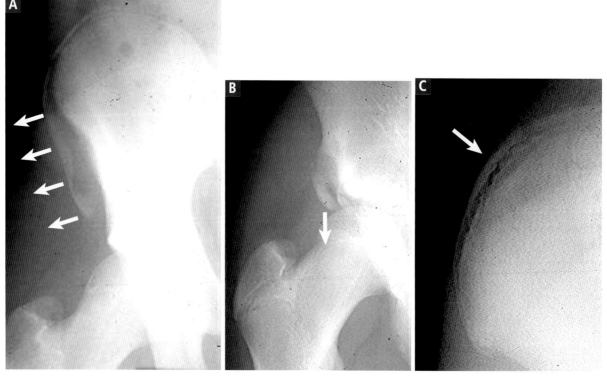

FIGURE 39.7 (A) Avulsion of the anterior superior iliac spine. (B) Avulsion of the anterior inferior iliac spine. (C) Avulsion of the iliac crest.

iliac spine, anterior inferior iliac spine, and lesser trochanter. With avulsions of the iliac crest and greater trochanter, abduction may be limited. Hip extension and knee flexion are limited with avulsions of the hamstring attachment on the ischial ramus.

Although diagnosis can be suggested by history and physical examination in a pubertal athlete, a plain AP of the pelvis should be obtained to confirm the diagnosis, to ascertain the presence of an unfused apophysis, and to evaluate the patient for fracture or displacement of the apophysis. If an avulsion of the anterior superior iliac spine or iliac crest is suspected, the physician ordering the radiograph must instruct the radiographer not to overpenetrate the film because the exposure normally used to visualize the center of the pelvis will cause the iliac crest to appear radiolucent.

The differential diagnosis of acute apophyseal injuries includes muscle strains, pelvic or femoral fractures, iliac crest contusions (hip pointer), and, rarely, hernias in the inguinal or abdominal area.

Treatment of apophyseal avulsion fractures depends on the amount of displacement of the avulsed fragment. In general, avulsion fractures that are not widely displaced can be treated nonsurgically, often with resolution of symptoms within 2 months. There is no consensus on what constitutes wide displacement. However, experience has shown that fragments displaced 1.5 cm or less usually heal with conservative treatment. The avulsion fracture that is most likely to displace widely is the avulsion of the ischial ramus apophysis. Surgical consultation is indicated for widely displaced fractures or fractures that do not resolve clinically within 2 months. In exceptional cases, surgical repair may be elected for quicker return to activity.

Treatment options for pelvic apophyseal avulsion fractures are summarized in **Table 39.2**. Although most avulsion injuries subside with conservative measures, return to full activity before complete bony union has been achieved may result in refracture or a chronic nonunion. Repeat plain films can confirm whether the avulsion has stabilized or healed. However, complete fusion of the apophysis may not occur until skeletal maturation has been reached. Follow-up x-rays are not necessary if the patient is doing well clinically. During the healing process, patients are usually able to tolerate low-impact aerobic exercise, such as cycling or swimming, and can work on improving general flexibility and strength. When patients have pain-free, normal motion, flexibility, and strength, they may be able to slowly resume impact activity and build up to higher speeds and more explosive movements as tolerated.

Muscle Strains

Muscle strains are acute injuries that involve varying degrees of muscle fiber or tendon disruption. Mild or grade I strains cause microscopic tears; moderate or grade II strains are partial tears; and severe or grade III strains involve gross rupture of the muscle. More severe grades of injury are associated with more bleeding and more obvious defects in the muscle.

TABLE 39.2

Stepwise Treatment of Pelvic Apophyseal Avulsion Fractures

PHASE	GOAL	PROTOCOL
Acute	Relieve pain	• Complete rest until pain subsides Crutches, if needed for pain-free ambulation • Ice 4-6 times a day • Analgesics
Subacute	Normalize ROM and flexibility	• Begin active ROM • When active ROM is near normal, begin gentle stretching of involved muscles

Protected functional activities	Normalize strength	• Begin muscle strengthening with isometrics, followed by:
		  Isotonic strengthening
		  Eccentric strengthening (later)
		• Address associated strength deficits

Advanced functional activities	Return to functional activity	• Graded return to running program
		  Plyometric and ballistic movements
		  Sport-specific training

ROM indicates range of motion.

Adductor Strain

Adductor strains occur in athletes who perform quick side-to-side movements, especially soccer and tennis players. Injuries typically occur when the athlete lunges laterally away from the side that becomes injured. With severe injuries, the athlete may report feeling a pop or snap. With severe injuries, there may be significant impairment of mobility and difficulty with walking, moving laterally, and running.

At examination, there is focal tenderness in the adductor muscle mass. The examiner should first palpate lightly to appreciate any focal swelling or defects in the muscle. Firmer palpation may be used to assess tenderness associated with mild injuries. Active and passive abduction are often limited. Adductor strength is reduced as a result of pain and/or muscle fiber disruption. Hip external rotation may be limited, but normal hip internal rotation and hip flexion can rule out intra-articular hip pathology. The differential diagnosis of adductor strain includes avulsion of the pubic ramus, osteitis pubis, entrapment of the ilioinguinal nerve, and a herniated lumbar disk with pain radiating into the groin.

Avulsion of the ischial ramus typically causes pain at the origin of the hamstrings, and is associated with bony tenderness. Osteitis pubis usually begins insidiously and causes pain with tenderness at the pubic symphysis. Inguinal hernia, especially if indirect, presents insidiously as a bulge or mass in the groin. Entrapment of the ilioinguinal nerve causes scrotal pain with an otherwise normal groin and scrotal examination. With testicular torsion and testicular contusion, there may be a history of direct trauma, and the scrotal examination is abnormal. Plain x-ray evaluation may be helpful to distinguish these injuries from avulsion fractures.

Generally, muscle injuries are initially treated with rest, ice, and compression. Limiting movement of the hip and applying ice frequently during the first 2 to 3 days after injury is usually enough for pain control. However, oral analgesics may be used for additional pain control. Spica strapping of the proximal thigh may benefit ambulation.

The treatment of muscle injuries progresses from limiting pain and further injury during the acute phase, restoring range of motion and strength in the subacute phase, and restoring function and sport-specific activities in the later phase. Return to play can occur when flexibility and strength are normal and the patient has successfully completed a functional progression that includes running, sprinting, and cutting without pain or limitation.

Iliopsoas Strain The iliopsoas is often injured acutely with a jumping or sprinting activity. The patient localizes pain to the inguinal creases–femoral triangle area. Because of the deep location of the muscle in the pelvis it may be difficult to palpate swelling or a defect in the muscle. Active hip flexion against resistance is weak and causes pain. Passive hip extension is also restricted and painful. The differential diagnosis of acute pain in the anterior hip includes avulsion of the anterior superior iliac spine or anterior inferior iliac spine, inguinal or femoral hernia, fascial hernia of the rectus femoris (sports hernia), or testicular torsion.

Gluteus Medius Strain The gluteus medius is the primary hip abductor and may be injured with a sudden lateral lunge. Muscle tenderness to palpation is most often found near the origin of the gluteus medius along the iliac crest, or near the insertion of the muscle immediately posterior and medial to the greater trochanter. There may be limitation of passive hip internal rotation. Hip abduction is weak and painful. Injuries that may resemble strain of the gluteus medius include avulsion of the greater trochanter or posterior iliac apophysis, pyriformis syndrome, and herniated lumbar disk with pain radiating into the buttock.

Gluteus Maximus Strain Strain of the gluteus maximus may occur with any forceful push-off. The pain is usually localized to the middle of the muscle, or occasionally to the origin near the sacroiliac joint. Hip flexion and extension are limited by pain, and hip internal rotation may also be slightly limited. Active hip extension is weak, but hip abduction remains strong. Differential diagnosis includes sacroiliac sprain, avulsion of the ischial apophysis, pyriformis syndrome, and herniated lumbar disk.

After the diagnosis has been confirmed, treatment for all muscle strains around the hip and pelvis follows similar principles: rest, protect from further injury, restore flexibility and strength, and gradually progress back to more demanding functional activities.

Sacroiliac Sprain

This injury is most commonly seen in straddle sports, such as equestrian, motocross, and cycling, and sports that require forceful push-off on one leg, such as jumping and vaulting. The sprain may begin with a single event or may develop insidiously. Maneuvers to provoke sacroiliac pain, such as the Patrick maneuver (**Figure 39.8**), should be carried out in an attempt to reproduce the pain. The individual may have difficulty finding a comfortable position for sitting. There may be pain with standing on one foot, with walking, or with hip abduction.

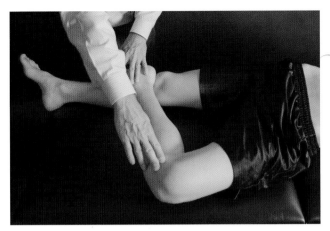

FIGURE 39.8 Maneuver to stress the sacroiliac joint.

At physical examination, there is tenderness to palpation of the affected sacroiliac joint. Range of motion of the hip joint is normal. Maneuvers to provoke sacroiliac pain should be carried out in an attempt to reproduce the pain. Hip abductors may be weak. X-rays are rarely diagnostic.

The differential diagnosis of sacroiliac pain includes ankylosing spondylitis, especially in boys; pyogenic arthritis, especially gonococcal arthritis in the adolescent; herniated lumbar disk with radiation into the buttock; and tumors.

Treatment involves avoiding painful activity, icing the affected area, strengthening the hip abductors, and possibly using a sacroiliac belt. Injection of corticosteroids into the most painful part of the joint may bring relief. Patients with sacroiliac sprain may seek the help of a manually trained therapist who can often provide relief by mobilizing the joint.

CHRONIC CONDITIONS AND OVERUSE INJURIES OF THE HIP AND PELVIS

Legg-Calvé-Perthes Disease

LCPD is an osteochondrosis of the femoral head. Also called avascular necrosis of the femoral head, it is thought to occur as a result of a disruption to the vasculature supplying the femoral head. It is not certain that this condition is associated with mechanical trauma or that it is more common among athletes. There is some evidence that a previous episode of aseptic synovitis of the hip increases the risk for development of LCPD. LCPD is included as a cause of chronic hip pain in athletes because most affected individuals are physically active.

LCPD usually manifests between the ages of 4 and 7 years with insidious onset of limping with some complaints of pain. Occasionally, a traumatic event will precipitate a medical consultation for hip pain caused by LCPD. The primary care provider should be aware that the patient with LCPD may experience referred pain to the medial knee. Classically, LCPD presents with more limp than pain. As such, the diagnosis of LCPD is often delayed by weeks to months after the onset of symptoms. Usually there are no constitutional symptoms, and the patient does not complain of other painful joints. Patients who have been previously diagnosed and treated for LCPD may continue to have symptoms later in life related to sports participation.

The physical examination of the child with LCPD usually reveals Trendelenberg gait. Weakness of the hip abductors forces the child to lean to the affected side while standing on the affected leg, then swing the affected leg around while standing on the unaffected leg. Despite the common complaint of medial knee pain, the knee examination is normal. Examination of the hip reveals a hip flexion contracture (positive Thomas test); a positive Perthes sign; limited internal and/or external rotation of the hip; and generalized weakness of the hip, especially in abduction. For the same reason, the Trendelenburg test is usually positive.

An AP x-ray of the pelvis and a frog's-leg view will reveal flattening of the femoral head, a moth-eaten appearance with areas of sclerosis alternating with areas or rarefaction, blurring of the physis, and loss of the normally smooth contour of the femoral head (**Figure 39.9**).

The differential diagnosis of LCPD includes arthritis and synovitis. Septic arthritis and toxic synovitis are

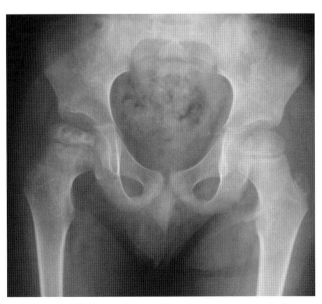

FIGURE 39.9 Radiographic appearance of Legg-Calvé-Perthes disease of the right hip.

accompanied by systemic symptoms of fever, chills, and body aches. Juvenile arthritis may affect the hip and involve other joints as well. Erythrocyte sedimentation rate and C-reactive protein are typically high in juvenile arthritis but not in LCPD. Children with congenital hip dysplasia have a long history of gait disturbance. X-rays or magnetic resonance imaging (MRI) may be needed to rule out tumor.

Children with LCPD should use crutches to limit weight bearing and they should be referred to an orthopedist. Favorable long-term outcomes from LCPD are associated with early detection and careful follow-up.

Iliac Apophysitis

Although apophysitis is possible at any of the secondary ossification sites about the pelvis, it is rare except for apophysitis of the iliac crest. Apophysitis is common at this site, probably because several large, powerful muscles either insert or originate on the iliac crest, including the iliac portion of the iliopsoas, the gluteal muscles, the tensor fascia lata, the lumbar paraspinous muscles, and the latissimus. As with other forms of apophysitis, iliac apophysitis most likely represents a stress fracture of the physis. Iliac apophysitis occurs primarily between the ages of 12 to 18 years, although some boys continue to be vulnerable into their early 20s. Although iliac apophysitis was originally described in runners, it may affect athletes in any sport that involves jumping; impact; or rapid acceleration, deceleration, and/or changes of direction. The onset may be gradual or sudden as a result of direct trauma to the area such as a blow or a fall. Although patients may complain of hip pain, they are usually able to localize the pain to the superior portion of the pelvis along the iliac crest. The symptoms are rarely present at rest. Low-impact activity, such as swimming, cycling, and weight lifting, may be more readily tolerated.

At physical examination, there is tenderness to palpation along the crest but no bony deformity. There may be pain or weakness associated with manual testing of the muscles that attach on the iliac crest, especially hip flexion and abduction.

X-rays usually reveal a normal-looking iliac apophysis (**Figure 39.10**) but may show fragmentation or slight separation of the physis (Figure 39.7C). The insidious onset of bony tenderness on the pelvis should also raise concern for tumors, including Ewing's sarcoma.

Initial treatment consists of limiting running as well as impact activities or anything that increases pain. Ice and anti-inflammatory medications can also relieve pain. Patients can maintain aerobic fitness by swimming, cycling, or using low-impact stair-climber or elliptical trainers.

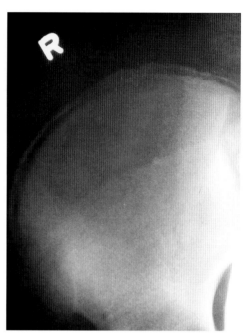

FIGURE 39.10 Normal appearance of the iliac crest apophysis.

Stretching the associated muscles is designed to relieve tension on the apophysis. Once strength deficits have been corrected, it is usually safe for the athlete to slowly resume running or impact activity.

Snapping Hip

Snapping or popping in the hip is a relatively common complaint that has a variety of potential causes. The most common cause is likely the result of the iliopsoas tendon snapping under the inguinal ligament or over the iliopectineal eminence. Snapping or popping over the anterior hip may also be a result of a torn acetabular labrum. In both cases, the symptoms occur with active hip flexion. On the lateral aspect of the hip, a tight iliotibial band may snap over the greater trochanter while the athlete is running or when the hip is repetitively flexed and extended. Pain may or may not accompany the snapping. With acetabular labral tears, there may be a sense of locking or catching in the hip or reports of a mechanical block to hip flexion. Patients will occasionally report a sensation of their hip going out of place.

Patients are usually able to reproduce their symptoms during the physical examination. Additional findings may include tenderness over the anterior hip or inguinal crease and pain with resisted hip flexion. Hip joint range of motion is normal. However, with a snapping iliopsoas, there may be tightness of the hip flexors. When the iliotibial band snaps over the greater trochanter, there may be tenderness just posterior to the greater trochanter and tightness of the iliotibial band as demonstrated by a positive Ober test (**Figure 39.6**). Hip joint motion should be normal. However, with an acetabular labrum tear, there may be pain or popping associated with passive hip flexion or the "scour test" when the hip is flexed, adducted, and rotated internally.

Plain radiographs of the hip are normal for these causes of snapping or popping in the hip. If a torn labrum is suspected, the diagnosis can be confirmed with an MRI-arthrogram of the hip.

The differential diagnosis for a snapping hip includes any structural abnormality that may permit subluxation of the hip joint or result in deformity of the joint. This may include congenital hip dysplasia, connective tissue disorders (Down syndrome, Ehlers-Danlos syndrome, or Marfan's syndrome), or generalized joint hypermobility.

Treatment requires a period of relative rest. Swimming and cycling may be more readily tolerated than running or jumping activities. Stretching exercises can relieve tightness in the iliopsoas or iliotibial band. For acetabular labral pathology, symptoms may subside by avoiding activity that requires maximum hip flexion or extension. For persistent pain or mechanical restrictions to hip motion, surgical consultation is appropriate.

Osteitis Pubis

An acute sprain to the pubic symphysis or repetitive shearing stresses across the joint may result in osteitis pubis. This injury is commonly seen in straddle sports or sports in which athletes do the splits. Excessive stress across the pubic symphysis causes increased osteoclastic resorption with erosive changes, joint widening, and instability of the joint. Affected patients present with pain in the hip adductors and pain at the pubic symphysis, or pubalgia, that occurs with abduction of the hip or stretch of the adductor muscles.

Physical examination reveals tenderness to palpation over the pubic symphysis. Associated findings include hip adductor tightness as well as pain and weakness with contraction of the hip adductors. X-rays reveal osteolysis (areas of sclerosis alternating with areas of rarefaction) of the pubic bone on one or both sides of the symphysis without periosteal reaction (**Figure 39.11**).

Other causes of pubalgia include bladder problems, sexually transmitted diseases, abdominal strains, and sports hernia. Stress fractures of the pubic rami are seen in adult athletes but are rare in children. The presence of periosteal

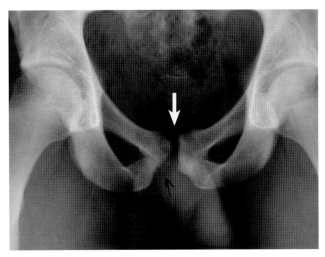

FIGURE 39.11 Osteitis pubis.

reaction should alert the clinician to the possibility of osteomyelitis or tumor.

Treatment involves avoiding painful activities, applying ice, and stretching the hip adductors. Return to play can occur when pain subsides and when flexibility and strength have been restored. X-rays may remain abnormal despite resolution of the pain.

DIFFERENTIAL DIAGNOSIS OF HIP, GROIN, AND PELVIS PAIN

Slipped Capital Femoral Epiphysis

Slipped capital femoral epiphysis, or SCFE, is an osteochondrosis of uncertain origin that affects the proximal femoral physis. Weakening of the physis causes the femoral head to slip off the femoral neck, effectively shortening the femoral neck (**Figure 39.12**). SCFE may present acutely or as a chronic condition. Most affected youngsters are preadolescent, overweight, and sedentary. Other risk factors include a history or family history of endocrinopathy such as diabetes or hypothyroidism. Pain begins insidiously and is often localized to the lateral hip or groin. Pain may radiate along the medial thigh to the knee. In some cases, patients with SCFE may have thigh or knee pain but no hip pain.

Physical examination reveals the characteristic somatotype, an antalgic gait, and tenderness over the hip. Hip range of motion is limited in internal rotation, external rotation, and flexion. A positive Perthes sign and a positive Trendelenburg test may also be observed. An AP and frog's-leg x-ray should be obtained. Positive x-ray findings, or a highly suggestive history and physical examination without obvious x-ray abnormalities, warrant referral to a pediatric orthopedist.

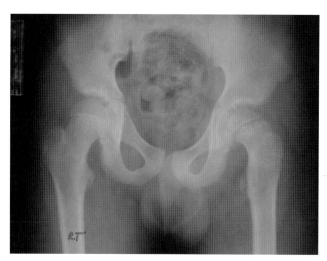

FIGURE 39.12 Slipped capital femoral epiphysis on left hip.

Hernias

Hernias are common causes of groin pain, especially among adolescent athletes. The indirect inguinal herniais most common and manifests with insidious onset of discomfort in the groin or scrotum and palpable swelling or a defect.

Sports hernias present with insidious onset of pain along the lateral margin of the distal rectus abdominis. Sports hernias have been reported to occur in hockey, soccer, baseball, and tennis players or in sports that require rapid rotation or lateral movement of the trunk. The pathology of the sports hernia has been described as a dehiscence of the rectus abdominis off the pubic ramus. A defect of the abdominal wall fascia may also be present. Results of physical examination are often nonspecific. Evidence of abdominal muscle strains or abdominal wall hernias should be ruled out. Imaging such as abdominal wall ultrasound or MRI may reveal a defect in the rectus. Management may include referral to a general surgeon who is familiar with this condition.

Scrotal Problems

In addition to hernias, groin pain can result from scrotal problems such as testicular torsion, epididymitis, or painful inguinal lymphadenopathy.

Herniated Lumbar Disk

A herniated lumbar disk can cause pain that radiates into the buttock and may mimic a strain of the gluteal muscles or sacroiliitis. Diagnosis of the herniated lumbar can be suspected when hamstring or buttock pain increases with flexion of the low back. An MRI of the lumbar spine can confirm the presence of a disk injury.

Nerve Entrapment Syndromes

Entrapment of the ilioinguinal nerve may occur after abdominal surgery or as a result of excessive abdominal strengthening exercises. The patient will present with pain in one hemiscrotum and the perineal area. Careful palpation just above and along the inguinal crease may reproduce the pain. Examination of the scrotum is normal. Treatment includes cessation of abdominal strengthening activity, local ice applications where the ilioinguinal nerve exits the abdominal wall, and occasionally, local corticosteroid injection.

ACUTE THIGH INJURIES

Quadriceps Contusion

Contusion of the quadriceps muscle can occur from colliding with another player; being hit by a projectile such as a pitched baseball; falling on a blunt object; or being struck with sports equipment such as a hockey stick, lacrosse stick, or soccer goal. Contusions result in intramuscular hemorrhage. Muscle swelling results in pain, spasm, and increasingly restricted motion.

At physical examination, there may be swelling, ecchymosis, and tenderness to palpation. The severity of the contusion can be graded according to the amount of passive knee flexion as tested when the patient is prone (**Figure 39.13**). A contusion is mild if the athlete is able to flex the knee beyond 90°, moderate if knee flexion is between 45° and 90°, and severe if knee flexion is less than 45°.

The differential diagnosis of a quadriceps contusion includes femur fracture, compartment syndrome, and myositis ossificans. Radiographs can rule out fracture and

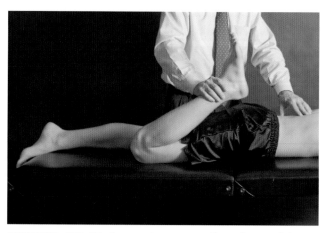

FIGURE 39.13 Assessing severity of quadriceps contusions.

soft tissue calcification seen with myositis ossificans (**Figure 39.15**).

Initial treatment for a quadriceps contusion includes ice and compression. Maintaining the quadriceps in an elongated position by bandaging the knee in flexion may reduce shortening from contracture. When the acute pain and swelling subsides, massage and gentle stretching can help restore the length of the quadriceps. Patients may return to activity when they have regained full flexibility and strength of the quadriceps.

Occasionally, liquefaction may occur in a large intramuscular hematoma. This presents as a fluctuant, nontender mass. These patients must be followed carefully for the development of pyomyositis. A hematoma that becomes hard, warm to touch, and tender should raise concerns for myositis ossificans.

Hamstring and Quadriceps Strain

Strains to the hamstrings or quadriceps usually occur with an eccentric contraction of the muscle. Sports that involve quick burst movements or frequent acceleration, deceleration, or change of direction are more commonly associated with strains. Injured athletes may report a history of muscle cramping, tightness, fatigue, or dehydration. Strains tend to occur centrally in the muscle or at the muscle-tendon junction. Pain or tenderness at the bony attachment may be a result of an apophyseal injury or avulsion fracture.

Palpation may reveal the presence of focal muscle swelling and/or a palpable defect in the muscle. Range of motion should be assessed for the injured muscle and compared with the uninjured side. X-rays are not usually helpful for strains unless the age of the individual and the location of the pain suggest an avulsion fracture.

Patients with symptoms of muscle tightness or spasm without a classic history for a strain should be evaluated for referred pain from the lumbar spine. The presence of tenderness deep in the thigh should raise concern for femoral stress fracture. A tender mass raises the possibility of myositis ossificans or soft tissue tumors such as a sarcoma.

The treatment of muscle strains begins with resting from the offending activity and providing ice and compression. When the acute pain and spasm subsides, gentle stretching and active range of motion exercises can commence. Weight bearing can begin when tolerated. Swimming or aquatic therapy can be done to maintain fitness in the early stage of recovery. Cycling or elliptical machines can be used once the available range of motion and strength permit. Because muscle strains are more

likely to occur with eccentric stresses, it is helpful to restore normal eccentric strength before returning to full activity. Surgical treatment for hamstring and quadriceps strains is generally not necessary unless the strain involves an avulsion with separation of the bony attachment site or a complete rupture of the tendon.

Rectus Femoris Herniation

The quadriceps, commonly the rectus femoris portion, can herniate through its fascia during exercise. The cause of this herniation is not clear. This muscle herniation may present with a pop, acute pain, and a visible area of swelling in the proximal third of the muscle. The pain does not necessarily prohibit continued activity. Unlike similar herniations that may occur in the tibialis anterior, these herniations are not usually associated with symptoms of elevated muscle compartment pressure or a compartment syndrome.

The herniated portion of muscle is soft, slightly tender, and can be manually reduced through the fascial defect. Restrictions of muscle flexibility and strength are not as common with hernias as they are with muscle strains. MRI can rule out soft tissue tumor, hemorrhage, or muscle fiber disruption.

Treatment includes use of ice and compressive wraps for symptom control. Surgical repair of the defect usually is not necessary to restore normal quadriceps function.

CHRONIC CONDITIONS AND OVERUSE INJURIES OF THE THIGH

Trochanteric Bursitis

Tightness of the iliotibial band may result in chronic lateral hip pain that is made worse with running activity. Pain and tenderness is localized to the posterior aspect of the greater trochanter where the iliotibial band crosses. There may be a popping or snapping sensation associated with activity and a dull, aching sensation after activity. Physical examination reveals point tenderness posterior to the greater trochanter, occasional swelling, and tightness of the iliotibial band as demonstrated by a positive Ober test. Patients with trochanteric bursitis may be noted to have varus alignment with a high-arched foot and/or varus alignment at the knees. Pain over the lateral hip can also be due to tendonitis of the gluteus medius or pyriformis muscle spasm due to a lumbar disk protrusion.

Treatment of trochanteric bursitis requires decreasing running, jumping, impact, or other pain-causing activities. Ice and anti-inflammatory modalities can reduce swelling in the trochanteric bursa, and stretching the iliotibial band can reduce tension and friction over the greater trochanter. Patients with varus alignment tend to have more tightness in the iliotibial band and less shock absorption capacity with running and impact activities. Adequate cushioning in the footwear may be a helpful adjunct to treatment of these individuals.

Femoral Stress Fracture

Femoral stress fractures present with a gradual onset of deep thigh pain. The pain is most pronounced with repetitive impact activity. Low-impact exercise and routine daily activities usually do not cause pain. Athletes involved with distance running and athletes who have osteopenia from dietary or hormonal causes are at increased risk. Given the mass of surrounding musculature, it may be difficult to palpate bony tenderness. However, application of a bending stress on the femur by way of the fulcrum test (**Figure 39.14**) may cause pain. Hip range of motion and muscle flexibility should be normal.

X-rays are indicated for suspected femoral stress fractures. If x-rays are normal, further testing may include a bone scan or MRI. If a bony abnormality is revealed, thin section computed tomography (CT) scanning can confirm that the abnormality is a stress fracture and can rule out other sources of bony pain such as an osteoid osteoma or tumor.

Treatment of a femoral stress fracture requires limiting impact activity for at least 6 weeks. For stress fractures in the femoral neck or for patients with persistent pain with weight bearing, crutches may be necessary. If dietary or hormonal factors are contributory, they should also be addressed. When healing is documented clinically and radiographically, the patient can gradually resume weight-bearing and impact activity. CT scanning limited to the

area of the stress fracture provides an objective measure of healing. The average time for recovery varies, but 3 to 6 months is not unusual.

CHRONIC THIGH PAIN

Myositis Ossificans

Myositis ossificans is a condition associated with the development of calcification in muscle tissue after trauma and intramuscular hemorrhage. It occurs most commonly in the quadriceps, but it can be seen in any large muscle mass exposed to direct trauma. The calcifications likely result from an exuberant inflammatory response within the muscle that is related to the amount of bleeding from the contusion.

Myositis ossificans usually manifests with a history of a contusion that becomes increasingly swollen, tender, hard in consistency, and warm to the touch. There may be increasing pain, loss of flexibility, and weakness despite rest and conservative treatment.

The diagnosis is confirmed by x-ray examination, which will reveal reticular or spicular calcifications within the muscle (**Figure 39.15**). These changes usually do not appear weeks to months after the onset of symptoms.

Treatment for myositis ossificans involves rest and anti-inflammatory medication and modalities, followed by gentle flexibility exercises. Any treatment that causes further muscle damage or bleeding in the muscle can worsen the condition. This includes forceful stretching, vigorous deep

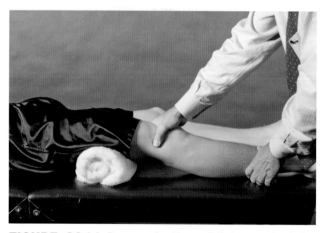

FIGURE 39.14 Demonstration of fulcrum test for suspected femoral stress fracture.

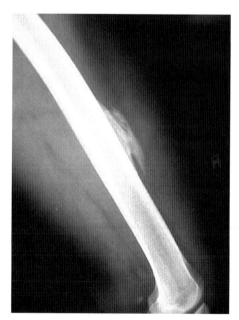

FIGURE 39.15 Myositis ossificans involving quadriceps.

tissue massage, or therapeutic ultrasound. Athletes may return to play when their flexibility and strength have returned to normal. Follow-up x-rays may reveal persistent calcification that appears layered or shingled over the femur. Surgical resection of these calcifications may precipitate more bleeding and calcification.

Meralgia Paresthetica

Meralgia paresthetica results from irritation of the lateral femoral cutaneous nerve as it passes over the anterior rim of the pelvis. It may be initiated by a direct blow to the anterior lateral thigh, friction from a gymnast bending over a bar, or repetitive hip flexion from cycling. It has also been reported to occur as a result of wearing tight slacks, hip huggers, and pistol belts, and it is also associated with pregnancy. The symptoms include a painful numbness or burning over the anterolateral thigh. Careful palpation in the proximal lateral thigh might localize a point of tenderness that is just medial and inferior to the anterior superior iliac spine. There may be a positive Tinel sign whereby pressure or percussion of the nerve produces paresthesias. Sensation may be diminished in the distribution of the nerve. Because the nerve supplies only sensation to the anterolateral thigh, motor deficits are not observed. Electromyography reveals abnormal somatosensory evoked potentials. This condition can usually be treated by avoiding the aggravating activity or apparel, by administering analgesics, and by injecting local corticosteroids. Recalcitrant cases may require surgical exploration and release of the nerve.

Lumbar Disk Herniation

Anterior or lateral thigh pain may be due to lumbar disc protrusions or herniations at the L3-4 level. Individuals typically have a history of back trauma and back pain. Referred pain to the thigh is characterized by the lack of local tenderness, swelling, or deformity. If thigh pain is coming from the back, symptoms will be worse with activities that stress the back rather than activities that stress the hip or thigh.

Pyomyositis

Pyomyositis is a rare complication that can develop days to weeks after blunt trauma to the muscle. These individuals may be previously healthy or have some condition causing immunocompromise, such as diabetes. Typically, individuals with pyomyositis manifest fever, chills, and worsening muscle pain. At physical examination, the thigh is warm or hot, swollen, and exquisitely tender to palpation. Muscle testing reveals muscle weakness and increased pain with muscle contraction. MRI is usually necessary to confirm the diagnosis. Surgical drainage is

often indicated. The infection must be treated with intravenous antibiotics against *Staphylococcus* and *Streptococcus.*

SUMMARY POINTS

- Injuries or conditions affecting the hip joint generally manifest as pain in the anterior hip and/or medial thigh. Patients are also likely to exhibit an antalgic gait or limp and restricted range of motion in the hip joint.

- Pain in the hip and pelvis that occurs posteriorly or laterally and permits normal hip joint motion may be referred from the low back or related to injury to muscles that attach to the pelvis.

- Diagnostic imaging of the hip is indicated for any patient with a history of major trauma, chronic joint pain, restricted joint motion, or a limp.

- Injury mechanisms that are likely to cause muscle strains in skeletally mature patients may cause avulsion of the muscle's attachment on the apophysis of a skeletally immature patient.

- Developmental conditions and osteochondroses can cause hip pain and hip joint degeneration in both athletes and nonathletes.

- A snapping hip could be a normal finding or could be due to bursitis, impingement of tight muscles on bony prominences, or a cartilage injury involving the acetabular labrum.

- Muscle contusions and muscle strains can both cause pain, swelling, loss of flexibility, and weakness. Despite different injury mechanisms and underlying pathology, treatment for both types of injury requires resolution of pain and swelling as well as restoration of normal flexibility and strength.

- Chronic pain in the hip, pelvis, and thigh can be due to tendonitis, stress fractures, and apophysitis, or due to less frequent conditions such as nerve entrapments, hernias, and referred problems from the lumbar spine.

SUGGESTED READING

Aronen JG, Chronister R, Ove PN. Thigh contusions; minimizing the length of time before return to full athletic activities with early immobilization in 120 degrees of knee flexion. *Orthop Trans.* 1991;15:77-78.

Hollingshead WH, Jenkins DB. *Functional Anatomy of the Limbs and Back.* 5th ed. Philadelphia, PA: WB Saunders; 1981.

Meyers WC, Foley DP, Garrett WE, et al. Management of severe lower abdominal or inguinal pain in high-performance athletes. *Am J Sports Med.* 2000;28:2-8.

Orava S, Ala-Ketola L. Avulsion fractures in athletes. *Br J Sports Med.* 1977;11:65-71.

Williams P, Terzl K. Management of meralgia paresthetica. *J Neurosurg.* 1991;74:76-80.

CHAPTER 40

Acute Injuries of the Knee

David T. Bernhardt, MD

Youth sports involving contact, collisions, running, jumping, and pivoting lead to a variety of acute injuries to the knee. Acute knee injuries may present for medical evaluation at an urgent care clinic, an emergency department, or a primary care provider's office. Providers in all of these settings need to recognize injury patterns, obtain appropriate histories, perform a focused knee examination, and prescribe appropriate treatment. The purpose of this chapter is to give a brief overview of knee anatomy, review the epidemiology of knee injures in athletes, highlight the unique aspects of the growing athlete, discuss the clinical evaluation, review common and unique diagnoses that tend to occur in young athletes, and outline treatment options.

ANATOMY

The knee is a pivotal hinge joint consisting of 4 bones (femur, tibia, fibula, patella) and 3 articulations (patellofemoral, tibiofemoral, tibiofibular). A combination of ligaments; a joint capsule; menisci; and large, dynamic muscle groups all provide stability (**Figure 40.1**). In skeletally immature patients, the epiphyses for the distal femur and proximal tibia are also an important part of the knee anatomy. An immature physis may be weaker than the surrounding ligaments. As a result, injury mechanisms that might result in a ligament sprain in a skeletally mature patient may produce a physeal injury in a skeletally immature patient.

The medial collateral ligament (MCL) provides stability to valgus stress and connects the femur and tibia on the medial side of the knee. The distal femoral epiphysis acts as the proximal attachment of the MCL in the skeletally immature athlete. The MCL and medial meniscus share

common fibers and can be injured concurrently. The lateral collateral ligament (LCL) connects the lateral femoral condyle to the proximal fibula but does not share fibers with the lateral meniscus. The LCL along with posterolateral musculotendinous restraints (lateral head of gastrocnemius, distal hamstring tendons, popliteus tendons, arcuate complex) provides protection against varus stress.

The anterior cruciate ligament (ACL) originates on the anterior portion of the tibial plateau and extends in a posterolateral direction to its attachment on the lateral portion of the intercondylar notch. The ACL primarily resists anterior displacement of the tibia on the femur. It acts as a stabilizer against rotational movement between the tibia and femur along with providing backup stability to medial and lateral stress.

The posterior cruciate ligament (PCL) courses from the posterior portion of the tibial plateau to its attachment anteriorly on the medial side of the interondylar notch. The PCL functions to prevent posterior translation of the tibia on the femur at all flexion angles and contributes to rotational stability.

The medial and lateral meniscus are C-shaped, collagenous structures that act as a force couple between the rounded surface of the distal femur and the flat tibial plateau. In addition to providing enhanced joint congruence between the tibia and femur, the menisci provide stability to the knee in the same way a chock block under the wheel of a car prevents it from rolling down a hill. The lateral meniscus covers more of the tibial plateau, and it is more circular and mobile than its medial counterpart. The medial meniscus is more firmly attached at the periphery to the deep fibers of the MCL. Most of the meniscus is avascular and receives nutrition through diffusion. The perimeniscal capillary plexus supplies blood to the outer

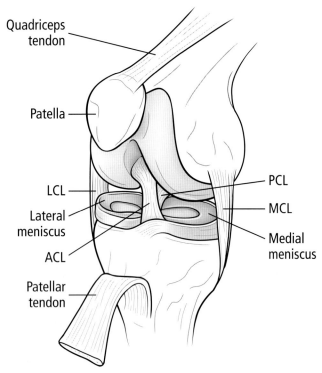

FIGURE 40.1 Knee anatomy showing major ligaments and menisci.

Flexion of the knee is the main function of the posterior and medial muscle groups, including the biceps femoris, semimembranosus, semitendinosus, gracilis, and sartorius. The semimembranosus, semitendinosus, and sartorius tendons all attach on the anterosuperior aspect of the medial tibia, forming the pes anserine tendinous complex. The pes tendon complex aids in knee flexion and contributes to dynamic stability of the knee.

EPIDEMIOLOGY

Knee injuries can occur from direct collisions with other players and by noncontact mechanisms such as jumping, pivoting, and hyperextension. Accordingly, sports such as football, basketball, soccer, lacrosse, hockey, wrestling, and alpine skiing are all high risk for acute injury.

Studies show that females are more likely to experience a knee injury compared with their male counterparts in the same sport. Particularly in basketball and soccer, females have 44% to 50% more injuries, with much of the difference related to ACL sprains. Such gender differences in knee injury rates do not exist for prepubertal athletes. Like overall injury rates, the incidence of knee injuries increases with age and skill level.

HISTORY

Determining the mechanism of injury is essential when trying to diagnose knee injuries. When a young patient does not recall how the injury occurred, witnesses such as parents, coaches, or teammates may help clarify the mechanism of injury. **Table 40.1** indicates injury mechanisms that are characteristic of specific injuries, and **Table 40.2** lists the questions clinicians should ask about acute knee injuries. An accurate history is especially important in the acute care

third of each meniscus (vascular zone). Injuries in the vascular zone of the meniscus may heal better because of the enhanced circulation. Meniscal injuries that can be surgically repaired also generally occur in the outer third of the meniscus.

Extension of the knee is provided by the quadriceps muscles, which combine to form the quadriceps tendon above the patella. The infrapatellar tendon inserts on the tibial tubercle and transmits quadriceps tension to the leg.

TABLE 40.1

Mechanism of Injury and Likely Diagnosis

Mechanism of Injury	Likely Diagnosis
Hyperextension	ACL ± meniscus tear
Hyperflexion	Medial meniscus tear
Valgus stress (direct force to outside of knee)	MCL ± medial meniscus ± ACL tear
Varus stress (direct force to inside of knee)	LCL tear
Twisting	ACL ± meniscus tear; dislocation of patella
Direct blow to anterior tibia with flexed knee	PCL tear
Direct blow to patella or femoral condyle	Patellar fracture; chondral fracture of articular cartilage

ACL indicates anterior cruciate ligament; LCL, lateral collateral ligament; MCL, medial collateral ligament; and PCL, posterior cruciate ligament.

Table 40.2

History for evaluation of acute knee injuries

- How did this injury occur?
- Was there swelling within 24 hours of the injury?
- Does your knee feel unstable or has it given out?
- Can you straighten or bend your knee all the way?
- Does your knee catch or get locked?
- Is there any history of previous injury to your knee?

setting, when the physical examination may be limited because of swelling, pain, or guarding. A running back who is tackled with a direct force to the outside of the knee (valgus stress) may sustain an injury to the MCL. A noncontact injury involving sudden stopping or pivoting (hyperextension) may result in an ACL injury.

Any injury that results in acute swelling suggests a hemarthrosis. Almost 50% of children aged 7 to 12 years and 65% of adolescents aged 13 to 18 years with a hemarthrosis have an ACL tear. Other possible causes of a hemarthrosis include patellar dislocation, fracture, or, more rarely, a meniscal tear.

Clinicians need to inquire about any previous knee injuries and prior episodes of knee instability or giving way. Recurrent instability suggests a preexisting injury from a ligament tear or patellar subluxation. Reflex quadriceps inhibition may lead to functional instability. This occurs when pain associated with patellar loading or knee movement causes inhibition of the quadriceps. The diminished quadriceps function can produce a feeling of instability or giving way. With functional instability, the knee performs as if it is more unstable than the integrity of knee ligaments would predict.

A history of catching or locking suggests a loose body, meniscal tear, or osteochondral lesion. A discoid meniscus is an anatomic variant of the lateral meniscus that occurs in 2% of the population. A discoid meniscus may produce symptoms and physical findings similar to a torn meniscus but without the typical history of a meniscal injury.

PHYSICAL EXAMINATION

The physical examination of the knee should include inspection and palpation, as well as tests of range of motion, strength, and ligamentous laxity. Because hip pathology may refer pain to the knee, hip range of motion should be examined.

The knee should be inspected for gross deformity or obvious effusion. If swelling is present, it should be determined whether the swelling is intra-articular or in the prepatellar bursa. An intra-articular effusion obscures the usual sulcus or dimple medial to the patella (**Figure 40.2**). Prepatellar swelling occurs anterior to the patella and tends to be more localized than intra-articular effusions (see Figure 40.14 later in this chapter).

Palpation should systematically evaluate key bony landmarks and assess for tenderness over the physis, joint line, and ligament attachment sites. Tenderness along the medial patellar border may indicate recent patellar subluxation or dislocation.

Strength can be assessed by observing isometric contractions, manual muscle testing, or testing strength against gravity. Strength may be difficult to assess in the acute setting because of pain and swelling. The presence of weakness after an acute injury is a relatively nonspecific finding unless the weakness is related to a specific muscle or movement. Inability to actively extend the knee may be the result of a quadriceps or patellar tendon rupture or an avulsion of the tibial tuberosity apophysis.

Ligamentous stability should be assessed for the 4 major ligaments of the knee, with particular emphasis placed on evaluation of the ACL and MCL. Because ligament stability varies among patients, an examination of the uninjured knee should be used as a baseline for comparison. The methods for assessing knee ligament stability are listed in **Table 40.3**. If pain, swelling, or guarding interfere with a reliable assessment of ligament stability, then the knee may be splinted and the examination repeated after the pain and swelling have subsided.

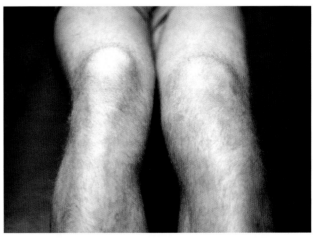

FIGURE 40.2 Appearance of intra-articular effusion in the left knee.

TABLE 40.3

Physical examination for ligamentous laxity

Ligament to Test	Maneuver	How to Perform	Other Tests
ACL	Lachman	Anterior translation of tibia with knee in 30° of flexion (see Figure 40.4)	Pivot shift
MCL	Valgus stress	Top hand acts as a fulcrum on lateral aspect of knee stressing MCL in both full extension and 20°-30° of flexion (see Figure 40.7)	…
LCL	Varus stress	Top hand acts as a fulcrum on medial aspect of knee stressing LCL in both full extension and 20°-30° of flexion	…
PCL	Tibial sag	Observe flexed knee from side view for evidence of posterior droop or sag of the tibia	Posterior drawer (see Figure 40.15)

ACL indicates anterior cruciate ligament; LCL, lateral collateral ligament; MCL, medial collateral ligament; and PCL, posterior cruciate ligament.

The McMurray test is used to determine injury to the meniscus. Internal and external rotation of the tibia with the knee maximally flexed places stress on the meniscus (**Figure 40.3**). A McMurray test that results in joint line pain, a click, or restricted motion when the knee is maximally flexed and rotated suggests a possible meniscus tear.

Patellar apprehension is often present after a patellar dislocation or with recurrent patellar subluxation. Patients will demonstrate apprehension or guarding when the examiner displaces their patella laterally (see Figure 40.11 later in this chapter).

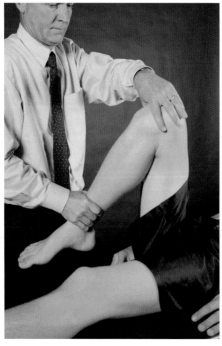

FIGURE 40.3 McMurray test.

IMAGING STUDIES

The standard radiographic series to evaluate a knee injury includes anteroposterior, lateral, and tunnel views along with a sunrise view of the patella. The anteroposterior and lateral views show fractures of the femur and tibial plateau, physeal injuries, condylar injuries, avulsion injuries of the tibial eminence, and displacement of the tibial tubercle apophysis. The tunnel view, which is an anteroposterior view done with the knee flexed to 45°, is the best way to look for an osteochondral lesion or loose bodies. A patellar view evaluates patellar alignment, patellar fracture, bipartite patella, and patellar osteochondral lesions.

Indications for radiographs include open fractures, penetrating trauma, intra-articular effusion, loss of joint motion, and inability to bear weight. Radiographs can also be used to assess skeletal maturity. Instability and swelling in a skeletally immature patient should raise concern for epiphyseal injury and avulsion fractures from where the ACL attaches to the tibial eminence. Plain films may also reveal tibial plateau fractures. The inability to bear weight for at least 4 steps at the time of the injury or in the emergency department is a good indication of possible fracture and the need for radiographs.

Magnetic resonance imaging (MRI) is often used to confirm clinical suspicion of ACL tears, PCL tears, and meniscal injury. MRI can also be used to rule out bone contusions, articular cartilage injuries, and strains of the quadriceps or patellar tendon.

ACL INJURIES

ACL tears are among the most common major knee injuries that young athletes experience, although they are rare before puberty. The frequency of ACL injuries increases with age and with participation in high-intensity, high-risk sports; female gender is also associated with higher incidence of noncontact ACL injuries in basketball and soccer. Although a single cause for the gender difference has not been shown, several theories have been proposed, including neuromuscular control, femoral notch size differences, limb alignment, and hormones. The degree of knee flexion while jumping or pivoting may also be a contributing factor. Female athletes who are more upright while pivoting or landing from a jump may be applying increased torsion to an extended knee. Since a straight knee is more vulnerable to torsional forces than a flexed knee, pivoting or landing from a jump with an extended knee may increase the risk for ACL injury.

The diagnosis of an ACL injury is usually suggested by a hyperextension or pivoting mechanism of injury and can be associated with hearing or feeling a pop in the knee. Noncontact injuries typically involve having the knee hyperextend while decelerating or changing direction. Contact injuries typically occur when the foot is planted and an anterior or lateral force to the knee causes it to hyperextend or give way. A valgus force may also commonly cause ACL injuries in combination with a sprain to the MCL and a meniscus tear. The terrible triad of an ACL, MCL, and meniscus injury should alert the clinician to look for all 3 injuries when any one of these injuries is found.

At examination, the Lachman test is the best way to determine laxity in the ACL (**Figure 40.4**). The Lachman test is done with the knee in approximately 30° of flexion. An intact ACL, or a negative Lachman test, is associated with a distinct stopping point when the tibia is pulled forward. A positive or abnormal Lachman test is noted when there is a clear increase in laxity compared with the uninjured knee or when the end point for the ACL on the injured knee is

not distinct. A pivot shift test can be used for assessment of rotatory instability of the knee. The pivot shift test may be more difficult to perform because of pain and guarding. The presence of a pivot shift is less critical to diagnosis and management than the presence of a positive Lachman test.

The anterior drawer test for diagnosing ACL injuries is limited by the fact that the hamstrings can restrict anterior translation of the tibia. Pain and guarding are more likely to interfere with interpretation of findings with an anterior drawer test. Furthermore, the anterior drawer test evaluates the ACL stability with the knee flexed to 90°. This is a relatively stable position of the knee and not a position in which the ACL is likely to be injured; nor is it a position in which ACL stability is a major contributor to knee stability. With ACL injuries, patellar tenderness and patellar apprehension are usually not present.

Diagnostic tests for suspected ACL injuries include initial plain radiographs to evaluate skeletal maturity, condylar injury, and tibial eminence fractures. MRI is often performed to confirm the diagnosis of an ACL sprain and to look for associated injuries to the meniscus or articular cartilage (**Figure 40.5**).

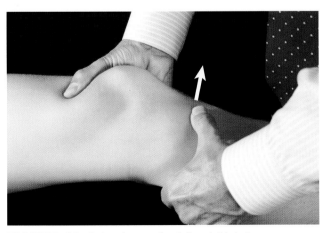

FIGURE 40.4 Lachman test for ACL injury.

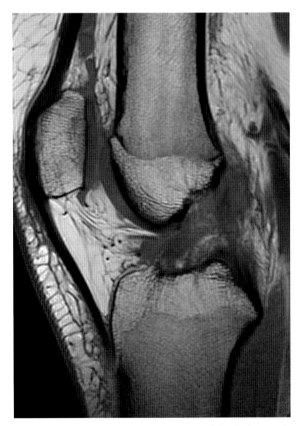

FIGURE 40.5 MRI demonstrating midsubstance tear of ACL.

The differential diagnosis in a patient with an acutely swollen and unstable knee includes patellar subluxation or dislocation, epiphyseal fracture, or tibial eminence fracture. These conditions can often be ruled out with an accurate history and physical examination along with plain radiographs. Tibial eminence fracture may be confused with an ACL injury because both have the same symptoms and physical findings. Plain radiographs of skeletally immature patients with acute knee injuries should be taken to rule out tibial eminence fractures and epiphyseal injuries (**Figure 40.6A-B**). A minimally displaced tibial eminence fracture may be effectively treated in a long leg cast with the knee in full extension. If the tibial eminence is further displaced, surgical fixation can be carried out. Although there is no particular medical urgency for treating midsubstance ACL tears in skeletally mature patients, fractures, tibial eminence avulsions, and epiphyseal injuries need prompt attention. Surgical consultation is appropriate for all of these injuries. Treatment options and outcomes may diminish with delays that go beyond 1 week from the time of injury. Although there is no particular medical urgency for treating ACL injuries, fractures and epiphyseal injuries need to be recognized and treated in a timely manner to optimize correct healing, preserve the full range of treatment options, and prevent further injury.

Treatment of the ACL tear in the skeletally immature athlete is controversial. Treatment options include managing the patient conservatively with rehabilitation and bracing or surgery. Referral to an orthopedist experienced in treating ACL injury who is experienced in physeal sparing reconstructions.

Athletes with an untreated ACL tear predictably experience functional limitations related to pivoting and jumping, further episodes of instability, and injury to secondary restraints such as the meniscus. Even with strengthening exercises and use of a protective knee brace, further episodes of instability can occur. ACL reconstruction affords the best option for restoring knee stability and minimizing the risk of additional injury. In patients with open physes, surgeons may suggest delaying ACL reconstruction because of the risk of the ACL graft disrupting growth in the physis. Therefore, skeletally immature patients with ACL tears are generally counseled to avoid high-risk activities and work with physical therapy to help restore full joint motion, strength, and proprioception. Wearing an ACL brace during activity may afford additional protection. Unfortunately, patients with ACL injuries who are treated with rehabilitation and bracing may still experience instability and functional limitations,

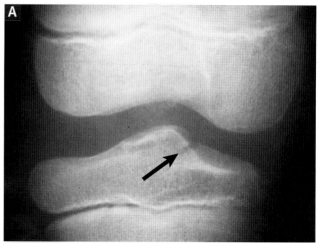
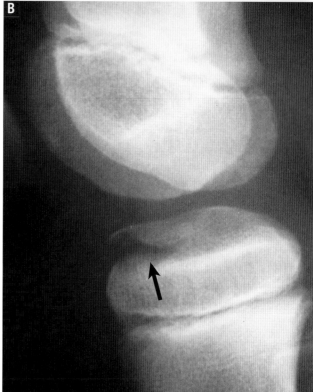

FIGURE 40.6 AP (A) and lateral (B) x-rays demonstrating tibial eminence fracture.

and they may still be at risk for further episodes of instability. Such patients may need to further modify or restrict their activities until they reach skeletal maturation and can undergo surgical reconstruction of the ACL.

For athletes with associated meniscus tears, early repair or resection of the meniscus tear may be necessary to restore motion and give rehabilitation a reasonable chance to be effective. Arthroscopic surgery to address a meniscal tear does not have to be deferred until physeal closure.

Most skeletally mature, active adolescent patients who participate in jumping or pivoting sports elect to undergo ligament reconstruction. There are no particular time constraints for undergoing ACL surgery. However, waiting 3 to 4 weeks after the original injury generally allows swelling to subside, allows range of motion to be restored, and permits some strengthening. This results in a faster recovery from surgery. Reconstructive surgery can still be effectively performed many years after the original ACL injury provided that further episodes of instability don't adversely impact function or cause irreversible damage to secondary structures such as the meniscus or articular cartilage.

Surgical reconstruction usually involves using a bone-patellar tendon-bone autograft, a hamstring tendon autograft, or an allograft from a tissue bank. Results are good or excellent more than 85% of the time and athletes can resume the sports they were participating in at the time of injury. With good surgical techniques and postoperative rehabilitation, patients can typically regain their range of motion and strength well before the 9 months of time required to allow the ACL graft to mature. Patients may feel ready to return to full sports activity before the reconstructed ligament is sufficiently strong to withstand the normal stresses associated with full activity. Even if a full return to sports is premature, there are usually some strengthening and conditioning exercises that can be done while waiting for the graft to mature. The general conditioning makes the waiting more tolerable and can help the athlete make a more rapid transition back to full activity once the graft has matured. Ongoing research and pilot programs are being developed for prevention of ACL injuries. Many of the principles underlying these programs, including proprioception exercises, running, jumping, and pivoting techniques, may prove beneficial to patients who are rehabilitating an ACL injury that has already occurred.

MCL INJURIES

Injury to the MCL occurs when a valgus force is applied to the knee of a planted or weight-bearing leg. This injury may be a direct result of blunt trauma to the lateral side of the joint. It may also occur if the knee buckles inward with cutting movements or when landing from a jump. The athlete may report a ripping or tearing sensation associated with pain over the medial aspect of the knee.

Isolated injury to the MCL rarely results in a large effusion. A large hemarthrosis associated with valgus stress is indicative of the terrible triad, which includes injuries to

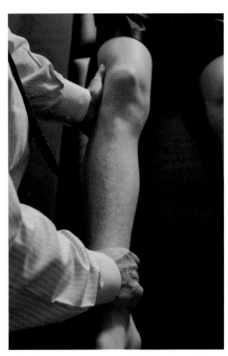

FIGURE 40.7 Physical examination for MCL stability.

the ACL and medial meniscus as well as the MCL. In the skeletally immature athlete, physeal injury or epiphyseal fracture must be considered in cases of medial pain, swelling, and instability.

Findings at physical examination include tenderness over the MCL, pain, and/or laxity with valgus stress. Valgus stress should be applied at 0° and 30° of flexion (**Figure 40. 7**). The severity of injury to the medial collateral ligament is based on the patient's response to valgus stress applied to the knee. A grade I injury is characterized by pain but no laxity with valgus stress testing. A grade II injury indicates a partial ligament tear. It is associated with increased medial laxity compared with the uninjured side, but an end point is present. A grade III injury represents a complete ligament disruption. With grade III injuries, pronounced medial laxity is present, and no end point can be discerned. Even though grade III injuries are the most severe, an examination that stresses a completely torn ligament may not be as painful as stressing a ligament that is only partially torn.

Injuries to the distal physis of the femur may be difficult to distinguish from MCL sprains. Patients with physeal injuries have medial pain and instability but also tend to have tenderness along the distal femoral physis that extends more anteriorly than the attachment site of the MCL. In skeletally immature patients with medial pain and findings suspicious of a physeal injury, plain radiographs are indicated to evaluate for physeal widening or displacement

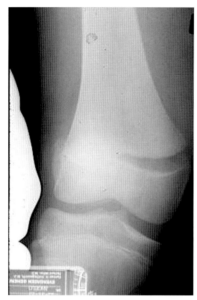

FIGURE 40.8 Stress x-ray demonstrating distal femoral physeal separation.

(**Figure 40.8**). Valgus stress to the knee during the physical examination or as part of a stress x-ray should be done with caution due to the risk of displacing the physis or related fracture fragments.

In addition to physeal injuries, the differential diagnosis for an MCL sprain includes a medial meniscal tear. The MCL and medial meniscus share common fibers. Twisting or a valgus blow can injure both structures. Occasionally, a patellar subluxation or dislocation can be confused with an MCL sprain.

Treatment for isolated MCL sprains usually is nonoperative. Initial treatment involves splinting for 1 to 4 weeks (depending on the severity of injury) with transition to a hinged brace to allow for ambulation and protected range of motion. Physical therapy can help restore joint motion, strength, and function. Treatment for a Salter-Harris fracture of the distal femoral physis requires immobilization with a cast or brace, crutches, and careful follow-up to ensure bony healing without deformity or growth disruption. Consultation with a pediatric orthopedic specialist is appropriate for management and follow-up of this and other physeal injuries.

Return-to-play criteria include completion of the physical therapy, including functional tasks such as running, pivoting, crossover steps, or grapevine exercises. An athlete who experiences pain or who favors the injured knee should be kept out of sports until more healing has taken place.

Parents may inquire about using knee braces to protect the MCL because many college and professional football teams have their players wear braces in attempt to prevent or reduce the severity of knee injuries. However, no conclusive evidence supports the use of prophylactic bracing; it may even increase the frequency of injury in selected positions of the knee.

MENISCAL INJURIES

The shape of the meniscus increases congruity between the flat tibial plateau and the round femoral condyle. The meniscus plays a fundamental role in load transmission, stability, lubrication, nutrition, and proprioception in the knee. A damaged meniscus that is untreated is likely to cause even greater problems with pain, swelling, stiffness, and arthritic change.

A discoid meniscus is a developmentally abnormal, thickened, misshapen lateral meniscus that can cause symptoms of locking or catching as a result of its abnormal shape. A discoid lateral meniscus may also be more prone to tearing or can produce symptoms of a torn meniscus without a history of acute injury.

A history of a twisting or hyperflexion injury may suggest a meniscus tear. Persistent mechanical symptoms (catching or locking), swelling, and pain also suggest the

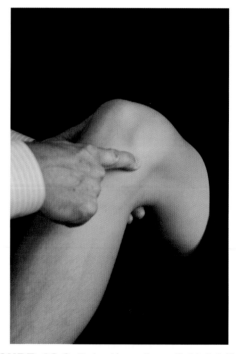

FIGURE 40.9 Palpation of medial joint line.

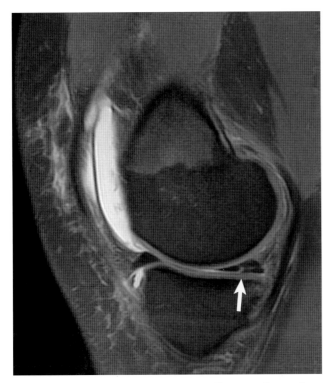

FIGURE 40.10 MRI demonstrating undersurface tear of posterior horn of medial meniscus.

diagnosis of a torn meniscus. Joint line tenderness and swelling are the most common signs (**Figure 40.9**). The McMurray test (**see Figure 40.3**) is not always positive with a torn meniscus. The diagnosis may rely on a history of swelling, locking, and catching after an acute injury or more subtle physical findings of pain or restricted motion with attempts to flex and rotate the knee. MRI has become the standard imaging modality to confirm the diagnosis of a torn meniscus (**Figure 40.10**).

The differential diagnosis of a torn meniscus includes osteochondritis dissecans, which can produce catching, locking, or swelling, either from an irregular joint surface or from a loose body. In osteochondritis dissecans, there are meniscal symptoms but usually no history of an acute injury.

A torn meniscus may heal if the tear is non-displaced and if the tear is in the vascular zone of the meniscus. Pediatric patients tend to have greater vascularity of their menisci than adults, and hence may have a slightly greater chance of healing a torn meniscus without surgical intervention. The enhanced vascularity may also improve prospects for meniscal repair. For a meniscus tear that warrants surgical treatment, the location and type of tear greatly influence the surgical treatment plan. Small vertical tears in the vascular third are usually amenable to surgical repair.

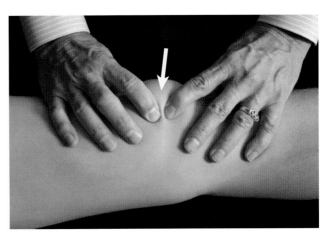

FIGURE 40.11 Patellar apprehension test.

Partial meniscectomies are usually necessary for tears that involve the avascular area of the meniscus or complex tears that involve multiple zones of the meniscus. Referral to an orthopedic surgeon experienced with knee arthroscopy is recommended.

PATELLAR INSTABILITY

With complete dislocations, the patella becomes laterally displaced from the femoral trochlea. With a patellar subluxation, the patella slides out of the femoral trochlea but reduces spontaneously. A twisting injury on a planted foot typically causes patellar dislocations or subluxations. Athletes often report a ripping or tearing sensation, followed by medial patellar pain and pronounced swelling. Physical examination usually reveals a large hemarthrosis with medial patellar tenderness, and apprehension if the patella is moved laterally (**Figure 40.11**).

When the patella is dislocated, the athlete is usually found holding the knee in a flexed position and complaining of severe pain. Reduction of the acute dislocation involves knee extension and gentle pressure to push the patella medially.

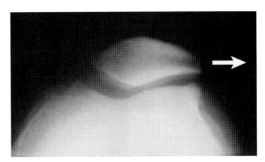

FIGURE 40.12 Sunrise radiograph demonstrating lateral subluxation of the patella.

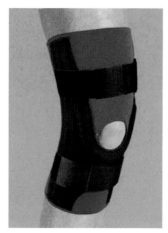

FIGURE 40.13 Patellar stabilizing brace.

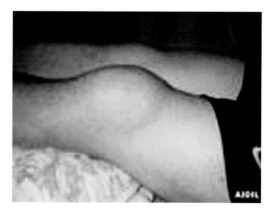

FIGURE 40.14 Knee swelling localized to prepatellar bursa.

Plain radiographs to evaluate a suspected fracture are warranted. However, radiographs are not always required prior to reducing a dislocated patella nor are they necessary to confirm that a dislocated patella has been successfully reduced. Patellar views may demonstrate subluxation, tilting of the patella, or a shallow femoral groove that predisposes the patella to tracking problems (**Figure 40.12**). Following patellar dislocation, patellar views may reveal an avulsion fracture of the medial border of the patella. MRI may be indicated to evaluate possible chondral injury or meniscal tear in athletes with persistent swelling or pain.

Treatment usually consists of immobilization for comfort, followed by rehabilitation. Restoring quadriceps strength is essential for restoring full function and stability but can be problematic if chondral injuries to the patella cause pain or become worse with quadriceps-strengthening exercises. Patellar stabilizing braces are often suggested to prevent recurrences in athletes returning to a twisting or pivoting sport, although little evidence supports their effectiveness in preventing recurrent patellar instability (**Figure 40.13**). Surgery to realign or stabilize the patella is an option for patients who experience repeated dislocations and whose injuries have failed to improve with nonsurgical treatment.

Recurrent patellar subluxation is marked by a transient, self-reducing, partial displacement of the patella from the femoral trochlea. Patellar hypermobility and apprehension are evident at physical examination. A more subtle finding is an abrupt lateral deviation of the patella as the leg is actively extended. Treatment is similar to that of acute dislocation, with aggressive rehabilitation and patella-stabilizing braces.

PREPATELLAR BURSITIS

Prepatellar bursitis is more common as an occupational overuse injury in adults who spend time on their knees (eg, roofers, carpet layers). In children, bursitis is encountered more frequently as an acute injury that results from a direct blow to the knee, from landing on a flexed knee, or from sports that involve kneeling, such as wrestling.

Physical examination usually reveals swelling localized to the prepatellar bursa. Flexion may be limited by pain and tightness due to swelling (**Figure 40.14**). Radiographs are not usually necessary to make the diagnosis but should be considered if there is suspicion for underlying patellar fracture.

Treatment consists of ice, compression, and, for more severe cases, immobilization in a splint. Range-of-motion exercise may be started when the swelling subsides and the pain improves. Physical therapy can be helpful if patellar pain is a barrier to restoring strength. Needle aspiration and drainage of the acutely swollen bursa may result in temporary relief of symptoms. Aspiration is associated with a risk of introducing infection, and the aspirated fluid often reaccumulates. Most cases of acute bursitis subside with rest and conservative care, but swelling and normal knee function may take several weeks to return to normal. Protection with a knee pad may decrease the risk of recurrent injury.

For patients with chronic symptoms or recurrent bursitis, referral to an orthopedist should be considered for possible bursectomy.

DIFFERENTIAL DIAGNOSIS OF ACUTE INJURIES

LCL Injuries

Injuries to the LCL are rare among young athletes. Injury occurs when a varus stress is applied to the knee. Like the MCL, the LCL is extra-articular, with little swelling associated with isolated injury. However, the LCL is not as closely opposed to the meniscus, and associated injury to the lateral meniscus is therefore rare. The differential diagnosis of acute lateral knee pain includes a torn lateral meniscus, sprain to the proximal tibiofibular joint, biceps femoris strain, popliteus strain, and tibial plateau fracture. Posterolateral knee pain can also be seen in conjunction with an ACL sprain. A complete tear of the LCL may require surgical treatment. Since many of the conditions seen in association with acute lateral knee pain may require surgical intervention, consultation with an orthopedic specialist may be beneficial prior to planning therapy or clearing the athlete to return to play.

PCL Sprain

Injury to the PCL is also rare in children and adolescents. The mechanism of injury is a direct posterior force to the anterior tibia with the knee flexed, such as a fall off a bicycle or when a baseball catcher is squatting to block home plate from a sliding baserunner. Severe hyperextension injuries may result in a PCL tear, although the ACL usually fails first. Physical examination may reveal a positive posterior drawer test or posterior sagging of the tibia (**Figure 40.15**).

Plain radiographs should be obtained to rule out epiphyseal or physeal fractures.

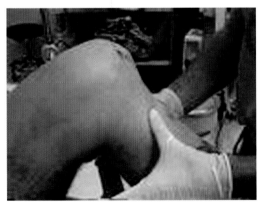

FIGURE 40.15 Posterior laxity associated with PCL sprain.

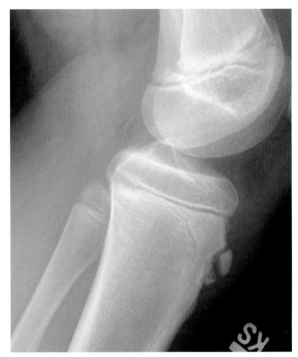

FIGURE 40.16 Tibial tuberosity avulsion fracture.

Suspicion of a PCL injury should result in a referral to an orthopedist. Unlike ACL injuries, PCL sprains are more likely to respond to nonsurgical treatment.

Tibial Tuberosity Avulsion Fractures

Tibial tuberosity fractures are rare injuries that affect patients whose tibial tubercle has not completely ossified (**Figure 40.16**). The mechanism of injury usually involves a forceful contraction of the quadriceps that occurs concurrently with knee flexion. At examination, the clinician may note swelling, tenderness over the tibial tubercle, and difficulty with active knee extension. Plain radiographs are diagnostic, with either partial or complete avulsion of the tuberosity. The knee should be splinted in extension, and the patient should use crutches. Referral to an orthopedic surgeon for further management is suggested to address fixation of the fracture and to assess possible injury to the tibial physis or articular surface.

DIFFERENTIAL DIAGNOSIS

Other acute knee injuries include patellar fractures, physeal injuries, chondral fractures, and sprains of the proximal tibiofibular ligament. Any knee injury resulting in acute swelling or difficulty bearing weight deserves a more thorough evaluation, including plain radiographs. Tenderness over the tibial or femoral physis raises concern for a Salter-Harris type 1 injury, even if plain radiographs are normal. MRI is warranted for athletes with persistent swelling, loss of range of motion, or significant disability.

RETURN TO PLAY

Before returning to play, athletes who experienced acute knee injuries must have resolved joint swelling, regained full range of motion, and restored symmetric strength. Prior to returning to play, patients should complete a course of functional rehabilitation. This includes the ability to run, pivot, jump, and perform sport-specific skills without pain, swelling or other limitation.

SUMMARY POINTS

- Understanding the mechanism of acute knee injuries helps focus the clinical evaluation, select appropriate diagnostic tests, and establish an accurate diagnosis.

- Physeal or epiphyseal injury needs to be considered in the differential diagnosis of all acute knee injuries in skeletally immature patients.

- A thorough physical examination will be sufficient to correctly diagnose most ligament sprains to the knee, patellar instabilities, and meniscal tears.

- Radiographs assess skeletal maturity, rule out fractures, and exclude physeal injuries. MRIs confirm suspected injuries to soft tissue structures such as ligaments, menisci, and articular cartilage.

- Many acute knee injuries can be effectively treated with conservative measures, including physical therapy.

- Return to play after an acute knee injury requires resolution of swelling, restoration of normal joint motion and strength, and ability to perform the functional tasks required by the sport.

- There is no single strategy, including prophylactic bracing, that has consistently proven to be effective in preventing acute knee injuries. Injuries may be reduced by limiting exposure to high-risk activities and through the use of preventive strategies that are still being investigated.

SUGGESTED READING

Albright JP, Powell JW, Smith W, et al. Medial collateral ligament knee sprains in college football: effectiveness of preventive braces. *Am J Sports Med.* 1994;22: 12-18.

Bjordal JM, Arnoy F, Hannestad B, et al. Epidemiology of anterior cruciate ligament injuries in soccer. *Am J Sports Med.* 1997;25:341-345.

Graf BK, Lange RH, Fujisaki CK, Landry GL, Saluja RK. Anterior cruciate ligament tears in skeletally immature patients: meniscal pathology at presentation and after attempted conservative management. *Arthroscopy.* 1992;8:229-233.

Louw QA, Manilall J Grimmer KA. Epidemiology for knee injuries among adolescents: a systematic review. *Br J Sports Med.* 2008;42(1):2-10.

McCarroll JR, Shelbourne KD, Porter DA, Rettig AC, Murray S. Patellar tendon graft reconstruction for mid-substance anterior cruciate ligament rupture in junior high school athletes: an algorithm for management. *Am J Sports Med.* 1994;22:478-484.

Moore BR, Hampers LC, Clark KD. Performance of a decision rule for radiographs of pediatric knee injuries. *J Emerg Med.* 2005;28:257-261.

Parkkari J, Pasanen K, Mattila VM, et al. The risk for a cruciate ligament injury of the knee in adolescents and young adults. a population-based cohort study of 46,500 people with a 9 year follow-up. *Br J Sports Med.* 2008;42(6):422-426.

Powell JW, Barber-Foss KD. Sex-related injury patterns among selected high school sports. *Am J Sports Med.* 2000;28:385-391.

Renstrom P, Ljungqvist A, Arendt E, et al. Non-contract injuries in female athletes: an International Olympic Committee current concepts statement. *Br J Sports Med.* 2008;42(6):394-412.

Stanitski CL, Harvell JC, Fu F. Observations on acute knee hemarthrosis in children and adolescents. *J Pediatr Orthop.* 1993;13:506-510.

Wroble RR, Henderson RC, Campion ER, et al. Meniscectomy in children and adolescents: a long-term follow-up study. *Clin Orthop Relat Res.* 1992;279:180-189.

CHAPTER 41

Overuse Injuries of the Knee

David T. Bernhardt, MD

Running or jumping sports such as track, cross-country, soccer, basketball, volleyball, and dance place excessive stresses on the extensor mechanism of the knee that can lead to pain and injury. Frequently, this pain is anterior in location and is the result of patellofemoral stress syndrome, Osgood-Schlatter disease, or patellar tendonitis. The excessive forces across the patellofemoral joint and excessive tension on the patellar tendon, combined with a myriad of biomechanical factors, play an important role in the cause of these problems. This chapter focuses on the most common causes of overuse-related knee pain. It reviews key aspects of the clinical evaluation, including history, physical examination, differential diagnosis, treatment, and prevention options.

ANATOMY AND BIOMECHANICS

Understanding the patellofemoral joint and the forces related to active extension of the knee is key to understanding overuse injuries. Active extension of the knee is provided by the quadriceps muscles, which transmit force through the quadriceps tendon, patella, and patellar tendon (**Figure 41.1**). The patella serves as a fulcrum to enhance the mechanical advantage of the quadriceps for extending the knee. The patella functions to improve power of the quadriceps by lengthening the lever arm from the quadriceps-tendon complex to the axis of knee flexion. Active flexion of the knee occurs primarily through the action of the hamstring muscles.

The patellofemoral joint is an area subjected to considerable frictional and compressive loads from activities that involve repetitive flexion and extension of the knee. The compressive forces on the patella are proportional to quadriceps tension and the degree of knee flexion (**Figure 41.2**). The patella normally glides smoothly through the femoral trochlea with flexion and extension of the knee. In full extension, the patella does not articulate with the femoral trochlea. At 20° of knee flexion, first contact is made across the medial and lateral facet of the patella. Joint reaction forces, or the force per unit area at the patellofemoral joint, increase in proportion to knee flexion and quadriceps tension. The depth of the patellar groove provides bony stability for the patella and a track in which the patella can move with knee motion.

When the patella tracks centrally in the patellar grove, there is a maximum surface area available for distributing compressive loads on the patella. When the patella tracks laterally or outside of the patellar grove, patellar compressive forces are concentrated to a smaller area of the patella and, hence, the patellofemoral joint reaction forces are increased (**Figure 41.3**). An abnormally shallow patellar groove contributes to patellar instability. The resultant tracking abnormalities cause uneven distribution of patellar compressive forces. With normal patellar tracking, the compressive forces and friction can lead to injury. However, when the patellar tracking is abnormal, the uneven distribution of forces can significantly lower the threshold for injury.

COMMON OVERUSE INJURIES

Areas of maximal tenderness frequently correlate with diagnosis (**Figure 41.4**). Overuse injuries of the knee tend to produce pain and tenderness near the location of the injured structure. Familiarity with surface anatomy can facilitate making a proper diagnosis.

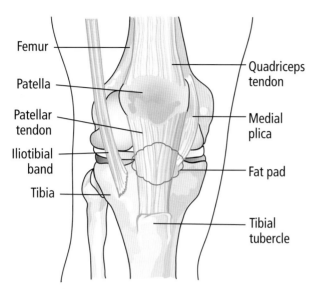

FIGURE 41.1 Anterior knee anatomy.

Femur

Patella

Patellar tendon

Iliotibial band

Tibia

Quadriceps tendon

Medial plica

Fat pad

Tibial tubercle

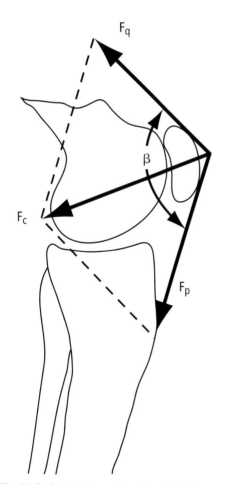

FIGURE 41.2 Determinants of patellofemoral compression forces. β, Angle of knee flexion; F_c, compression force on patellofemoral joint; F_p, patellar tendon force; F_q, quadriceps force.

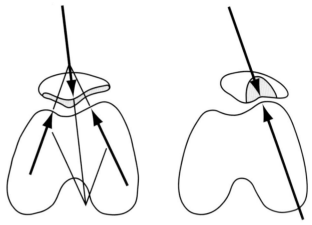

FIGURE 41.3 Distribution of compressive forces on patella with normal tracking and lateral tracking.

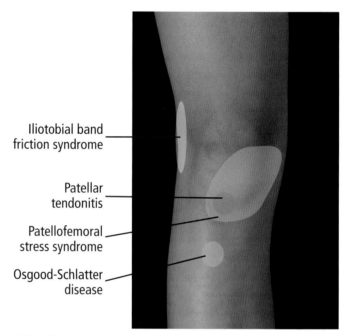

Iliotobial band friction syndrome

Patellar tendonitis

Patellofemoral stress syndrome

Osgood-Schlatter disease

FIGURE 41.4 Areas of maximal tenderness for specific diagnoses.

Patellofemoral Stress Syndrome

Patellofemoral stress syndrome (PFSS) is among the most common overuse conditions that bring athletes to see their primary care provider. This condition has historically been referred to as chondromalacia patella. Chondromalacia means "softened cartilage." While softened, thinned, or irregular cartilage may be seen in association with PFSS, chondromalacia patella is a pathologic diagnosis and should be reserved for patients who have radiologic or surgical evidence of softening of cartilage. The clinicopathologic correlation between cartilage softening and patellofemoral pain is poor. It is possible to have patellofemoral pain with no pathologic evidence of chondromalacia, and it is possible for the patient to have chondromalacia without patellofemoral pain.

The history and physical examination are crucial to establishing an accurate diagnosis and identifying the specific factors that may be contributing to the problem. There is no single cause of PFSS. A variety of intrinsic and extrinsic factors can be associated with this problem and the causes may differ among different individuals despite having the same diagnosis. Intrinsic factors may include malalignment, patellar hypermobility, inadequate flexibility, or strength imbalances. Malalignment problems that have been associated with this condition include femoral anteversion, tibial torsion, and foot hyperpronation. Lower extremity malalignment contributes to abnormal patellar tracking and increased forces at the patellofemoral joint.

Extrinsic factors include abnormalities related to training, equipment, and terrain. Training errors, such as rapid increases in the intensity, duration, frequency, or type of workouts (eg, sprinting and hill work), may lead to increased stress across the patellofemoral joint. Shoes that provide inadequate arch support or hindfoot cushioning may be a contributing factor. Equipment problems, including a bicycle with the seat too low, can contribute to patellofemoral pain.

The most common manifestation of PFSS is insidious onset of dull, diffuse, aching anterior knee pain with activity. The pain may manifest bilaterally or unilaterally. The pain is often worse with prolonged sitting or squatting, or with direct pressure from kneeling. Some patients report mild swelling or a sense of the knee feeling weak or unstable. Reports of crepitation or grinding are also common.

The physical examination begins with an inspection of the lower extremities in the standing position looking for malalignment (**Figure 41.5**). The quadriceps angle (Q angle) is measured in the standing position and is formed by the angle between a line from the midportion of the patella through the tibial tubercle and a line from the midpoint of the patella to the anterior superior iliac spine. Normally, this angle should measure up to 10° for boys and 15° for girls. An increased Q angle creates a vector for lateral patellar tracking and abnormal patellofemoral loads. Patients with internal femoral rotation and/or external tibial rotation tend to have an increased Q angle. On inspection, patients with increased femoral anteversion may appear to have "squinting patella." In this condition, the patellae tend to face inward rather than straight ahead. Hyperpronation can also contribute to an increased Q angle and should be evaluated as part of the assessment for malalignment (**Figure 41.6**).

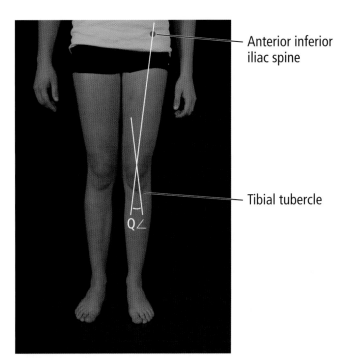

FIGURE 41.5 Lower extremity malalignment.

Anterior inferior iliac spine

Tibial tubercle

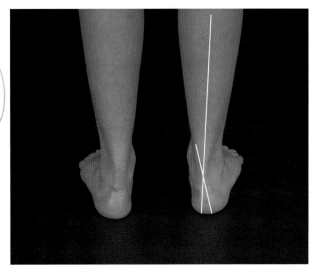

FIGURE 41.6 Appearance of hyperpronation (posterior view).

A high-riding patella is another form of patellar alignment that can be associated with PFSS. A high-riding patella or "patella alta" is associated with patellar hypermobility since the patella sits above the femoral sulcus. Without the benefit of the stability that is conferred by articulation in the femoral sulcus, the patella tends to track erratically. Finally, a patella that rests lateral to the femoral sulcus can also be associated with PFSS. Laterally positioned patellae have been described as "grasshopper eyes" because they face outward rather than straight ahead.

Patellar tracking can be observed by having patients extend their knee from a seated position. In patients with abnormal tracking or a tight lateral retinaculum, the patella may abruptly move laterally as the knee moves into extension. After assessing patients for lower extremity alignment and patellar tracking, the examination continues with an inspection for swelling, erythema, or increased warmth. Quadriceps atrophy or diminished vastus medialis definition may be noted. Knee range of motion and ligamentous stability should be evaluated. Palpation may reveal tenderness under the medial patellar facet or with compression of the patella. Plain radiographs are often normal but may reveal conditions in the differential diagnosis, such as osteochondritis dissecans or a bipartite patella (**Figure 41.7**).

Treatment of PFSS should focus on modifying or correcting the intrinsic and extrinsic factors that have been identified as causes. Usually rest or activity modification is required. It may be helpful to suggest alternate forms of conditioning that do not require repetitive knee flexion. Swimming, in-line skating, or elliptical machines may be tolerated as options to maintain fitness. Training errors need to be specifically addressed with the athlete, his or her parents, and the coach. Ice and anti-inflammatory medications may be helpful in

controlling pain or inflammation associated with the injury. Physical therapy can be helpful in addressing intrinsic factors such as core and hip weakness, hamstring tightness, strength imbalances, and patellar tracking dysfunction.

Biomechanical abnormalities that appear to contribute to abnormal patellar tracking should also be addressed. Correction of hyperpronation with either over-the-counter or custom orthotics may be helpful in reducing stress on the patella from abnormal tracking. For the athlete who demonstrates patellar hypermobility or tracking problems, a patellar stabilization sleeve may be prescribed. Patellar taping can also relieve pain from abnormal patellar tracking. In the child or adolescent with refractory pain, compliance with activity guidelines and treatment should be verified. When treatment guidelines are followed, persistent pain raises concern for alternative diagnoses or for more advanced cases of PFSS. Surgical treatment for PFSS is rarely necessary and not always effective when carried out. Surgical shaving of rough cartilage from chondromalacia unfortunately does not restore normal cartilage and does not improve the capability of the patellofemoral joint to handle compressive loads. A lateral release or patellar realignment surgery may be done in attempt to improve patellar tracking, but many patients still have pain due to the damage sustained prior to the surgery.

Osgood-Schlatter Disease

Osgood-Schlatter disease, or tibial tubercle apophysitis, is a common cause of knee pain in the skeletally immature athlete. This condition is not really a disease. Rather, it results from repetitive tension causing microavulsions of the apophyseal cartilage where the patellar tendon inserts on the tibial tuberosity apophysis.

Typically, Osgood-Schlatter disease begins as an insidious onset of achy knee pain over the tibial tubercle. Patients are typically boys aged 11 to 15 years, but girls in a slightly younger age range can also be affected. There is usually a history of high levels of running or jumping activity or a recent increase in the overall activity level. The pain may become more severe with activity and can be worsened by direct impact or a fall on a hard surface. Physical examination reveals point tenderness directly over a prominent, swollen tibial tubercle. Radiographs are not necessary to make the diagnosis but can be helpful to assess the degree of bony maturation; to look for separation or avulsion of the apophysis; and to rule out other conditions in the differential diagnosis such as a bone cyst, tumor, or infection (**Figure 41.8**).

Like PFSS, Osgood-Schlatter disease is best managed with activity modification, ice, and time. The symptoms from Osgood-Schlatter disease will resolve when the tibial tubercle

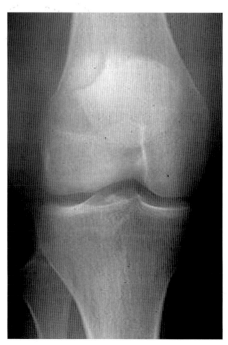

FIGURE 41.7 Bipartite patella.

apophysis matures and fuses to the tibia. However, if the tension on the immature apophysis can be relieved, it is possible to resume activity before skeletal maturity is reached. Flexibility exercises for the hamstrings and quadriceps can reduce tension on the quadriceps and patellar tendon. Tight hamstrings provide resistance for knee extension. The additional quadriceps work to overcome hamstring resistance can unnecessarily increase tension on the tibial tubercle apophysis and contribute to further pain.

An infrapatellar strap may be helpful in providing symptomatic relief by changing the tension of the tendon on its insertion. When pain has subsided, flexibility has been improved, and light or moderate forms of exercise are tolerated, it may be possible for the patient to gradually resume running and jumping activities. Specific suggestions for a safe rate of activity increase are helpful, and the rate of increase may need to be altered according to pain.

Patellar Tendonitis

Patellar tendonitis, or jumper's knee, is another common condition related to running or repetitive jumping. Patellar tendonitis is more likely to occur after the tibial tubercle apophysis matures. Studies suggest that between 7% and

14% of adolescent volleyball and basketball players may experience this condition during a season. Although the term *tendonitis* suggests an inflammatory condition of the tendon related to overuse, its cause may instead be related to microscopic tearing or damage to the collagen, along with neovascularization.

Patellar tendonitis manifests as an achy to sharp pain localized over the proximal portion of the tendon with focal tenderness directly over the inferior pole of the patella (**Figure 41.9**). The patellar tendon is vulnerable to excessive tension as well as torsion. Therefore, hamstring and quadriceps flexibility should be assessed to look for sources of excessive tension on the patellar tendon. Lateral patellar tracking, hyperpronation, and patellar hypermobility may all contribute to increased torsion on the patellar tendon. Plain radiographs are usually normal. Occasionally, a traction spur at the tendon attachment can be seen. MRI is useful for evaluating more advanced forms of patellar tendonitis where microscopic tears coalesce to form a swollen, cystic, degenerative nidus of necrotic tissue at the inferior patellar pole (**Figure 41.10**).

Treatment should focus on reducing activities that cause pain as well as on correcting intrinsic and extrinsic factors that contribute to patellar tendon overload. Ice and judicious nonsteroidal anti-inflammatory medications may be used. Physical therapy focusing on hamstring, quadriceps, and hip flexor flexibility is often helpful. Biomechanical abnormalities, particularly those that contribute to increased torsion on the patellar tendon, should also be addressed. As the pain subsides, exercises focusing on strengthening the core, hip abductors, and quadriceps can ensue. Patellar tendon straps or knee sleeves with inferior buttresses can also be helpful in addressing biomechanical abnormalities

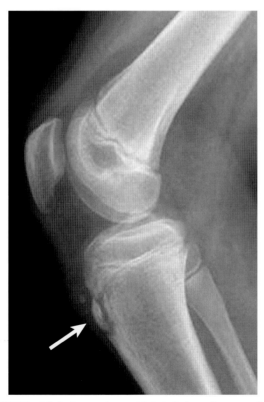

FIGURE 41.8 Immature tibial tubercle apophysis with Osgood-Schlatter disease.

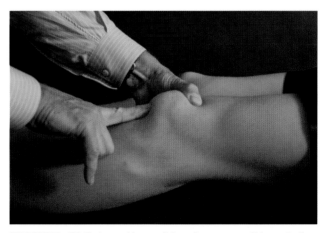

FIGURE 41.9 Location of tenderness with patellar tendonitis.

should be no evidence of swelling, joint line tenderness, or pain with McMurray's test. If the history and physical examination are consistent with a diagnosis of ITBFS, radiographic testing, including MRI, is not necessary.

Treatment for this condition should focus on limiting impact activities and on anti-inflammatory care with ice and nonsteroidal anti-inflammatory drugs. Stretching the iliotibial band and hamstrings (**Figure 41.13**) may also relieve friction over the lateral femoral condyle, and strengthening the gluteal and hip abductors may help with shock absorption associated with heel strike. Biomechanical factors should also be addressed, including correction of leg length discrepancy and providing adequate shock absorption in the form of a more cushioned shoe or a shoe insert. Finally, patients need to be educated on training errors; in particular, they should be counseled to avoid hard surfaces, excessive downhill running, or a rapid increase in activity.

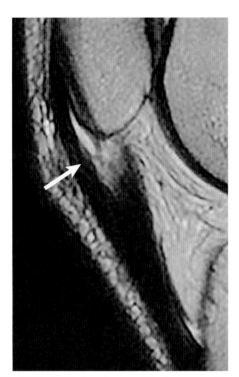

FIGURE 41.10 MRI showing cystic degenerative changes associated with advanced patellar tendonitis.

and relieving pain. Return to sports must be gradual to avoid recurrence.

Iliotibial Band Friction Syndrome

Iliotibial band friction syndrome (ITBFS) is a common cause of lateral knee pain in runners. The syndrome results from the iliotibial band sliding over the lateral femoral condyle as the knee moves between flexion and extension. This syndrome is characterized by pain over the posterolateral aspect of the knee and is usually described as dull or achy in quality. The pain is typically worse when running downhill, running on hard surfaces, or running in shoes that lack shock absorption. Runners who stop, start, and change directions are less likely to experience ITBFS than those who run continuously. The pain associated with ITBFS can be severe enough to prevent running, but it typically subsides rapidly with rest or if knee flexion is avoided.

Physical examination commonly reveals varus alignment where the patient is bowlegged and has a high-arched, cavus foot. Leg length discrepancies may be noted; ITBFS occurs most commonly on the shorter leg. A tight iliotibial band can be demonstrated by a positive Ober's test (**Figure 41.11**). If tenderness is present, it is usually found over the posterior fibers of the iliotibial band at the level of the lateral femoral condyle (**Figure 41.12**). There

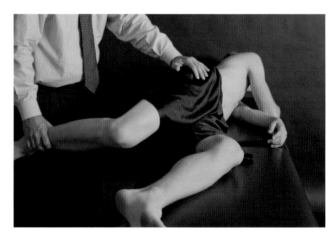

FIGURE 41.11 Ober's test for tightness of iliotibial band.

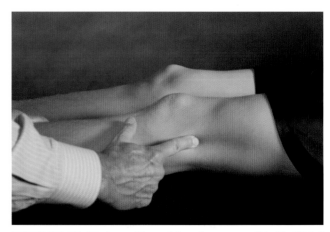

FIGURE 41.12 Location of tenderness with iliotibial band friction syndrome.

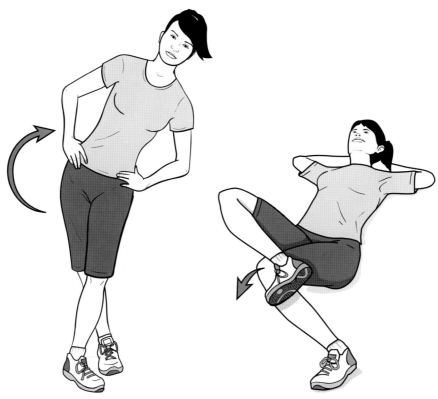

FIGURE 41.13 Stretches for the IT band.

DIFFERENTIAL DIAGNOSIS OF OVERUSE KNEE INJURIES

PFSS is the most common overuse injury to the knee, but there are other conditions in the differential diagnosis that have different causes and different treatments.

Discoid Meniscus

A discoid meniscus is an abnormally shaped meniscus where meniscal tissue covers most of the tibial plateau. A discoid meniscus most commonly involves the lateral meniscus. Although it is usually asymptomatic, this anatomic variant may cause clicking, popping, or catching. A discoid meniscus may also become torn in circumstances that would not be expected to cause a tear in a normal meniscus. If a discoid lateral meniscus becomes torn, it causes symptoms and physical findings similar to a tear in a normal meniscus, including swelling, catching, and/or locking of the knee. Examination reveals tenderness over the lateral joint line.

There may be a painful catch or clunk associated with active knee extension. Diagnosis is based on an MRI or diagnostic arthroscopy (**Figure 41.14**). An asymptomatic discoid meniscus that has been identified as an incidental

finding warrants no restrictions to activity or formal treatment. A symptomatic discoid meniscus that is not torn can be treated with activity modification and observation. If it becomes increasingly symptomatic, causes locking in the knee, or becomes torn, arthroscopic surgical evaluation should be considered.

Osteochondritis Dissecans

Osteochondritis dissecans is a developmental condition that occurs in skeletally immature patients. While osteochondritis dissecans is not an overuse injury, it frequently presents in the context of knee pain that develops gradually. The pathologic changes involve focal areas of hypovascularity that can lead to necrosis of the bone, bony collapse, and ultimately, detachment of a fragment of bone and the overlying cartilage. Osteochondritis dissecans most commonly occurs on the lateral aspect of the medial femoral condyle.

Patients with osteochondritis dissecans may be asymptomatic, or they may have symptoms of pain, swelling, catching, or locking in the knee. There is usually no history of acute or overuse injury. Physical examination may reveal intra-articular swelling, joint line tenderness, restricted joint motion, and occasionally, a positive

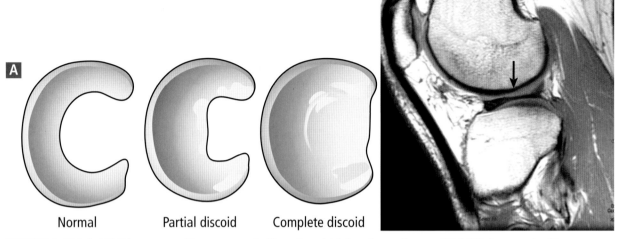

FIGURE 41.14 (A) Diagrammatic representation discoid lateral meniscus. (B) MRI demonstrating same.

Normal   Partial discoid   Complete discoid

McMurray's test. Ligament testing is normal. Plain radiographs, including an AP, lateral, and notch view, are usually sufficient to make the diagnosis. In the early stages, osteochondritis dissecans may appear as a hyperlucency in the interchondylar notch (**Figure 41.15**). In later stages, there may be deformity of the joint or a visible loose body (**Figure 41.16**).

The differential diagnosis for osteochondritis dissecans includes a torn meniscus, a symptomatic discoid meniscus, medial plica syndrome, and patellofemoral stress syndrome. If osteochondritis dissecans is diagnosed in the early stages, healing may occur with conservative measures such as limiting impact activity and protecting the knee with a brace or use of crutches. Activities can gradually be resumed when

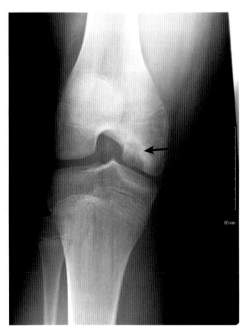

FIGURE 41.15 Early changes of osteochondritis dissecans in knee.

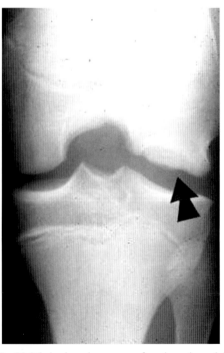

FIGURE 41.16 Late changes of osteochondritis dissecans in knee (involving lateral femoral condyle).

there is evidence of clinical and radiographic healing. The prognosis is improved if the patient is skeletally immature at the time of diagnosis and if treatment commences before the osteochondritic lesion has collapsed or become detached. If the patient doesn't improve with conservative measures, if the diagnosis is made at a more advanced stage, or if the patient is approaching skeletal maturity, surgical consultation is advisable. Surgical treatment can include arthroscopic drilling of the lesion in an attempt to stimulate blood flow and promote healing. If there is a detached osteochondral fragment, surgical fixation or resection may be indicated.

Medial Plica Syndrome

Medial plica syndrome is another cause of anteromedial knee pain in runners. The plica is a synovial septae remnant that can become irritated with repetitive knee flexion or direct trauma to the medial retinaculum. The medial plica extends from around or under the medial facet of the patella and extends medially and distally toward the medial fat pad and the medial joint space (**Figure 41.17**). The plica is a normally existing structure. However, if it becomes inflamed, patients will develop symptoms, including a vague medial knee pain that worsens with knee flexion. They may also experience a snapping or catching sensation that mimics a meniscus tear. Physical examination reveals tenderness directly over the palpably thickened medial plica. Treatment focuses on anti-inflammatory measures, mobilization of the tight and thickened plica, patellar taping or a patellar sleeve, and correction of any biomechanical abnormalities that may contribute to patellar tracking dysfunction. Surgical excision of a pathologic plica can be effective at relieving symptoms if other potential sources of pain have been ruled out.

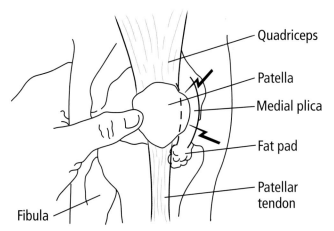

FIGURE 41.17 Diagrammatic representation of inflamed medial plica.

Fat Pad Impingement

Fat pad impingement or Hoffa disease is characterized by vague, achy pain deep to the patella tendon. Unlike other causes of anterior knee pain, where the symptoms are worse with knee flexion, fat pad impingement pain is worse with terminal extension of the knee. Ballet dancers, gymnasts, swimmers, or other athletes who repeatedly kick or maximally extend their knees are at increased risk for fat pad impingement. Even the most lean patients have fatty tissue in the intercondylar notch. This tissue acts as a shock absorber and provides lubrication to the knee. Physical examination demonstrates tenderness directly over the lateral and/or medial fat pad, and there may be a visible fullness around the patellar tendon that is most obvious when the knee is extended. Patients typically experience pain with active or passive extension of the knee. Full knee extension may be limited. In patients with genu recurvatum, there may be full extension, but the symptomatic knee may lack the hyperextensibility of the asymptomatic knee. Treatment for fat pad impingement involves measures to decrease swelling and inflammation in the fat pad and avoidance of activity associated with rapid or forceful knee extension. Bicycling is usually well tolerated because the knee does not fully or rapidly extend with this activity. Symptomatic relief with a corticosteroid injection can help confirm the diagnosis and can also be used to treat problematic cases. Inadvertent corticosteroid injection into or near the patellar tendon can result in tendon rupture. Surgical resection of the fat pad is rarely necessary.

Sinding-Larsen Johansson Disease

Sinding-Larsen Johansson disease, or patellar apophysitis, is a result of repetitive traction forces exerted by the patellar tendon pulling on the inferior patellar apophysis. Sinding-Larsen Johansson disease manifests much like Osgood-Schlatter disease but tends to occur in a younger age group (10-13 years) and involves an apophysis at the proximal end of the patellar tendon rather than the distal end. Patients often report infrapatellar pain that is exacerbated by running, climbing, and kneeling. Physical examination reveals focal tenderness at the distal pole of the patella in a similar location to where patellar tendonitis occurs. Plain radiographs demonstrate irregular calcification at the distal pole of the patella (**Figure 41.18**). Treatment is similar to that of Osgood-Schlatter disease; activity modification, anti-inflammatory care, flexibility exercises, and a gradual resumption of activity are suggested. A knee sleeve with an infrapatellar buttress or a patellar strap may also be a helpful adjunct to treatment.

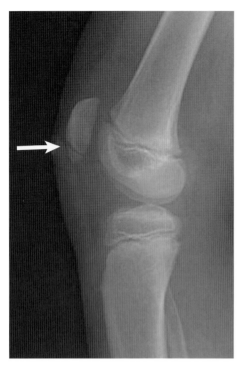

FIGURE 41.18 X-ray finding of Sinding-Larsen Johansson disease.

SUMMARY POINTS

- Overuse injuries of the knee are typically caused by a combination of extrinsic and intrinsic risk factors.

- A careful history is necessary to identify abnormalities of training and equipment that may be contributing to the injury, and the physical examination should include assessment of flexibility, strength, and lower extremity biomechanical abnormalities.

- PFSS is the most common overuse injury to the knee. PFSS results from excessive forces of compression and friction at the patellofemoral joint. Treatment depends on proper identification of relevant risk factors, and the treatment for this diagnosis may vary between individuals according to the specific underlying causes.

- Diagnostic imaging for overuse knee injuries includes radiographs to evaluate skeletal maturation, bony abnormalities, and apophyseal injuries. MRI evaluates soft tissue abnormalities, including chondromalacia, meniscal pathology, and tendonitis.

- Developmental variants and growth-related conditions contribute to many overuse knee injuries.

- Treatment of overuse injuries to the knee requires identification and correction of the underlying causes as well as outlining suitable options for maintaining fitness during the rehabilitation process and providing guidelines to allow for a gradual resumption of activity once treatment has been completed.

SUGGESTED READING

Bloom OJ, Mackler L. What is the best treatment for Osgood-Schlatter disease? *J Family Pract.* 2004;53:153-156.

Fredericson M, Weir A. Practical management of iliotibial band friction syndrome in runners. *Clin J Sports Med.* 2006;16:261-268.

Gisslen K, Alfredson H. Neovascularization and pain in jumper's knee: a prospective clinical and sonographic study in elite junior volleyball players. *Br J Sports Med.* 2005;39:423-428.

Kujala UM, Kvist M, Heinonen O. Osgood-Schlatter's disease in adolescent athletes: retrospective study of incidence and duration. *Am J Sports Med.* 1985;13:236-240.

LaBellla CR, Huxford MR, Smith TL, Cartland J. Preseason neuromuscular exercise program reduces sports-related knee pain in adolescent athletes. *Clin Pediatr.* 2009; 48:327-330.

Medlar RC, Lyne ED. Sinding-Larsen-Johannson: its etiology and natural history. *JBJS.* 1978;60:1113-1116.

Wall EJ, Vourazeris J, Meyer GD et al. The healing potential of stable juvenile osteochondritis dissecans knee lesions. *J Bone Joint Surg Am.* 2008;90(12):2655-2664.

CHAPTER 42

Lower Leg

Michael C. Koester, MD

The lower leg, including the tibia and fibula, is subject to injury from both acute forces and chronic repetitive stresses. Injuries include fractures, contusions, muscle strains, periostitis, stress fractures, and compartment syndromes. This chapter reviews common acute injuries as well as the most frequent causes of chronic leg pain. Biomechanical factors that predispose athletes to overuse injuries of the lower legs are also discussed, as are treatment options that address specific biomechanical abnormalities.

ANATOMY

The lower leg consists of the tibia and fibula, which are bound together by syndesmotic ligaments proximally and distally and an interosseous membrane spanning the distance between them. Although the fibula is critical in providing lateral stability to the ankle joint and ligamentous stability to the knee, it bears only approximately 15% of the weight borne by the lower leg.

Except for the anteromedial aspect of the tibia, the bones of the lower leg are surrounded by muscles. These muscles are divided into 4 distinct compartments: anterior, lateral, superficial posterior, and deep posterior (**Figure 42.1**). The compartments are enclosed by fascia. Each compartment contains muscles as well as nerves and vascular structures traveling distally to the foot. Limited compliance of the enveloping fascia restricts swelling within the compartments. High pressure within a muscle compartment may compromise muscle, nerve, and/or vascular function, leading to acute or exertional compartment syndromes.

The muscles of the leg also have attachments to the periosteum of the tibia and fibula (**Figure 42.2**). This anatomic arrangement helps the muscle shield the bones from stress and dissipate impact forces. Microscopic tears of the muscle attachment on the periosteum occur with medial tibial

stress syndrome (MTSS), also known as shin splints. If the protective role of these muscles is compromised, continued impact activities can lead to stress fracture.

BIOMECHANICS

The elements of gait associated with normal walking and running include a stance phase and a swing phase. The stance phase includes heel strike, midstance, and push-off. The swing phase is non–weight-bearing and essentially allows the leg to recover and prepare for the next step. Most overuse injuries are related to events that take place during the stance phase.

When the foot comes in contact with the ground at heel strike, the subtalar joint begins to pronate. Pronation allows the foot to adapt to the surface and helps absorb shock by dissipating impact forces. Between midstance and push-off, the subtalar joint supinates. Supination allows the foot to assume a more stable configuration and allows the foot to function as a rigid lever for push-off. Pronation and supination are normal components of gait, although injuries may occur with excessive pronation or supination.

An excessively pronated foot remains flexible and somewhat unstable. This places increased demands on the muscles of the leg to stabilize the foot for push-off. Excessive pronation also is associated with increased internal rotation of the tibia. This can contribute to patellar tracking abnormalities and malalignment at joints proximal to the foot.

An excessively supinated foot appears as a high-arched, cavus foot. Because a supinated configuration is more rigid, this foot type may be associated with stress fractures and other injuries related to repetitive impact stresses.

Biomechanical variations play a role in the way structures in the leg respond to repetitive stress. The term *miserable*

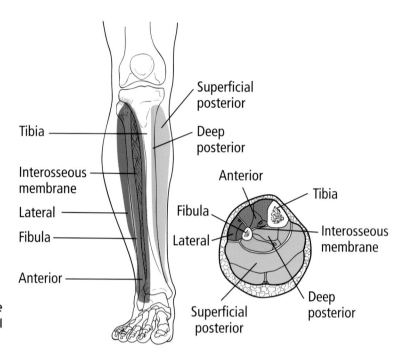

FIGURE 42.1 The leg has 4 major muscle compartments: anterior, lateral, superficial posterior, and deep posterior.

malalignment syndrome refers to a pattern of anatomic variations that includes femoral anteversion, an increased Q angle, genu valgus and hyperpronation of the foot. However, the effect of many of these variations may be mitigated by modifications in footwear and by specific strengthening programs.

An important muscle that influences biomechanics during running is the gluteus medius, which is the primary hip abductor. Weakness in this muscle may have implications for the entire leg during the running gait. When the runner is in the stance phase of running, the gluteus medius prevents the femur from excessive adduction and internal rotation, as well as preventing the knee from falling into a valgus position. This secondarily limits excessive internal rotation of the tibia relative to the foot and limits weight transfer to the medial aspect of the foot.

Weakness of the gluteus medius permits excessive internal rotation of the leg. This is associated with increased strain on the tibialis posterior and soleus from excessive rotation as well as greater demands on these muscles to control the additional pronation that is associated with internal tibial rotation.

Normally, the posterior tibialis muscle is able to control the midfoot, bringing it back into supination as push-off occurs. In the overpronated foot, these muscles are overstretched as they contract eccentrically in an attempt to limit the amount of pronation and bring the foot back into supination. The excessive force of these eccentric contractions also contributes to the development of MTSS and tibia stress fractures.

Excessive pronation may be modified through the use of orthotics or stabilized running shoes. Orthotics, both custom and off the shelf, limit the excessive motion of the overpronating foot. They can attenuate the forces of the repetitive eccentric contractions of the soleus and posterior tibialis muscles, lessening the risk for the development of MTSS and tibial stress fracture.

The opposite of the overpronating foot is the high-arched or cavus foot. The presence of a cavus foot should alert the clinician to the possibility of an underlying neurologic disorder. However, most highly arched or cavus feet are part of the normal spectrum of foot types. Because a cavus foot has limits pronation, the foot is less able to attenuate ground reaction forces. These impact forces are then transmitted through the foot to the lower extremity. Athletes with a cavus foot are at a higher risk for developing stress fractures in the metatarsals and tarsals, in addition to being at risk for MTSS and tibial stress fractures. When considering orthotics for a cavus foot, it must be remembered that this foot type has greater intrinsic stability but lacks shock-absorbing capacity. Shoes or inserts that add cushion may be helpful; shoes or arch supports that add stability may compound problems related to diminished shock absorption.

Although there are a variety of shoes available to the runner, the ability of the shoe itself to control hind-foot motion is debatable. Shoes made for overpronating feet have a reinforced medial heel that wears down less rapidly than nonreinforced shoes. Shoes should fit the foot comfortably

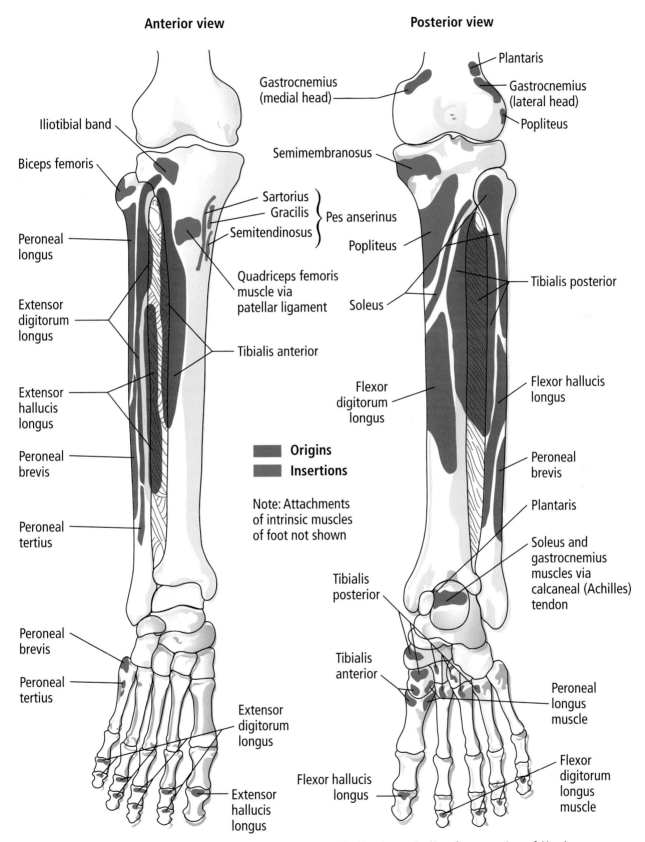

FIGURE 42.2 Highlighted areas indicate broad-based attachment sites for muscles of the leg.

and should be replaced about every 300 running miles or every 6 months.

Soccer cleats generally have poor arch support and poor cushioning. Inserts in cleated shoes may be helpful to provide support for athletes with overpronation or cushion for athletes who have a supinated foot.

EVALUATION

History

In evaluating acute injuries, the mechanism of injury is critical to making an accurate diagnosis. If the foot is firmly planted on the ground when the lower leg is struck, the risk of a fracture is greater than if the foot is not fixed on the ground. If the athlete was able to immediately bear weight or quickly return to play, a significant injury to a bone or joint is unlikely. Inquiries should also be made about the occurrence of an audible pop and the sudden onset of swelling.

Lower leg pain without a definitive injury typically suggests an overuse injury such as MTSS, stress fracture, or exertional compartment syndrome. Overuse injuries can result from training errors, such as rapid increases in training volume, changes in training surface or terrain, concurrent participation in multiple sports, or changes in equipment such as new running shoes. The history of an overuse injury should also include inquiries about the location of pain, timing of pain in relationship to activity, and the effect of pain on continued training. The history should also include identification of what makes the pain worse, what makes the pain better, and whether there are activities that can be continued without pain. The results of any previous evaluations and treatments should also be elicited. Table 42.1 lists factors contributing to MTSS and stress fractures.

Pain that is constant, pain that does not change with activity, or pain that disrupts sleep should raise concerns about an infection or neoplasm. Constitutional symptoms, including weight loss and fever, also imply more serious pathology.

Physical Examination

The approach to examining an athlete with a suspected overuse injury varies greatly from the acute injury evaluation. The acute injury evaluation must first focus on the presence of swelling, ecchymosis, open wounds, and angular or rotational deformities. Palpation should include an assessment of bone, epiphysis, apophysis, muscle, tendon, syndesmosis, and ligamentous structures for

TABLE 42.1

Extrinsic and Intrinsic Factors Contributing to MTSS and Stress Fractures

Extrinsic Factors	Intrinsic Factors
Rapid increase in training intensity or volume	Lower extremity malalignment
Sustained levels of high-impact activity	Foot type (hyperpronated, supinated)
Hard surfaces	Tibial varum
Inadequate footwear	Femoral anteversion
Inadequate cushion	Hip abductor weakness
Inadequate support/stability	Amenorrhea
Orthotics	Osteopenia
Inappropriate prescription	
Inadequate fit	
Material breakdown/failure	

tenderness or swelling. Vascular status should be assessed by palpating the dorsalis pedis and posterior tibial artery pulses. A neurologic evaluation should also be performed by evaluating the athlete's sensation distal to the site of injury.

In cases of a suspected overuse injury, a thorough evaluation of the lower extremity alignment should be conducted. The athlete should be evaluated while standing barefoot and while walking. The foot type should be characterized as neutral, pronated, or supinated. Overall alignment of the lower extremities should also be assessed, including the amount of femoral anteversion, Q angle, and presence of tibia varum (**Figure 42.3**). For runners, the running shoe should be evaluated to ensure that it is in good condition and that it provides the stability and cushioning appropriate for the athlete's foot type.

The anterior tibial border, medial tibial border, and fibula should be palpated for tenderness. Strength of the hip abductors can be judged by manually resisting hip abduction or having the athlete balance on each leg (**Figure 42.4**). If the contralateral hip drops compared with the level of the hip on the leg in single stance, weakness of the hip abductors is implied. Pain with a single-leg hop on the involved extremity may signal a stress fracture.

Imaging Studies

Even the most detailed physical examination cannot always rule out the presence of a fracture or other bony lesion. If bony pathology is suspected, evaluation should include anteroposterior and lateral radiographs of the entire tibia and fibula. Normal-appearing radiographs exclude an acute

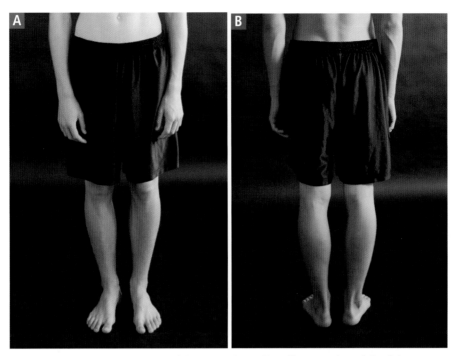

FIGURE 42.3 Inspection of lower extremity alignment and foot type.

fracture. However, stress fractures and osteomyelitis may not be visible for several weeks after the onset of pain.

If a stress fracture is strongly suspected, radiographs can be repeated in 2 weeks to look for the development of a fracture callus. If a more immediate diagnosis is needed, or if more serious pathology is suspected by history (eg, fever, night pain, weight loss), further imaging studies should be obtained. Bone scans were long considered the standard for evaluating suspected stress fractures, but they are limited by their high sensitivity to any increased metabolic activity in the bone. Thus, acute fractures, stress fractures, stress reactions, infections, and tumors are difficult to differentiate on bone scan. Magnetic resonance imaging (MRI) is increasingly being accepted as the standard for the evaluation of stress fractures and other skeletal pathology such as suspected tumors or infection. One important advantage to MRI is the ability to provide a detailed anatomic evaluation of both the bone and the surrounding soft tissue. MRI also takes less time and results in less radiation exposure than bone scans.

ACUTE INJURIES

Fractures

Acute fractures are more common in contact and collision sports but can occur from noncontact forces related to jumping or twisting. Because of the tremendous force

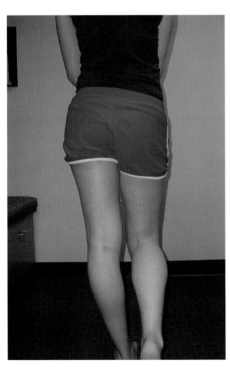

FIGURE 42.4 Evaluation of hip abductor strength. Weakness results in dropping of contralateral hip.

required to fracture the tibia, such fractures are usually obvious. Tibial fractures manifest with immediate onset of swelling, deformity, and inability to weight bear. As a result, initial evaluation and treatment are more likely to occur in the emergency department than the primary care provider's office. Treatment for tibial fractures typically involves a long leg cast with crutches. Fractures that are angulated, unstable, or involve a physis may need surgical fixation.

Fibular fractures can be much more difficult to diagnose clinically and may occur from a variety of mechanisms. In instances of blunt force trauma to the lower leg, the fibula is often fractured in conjunction with a tibial fracture. Direct blows to the lateral leg are a common cause of an isolated fibular fracture. For isolated fibular fractures due to blunt trauma, athletes may be able to walk and tolerate weight-bearing activity.

Fibular fractures may also result from rotational forces on the foot and ankle and inversion ankle injuries. If the talus rotates in the ankle mortise, the syndesmosis and interosseus membrane may be disrupted. This results in a diastasis of the ankle mortise and can permit transmission of forces proximally, causing a fibular fracture (**Figure 42.5**). Because of the disruption of integrity of the ankle mortise, a fibular fracture occurring in conjunction with a syndesmosis sprain should be treated initially with a splint and crutches, and the athlete should promptly be referred to an orthopedic surgeon.

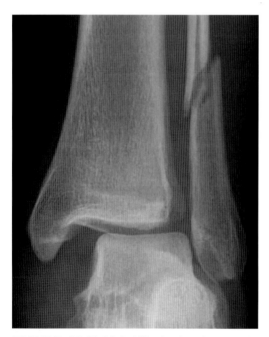

FIGURE 42.5 Distal fibular fracture. Note widening of ankle mortise.

If a significant ankle syndesmosis injury is not present, a nondisplaced fibular fracture can be treated with a short leg walking cast or walking boot for 4 to 6 weeks. An intact syndesmosis and interosseus membrane provide support, internal bracing, and protection for the fractured fibula.

Compartment Syndrome

Tibial fractures are the most common cause of acute compartment syndrome in the leg. However, compartment syndrome may be caused by soft tissue injury or hemorrhage that produces sudden increases in muscle compartment pressure. The possibility of compartment syndrome should be suspected when there is increasing pain, swelling, weakness, or muscle dysfunction after an injury. Physical examination reveals an exquisitely tender and firm leg, pain with passive calf stretching, and distal neurovascular compromise. Immediate surgical consultation should be obtained. An emergency fasciotomy is required for abnormally elevated compartment pressures.

Muscle Strains

Strains of the calf muscles are relatively rare in young athletes. The most commonly injured muscle is the gastrocnemius. In most instances, the strain will occur at the musculotendinous junction of the medial head of the gastrocnemius. The onset of pain is sudden, and the athlete may feel a pop or a tearing sensation. There may be swelling, ecchymosis, and a palpable defect at the musculotendinous junction. Initial treatment should consist of ice, compression, and either crutches or a walking boot. Physical therapy can help the athlete regain normal flexibility and strength before returning to activity. Injuries to the peroneal muscles are rare because inversion of the ankle is more likely to cause a ligament sprain than a peroneal strain.

Contusions

Contusions to the anterior and anteromedial tibia may result in significant bony pain because this area is not protected by overlying muscle or soft tissue. A subperiosteal hematoma can cause a visible, tender prominence with a hard, bonelike consistency. The level of pain and bony tenderness may raise concern for fracture, but the mechanism of injury and the athlete's ability to bear weight are not typical for fractures. With fractures, tenderness can be appreciated around all sides of the bone, and pain may occur with a fulcrum test. Radiographs may still be necessary to distinguish between bone contusions and fractures. Athletes and their caregivers should be forewarned that a visible or palpable nodule may persist on the tibia for several months after a contusion.

OVERUSE INJURIES

Medial Tibial Stress Syndrome

The most common cause of chronic lower leg pain in young athletes is MTSS, or shin splints. The exact cause of MTSS is unknown, but the soleus muscle where it attaches to the periosteum of the posteromedial tibia is likely involved. The tendinous origin of the posterior tibialis muscle along the posteromedial tibial border has also long been implicated as a potential source of pain. The repetitive tension of muscular contractions, coupled with the impact forces of running, causes microscopic tears and subsequent inflammatory change along the periosteum.

MTSS is often seen early in a sports season when the athlete undergoes a rapid increase in impact activity. Many affected athletes will have increased foot pronation. Diffuse tenderness along the posteromedial tibia points toward the diagnosis of MTSS (**Figure 42.6A**). The differential diagnosis includes stress fractures (**Figure 42.6B**), which are characterized by focal bony tenderness, and exertional compartment syndrome, which may present without tenderness or

may manifest with diffuse tenderness and tightness over the anterior compartment.

The diagnosis of MTSS can be confirmed by ruling out other conditions in the differential diagnosis. Plain films have insufficient sensitivity to rule out stress fractures. However, a bone scan or MRI can detect more subtle bony changes seen in both MTSS and stress fractures. **Figure 42.7A** shows the patchy and diffuse uptake seen with MTSS, and **Figure 42.7B** shows the more concentrated and focal increased uptake associated with stress fracture.

MTSS often resolves with reducing impact activity, followed by a slow return to activity once symptoms have

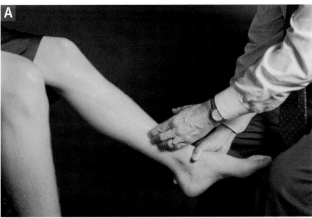

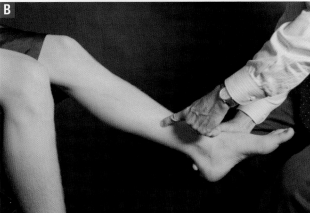

FIGURE 42.6 (A) Location of tenderness with MTSS. (B) Location of tenderness with tibial stress fracture.

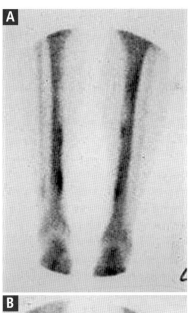

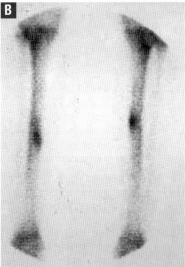

FIGURE 42.7 (A) Bone scan showing diffuse uptake consistent with medial tibial stress syndrome. (B) Bone scan demonstrating focal increased uptake consistent with bilateral tibial stress fracture.

subsided. A strategy to prevent further occurrences should involve the use of more supportive shoes or arch supports in overpronated feet. Physical therapy can help restore flexibility and strength of the posterior tibialis and soleus muscles as well as strengthen the hip abductors if any weaknesses are identified. Treatment should also address training errors, including sudden increases in training volume.

Stress Fractures

Tibial stress injuries evolve along a continuum, beginning with MTSS and culminating in a stress fracture. Although not everybody with stress fractures will first have symptomatic MTSS, identifying and treating MTSS could prevent the development of stress fractures. Tibial stress fractures occur most commonly along the posteromedial tibial border and are related to repetitive compression. Anterior tibial stress fractures are less common. They are related to tension, rather than compression, on the tibia. Athletes who repeatedly plant their foot to jump, decelerate, or change direction are more likely to have a tension-related anterior tibial stress fracture.

Stress fractures of the medial malleolus are also less common and may require more specialized treatment. Fibular stress fractures are less common than tibial stress fractures. They are usually seen in distance runners or athletes with varus alignment. Stress fractures can occur at multiple sites and can be bilateral.

A diagnosis of stress fracture should be suspected when an athlete has point bony tenderness (see Figure 42.6B) and a history of repetitive impact activity. Athletes whose diets are deficient in calcium, athletes with eating disorders, and athletes with amenorrhea may develop stress fractures more easily than other athletes. The diagnosis of stress fracture is confirmed through imaging studies. Plain films are often negative for stress fracture, even when the films are repeated a few weeks later. Anterior tibial stress fractures are an exception. An area of cortical elevation and/or a transverse lucency are often seen in a patient who has bony tenderness and a visible or palpable bony prominence (**Figure 42.8**). When plain films show no abnormalities, bone scan and MRI are options that afford more sensitivity than plain films. MRI is emerging as the favored diagnostic test because it can quantify the degree of reactive change within the injured bone, including early stress reactions that may manifest only as periosteal edema. In more serious injuries, edema within the bone marrow will develop, with repeated stress culminating in the development of a visible fracture line through the cortex (**Figure 42.9**).

An athlete with an anterior tibial stress fracture should be splinted, placed on crutches, and referred to a sports

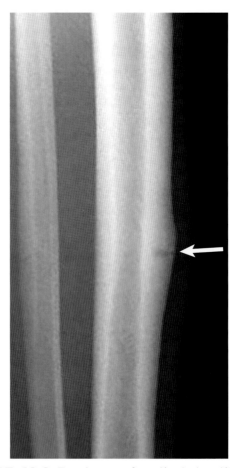

FIGURE 42.8 Focal area of cortical elevation seen with anterior tibial stress fracture.

medicine specialist. In some cases, intramedullary rodding of the tibia is indicated. Medial malleolar stress fractures should also be referred to a sports medicine specialist for further management.

Posteromedial tibial stress fractures are treated with relative rest and nonimpact cross training to maintain aerobic fitness. There is some evidence that the use of a long pneumatic splint speeds recovery time. If diagnosed early, most tibial stress fractures will heal within 4 to 6 weeks of the initiation of conservative treatment. However, additional time for healing may be required in patients with dietary or hormone deficiencies. Treatment should also address contributing biomechanical abnormalities and training errors. Once the bone has healed, another 2 to 3 months may be required for the athlete to gradually resume a full training regimen.

In most cases, athletes may be cleared to resume activity once the tenderness has resolved and contributing training and biomechanical factors have been addressed. Confirmation

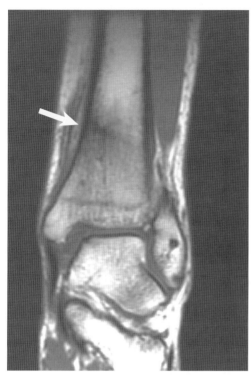

FIGURE 42.9 Distal tibial stress fracture shown by MRI.

of healing with x-rays or other imaging modalities can be problematic. If plain films did not originally show the stress fracture, follow-up plain films will not be useful to confirm healing. Abnormalities may persist on bone scan or MRI after clinical healing has occurred. If radiologic confirmation is necessary to confirm healing of a stress fracture, a computed tomography (CT) scan may be the most reliable option.

Exertional Compartment Syndrome

Exertional compartment syndrome is a rare but disabling condition that may occur in runners of all ages. With exertional compartment syndrome, the exercising muscle becomes engorged with blood and the enveloping fascia does not have the elasticity to accommodate this increase in muscle volume. As the pressure increases within the affected compartment, the arteries and nerves are compromised, resulting in pain and cramping. Numbness and tingling corresponding to the dermatomal distribution of the affected nerve may also occur. The anterior compartment is the most common location for exertional compartment syndrome because noncompliant bony structures (ie, the tibia and fibula) make up 2 walls of the compartment.

Exertional compartment syndrome will manifest as pain, tightness, and cramping in the muscles and usually arises after a predictable amount of elapsed time into a bout of

exercise. The pain usually subsides predictably with rest and tends not to occur with low-impact activity such as cycling or swimming. Discontinuous running, such as in soccer or basketball, is less likely to cause exertional compartment syndrome than continuous distance running.

In cases of exertional compartment syndrome, the physical examination will typically be normal at rest. Occasionally there will be a sense of fullness or increased pressure diffusely over the anterior compartment. A small muscle hernia and/or fascial defect may also be detected distally. When physical examination reveals nothing abnormal, an exercise challenge that includes running or repetitive plantarflexion-dorsiflexion exercises may reproduce the symptoms.

The diagnosis is confirmed by compartment pressure testing. An abnormal compartment pressure study may reveal high pressures at rest, abnormal increases with exercise, abnormally delayed recovery of pressure with rest, or some combination of these abnormal measurements. Once the diagnosis is made through compartment pressure testing, treatment options include modifying activity or undergoing fasciotomy. Physical therapy and/or shoe modifications are not particularly effective for this condition.

Differential Diagnosis of Chronic Leg Pain

A variety of other conditions may cause lower extremity pain in the young athlete. Referred pain and radiculopathy must always be considered potential causes of lower extremity pain. Although hip pathology typically results in knee pain, it occasionally manifests in the calf or shin. Lumbar radiculopathy may also cause calf or foot pain. Although spinal stenosis and disk herniations are rare in young athletes, low back pathology should be considered when leg pain is not otherwise explained. Foraminal stenosis due to a lateral disk protrusion or spondylolisthesis can also cause referred pain to the leg. With foraminal stenosis, there may or may not be associated back pain.

Peripheral nerve entrapments can cause leg pain as well as numbness, tingling, and burning in the distribution of the affected nerve. The common peroneal nerve is the most likely nerve to be involved, and the source of nerve irritation is most commonly at the fibular head. The tendinous origin of the peroneal longus muscle stretches around the fibular head and can compress the nerve. Instability from a sprain of the proximal tibiofibular joint can also result in peroneal nerve injury. The superficial sensory peroneal nerve can become entrapped as it exits the muscle compartment proximal to the lateral malleolus. The entrapment typically occurs at the same site where muscle hernias are seen with exertional compartment syndromes.

Popliteal artery entrapment syndrome may manifest in a very similar way as exertional compartment syndrome and can be difficult to diagnose. The condition is caused by an entrapment of the popliteal artery and results in compromised blood flow to the lower leg. With increasing exercise, the artery is compressed, leading to ischemia and pain in the muscles of the lower leg. The entrapment may by anatomic (abnormal course of the artery or abnormal displacement of the heads of the gastrocnemius) or functional (hypertrophy of the heads of the gastrocnemius).

Physical examination for popliteal artery entrapment is typically normal. However, decreased pulses at the dorsalis pedis and posterior tibialis arteries may be seen when the ankle is plantarflexed. As with the examination for exertional compartment syndrome, the clinician should consider having the athlete run or use tubing for resistance in an attempt to reproduce the symptoms. Foot pulses should be assessed with the foot neutral and plantarflexed. Definitive diagnosis may be made with magnetic resonance angiography, duplex ultrasonography, or standard angiography. All studies must be dynamic, assessing the popliteal artery with the ankle moved from neutral to plantarflexion. Surgical release of the artery may be required.

Osteomyelitis and Neoplasm

Infection and tumor must be in the differential diagnosis when encountering any young athlete with pain in an extremity. When a history of athletic activity or trauma is reported, clinicians may be biased to look for a musculoskeletal injury rather than a serious or potentially life-threatening medical problem. Infections and tumors can manifest like an overuse injury, with a gradual onset of pain that increases with activity. Unlike pain from an overuse injury, the pain from infection or tumor does not typically subside with rest or respond to simple treatment measures. There may be pain at night as well as constitutional symptoms such as fever, sweats, chills, or weight loss.

X-rays are indicated as part of the evaluation for unexplained extremity pain. Plain radiographs may not initially show any abnormalities, particularly in the case of osteomyelitis. Blood work may show high white blood cell count, sedimentation rate, or C-reactive protein. MRI is indicated to further investigate suspicious radiographs or persistent pain. In some cases, malignant neoplasm cannot be distinguished from osteomyelitis by MRI, and an open biopsy must be performed. Suspected osteoid osteoma is best diagnosed by CT scan. An osteoid osteoma appears as a small, sclerotic lesion with a central nidus (**Figure 42.10**). Osteoid osteoma classically manifests as pain that is worse

at night but is relieved by nonsteroidal anti-inflammatory medication. Ewing sarcoma and osteogenic sarcoma are the 2 most common bony malignancies seen in children and adolescents.

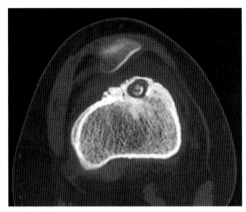

FIGURE 42.10 CT appearance of osteoid osteoma in the distal femur.

SUMMARY POINTS

- Lower leg injuries in young athletes range from acute fractures requiring emergent orthopedic surgical care to overuse syndromes requiring careful identification and treatment of the underlying causes.

- Training errors, including sudden increases in training volume or participation in multiple sports, can be a significant contributor to overuse injuries.

- Strength imbalances, including weakness in the gluteus medius, may result in a variety of problems affecting the entire leg during the running gait.

- MRI is increasingly being accepted as the standard for the evaluation of stress fractures and other skeletal pathology such as tumors or infection.

- Biomechanical and anatomic abnormalities contribute to a variety of overuse injuries. Available treatments, such as therapeutic exercises and orthotics, do not eliminate these abnormalities but can mitigate their effect on injury.

- MTSS causes diffuse tenderness along the posteromedial border of the tibia. The findings are often bilateral and are the result of a combination of training error and biomechanical abnormalities. Continued activity without treatment may lead to stress fracture.

- Sudden increases in pressure in a muscle compartment can cause an acute compartment syndrome. Compartment pressure increases associated with exercise cause an exertional compartment syndrome. Acute compartment syndromes may require emergent surgical attention; exertional compartment syndromes may subside with rest or benefit from nonemergent surgical treatment.

- Leg pain in athletes can be referred from the lumbar spine or can be due to non–sports-related problems, such as infection or tumor.

SUGGESTED READING

Fredericson M, Cookingham CL, Chaudhari AM, Dowdell BC, Oestreicher N, Sahrmann SA. Hip abductor weakness in distance runners with iliotibial band syndrome. *Clin J Sport Med.* 2000;3:169-175.

James SL, Bates BT, Osternig LR. Injuries to runners. *Am J Sports Med.* 1978;6:40-50.

Krivackas LS. Anatomical factors associated with overuse sports injuries. *Sports Med.* 1997;24:132-146.

Loud KJ, Micheli LJ, Bristol S, Austin SB, Gordon CM. Family history predicts stress fracture in active female adolescents. *Pediatrics.* 2007;120:e364-e372.

Sofka CM. Imaging of stress fractures. *Clin Sports Med.* 2006;25:53-62.

Swenson EJ Jr, DeHaven KE, Sebastianelli WJ, Hanks G, Kalenak A, Lynch JM. The effect of a pneumatic leg brace on return to play in athletes with tibial stress fractures. *Am J Sports Med.* 1997;25:322-328.

Willems TM, Witvrouw E, De Cock A, De Clercq D. Gait-related risk factors for exercise-related lower-leg pain during shod running. *Med Sci Sports Exerc.* 2007;39:330-339.

CHAPTER 43

Acute Foot and Ankle Injuries

Steven J. Anderson, MD

Acute ankle and foot injuries are common in athletes and other active young people. Sprains account for the greatest number of acute injuries. However, fractures and injuries related to skeletal immaturity are also an important part of the differential diagnosis. To properly diagnose and manage these conditions, physicians should be familiar with ankle anatomy and how anatomy dictates specific injury patterns. When the injury pattern points to an ankle inversion sprain, evaluation and treatment are relatively straightforward. However, when the injury pattern suggests a diagnosis other than a sprain, bony or growth plate injuries are more likely, as is the need for more detailed radiographic evaluation and/or surgical consultation.

ANKLE INJURIES

The ankle joint is made up of the talus, which articulates in a bony mortise formed by the distal tibia and fibula. The joint gains its stability from a combination of bony architecture, ligamentous support, and musculotendinous reinforcement (**Figure 43.1**). The tibia and fibula are held together by the anterior and posterior tibiofibular ligaments as well as the interosseous membrane. The medial and lateral collateral ligaments limit eversion and inversion of the ankle, respectively. The medial and lateral malleoli are extensions from the distal tibia and fibula and contribute to the integrity of the bony ankle mortise. In skeletally immature patients, an open physis separates the malleoli from the shaft of the tibia and fibula. Because the physis is weaker than the surrounding ligaments, skeletally immature patients are uniquely susceptible to physeal injury. Musculotendinous structures allow for movement of the ankle and foot and provide additional support and stability.

Acute ankle injuries can affect any of the aforementioned structures individually or in combination. Because sprains are the most common acute ankle injury, sprains are the primary focus of this discussion and serve as a reference point for identifying other problems in the differential diagnosis, including fractures, physeal injuries, and strains.

Sprains

The primary ligamentous support for the ankle includes the 3-part lateral ligament complex and the 5-part medial or deltoid ligament complex. The 3 lateral ligaments include the anterior talofibular ligament (ATFL), the calcaneofibular ligament (CFL), and the posterior talofibular ligament (PTFL) (**Figure 43.1**). Distinguishing the 5 parts of the deltoid ligament complex is less relevant clinically because injuries to a single component of the deltoid are rare.

Musculotendinous structures provide additional stability to the bony and ligamentous structures. The peroneal muscles laterally provide resistance to inversion stress. On the medial aspect of the ankle, the posterior tibialis muscle provides resistance to eversion stresses, and the tibialis anterior resists plantarflexion and eversion. Proprioception is an important component of stability in that the awareness of joint position helps activate the musculotendinous structures responsible for maintaining joint stability.

Ligament sprains in the ankle are most likely to occur when the joint is in a position that provides the least amount of bony stability. For the ankle, the position of least bony stability is plantarflexion and inversion. In plantarflexion, the narrower posterior portion of the talus engages in the ankle mortise. This results in more space around the talus, and hence more laxity of the joint (**Figure 43.2**). With dorsiflexion, the wider anterior

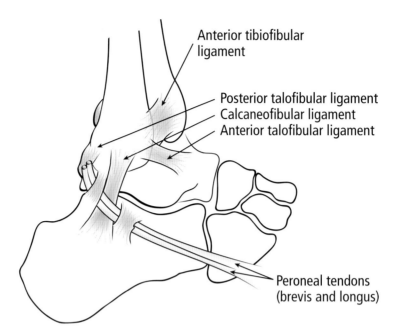

FIGURE 43.1 Lateral view of ankle showing lateral ligament complex and peroneal tendons. Reprinted with permission from Griffin LY, ed. *Essentials of Musculoskeletal Care.* 3rd ed. Rosemont, IL: American Academy of Orthopaedic Surgeons; and Elk Grove Village, IL: American Academy of Pediatrics; 2005:593.

portion of the talus engages in the ankle mortise, resulting in a tighter fit and greater bony stability.

Inversion is a less stable position for the ankle than eversion because the lengths of the medial and lateral malleoli differ (**Figure 43.3**). Compared with the medial malleolus, the lateral malleolus extends farther distally and blocks the talus from moving laterally or everting. This feature of the ankle's bony architecture makes it easier for the ankle to invert than evert. Therefore, as a result of the shape of the talus and the difference in length of the malle-oli, plantarflexion and inversion together is the position of least bony stability in the ankle and the position in which ligamentous structures must play a greater role in stabiliz-ing the joint. Ligamentous injuries are most likely to occur when the ankle is in a plantarflexed and inverted position, and bony injuries are more likely when the ankle is dorsi-flexed and everted.

When the ankle is plantarflexed and inverted, the ATFL assumes a vertical orientation and becomes the primary lateral stabilizer for the ankle (**Figure 43.4**). If the ATFL is injured or fails, the CFL is subjected to inversion stresses. If both the ATFL and CFL fail, the PTFL may be injured. The anatomy of the ankle establishes a predictable pattern of injury in which the lateral ligaments are at risk in descending order from anterior to posterior. Because of anatomically determined susceptibilities, it is difficult to

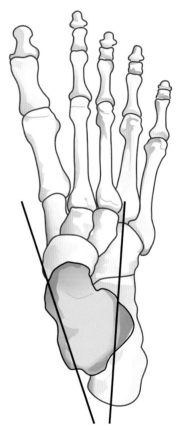

FIGURE 43.2 View of superior articular surface of talus showing the wider anterior portion.

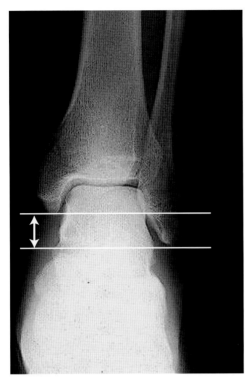

FIGURE 43.3 Bony anatomy of ankle mortise with lines indicating relative difference in length between medial malleolus and lateral malleolus with the latter malleolus extending more distally.

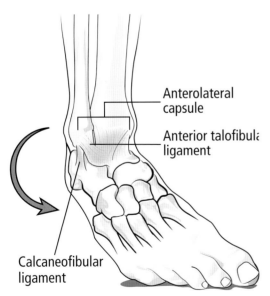

Anterolateral capsule

Anterior talofibula ligament

Calcaneofibular ligament

FIGURE 43.4 Mechanism of injury with inversion ankle sprain.

injure the CFL or the PTFL without first injuring the ATFL. Injuries to the medial ligaments are overall less common because of more prominent bony barriers to eversion. When the mechanism of injury or physical findings deviate from the typical pattern for inversion sprains, fractures or other diagnoses should be considered. Similarly, swelling and pain that is more pronounced on the medial portion of the ankle should raise suspicion for fracture. Because dorsiflexion and eversion afford greater bony stability to the ankle, injuries in this position are more likely to be bony in nature. Finally, if there is an injury to a ligament that is normally protected by bony structures, a bony injury should also be suspected.

Clinical Evaluation

History A history of the mechanism of injury is extremely helpful in diagnosing acute ankle injuries. It is important to determine the position of the foot at the time of injury and how the force was applied. If patients describe having the ankle "turn in" or "turn out," they should still demonstrate what they mean by turning in or out. The history should also include reports of the location of pain, swelling, functional restrictions, and previous injuries, as well as questions about instability, stiffness, weakness, pain at rest, concurrent injury, and other musculoskeletal problems.

Determining the location of pain and swelling is more useful clinically than the magnitude of pain and swelling. Inversion sprains should have pain and swelling that is most pronounced over the ATFL and CFL. Findings that suggest a diagnosis other than sprain include pain and/or swelling that is more pronounced medially or posteriorly rather than anteriorly or laterally. Pain and/or swelling in the midfoot, forefoot, or upper leg may indicate something other than an ankle sprain.

Functional restrictions tend to be more reliable indicators of the severity of injury than the severity of pain. Functional limitations may include the inability to stand, walk, run, jump, change directions, or pivot.

Finally, a sports history should be obtained as part of the evaluation. An understanding of the demands of the athlete's sport will help determine specific rehabilitation goals, suitable activities for cross training, and requirements for return to play.

Physical Examination The physical examination consists of inspection, palpation, and tests for ligament stability. The physical examination should always begin with a baseline evaluation of the uninjured ankle. The examination should also include the joints proximal and distal to the injury.

Inspection can identify swelling, ecchymosis, and deformity. Swelling will be localized over the injured structure initially but becomes more diffuse over time. Swelling and bruising around the heel, forefoot, or between the toes may appear days to weeks after an ankle sprain or fracture.

Palpation starts with bony landmarks, including the medial and lateral malleoli, the talus, the calcaneus, the fifth metatarsal, and the proximal fibula. To enhance patient cooperation, palpation should begin in the least painful areas. If there is bony tenderness over the lateral malleolus, an effort should be made to distinguish tenderness limited to a ligament attachment site from tenderness that traverses the malleolus or an open physis.

Important ligaments to palpate include the ATFL, CFL, PTFL, anterior tibiofibular ligament, and deltoid ligament (**Figure 43.5**). Tenderness over the anterior joint line or anterior tibiofibular ligament warrants a more detailed evaluation for tenderness in the syndesmosis or interosseous membrane. Also, the peroneal tendon and Achilles tendon should be evaluated for signs of injury. Any positive findings should be analyzed for consistency with the reported mechanism of injury and the expected pattern for ligament sprains. The particular structures that are most tender on palpation are more relevant to establishing an accurate diagnosis than the degree of tenderness.

Testing to assess for ligament stability can be limited by swelling and guarding in the acute phase of an ankle injury. Fortunately, injuries to the ATFL can be reliably assessed, even in the acute phase, with the anterior drawer test. To perform the anterior drawer test, grasp the heel and hold the ankle in a neutral (90°) or slightly plantar-flexed position with one hand and use the other hand to stabilize the distal tibia and fibula. Then, pull the heel forward and assess the degree of excursion (**Figure 43.6**). The integrity of

the end point and the degree of difference from the uninjured ankle should be noted. Differences of 5 mm or more have been reported to be significant. However, accurate assessment of millimeters of ankle joint motion is difficult. If the ankle used for comparison has been previously injured, the relative difference in ligamentous laxity may be less than the severity of injury would predict.

The talar tilt test is performed by first grasping the heel while stabilizing the tibia. The ankle is then inverted and everted while maintaining a neutral (90°) position (**Figure 43.7**). Laxity is again compared with the uninjured ankle. The degree of instability measured by the talar tilt test is often limited by pain and guarding. Attempts to accurately measure degrees of talar tilt are fraught with the same limitations associated with measuring millimeters of joint motion with the anterior drawer test. Fortunately, the diagnosis and initial management of ankle injuries depend less on talar tilt than on other factors such as the mechanism of injury, the location of maximal swelling and tenderness, and the presence of bony tenderness. Accordingly, examination under anesthesia or a stress test is not necessary in the evaluation of acute inversion sprains.

The value of strength testing in the acutely injured ankle is limited because of pain inhibition and guarding. However, athletes with chronic instability or recurrent injury may have calf or peroneal weakness. If strength testing of the peroneals results in pain or snapping of the peroneal tendon, a peroneal tendon strain or subluxation should be considered in the differential diagnosis.

A modified Romberg test can identify proprioceptive deficits commonly seen with sprains (**Figure 43.8**). To perform the test, the athlete stands and balances on one foot with his or her eyes closed. The balance on the affected

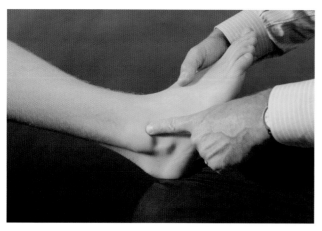

FIGURE 43.5 Palpation of anterior talofibular ligament.

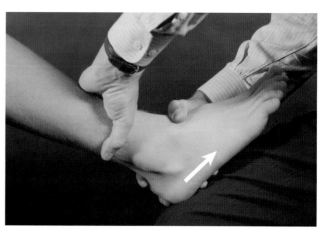

FIGURE 43.6 Anterior drawer test.

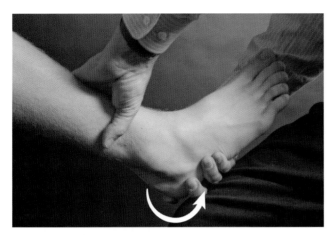

FIGURE 43.7 Talar tilt test.

foot is typically impaired, even after the initial pain, swelling, and weakness have resolved.

Radiologic Evaluation Radiographic evaluation of acute ankle injuries should include anterior, lateral, and mortise views. Bony tenderness over the foot or upper leg should be evaluated with additional views. Tenderness or radiographic irregularities over a physis warrant close scrutiny for physeal widening or displacement. Comparison views may be helpful in evaluating suspected changes in the physis. If there is physeal tenderness and suspicious radiographic findings, the patient should be treated as if he or she has a fracture.

Determining when to obtain radiographs is a greater challenge than determining which views to order. In general, radiographs are most useful when bony injuries are probable. Common indications of possible bony injury include an eversion or dorsiflexion mechanism of injury; pain or tenderness that is more pronounced medially than laterally; tenderness over the distal tibial or fibular physes; bony tenderness that extends beyond the ligament attachment sites; bony tenderness in the proximal fibula, the midfoot, or the forefoot; and pain and/or swelling that has not subsided in a reasonable time frame, even if original radiographs were normal.

Although not all patients with ankle injuries need radiographic evaluation, it is better to err on the side of obtaining the radiograph rather than missing a fracture. Stress radiographs, bone scans, arthrography, and/or magnetic resonance imaging (MRI) are not routinely indicated in the initial evaluation of a sprained ankle. However, more detailed imaging may be helpful in evaluating persistent ankle symptoms in patients who have already had normal plain films or in patients with findings that suggest something other than an inversion sprain.

Differential Diagnosis Acute ankle injuries that occur with a plantar flexion and inversion mechanism are most

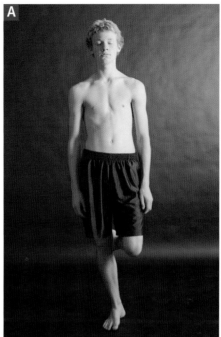

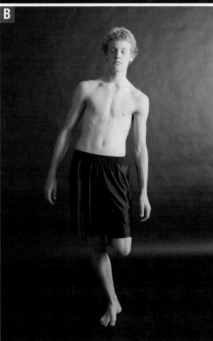

FIGURE 43.8 Modified Romberg test. (A) Patient balances on 1 leg wth eyes closed. (B) Patient tries to maintain balance. Compare ability to maintain balance between injured and uninjured sides.

likely to be ligament sprains. Athletes who experience an inversion injury but have pain and tenderness over the posterolateral ankle should be evaluated for peroneal tendon strains or subluxation. An athlete with an injury caused by ankle dorsiflexion, with or without rotation, may sprain the interosseous membrane. This results in a syndesmosis sprain, or what is referred to as a high ankle sprain. This same mechanism may tear the syndesmosis from distal to proximal and cause a proximal fibular (Maisonneuve) fracture (**Figure 43.9**). Syndesmosis sprains and Maisonneuve fractures are both associated with disruption of the connection between the tibia and the fibula. This results in an unstable ankle mortise and often requires surgical treatment to restore integrity to the mortise.

Some injuries that are initially diagnosed as sprains may have persistent pain, swelling, and/or instability, despite treatment. Under these circumstances, alternative diagnoses should be considered, including talar dome fracture, tibial plafond fracture, or an unstable ankle mortise. In these patients, repeat radiographs are indicated. With an inversion mechanism, there are distraction forces along the lateral portion of the ankle and compression forces medially. The compressive force on the medial talar dome can cause a small chondral fracture or an area of focal osteonecrosis that may appear to be normal on initial radiographs but shows up as an area of hyperlucency or deformity on subsequent x-rays (**Figure 43.10**). Talar dome fractures require immobilization, crutches, and surgical consultation.

Persistent pain and hypersensitivity in association with vasomotor changes may indicate reflex sympathetic dystrophy. Finally, conditions such as tarsal coalitions and/or osteochondritis dissecans of the talus may cause the ankle to become painful or functionally unstable without a history of inversion injury or commensurate degrees of ligament instability.

Rehabilitation Effective treatment of ankle sprains depends on an accurate diagnosis. Nonoperative therapy is effective for most ankle sprains. Even with pronounced ligamentous laxity, most athletes can return to play with proper rehabilitation and the use of ankle braces or tape. Referral to an orthopedic specialist is indicated for fractures of the malleolus, growth plate, fibula, or talar dome and for any injury that disrupts the integrity of the ankle mortise, including a syndesmosis sprain. Likewise, recurrent peroneal tendon dislocations and severe ligamentous laxity with chronic instability that does not respond to nonoperative treatment may also require surgical consultation.

Once other diagnoses have been ruled out, ankle sprains—regardless of their severity—can be treated in 5 phases (**Table 43.1**). More severe sprains require additional time in each phase. The phases of treatment should progress sequentially. Moving on to the next phase of treatment depends on the successful completion of the previous phase.

Phase I treatment involves resting and protecting the ankle to permit healing, to prevent further injury, and to control pain and swelling. The choice of cast boots, splints, taping, bracing, and/or crutches depends on the severity of injury and the comfort level of the patient. More severe sprains may require the use of a cast boot or splint. Traditional short leg casts are better for treating ankle and foot fractures. With sprains, a cast prevents using ice to treat swelling and will become loose when swelling subsides. A cast also restricts early weight bearing. Early weight bearing is beneficial for sprains but potentially harmful for fractures. Crutches should also be used if the patient is unable to

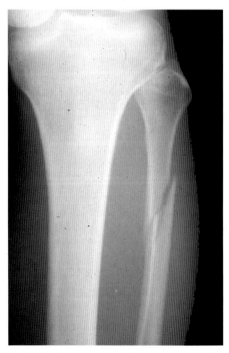

FIGURE 43.9 Maisonneuve fracture of proximal fibula.

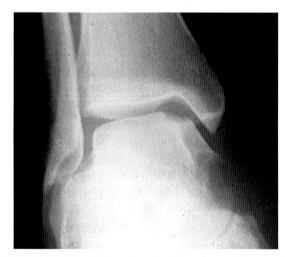

FIGURE 43.10 Osteochondral fracture of superior-medial talar dome.

TABLE 43.1

Phases of Rehabilitation for Ankle Sprains

Phase	Description
I	• Rest, protection (brace, wrap, splint, cast, and/or crutches) • Control inflammation (ice, compression, elevation) • Early weight bearing as tolerated
II	• Reduce residual swelling • Restore flexibility and joint range of motion • Restore strength (with emphasis on peroneals and calf) • Resume low-impact aerobic training; maintain general fitness
III	• Restore proprioception • Restore agility/coordination
IV	• Functional progression (jogging, running, sprinting, cutting, jumping; sport-specific skills)
V	• Gradual return to practice and competition • Maintenance exercises and long-term protection

Phase II treatment begins once pain and swelling have subsided to the point where the athlete can comfortably bear weight and ambulate. In this phase, active exercises are initiated to help restore range of motion and strength that were lost as the result of injury and subsequent immobilization. Range of motion can be restored by actively moving the ankle in all planes of motion, such as drawing letters of the alphabet with the toes. Adequacy of motion can be assessed by having the patient perform a single-legged squat. If ankle dorsiflexion is restricted and the depth of squat is limited by swelling or pain, it will be difficult for the patient to successfully progress with other aspects of rehabilitation.

Exercises that use elastic tubing can help restore strength to the muscles of the leg and calf (**Figure 43.12**). Peroneal strength is particularly important because the peroneals are the primary muscular backup to the lateral ligaments. Calf

comfortably bear weight, even with protection and support. Commercial splints and braces are available to provide the various degrees of protection and support that might be necessary. A milder sprain may require only a figure 8 brace or elastic bandage for protection (**Figure 43.11**). The lighter-weight rehabilitation braces may also be used for extra protection when patients are ready to resume their sport.

If diagnoses such as fracture or syndesmosis sprain have been ruled out, early weight bearing as tolerated is permitted and encouraged. Ice, elevation, and compression can be used to control swelling and pain. Heat has no role in the initial treatment of acute ligament injuries. Anti-inflammatory medications can help reduce swelling and pain but do not promote ligamentous healing.

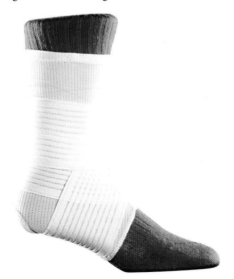

FIGURE 43.11 Figure 8 ankle brace.

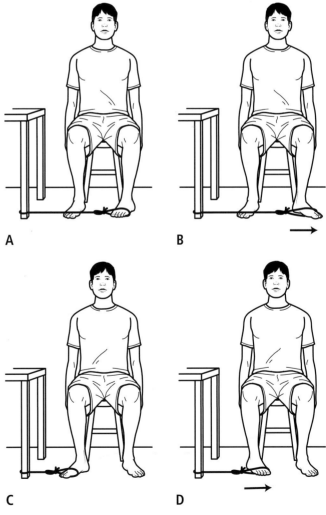

FIGURE 43.12 Peroneal strengthening using elastic tubing.

strengthening can also be performed by toe raises, with or without added weight, and toe raises on the edge of a step (**Figure 43.13**). For more severe sprains, or to ensure that exercises are being carried out appropriately, the athlete may benefit from the assistance of a certified athletic trainer or a physical therapist.

Most athletes in phase II of rehabilitation can resume some form of cross training or general conditioning to maintain fitness while the ankle heals. Upper body exercises, such as weight lifting, may be tolerated; so will low-impact aerobic exercises such as swimming, deep water pool running, cycling, stair climbing, and using elliptical trainers and rowing machines.

Phase III treatment focuses on restoring ankle proprioception as well as agility and coordination. This phase begins once the athlete has regained joint motion and strength and has demonstrated tolerance to low-impact aerobic activities. During this phase of rehabilitation, exercises are designed to restore balance, agility, coordination, and proprioception. Exercises to restore proprioception are performed on a balance board, a wobble board, or a minitrampoline, or simply by standing on one leg while playing catch with a ball or doing some other distracting activity (**Figure 43.14**). As proprioception improves, agility exercises can be added, including jumping forward, backward, and sideways with one or both feet.

In phase IV of treatment, athletes make the transition back to their sport through what is known as a functional progression. For running sports, athletes may progress from jogging or running straight ahead on a flat surface to sprinting. If straight-ahead activity is tolerated without pain or limitation, patients can introduce lateral movements by running in circles or figure 8s. They can increase speed and progress to tighter turns. This can be followed by running with gentle cuts of 30° to 45° and progressing to more severe

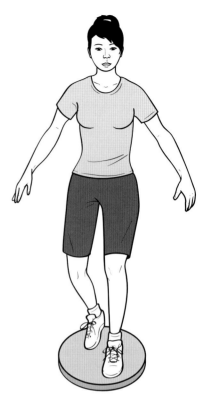

FIGURE 43.14 Use of balance board for proprioception exercises.

cuts (90° to 135°) with increasing speed. Running grapevines or crossover steps can also be performed. Sport-specific drills (eg, passing or dribbling a soccer ball, running backward) can also be carried out once running and cutting can be done. During the functional progression, an ankle brace or tape can be used to provide extra support, even if extra protection is no longer required for daily activity.

In phase V, the athlete has completed the functional program and should be ready to return to practice. Once patients progress to the point where they can carry out full activities in practice, they may be cleared to resume competition. Rehabilitation exercises, including strengthening and proprioception, should be continued on a maintenance basis until the athlete has been symptom free with full activities for at least 1 month.
Return-to-Play Criteria Physicians are often pressured to project a time when an athlete will be able to return to play after an ankle sprain. Because injuries and recovery rates are variable, it is difficult to estimate an exact date or time when return to sports will be safe. However, by outlining the sequential phases of rehabilitation, athletes will know the necessary steps for recovery and will be able to measure their progress against this standard. As a rough estimate, if an ankle sprain requires 2 weeks for the swelling and pain to subside, it will take another 2 weeks to restore joint motion and strength,

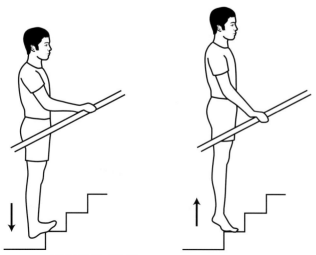

FIGURE 43.13 Calf strengthening.

then another 2 weeks to restore proprioception and the ability to perform functional tasks such as running, jumping, and pivoting. This hypothetical scenario would translate to a 6-week recovery. An injury that required only a week to go through each phase of rehabilitation would be a 3-week injury. When patients are invested in their recovery process, they are less likely to see the physician as a barrier to returning to play, and the criteria for return to play can be based on objective measurements rather than arbitrary time frames.

Functional testing provides an objective means to determine readiness to return to play. Functional testing is based on the functional tasks that the ankle performs in a given activity or sport. The ankle joint motion required to adequately perform the various functional tasks of each sport or activity may differ. Comparing the available ankle motion with the required motion for a given sport or sports is an important functional parameter that can be measured and factored into a return to play decision. If a sport requires the athlete to run, jump, or pivot, athletes should be able to perform these functional tasks without pain or limitation before return to play. If athletes can test their ankle and reestablish full function in a noncompetitive, controlled setting, they are less likely to encounter functional limitations or further injury when they return to their sport.

Prevention of Ankle Sprains The use of tape, braces, and high-top shoes has been suggested to prevent ankle sprains. However, no studies have proved that these measures are effective in preventing sprains or physeal injuries. External support may be more effective for chronic ankle instability or for prevention of recurrent sprains. Taping is considered the most secure means of ankle protection after a sprain, but even with the optimal taping, the tape will become loose during play. Because many ankle sprains are recurrent, proper treatment and rehabilitation of previous ankle sprains can prevent many subsequent sprains.

Ankle Fractures

Small avulsion fractures at the tip of the lateral malleolus or medial malleolus typically do not require treatment any different from treatment for sprains. Fractures that are intra-articular, involve a physis, or allow for widening of the ankle mortise are of greater clinical concern. Salter-Harris type I and II fractures of the fibula can be caused by an inversion force. If the patient has tenderness and swelling over the distal fibula, the physician should carefully examine the radiograph for widening of the fibular physis (**Figure 43.15**).

Signs of this injury can be subtle and hard to detect. If there is suspicion or proof of physeal separation, the leg should be immobilized in a short leg walking cast for 3 to 4 weeks.

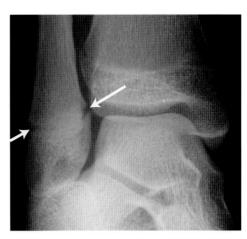

FIGURE 43.15 X-ray showing slight widening at margins of distal fibular physis. Note that the distal tibial physis is narrowed.

Follow-up evaluation and x-ray are also suggested to ensure normal healing and to rule out disrupted growth. Fractures involving a physis should be monitored for 2 years or until skeletal maturity is reached. If a twisting injury causes a fracture of the fibula proximal to the physis, the syndesmosis is typically disrupted. This results in an unstable mortise and problems with chronic instability or arthritis unless the fracture is stabilized surgically. Occasionally, fractures of the distal fibula occur from a direct blow, such as getting kicked in soccer or getting hit by a baseball. Because this mechanism does not disrupt the syndesmosis or destabilize the mortise, such fractures can usually be treated without surgery.

Salter-Harris type II fractures of the tibia are caused by an abduction external rotation force, and they are accompanied by an associated fracture of the fibula above the level of the syndesmosis. Examination will reveal gross displacement, and the metaphyseal fragment may be tenting the skin medially. As the athlete approaches skeletal maturity, the physes begin to close and the injury pattern for ankle fractures changes. The distal tibial physis closes first medially. Fractures occur through the lateral aspect of the physis and propagate proximally through the physis and/or distally through the articular surface. This produces the triplane fracture. The key to diagnosis of a triplane injury is that it will appear as a Salter-Harris type III fracture on the anteroposterior radiograph; on the lateral radiograph, it will appear as a Salter-Harris type II fracture (**Figure 43.16**). A computed tomography (CT) scan will most likely be needed to define the fragments and to plan treatment. Surgery is usually needed to restore the articular alignment and to minimize the risk of posttraumatic arthritis. Surgical consultation is appropriate for any ankle fracture, particularly fractures that involve the physis.

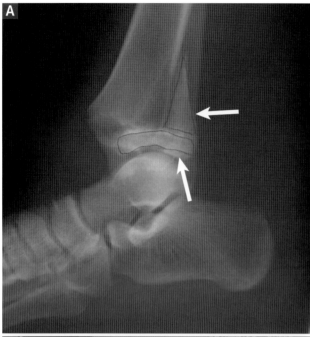

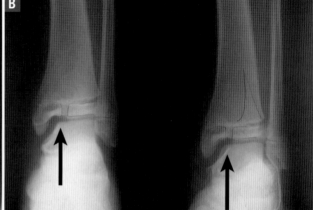

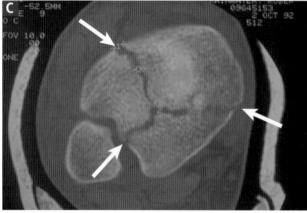

FIGURE 43.16 Triplane fracture. (A) On the lateral view, the entire epiphysis appears displaced with the metaphyseal fragment. (B) On the anteroposterior view, the epiphysis is fractured into at least 2 fragments, and the joint surface is involved. (C) A CT scan shows at least 3 fracture lines through the epiphysis.

FOOT INJURIES

The foot consists of 7 tarsals, 5 metatarsals, and 14 phalanges. The hindfoot consists of the talus and calcaneus; the midfoot consists of the navicular, cuboid, and cuneiforms. The forefoot includes the metatarsals and phalanges (**Figure 43.17**). Ligamentous structures provide support for the tarsals, metatarsals, and phalanges. Intrinsic and extrinsic muscles of the foot provide for movement and additional dynamic stability.

Foot Sprains

An inversion injury to the foot can result in a sprain of the calcaneal-cuboid joint or midfoot sprain. Patients manifest tenderness and swelling over the lateral portion of the midfoot at the calcaneal-cuboid joint and experience pain with passive inversion of the foot. Radiographs are typically normal but may show a small avulsion fracture off the cuboid.

The differential diagnosis includes a peroneal tendon strain, fifth metatarsal fracture, and cuboid fracture. Treatment requires stabilization of the foot with a rigid-sole cast shoe or cast boot. Taping may help stabilize the midfoot when the patient is ready to resume running, jumping, or cutting activity.

A sprain to the second tarsometatarsal joint is referred to as a Lisfranc sprain. This injury was originally described in soldiers in Napoleon's army who fell off their horses with a foot caught in the stirrup. Examination reveals tenderness and swelling over the proximal aspect of the second metatarsal and pain with passive abduction of the forefoot. Weight-bearing x-rays show a diastasis between the first and second metatarsals and occasionally a small avulsion fracture between the second metatarsal and the medial cuneiform. Treatment of a Lisfranc sprain requires cast immobilization and restricted weight bearing for at least 6 weeks. If

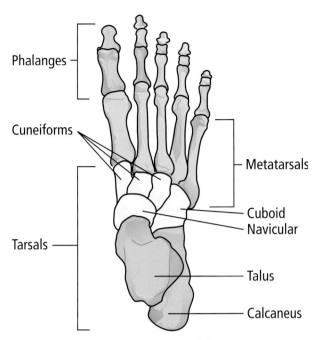

FIGURE 43.17 Bony anatomy of the foot.

Phalanges

Cuneiforms

Metatarsals

Cuboid
Navicular

Tarsals

Talus

Calcaneus

there is a fracture or lateral displacement of the second metatarsal, surgical stabilization should be performed. Sprains to the first metatarsal-phalangeal joint, or turf toe, can occur from a forced plantarflexion or dorsiflexion injury to the great toe. Patients experience pain and swelling at the first metatarsophalangeal joint and have difficulty flexing the toe as well as pushing off with walking or running. There is tenderness over the collateral ligaments and pain with passive motion in all planes. Radiographs may be normal but may be necessary to rule out a fracture of the base of the proximal phalanx or an avulsion fracture at the attachment of the collateral ligaments. Treatment of turf toe includes use of taping, a splint, and/or a rigid-soled shoe to stabilize the joint. When pain and swelling subside, selected forms of exercise may be slowly resumed. Activities such as cycling, using stair-climber or elliptical machines, rowing, skating, and weight lifting may initially be more readily tolerated because dorsiflexion or pushing off with the great toe is not required. When the patient returns to running, continued use of tape or a stiff-soled shoe can help relieve pain and protect the injured joint. It may be difficult for patients to regain preinjury running speed until the full joint range of motion has been restored.

Foot Strains

The muscular support of the foot comes from intrinsic and extrinsic sources. The smaller, intrinsic muscles of the foot (interossei, lumbricals, flexor/extensor digitorum brevis,

flexor/extensor hallucis brevis, abductor hallucis, peroneus tertius) rarely become the focus of an isolated injury. However, the larger extrinsic muscles do become injured and can produce clinically significant deficits.

The flexor hallucis longus (FHL) may be strained from a forceful contraction of the FHL that occurs while the great toe is in a dorsiflexed position. Ballet dancers and gymnasts are at particular risk for this injury because they frequently push off from a dorsiflexed great toe without the protection of a stiff-soled shoe. Prior FHL tendonitis or prior cortisone injections for tendonitis may increase the risk of an FHL strain.

The tendon may fail near the great toe, in the arch, or at the posteromedial ankle. The location of tenderness and swelling will vary according to the location of the strain. The critical finding at physical examination is pain and weakness associated with active flexion of the great toe. Treatment for an FHL strain should initially include crutches and immobilization in a splint with the ankle plantarflexed. Surgical consultation is warranted for higher-grade strains.

The tibialis posterior tendon supports the medial portion of the midfoot and assists with active adduction of the forefoot. The tibialis anterior also attaches to the medial portion of the midfoot and works to dorsiflex the ankle and adduct the forefoot. Injuries to either of these tendons produce local tenderness as well as pain and weakness associated with active contraction of the respective muscles. MRI may be required to confirm the diagnosis. Preliminary treatment should include splinting the foot and ankle or immobilization in a cast boot with crutches. High-grade partial or complete (ie, grades II–III) strains should be referred for surgical consultation.

Foot Fractures

The foot is anatomically divided into the hindfoot, midfoot, and forefoot. Hindfoot fractures include fractures of the talus and calcaneus. Talar dome fractures that occur in conjunction with ankle sprains have been previously discussed. Fractures of the talar neck or calcaneal fractures typically occur from high-impact loads, such as a motor vehicle accident or the impact from landing on a hard surface. The hallmarks of a talus or calcaneal fracture include swelling, ecchymosis, difficulty with weight bearing, and bony tenderness. Plain radiographs may appear normal, particularly if there is no deformity. A CT scan may be necessary to confirm the diagnosis and to appreciate the location, extent, and deformity associated with the injury. Immobilization and crutches should be used for initial therapy. Surgical consultation is suggested, and surgical treatment may be necessary for fractures with significant deformity.

The bones of the midfoot include the navicular, cuboid, and cuneiforms. Midfoot fractures can occur with direct impact or through a twisting mechanism. Again, the hallmarks of fracture are pain, swelling, ecchymosis, difficulty bearing weight, and point bony tenderness. As is the case with hindfoot fractures, the bones of the midfoot may be compressed rather than separated or displaced. This can make diagnosis by plain radiographs difficult. A bipartite navicular, accessory navicular, or os peroneum can appear to be a fracture but actually represents preexisting anatomic variants. Initial treatment for midfoot fracture also involves immobilization and crutches. Surgery may be indicated for deformity or nonunions.

The bones of the forefoot include the metatarsals, phalanges, and sesamoids. Metatarsal fractures and phalangeal fractures are the most common foot fractures. Fractures of the fifth metatarsal typically occur from an inversion injury and can be overlooked when an ankle sprain is suspected. Proximal fifth metatarsal fractures (**Figure 43.18**) as well as avulsion injuries to the peroneal brevis attachment can easily be confused with apophysitis of the fifth metatarsal or Iselin disease (**Figure 43.19**). If the bony fragment on the proximal fifth metatarsal is oriented parallel to the long access of the bone or is present on the contralateral side, an apophysis should be suspected. An avulsion fracture or a painful apophysis can be treated like a peroneal tendon strain. Immobilization followed by a rehabilitation program is appropriate. The fracture fragment may not fully heal or unite on follow-up x-ray, but a normal-appearing x-ray is not essential for a satisfactory clinical outcome.

A fracture that occurs at the metaphyseal-diaphyseal junction of the fifth metatarsal is known as a Jones fracture (**Figure 43.20**). A Jones fracture should be immobilized in a splint, a cast, or a cast boot, and the patient should initially be placed on crutches. Because there is a high incidence of nonunion with Jones fractures, surgery may need to be done. It is difficult to predict who will heal and whose injury will result in nonunion. Early surgical consultation may be appropriate for patients who may want to consider surgery over the risk of lengthy time delays associated with nonunions.

Fractures in the distal or midshaft portion of the fifth metatarsal are known as dancer's fractures (**Figure 43.21**). Most of these fractures can be treated conservatively with immobilization and crutches for 3 to 4 weeks followed by a

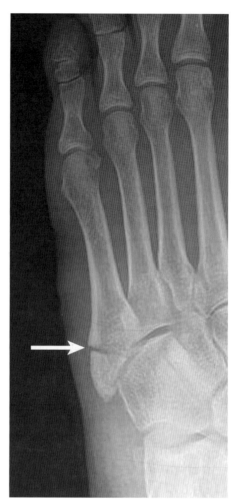

FIGURE 43.18 Avulsion fracture of proximal fifth metatarsal.

walking cast and weight bearing for another 3 to 4 weeks. However, initial surgical consultation is also appropriate.

Fractures of the second to fourth metatarsals can occur from direct blows to the foot or by twisting the foot. An isolated metatarsal fracture of the second, third, or fourth metatarsal is surrounded by intact metatarsals that provide an internal splinting mechanism. Treatment for such fractures usually requires a cast shoe or cast boot and crutches for 3 to 4 weeks, followed by protection in a rigid-soled shoe and protected weight bearing for another 3 to 4 weeks.

Fractures of the first metatarsal are rare in sports. Because of the load-bearing responsibilities of the first metatarsal, injuries should initially be immobilized, and crutches should be used. Early surgical referral is also appropriate.

The phalanges can readily be fractured, particularly in athletes who participate in sports with no shoe or foot

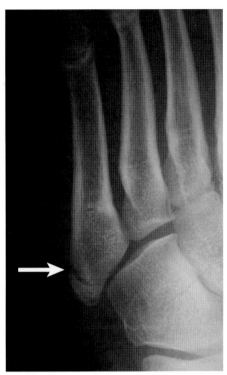

FIGURE 43.19 Apophysis at proximal fifth metatarsal in a patient with Iselin disease.

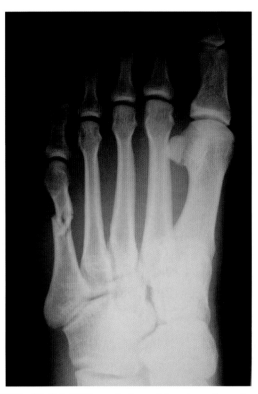

FIGURE 43.21 Fifth metatarsal fracture in a dancer.

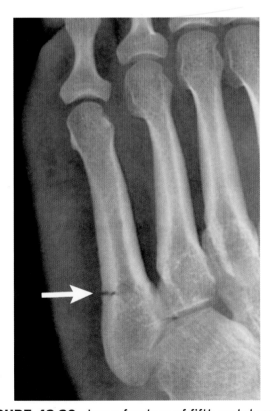

FIGURE 43.20 Jones fracture of fifth metatarsal.

protection. For the most part, phalangeal fractures that are minimally displaced can be treated with buddy taping and the use of a stiff-soled shoe or cast shoe. Fractures of the great toe typically require a greater degree of protection and a longer period of recovery.

Sesamoid fractures occur from heavy impact to the ball of the foot. Because the sesamoid bones are often bipartite or tripartite, it can be difficult to distinguish a sesamoid fracture from a preexisting variation. The presence of tenderness and swelling in the sesamoids after a plausible injury history warrants immobilization in a cast shoe or cast boot as well as use of crutches. Clinical standards for recovery and return to play are used because an injured sesamoid may remain abnormal in radiographic appearance, even in patients who have become symptom free.

OTHER ACUTE FOOT AND ANKLE INJURIES

Occasionally, a bony injury to the foot or ankle is insufficient to cause a fracture but can cause a bone bruise or contusion. This occurs most commonly in the heel. A heel bruise has a normal x-ray and bone scan but may show marrow edema on an MRI. Soft tissue contusions as well as lacerations, abrasions, acute bursitis, puncture wounds, and foreign bodies from puncture wounds may manifest as acute foot or ankle pain. Lacerations, blisters, or other wounds to the plantar aspect of the foot are particularly concerning because of the risk of infection and the difficulty in achieving proper wound healing while bearing weight.

SUMMARY POINTS

- Ankle sprains are the most common acute ankle injury. Ankle inversion sprains typically occur from an inversion plantarflexion mechanism and manifest as pain, swelling, tenderness, and laxity of the lateral ligament complex.

- When acute ankle injuries *do not* follow the clinical pattern for an inversion sprain, there is a far greater chance of fracture. Accordingly, when ankle injuries occur from eversion dorsiflexion mechanisms and produce pain and swelling that is more prominent medially, x-rays are more likely to show bony abnormalities.

- Nonoperative treatment is effective for most ankle sprains, and return to sports participation is possible once ankle function has been restored. Ankle fractures and growth plate injuries are more likely to need surgical intervention.

- Acute foot injuries include fractures, sprains, and strains. Anatomic variants and growth-related conditions can easily be confused with the effects of injury.

SUGGESTED READING

Anderson SJ. Acute ankle sprains: keys to diagnosis and return to play. *Phys Sports Med.* 2002;30:29-40.

Anderson SJ. Lower extremity injuries in youth sports. *Pediatr Clin North Am.* 2002;49:627-641.

Chambers HG. Ankle and foot disorders in skeletally immature athletes. *Orthop Clin North Am.* 2003;34:445-459.

Frost SC, Amendola A. Is stress radiography necessary in the diagnosis of acute or chronic ankle instability? *Clin J Sport Med.* 1999;9:40-45.

Gross JT, Liu HY. The role of ankle bracing for prevention of ankle sprain injuries. *J Orthop Sports Phys Ther.* 2003;33;572-577.

Hopkins JT, Palmieri R. Effects of ankle joint effusion on lower leg function. *Clin J Sport Med.* 2004;14:1-7.

Judd DB, Kim DH. Foot fractures frequently misdiagnosed as ankle sprains. *Am Fam Physician.* 2002;66:785-794.

Kerkhoffs GM, Rowe BH, Assendelft WJ, Kelly KD, Struijs PA, van Dijk CN. Immobilisation for acute ankle sprain: a systematic review. *Arch Orthop Trauma Surg.* 2001;121: 462-471.

Lin CF, Gross ML, Weinhold P. Ankle syndesmosis injuries: anatomy, biomechanics, mechanism of injury, and clinical guidelines for diagnosis and intervention. *J Orthop Sports Phys Ther.* 2006;36:372-384.

McGuine TA, Keene JS. The effect of a balance training program on the risk of ankle sprains in high school athletes. *Am J Sports Med.* 2006;34:1103-1111.

Merrill KD. The Maissonneuve fracture of the fibula. *Clin Orthop.* 1993;287:218–223.

Niemi WJ, Savidakis J Jr, DeJesus JM. Peroneal subluxation: a comprehensive review of the literature with case presentations. *J Foot Ankle Surg.* 1997;36:141-145.

Nunley JA, Vertullo CJ. Classification, investigation, and management of midfoot sprains. Lisfranc injuries in the athlete. *Am J Sports Med.* 2002;30:871-878.

Olmsted LC, Vela LI, Denegar CR, Hertel J. Prophylactic ankle taping and bracing: a numbers-needed-to-treat and cost-benefit analysis. *J Athl Train.* 2004;39:95-100.

O'Malley MJ, Hamilton WG, Munyak J. Fractures of the distal shaft of the fifth metatarsal: "dancer's fracture." *Am J Sports Med.* 1996;24:240-243.

Osborne MD, Rizzo TD. Prevention and treatment of ankle sprain in athletes. *Sports Med.* 2004;39:95-100.

Richie DH. Functional instability of the ankle and the role of neuromuscular control: a comprehensive review. *J Foot Ankle Surg.* 2001;40:240-251.

Schachter AK, Chen AL, Reddy PD, Tejwani NC. Osteochondral lesions of the talus. *J Am Acad Orthop Surg.* 2005;13:152-158.

Stiell IG, Breenberg GH, McKnight RD, et al. Decision rules for the use of radiography in acute ankle injuries: refinement and prospective validation. *JAMA.* 1993;269: 1127-1132.

Thacker SB, Stroup DF, Branche CM, Gilchrist J, Goodman RA, Weitman EA. The prevention of ankle sprains in sports. A systematic review of the literature. *Am J Sports Med.* 1999;27:753-760.

Trojian TH, McKeag DB. Single leg balance test to identify risk of ankle sprains. *Br J Sports Med.* 2006;40:610-613.

Verhagen E, van der Beek A, Twisk J, Bouter L, Bahr R, van Mechelen W. The effect of a proprioceptive balance board training program for the prevention of ankle sprains: a prospective controlled trial. *Am J Sports Med.* 2004;32:1383-1384.

CHAPTER 44

Chronic Foot and Ankle Injuries

Daniel E. Kraft, MD

With more organized, specialized, and intensive sports activities available to young people today, overuse injuries, including those to the foot and ankle, are being seen by medical professionals with increasing frequency. The foot and ankle are the primary points of impact in most sports, and foot and ankle overuse injuries are seen across the spectrum of athletic endeavors. Many of the injuries are a result of an increase in activity level that exceeds the adaptive capacity of the body to handle the repetitive loads. In the foot and ankle, these overuse injuries may involve the apophysis, tendon, or bone. This chapter discusses the clinical evaluation, diagnosis, and treatment of nonacute foot and ankle injuries.

ANATOMY/BIOMECHANICS

The ankle joint comprises the talus and its articulation in the bony mortise formed by the distal tibia, fibula, medial malleolus, and lateral malleolus. The foot can be anatomically divided into the hind foot, midfoot, and forefoot (**Figure 44.1**). The tarsal bones of the hind foot include the talus and calcaneus. The midfoot includes the navicular, cuboid, and cuneiforms. The forefoot includes the metatarsals, phalanges, and sesamoids. Accessory ossicles are commonly found near the navicular, in the peroneal tendon, and posterior to the talus (os trigonum). Ligaments provide support for bony structures in the foot but are rarely involved with overuse injuries. The plantar fascia extends from the base of the calcaneus to the proximal phalanges. It helps maintain the longitudinal arch of the foot. Muscular support for the longitudinal arch comes from intrinsic muscles of the foot and extrinsic muscles of the calf and leg that connect to the foot by long tendons. Growth centers, or apophyses, serve as attachment sites for the Achilles tendon on the calcaneus and the peroneal brevis tendon on the fifth metatarsal.

Pronation and supination occur at the subtalar joint (**Figure 44.2**). As a result of the axis rotation of the subtalar joint, pronation is actually a combination of ankle eversion, dorsiflexion, forefoot abduction, and internal rotation of the tibia. Supination is a combination of ankle inversion, plantarflexion, forefoot adduction, and external rotation of the tibia. The angle of rotation around the subtalar joint allows movement in the foot to be translated to rotation in the leg.

With each gait cycle, the subtalar joint alternates between pronation and supination. At heel strike, the subtalar joint pronates. A pronated foot is flexible and adaptable, and it is effective at absorbing impact. As the foot progresses from midstance to push-off, the subtalar joint supinates. A supinated foot is more stable, and it allows the foot to function as a rigid lever to allow for push-off. A foot that is excessively pronated places additional demands on extrinsic musculature to provide needed stability.

The increased internal tibial rotation associated with excessive pronation can contribute to malalignment problems proximally. A foot that is excessively supinated has diminished shock-absorbing capacity and is associated with impact-related injuries such as stress fractures. Restricted or painful motion at the subtalar joint can be the result of a bony bridge or fusion at the subtalar joint or tarsal coalition.

In addition to bony and musculotendinous injury, overuse problems in the foot-ankle area can involve a subcutaneous bursa, peripheral nerve, plantar interdigital nerve, or arteries. Injuries to these structures produce bursitis, neuritis, Morton neuroma, and vasospasm, respectively.

EVALUATION

History

As is the case with other overuse injuries, the history should begin with a review of the athlete's current training patterns, recent changes or increases in training, and changes in equipment, such as shoes. The timing, location, quality, and severity of pain should be determined, as should the presence of swelling, stiffness, clicking, popping, instability, weakness, numbness, and tingling. The effect of

Bones of the ankle and foot

Dorsal view

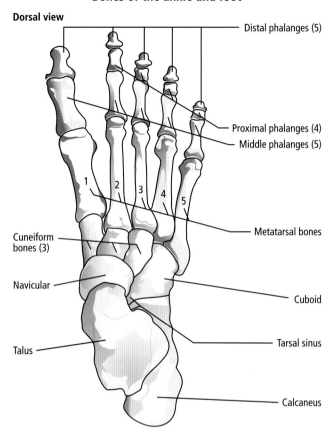

Distal phalanges (5)

Proximal phalanges (4)

Middle phalanges (5)

1 2 3 4 5

Cuneiform bones (3)

Metatarsal bones

Navicular

Cuboid

Talus

Tarsal sinus

Calcaneus

FIGURE 44.1 Bony anatomy of foot and ankle.

the condition on activity should be investigated, including which activities can be continued without symptoms. Details of prior or concurrent injury should be elicited, as should the results of previous tests and treatment.

Physical Examination

The physical examination for overuse injuries in the foot and ankle should begin with an inspection of gait and lower extremity alignment. Knowing the foot type can help the clinician understand the cause of the injury and the plan for treatment of specific injuries (**Figure 44.3**). A hyperpronated or flat foot appears with the calcaneus everted, forefoot abducted, ankle dorsiflexed, and tibia internally rotated with respect to the foot. A supinated or high-arched foot appears with an inverted calcaneus, adducted forefoot, plantarflexed ankle, and externally rotated tibia. With a flexible flat foot, the calcaneus will invert, and an arch will develop when the patient stands on his or her toes. With a rigid flat foot (as seen with subtalar tarsal coalitions), the arch will remain flat and the calcaneus will remain everted with a toe raise.

The foot and ankle should be inspected for swelling, abnormal bony prominences, and general configuration. A Morton's foot type has a second metatarsal that is longer than the first metatarsal. A bunion is associated with hallux valgus or a great toe that deviates laterally at the first metatarsal phalangeal joint. Metatarsus adductus or a varus forefoot implies that all the metatarsals point medially. Inspection of the callus pattern on the plantar aspect of the foot can reveal where most of the weight-bearing stress has occurred. Inspection of the patient's athletic shoes and other footwear may also provide insights into the cause of foot or ankle pain.

Medial view

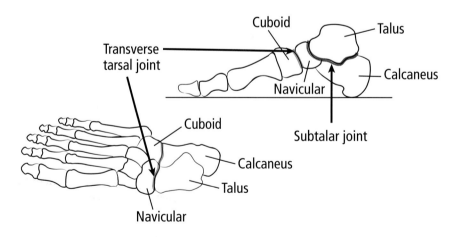

Cuboid

Talus

Transverse tarsal joint

Calcaneus

Navicular

Subtalar joint

Cuboid

Calcaneus

Talus

Navicular

Superior view

FIGURE 44.2 Location of subtalar and midtarsal joints.

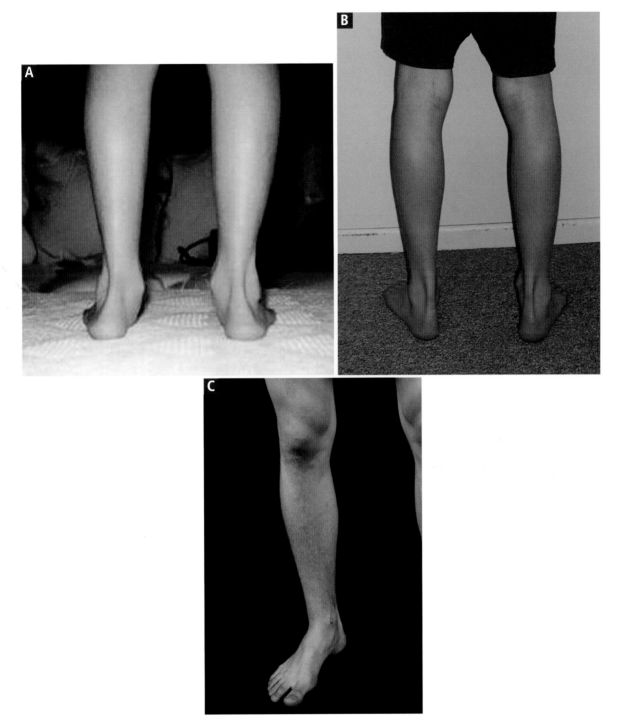

FIGURE 44.3 (A) Pronated foot. (B) Neutral foot. (C) Supinated foot.

Palpation should evaluate bony tenderness over the tarsals, metatarsals, sesamoids, and ankle. Bony tenderness may also be found over an apophysis at the heel or fifth metatarsal. Superficial tenderness with or without localized swelling may be due to bursitis over any bony prominence. With tendonitis, there may be tenderness and/or swelling involving the

Achilles tendon, tibialis posterior, or peroneal tendons. The interdigital space between the metatarsals should be palpated for tenderness or swelling involving an interdigital nerve.

Testing joint range of motion and stability can reveal abnormalities from prior ligamentous or bony injuries and can help identify restrictions that may alter normal foot mechanics. For example, restricted dorsiflexion of the ankle may place additional demands for dorsiflexion on the midfoot. Hypermobility of the first metatarsal may shift more load-bearing demands on the lateral portion of the foot. Loss of ankle dorsiflexion could be due to chronic bony changes on either the anterior talus or on the anterior distal tibia. Loss of ankle plantarflexion could be due to an accessory ossicle (os trigonum) causing bony impingement posterior to the talus.

Strength testing can reveal specific patterns of weakness or serve as a provocative test for specific tendon injuries. Pain or weakness with flexion of the great toe may indicate tendonitis of the flexor hallucis longus. Pain, weakness, and/or a snapping sensation may indicate tendonitis or subluxation of the peroneal tendons.

Sensory deficits can be seen with lumbar radiculopathy as well as peripheral nerve injuries to the sural nerve, medial or lateral plantar nerve, deep peroneal nerve, or the superficial sensory peroneal nerve. Skin color or temperature changes could be seen with peripheral vascular disease, Raynaud disease, or sympathetic dysfunction.

Imaging Studies

Plain radiographs of the foot and/or ankle are indicated for any patient with bony pain, tenderness, or restricted motion in the foot or ankle. Anteroposterior (AP), lateral, and oblique views can reveal abnormalities related to foot structure and alignment, as well as growth centers, accessory ossification centers, and selected abnormalities such as stress fractures and bone cysts. Magnetic resonance imaging (MRI) is useful for suspected soft tissue injuries such as tendonitis or for chondral or osteochondral lesions. Bone scans are still an option for evaluating stress fractures. However, it is not unusual for bone scans performed on active individuals to reveal multiple areas of increased radiotracer uptake in the foot and ankle. Careful clinical correlation is necessary to determine which areas of increased uptake on bone scan are clinically important. Computed tomography (CT) scans are useful in clarifying complex bony abnormalities such as a tarsal coalition, in evaluating healing of stress fractures, and in defining pathology in bone cysts or tumors.

APOPHYSITIS

Calcaneal Apophysitis (Sever's Disease)

One of the most common overuse injuries affecting young athletes is calcaneal apophysitis, or Sever's disease. Calcaneal apophysitis was first described in 1912 as a case of posterior heel pain. This pain is caused by a traction-related stress reaction at the insertion sites of the Achilles tendon and the plantar

fascia on the calcaneal apophysis (**Figure 44.4**). The calcaneal apophysis appears radiographically between ages 8 and 9 years and fuses between ages 12 and 15 years. Calcaneal apophysitis clinically manifests during this interval. Because skeletal maturation generally occurs later in boys than girls, boys who develop calcaneal apophysitis tend to be slightly older than girls.

Athletes with calcaneal apophysitis will experience heel pain in one or both heels. The pain initially occurs after sports activities, but as the problem progresses, the pain may occur during activity; ultimately, the pain may limit activity. A limp or altered running style may be observed. The symptoms usually resolve with rest but quickly reappear when activity resumes. Running and high-impact activities, such as soccer, basketball, and football, are commonly associated with calcaneal apophysitis. Use of athletic cleats has been implicated as a contributing factor because the cleats generally lack a cushion, arch support, or a heel lift to protect the apophysis.

At physical examination, athletes with calcaneal apophysitis will have point tenderness over the calcaneal apophysis, which can be palpated either medially or laterally on the calcaneus (**Figure 44.5**). Tenderness may also be appreciated near the insertion of the Achilles tendon. A tight calf and Achilles tendon may contribute to increased tension on the calcaneal apophysis. A hyperpronated or flat foot is associated with increased tension on the plantar fascia, which further contributes to tension on the apophysis.

Radiographs are not necessary to diagnose calcaneal apophysitis when the clinical findings are consistent with the diagnosis. X-rays can be performed to exclude other bony abnormalities and to determine the maturation of the apophysis (**Figure 44.6**).

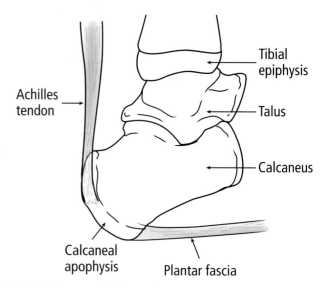

FIGURE 44.4 Calcaneal apophysis with attachment of Achilles tendon and plantar fascia.

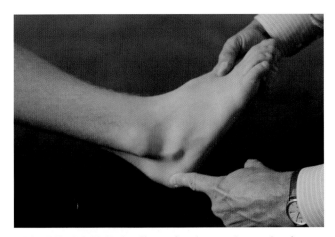

FIGURE 44.5 Palpation of calcaneal apophysis.

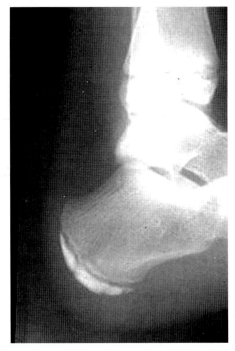

FIGURE 44.6 Lateral radiograph in patient with calcaneal apophysitis.

The calcaneal apophysis normally has an irregular and fragmented appearance. The radiographic appearance of a symptomatic calcaneal apophysis is not distinguishable from an asymptomatic calcaneal apophysis.

The differential diagnosis for heel pain includes Achilles tendonitis, os trigonum/posterior impingement, plantar fasciitis, and calcaneal stress fractures. Achilles tendonitis occurs more commonly in skeletally mature patients and it is associated with tenderness in the distal Achilles tendon rather than on the apophysis. A symptomatic os trigonum causes pain and tenderness posterior to the talus and

symptoms that are worse when the os trigonum is compressed with active or passive plantarflexion of the ankle. The presence of an os trigonum or an elongated posterior talar process can be confirmed by plain films.

Plantar fasciitis is rare in skeletally immature patients. However, if the calcaneal apophysis has matured and if there is tenderness on the plantar aspect of the calcaneus, plantar fasciitis may be diagnosed. Calcaneal stress fractures cause pain and tenderness in the body of the calcaneus rather than just the apophysis. A calcaneal stress fracture can be diagnosed by bone scan or MRI.

Calcaneal apophysitis is a self-limited problem that will resolve when the apophysis matures but can become asymptomatic much earlier with proper treatment. Long-term problems from calcaneal apophysitis are rare. Treatment is designed to relieve tension and compression on the apophysis. Usually patients need to reduce running, jumping, and impact activity. However, low-impact activities, such as cycling, swimming, skating, or weight lifting, can often be continued in a pain-free manner. Ice treatments can be used after activity or if there is pain. Stretching the calf and Achilles tendon can also relieve tension on the calcaneal apophysis. A heel lift, approximately three-eighths of an inch in height, is used in the shoes to further decrease tension on the apophysis and reduce pain during activity. A felt or rubber heel lift or a heel cup can provide both lift and cushion. Inserts that protect the heel should be used in both shoes, even if only one heel is symptomatic. It may also be possible to use an orthotic insert to provide arch support as long at the heel can be built up to allow for relief of tension on the Achilles tendon.

When the pain subsides and when flexibility has been increased, it may be possible for the athlete to gradually resume running and other impact activities. Symptoms of heel pain should determine the rate of increase.

Iselin Disease (Fifth Metatarsal Apophysitis)

Another traction apophysitis that affects the foot and ankle area of young athletes is Iselin disease. This traction apophysitis involves the attachment of the peroneal brevis tendon at the base of the fifth metatarsal.

Pain is produced with high levels of impact activities and activities that cause repetitive peroneal muscle action, such as performing lateral movements and cutting. Iselin disease occurs in a similar age range as calcaneal apophysitis. Athletes typically experience lateral foot pain and point tenderness over the base of the fifth metatarsal (**Figure 44.7**). Iselin disease is a clinical diagnosis, and x-rays are mainly used to confirm the presence of an apophysis and to rule out other bony problems (**Figure 44.8**).

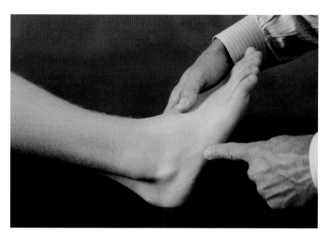

FIGURE 44.7 Location of tenderness in Iselin disease.

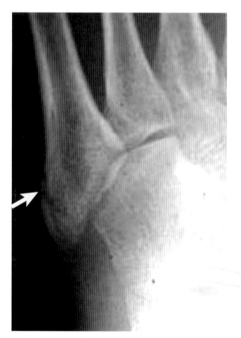

FIGURE 44.8 Iselin apophysitis.

The differential diagnosis for Iselin disease includes stress fractures of the fifth metatarsal, avulsion fractures, the Jones fracture, and os peroneum. (**Figure 44.9A-C**). Careful palpation of the fifth metatarsal to determine point tenderness at the base of the fifth metatarsal versus the shaft will help differentiate these diagnoses. Stress fractures are also more commonly seen in older adolescent athletes. Acute avulsion of the base of the fifth metatarsal will have similar tenderness as Iselin disease during physical examination, but the athlete will have a history of a specific inversion injury versus a more chronic history, as seen with Iselin disease. Plain films can also be used to help differentiate stress fractures and

avulsion fractures from Iselin disease. A comparison plain film of the opposite foot will help prove whether the patient's film is actually showing a physis or an avulsion injury.

Iselin disease can be more stubborn and less responsive to treatment than calcaneal apophysitis. Initial conservative treatment includes modifying activity, applying ice, and stretching and strengthening the peroneals. Orthotics can also help these patients, but measures to diminish tension on the peroneals may shift the foot into pronation. If pain continues, immobilization with a walking boot may be indicated. Iselin is usually a self-limited problem, like calcaneal apophysitis. Rare cases of apophyseal nonunion related to Iselin disease have been reported.

BONE PROBLEMS

Metatarsal Stress Fractures

The most common stress fracture occurring in the foot is the metatarsal stress fracture. Repetitive stress across the midshaft of the metatarsal bone from impact activities like running and jumping is the major cause of injury. This type of stress fracture is commonly seen both in boys and girls. The second, third, and fourth metatarsals are the most commonly affected.

Athletes will experience a gradual onset of midfoot pain that increases with impact activities. Commonly, athletes will have a history of 2 to 3 weeks of increasing pain before they seek medical attention. Short periods of rest, such as 3 to 5 days, will temporarily alleviate the pain symptoms, only to have them recur when the athlete returns to the offending activity.

Careful palpation at physical examination will yield point tenderness over the metatarsal bone. It may be possible to palpate a swollen area of callus formation in the midshaft of the metatarsal. Athletes will also complain of pain in the foot when performing the single-leg hop test.

Plain radiographs should always start the diagnostic workup for a suspected metatarsal stress fracture. Plain films may be normal or show cortical callus formation along the affected metatarsal cortex, which usually indicates new bone healing a stress fracture (**Figure 44.10**). If plain films are normal and the possibility of a metatarsal stress fracture is still being considered, further testing by either MRI or bone scan can confirm the diagnosis of a stress fracture.

Nerve-related problems, such as impingement of the deep peroneal nerve or a Morton's neuroma, can mimic symptoms of a metatarsal stress fracture. Both of these problems can be differentiated from a stress fracture with careful palpation of the midfoot and forefoot. Deep peroneal nerve

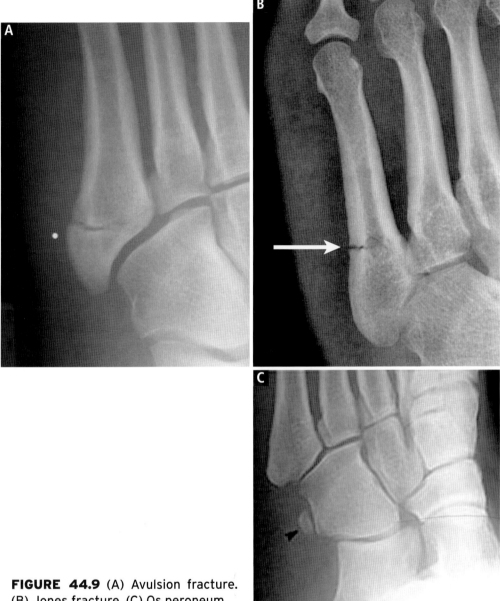

FIGURE 44.9 (A) Avulsion fracture. (B) Jones fracture. (C) Os peroneum.

pain will be elicited by palpating the route of the nerve, most typically at the area of the first and second cuneiform bones. This pain will also often refer into the 1 to 2 web space when symptomatic. Morton's neuroma pain most commonly is located between the third and fourth metatarsal heads. There may be visible swelling and pain elicited by squeezing the metatarsal heads. With a symptomatic neuroma, imaging studies (plain film, bone scan, MRI) can rule out a bony source for the pain but cannot confirm the diagnosis of a symptomatic neuroma.

Metatarsalgia is a nonspecific pain of the metatarsal head and can have symptoms like a stress fracture. Patients with metatarsalgia will also have normal plain films and normal MRI or bone scan.

Initial treatment for metatarsal stress fractures begins by restricting the athlete from impact activities. Many physicians will immobilize the foot in a walking boot for 2 to 4 weeks. The boot affords protection for the stress fracture while permitting pain-free ambulation without the need for crutches. The boot also allows athletes to transition more quickly into cross training with nonimpact activities, such as riding a stationary bike or using an elliptical trainer.

To help get athletes back to play and help prevent recurrence of the stress fracture, custom orthotics can be used to

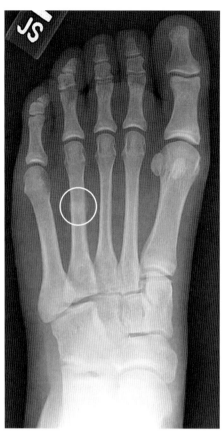

FIGURE 44.10 Fourth metatarsal stress fracture.

unload the affected metatarsal bone. This type of custom orthotic will decrease the impact stress across the fracture site and help the athlete experience less pain when returning to play. The orthotic can also decrease the chance of recurrence.

Metatarsal stress fractures involving the second, third, and fourth metatarsals require a minimum of 6 weeks to heal. Athletes may be able to return to low-impact conditioning or cross training as early as 3 to 4 weeks. Athletes need to continue to cross train with nonimpact activities until the stress fracture has healed completely. Training errors, including "too much, too soon, too fast," also need to be addressed. Dietary issues (total caloric and calcium intake) and menstrual irregularities should also be addressed, if applicable.

If an athlete with a metatarsal stress fracture is allowed to return to play too early or not followed closely, the sequelae can include complete fracture of the metatarsal or nonunion. Pain is an excellent indicator of the status of a healing metatarsal stress fracture. Therefore, athletes should avoid anti-inflammatories or other pain medicines during their return to play so as not to block their symptoms of pain. Follow-up radiographs can also confirm that healing has occurred.

Jones Fracture

Fractures at the metaphyseal-diaphyseal junction of the fifth metatarsal are known as Jones fractures (**Figure 44.11**). This terminology may be applied to an acute fracture at this area or a more chronic injury such as a stress fracture or nonunion of an acute fracture. Whether the injury occurs acutely or from repetitive stress, delayed healing is common as a result of the tenuous blood supply to this area of the bone. Fibrous unions or nonunions are much more common in the proximal fifth metatarsal than in the other metatarsals. As a result, short periods of rest or immobilization in a cast boot may be insufficient to achieve complete bony healing. Surgical consultation is indicated to address options for internal fixation and possible bone grafting when healing is delayed. Given the high rate of delayed healing or non-union, it may also be appropriate to address surgical options earlier in the course of treatment.

Navicular Stress Fracture

Although less common than metatarsal stress fractures, navicular stress fractures can also occur in sports involving repetitive impact. The athlete will seek care for activity-related midfoot pain or anterior ankle pain. A high-arched, cavus foot may contribute to increased stress concentrated in the navicular. Point tenderness over the dorsal aspect of

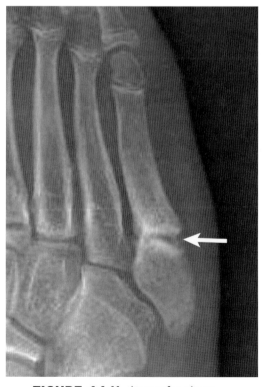

FIGURE 44.11 Jones fracture.

the navicular should warrant further evaluation for a stress fracture.

Diagnostic tests should start with plain films of the foot and move to a bone scan (**Figure 44.12**) or MRI if plain films are normal. If a bony abnormality is diagnosed, a CT scan can be performed to confirm the extent of injury and then used as a baseline to document healing during follow-up care.

Treatment for navicular stress fractures starts with 6 weeks of non–weight bearing while wearing a cast boot. If the CT scan shows evidence of healing, the athlete may require another 4 to 6 weeks of weight bearing while still wearing a cast boot. If there is clinical and radiographic evidence of continued healing, the athlete may be fitted with a custom orthotic and gradually transitioned back to weight bearing and, eventually, impact activities. Nonunions can occur with navicular stress fractures and need surgical intervention with screw fixation.

Accessory Navicular

Accessory bones about the foot and ankle are normal variants and represent secondary centers of ossification (**Table 44.1, Figure 44.13**). Approximately 22% of all individuals 16 years and younger have at least one accessory ossicle. These variants are usually asymptomatic but can become symptomatic with sports activity. Athletes with a painful accessory navicular have medial foot pain that is worse with impact activities or tight-fitting shoes. At physical examination, they have a bony prominence over the medial aspect of their navicular, and they tend to be flat-footed. Point tenderness can be elicited over the medial navicular.

Plain radiographs can verify the diagnosis. AP, lateral, and oblique views of the foot are obtained to evaluate the accessory navicular (**Figure 44.14**). The accessory navicular appears medial and proximal to the navicular. Clinical symptoms, along with a positive plain film, are usually diagnostic of a painful accessory navicular.

Other possibilities for medial foot pain include a navicular stress fracture, bipartite navicular, tibialis posterior tendonitis,

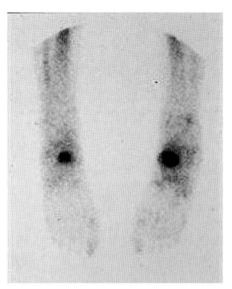

FIGURE 44.12 Bone scan showing bilateral navicular stress fractures.

plantar fasciitis, and deep peroneal nerve entrapment pain. Careful palpation of the foot will help differentiate navicular stress fracture from a symptomatic accessory navicular. As noted previously, the navicular stress fracture will more commonly have tenderness over the dorsum of the navicular, whereas the accessory navicular will have more medial tenderness. A bipartite navicular may appear radiographically similar to a non-union stress fracture through the central portion of the navicular. However, a bipartate navicular typically appears without the lengthily clinical history of stress fracture pain. The presence of similarly appearing radiographic findings on the asymptomatic foot can confirm the diagnosis of bipartite navicular. Tibialis posterior tendonitis manifests as pain and tenderness along the course of the tendon proximal to the navicular. Plantar fasciitis manifests as heel or arch pain with tenderness along the proximal portion of the plantar fascia as it attaches to the medial aspect of the

Table 44.1		
Location and Frequency of Common Accessory Bones of the Foot		
Common Accessory Bones	**Location**	**Frequency**
Os tibiale externum (accessory navicular)	Medial aspect of navicular	4%-21%
Os peroneum	Lateral aspect of cuboid	5%-20%
Os trigonum	Posterior to talus	3%-14%
Os vesalianum	Base of fifth metatarsal	6%
Os supranaviculare	Superior aspect of navicular	1%-3%
Os intermetatarseum	Between first and second metatarsal	1%
Os subfibulare	Distal portion of lateral malleolus	2%
Os subtibiale	Distal portion of medial malleolus	1%

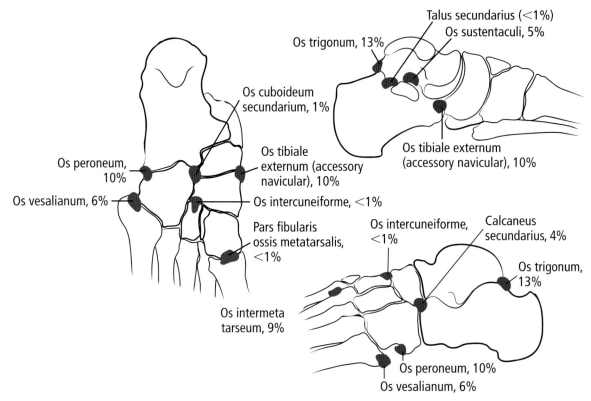

FIGURE 44.13 Location and frequency of accessory ossification centers of foot.

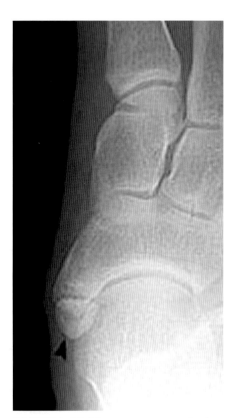

FIGURE 44.14 Accessory navicular.

calcaneus. Deep peroneal nerve pain is most commonly over the dorsum of the midfoot, which differs from the medial pain seen with the accessory navicular.

Because many athletes with a painful accessory navicular have flat feet, treatment usually begins with orthotics to support the arch. Rehabilitation will also focus on improving Achilles tendon flexibility, which can improve ankle-foot mechanics and decrease medial foot stress. Athletes' return to play will be tempered by pain. If pain continues with conservative treatment, some athletes may be candidates for surgical intervention where the accessory navicular is excised. Athletes with a painful accessory navicular who participate in barefoot sports like gymnastics and dance generally do not respond well to conservative treatment. Taping the arch during activity may provide some relief. Surgical treatment may be sought to treat persistent symptoms.

Os Trigonum

Athletes who experience posterior ankle pain but who have no known injury can have a symptomatic os trigonum. The os trigonum is a bony ossicle off the posterior aspect of the talus. Repetitive or forced plantarflexion activities in sports are the most common cause for an os trigonum becoming symptomatic. This occurs in ballet dancers from pointing their toes, soccer players from striking the ball, and swimmers from kicking or using fins.

At physical examination, palpation of the posterior talus anterior to the Achilles tendon will produce pain. The athlete will also experience posterior pain with active or passive plantarflexion of the ankle. Plain radiographs can be diagnostic for the presence of an os trigonum (**Figure 44.15**). The differential diagnosis of posterior talar pain includes flexor hallucis longus tendonitis, tibialis posterior tendonitis, and posterior talar impingement without associated bony pathology. Treatment for a symptomatic os trigonum starts with modifying activity to reduce plantarflexion, icing, and anti-inflammatory medications. Taping may reduce plantarflexion. Corticosteroid injection may reduce swelling in the surrounding soft tissues. If symptoms do not respond to conservative treatment, surgical excision of the symptomatic os trigonum may be needed.

Sesamoiditis

The location of the sesamoid bones on the plantar aspect of the foot and their function in the mechanics of the great toe expose the sesamoids to overuse injuries. Sports cleats with stress points directly over the sesamoids and barefoot activities like dance have been contributing factors in cases of sesamoiditis. Athletes will complain of pain over the ball of the foot with impact or with pushing off from the toes. Sesamoiditis, which is inflammation of soft tissue around sesamoids, and a sesamoid stress fracture will manifest as similar pain over the ball of the foot.

Plain radiographs of the foot, including the sesamoid view, can help with the initial assessment (**Figure 44.16**). Sesamoid fractures may be difficult to differentiate from anatomic variants such as bipartite sesamoid bones.

Sesamoid stress fractures may require a bone scan or MRI to confirm the diagnosis.

Treatment for sesamoiditis typically starts with restriction of impact activities and the use of a dancer's pad to decrease stress across the sesamoid. Once patients are asymptomatic, they can try a gradual return to sports activity while still using the dancer's pad. If pain continues, then immobilization in a walking boot may be required.

Sesamoid stress fractures, on the other hand, are treated with immobilization in a walking boot for 4 to 6 weeks. A plan of gradual return to impact activities is then followed to return athletes to play. Use of a dancer's pad or custom orthotic with relief for the sesamoids can help ensure a safe return to full activity.

Tarsal Coalition

Tarsal coalition is a congenital bridging of at least 2 tarsal bones in the foot. The coalition is initially cartilaginous and not seen with plain radiographs. As bones become ossified with skeletal maturity, the coalition becomes more rigid, more painful, and more likely to be seen on plain x-rays. Three percent to 5% of the general population has this variant. The 2 most common coalitions are calcaneonavicular and talocalcaneal.

The athlete's symptoms may be initiated with an acute injury or may develop over time. Athletes will experience symptoms of midfoot and/or hind foot pain; the most common age range of affected athletes is 8 to 16 years, the age at which the tarsal bridging starts to ossify, causing painful restriction of subtalar motion. Also, this is an age when many athletes increase the level and intensity of their sports participation. The combination of these 2 factors

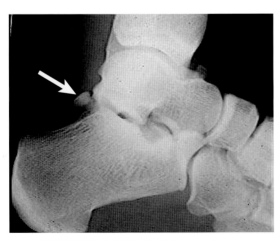

FIGURE 44.15 Os trigonum.

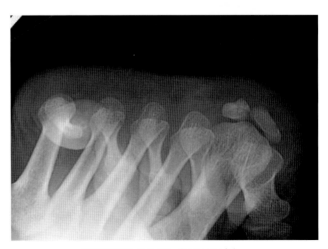

FIGURE 44.16 Sesamoids.

likely plays a major role in the development of symptoms in athletes with tarsal coalition during this stage of life.

The physical examination will reveal a valgus hind foot with increased foot pronation. Subtalar motion will be restricted when tested in a plantarflexed position. Patients with subtalar tarsal coalitions can have a rigid, painful flat foot. Peroneal spasm may be seen with tarsal coalitions. This may be a compensatory response that helps restrict painful subtalar motion.

Plain film evaluation should include AP, lateral, and oblique views of the foot and a tangential view of the calcaneus (**Figure 44.17**). CT scan is still considered the gold standard for diagnosis of tarsal coalitions (**Figure 44.18**).

Conservative treatment includes stretching the Achilles tendon and wearing custom orthotics to support the arch and reduce painful motion at the subtalar joint. Surgical intervention may be necessary to remove the coalition. Controversy exists regarding the optimal timing of surgery. Many surgeons now suggest surgical treatment during adolescence to help prevent more advanced degenerative changes in the subtalar area.

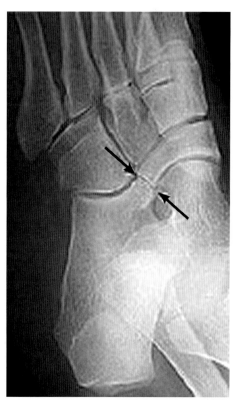

FIGURE 44.17 Calcaneonavicular tarsal coalition.

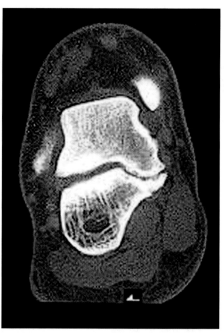

FIGURE 44.18 CT scan showing talocalcaneal coalition.

Osteochondritis Dissecans of Talus

Osteochondral lesions of the talar dome can cause ankle pain in adolescent athletes. This problem should be suspected in an adolescent athlete with a history of an ankle sprain that does not improve with appropriate conservative treatment. Osteochondritis dissecans should also be suspected in an athlete who experiences symptoms of joint swelling and pain with no significant injury. These athletes will often have increasing pain or symptoms of instability with activity.

Plain films may show hyperlucency in the talar dome and occasionally a bony defect or loose body. MRI is used to both diagnose and evaluate the extent of the lesion (**Figure 44.19**). Treatment requires limiting impact activity and following the patient clinically and radiographically for evidence of healing. Surgical consultation is advisable and persistent pain, swelling, or mechanical symptoms may warrant surgical intervention.

TENDON PROBLEMS

Achilles Tendonitis

Athletes diagnosed with Achilles tendonitis typically have symptoms of pain, burning, and/or tightness in the distal Achilles tendon associated with running or jumping activities.

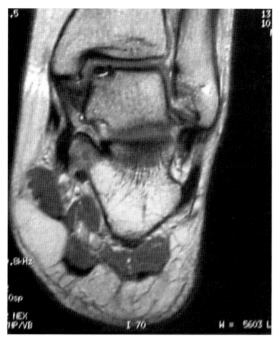

FIGURE 44.19 MRI showing osteochondritis dissecans of the superior-medial talar dome.

Their history will be similar to that of athletes with calcaneal apophysitis, but patients with Achilles tendonitis are older and usually have fused calcaneal apophyses. At physical examination, tenderness can be elicited over the Achilles tendon 3 cm to 4 cm proximal to the insertion on the calcaneus. There may also be mild swelling, crepitation, and pain with passive stretch or resisted contraction of the calf.

Treatment for Achilles tendonitis starts with modifying activity to reduce tension on the Achilles tendon. Running on hills, jumping, sprinting, or performing explosive movements subject the Achilles tendon to additional tension. Conversely, activities such as cycling, using elliptical trainers, stair climbing, or swimming can usually be tolerated without overloading the Achilles tendon. Treatment includes icing to relieve pain and inflammation and following a stretching program for the calf and Achilles tendon. The use of heel lifts can further reduce tension on the Achilles tendon. For patients who have hyperpronation contributing to excessive torsion on the Achilles tendon, the use of a more supportive shoe or orthotic can help.

Athletes can gradually increase the volume and intensity of their sports activities as symptoms allow. Throughout their return-to-play process, cross training is used until the desired level of running has been achieved.

Flexor Hallucis Longus Tendonitis

Flexor hallucis longus (FHL) tendonitis is a form of tendonitis most commonly seen in ballet dancers. The symptoms include medial or posteromedial ankle pain associated with flexion of the great toe. The inflammation most commonly affects the FHL tendon just posterior to the medial malleolus but can also be felt along the medial arch up to the sesamoids. Dancers will complain of pain and tightness with occasional episodes of popping or catching that result from swelling and trapping of the tendon sheath.

The differential diagnosis of FHL tendonitis includes tibialis posterior tendonitis, peroneal tendonitis, posterior talar impingement and a symptomatic os trigonum. With tibialis posterior tendonitis, the tenderness is more medial and the patient is often flat-footed. With peroneal tendonitis, the tenderness is just posterior to the lateral malleolus, and the patient commonly has a high-arched foot with a varus hind foot.

Initial treatment for FHL tendonitis should focus on icing and restricting dance activities to allow symptoms to improve. Rehabilitation focuses on FHL strengthening. Dance mechanics also need to be evaluated to help the athlete eliminate technique problems that might contribute to the problem.

SUMMARY POINTS

- The radiographic changes associated with skeletal immaturity and the presence of common anatomic variants create unique, and sometimes confusing, injury patterns in young athletes.

- Understanding the pattern of stresses associated with various foot types can help physicians provide better advice on footwear and orthotics as they apply to injury treatment and prevention of reinjury.

- Apophysitis in the heel and foot can be treated effectively by using measures such as activity modification, stretching, and/or shoe inserts to relieve traction on the apophysis.

- Stress fractures in the tarsals and metatarsals are more likely in endurance athletes, athletes participating in repetitive impact activities, or athletes with dietary or hormonal deficiencies. Proper treatment requires correction of the underlying risk factors for stress fracture and documentation of bony healing before returning to full activity.

- Accessory ossification centers may become painful with sports activity, may be confused with avulsion fractures, or may be entirely asymptomatic. A careful clinical examination and imaging studies are necessary to determine the clinical significance of an accessory ossification center and to determine which form of treatment, if any, is appropriate.

- Developmental conditions, such as tarsal coalition and osteochondritis dissecans, should be considered in athletes with ankle pain but no clear history of injury.

- Tendonitis is a less common cause of foot and ankle pain in patients with open apophyses. However, like all overuse injuries, effective treatment of tendonitis requires careful evaluation and correction of abnormal training patterns and biomechanics.

SUGGESTED READING

Chambers HG. Ankle and foot disorders in skeletally immature athletes. *Orthop Clin North Am.* 2003;34:445-459.

Hurwitz SR, ed. Athletic foot and ankle injuries. *Clin Sports Med.* 2004;23:1-174.

Kraft D, Zippin J. Pediatric problems and rehabilitation geared to the young athlete. In: Porter DA, Schon LC, eds. *Baxter's the Foot and Ankle in Sport.* 2nd ed. Philadelphia, PA: CV Mosby; 2008:chap 27.

Manusov EG, Lillegard WA, Raspa RF, Epperly TD. Evaluation of pediatric foot problems, part I: the forefoot and the midfoot. *Am Fam Physician.* 1996;54:592-606.

Manusov EG, Lillegard WA, Raspa RF, Epperly TD. Evaluation of pediatric foot problems, part II: the hindfoot and the ankle. *Am Fam Physician.* 1996;54:1012-1026, 1031.

Micheli LJ, Ireland ML. Prevention and management of calcaneal apophysitis in children: an overuse syndrome. *J Pediatr Orthop.* 1987;7:34-38.

Porter DA, Schon LC, eds. *Baxter's the Foot and Ankle in Sport.* 2nd ed. Philadelphia, PA: CV Mosby; 2008.

Stanitski, DeLee, Drez. Overuse injuries. In: *Pediatric and Adolescent Sports Medicine.* Vol 3. WB Saunders; 1994:162-174.

Tsuruta T, Shiokawa Y, Kato A, et al. Radiological study of the accessory skeletal elements in the foot and ankle. *Nippon Seikeigeka Gakkai Zasshi.* 1981;55:357-370.

CHAPTER 45

Nontraumatic Causes of Musculoskeletal Pain

Claire M. A. LeBlanc, MD

Kristin Houghton, MD

Eric Small, MD

The physician caring for young athletes should recognize that not all joint pain and swelling will be directly related to injury. Children with pain, warmth, swelling, and limitation of function may have medical disorders masquerading as traumatic or mechanical conditions. The differential diagnosis includes acute and chronic inflammatory diseases and pain amplification syndromes. (**Table 45.1**)

ACUTE INFLAMMATORY CONDITIONS

Infectious Causes of Musculoskeletal Pain

Viral Arthritis Many viruses can be associated with arthralgia and, less commonly, arthritis. Joint pain and/or swelling from viral arthritis is generally migratory, is short lived (1-2 weeks), and disappears without permanent damage. Viruses that cause arthralgia and arthritis include parvovirus B19; rubella; hepatitis B; alpha viruses (eg, Ross River virus); and less commonly, Epstein-Barr virus, adenovirus, cytomegalovirus, varicella, mumps, and enterovirus. Rubella, hepatitis B, and alpha viruses typically result in polyarthritis (arthritis in 5 or more joints), whereas mumps, varicella, and other viruses affect 1 or 2 large (eg, knee) joints.

Transient or toxic synovitis of the hip is a benign, self-limited disorder presumably related to viral illness since it may be preceded by a nonspecific upper respiratory tract infection. This condition is most common in boys between 3 and 10 years of age; moderate hip pain is the chief complaint. A low-grade fever may occur, but the ESR and WBC count are usually normal. Complete resolution occurs with rest, analgesics, or nonsteroidal anti-inflammatory medication for 7 to 10 days.

Septic Arthritis Septic arthritis usually arises by the hematogenous spread of infection from a focus elsewhere in the body but may also occur from a penetrating injury or contiguous spread of osteomyelitis. Fever and other systemic symptoms are common. Monoarthritis (1 joint) is typical, particularly in the lower extremities (eg, knee, hip, and ankle). The affected joint is swollen, hot, red, and very painful, especially with movement. Radiographic imaging may reveal a nonspecific joint effusion in early stages. Proteolytic enzymes released from intra-articular inflammatory cells can rapidly destroy articular cartilage, resulting in permanent joint damage within 3 days. The accumulation of infected fluid in the joint leads to a rise in intra-articular pressure, which may impair blood flow to the epiphysis (especially hip), leading to avascular necrosis. Immediate joint aspiration is critical for diagnostic purposes. Synovial fluid analysis usually reveals a white count of over 50 000/mm^3, primarily neutrophils. Blood and synovial fluid cultures identify the causative agent in up to 50% and 70% of cases, respectively. In children, the usual organisms are *Staphylococcus aureus, Streptococcus pneumoniae,* and group A *Streptococcus* (GAS). In sexually active youth, gonococcal arthritis is a consideration; typically multiple joints are involved. All individuals with septic arthritis of any cause urgently require intravenous antibiotics. Surgical consultation should take place concurrently with initiation of antibiotic

TABLE 45.1

Nontraumatic Causes of Musculoskeletal Disease

Diagnosis	MSK Pain	Redness, Warmth	Joint Number	Back Pain	Constitutional Symptoms	Organs Affected	Enthesitis	Muscle
Viral arthritis	Arthralgia	Warm joints, swelling	Few to many	+/-	URI, fever, gastroenteritis, myalgia	No	No	Myalgia
Septic arthritis	+++ Joint	Red, hot joint, swelling	One	No	Fever, septic	No	No	No
Lyme arthritis	Minimal	Warm, joint swelling	One to two	No	Early findings: arthralgia, myalgia	CNS, skin	No	No
Osteomyelitis	+++ Bone	Red, warm bone	One bone	Vertebral	Fever, septic	No	No	No
Reactive arthritis	++ Joints	+/- Red, warm joints	Few	+/- in chronic cases	Fever, fatigue, gastroenteritis, URI, mouth ulcers, sore throat	Eyes, skin, GI, GU, CVS, lymph nodes	Yes	Chronic forms: muscle wasting
Drugs	++ Joints	Warm joints, ⇩ swelling	Few to many	+/-	Fever, malaise, myalgia	Skin, other	No	Myalgia
Henoch-Schönlein purpura	++ Pain periarticular	Warm joints, periarticular swelling	Few	No	Fever, malaise	Skin, GI, GU	No	Myalgia
Tumors	+++ Bone Bone marrow: night pain	+/- Warm bone	Usually one	Yes	Fever, weight loss, sweats	Skin, lymph nodes, Other	No	Myalgia
Juvenile idiopathic arthritis	Minimal pain; AM joint stiffness	Warm joints	Few to many	No	Malaise, fever, fatigue, anorexia, failure to thrive	Eyes, CVS, skin, lymph nodes	Yes	Muscle wasting
ERA	+ AM pain stiffness joints; SI; +/- back	+/- Redness warm joints	Few; lower limbs	Yes	Gastroenteritis	Eyes, heart, GI, GU, skin	Yes	Muscle wasting
Systemic lupus erythematosus	++ Joint pain > stiffness and swelling	Warmth uncommon	Few to many	Decreased bone density	Fever, malaise, weight loss	CNS, heart, kidney, other	No	Myalgia
Juvenile dermatomyositis	+ Joints	Warmth uncommon	Few to many	Decreased bone density	Fever, fatigue, malaise	Skin, muscle, other	No	Myositis
Local AMPS	++++ Regional	Cool, mottled limb	Few	No	No	No	No	No
Generalized AMPS	+++ Nonspecific	No	Many	Yes	Fatigue, malaise	No	No	Myalgia

AMPS indicates amplified musculoskeletal pain syndrome.

therapy. Surgical drainage may be necessary to effectively treat the infection and reduce complications. Once clinical improvement occurs, treatment can be changed to oral antibiotics for an additional 3 weeks. Individual variation may occur depending on the timing of diagnosis, initiation of treatment, and factors specific to the host and microbe; hence, therapy should be modified accordingly.

Osteomyelitis In children, osteomyelitis is typically acute, with bacteria reaching bone from hematogenous dissemination or direct invasion. The metaphyses of rapidly growing bones in the lower extremity (especially distal femur and proximal tibia) are most commonly affected. Fever, severe bone pain, and tenderness with or without localized swelling are typical features. A joint effusion may be adjacent to the site of bone infection. This may reflect associated septic arthritis, especially if the metaphysis resides within the joint capsule. Soft tissue swelling is an early finding on plain radiographs, but mottling of the bone and periosteal elevation take 7 to 14 days to occur. Although imaging with radionuclide scanning, CT, and MRI may identify the bony lesion earlier, these findings are nonspecific. Infection can be confirmed by identifying the causative organism through aspiration of subperiosteal pus (positive in 80% of patients), blood (positive in up to 60% of patients), and sometimes synovial fluid. Typically, the infectious agents are similar to those that cause septic arthritis and include *Staphylococcus aureus, Streptococcus pneumoniae,* and group A *Streptococcus.* Appropriate intravenous antibiotics should be initiated as soon as possible and once the patient has improved clinically, oral antibiotics may be prescribed for a total of 4 to 6 weeks. Each patient may have a variable presentation, so the duration of therapy and selection of antibiotic should be individualized. Surgical intervention for acute osteomyelitis may be indicated if an abscess has formed, if there is impending spinal instability due to the destructive effects of the infection, or if clinical improvement has not occurred using intravenous antibiotics. Surgical treatment is commonly indicated for chronic osteomyelitis. Debridement of a sequestrum of necrotic bone may be indicated to resolve the infection.

Lyme Disease Athletes may travel to or live in regions where Lyme disease is endemic, including the northeast, mid-Atlantic, and north-central United States and parts of central Europe. Lyme disease is caused by *Borrelia burgdorferi,* which is transmitted by deer tick bites. Within days or weeks of the tick bite, children may develop erythema chronicum migrans, headache, neck stiffness, or arthralgias/myalgias. Several weeks later, multiple erythema migrans lesions may appear along with cranial nerve palsies, occasionally central nervous system disease, and rarely carditis. Untreated, 50% develop an almost painless arthritis, usually of the knee. Late disease is characterized typically by recurrent arthritis affecting a few large joints. Diagnostic testing includes serologic screening using ELISA and western blotting techniques and more specifically a synovial biopsy to detect the organism by polymerase chain reaction (PCR). Treatment of the arthritis consists of either oral amoxicillin, doxycycline, or cefuroxime for 28 days. Persistent or recurrent arthritis may require intravenous ceftriaxone or penicillin for 14-28 days. When traveling to endemic regions, athletes should be reminded to wear light-colored long pants tucked into their socks and tick repellents that contain N, N-diethyl-3-methylbenzamide (DEET), and to remove ticks promptly in an appropriate manner for best disease prevention.

Reactive Arthritis Children may develop arthritis. Several weeks after infection with GAS (acute rheumatic fever; poststreptococcal reactive arthritis), certain gastrointestinal organisms (*Salmonella, Shigella, Yersinia,* or *Campylobacter*), and some sexually transmitted diseases (*Chlamydia*). This form of rheumatic disease (reactive arthritis) is common, and physicians should expect to encounter athletes who are affected. The pathogenesis is similar in all forms of reactive arthritis regardless of the triggering agent. The arthritis develops as a result of molecular mimicry, when the patient's immune system cross-reacts with proteins in the infecting organism and in human tissue.

Acute Rheumatic Fever Acute rheumatic fever (ARF) used to be a common disease worldwide until industrialization and improved public hygiene. Currently, ARF is typically found in developing countries (incidence 200/100000) annually) but is still documented in the United States (incidence 3/100000). Two to three weeks following pharyngitis with a rheumatogenic strain of GAS, children may develop the clinical features of ARF. The diagnosis is confirmed by fulfilling the Jones criteria, including 2 major features (carditis, polyarthritis, chorea, erythema marginatum, subcutaneous nodules) or 1 major and 2 minor features (arthralgia, fever, previous acute rheumatic fever or rheumatic carditis, elevated acute phase reactants, prolonged PR interval). Evidence of antecedent GAS infection is essential. Typically, a migratory polyarthritis of larger joints occurs in 70% of cases, and these are usually red, swollen, hot, and very painful. Arthritis persists for about 3 weeks without treatment. Management consists of a therapeutic course of penicillin and aspirin for several weeks followed by prophylactic penicillin for at least 5 years or until age 21 years if there is no associated carditis. Patients with carditis require penicillin prophylaxis for 10 years or well into adulthood, whichever is longer. Should the patient have carditis with persistent valvular disease, such treatment should be given at least until age 40 years and sometimes lifelong.

Poststreptococcal Reactive Arthritis Some children develop arthritis after GAS pharyngitis without meeting the Jones criteria; this is called poststreptococcal reactive arthritis (PSRA). Many believe PSRA is an extension of the spectrum of ARF, considering that the affected age is similar (5-16 years), it is not triggered by GAS pyoderma, and a similar carditis may occur in about 6% of cases. Several features are different, including the lack of features (not symptoms, because not all of the Jones criteria are symptoms), outlined in the Jones criteria, a shorter latency period between throat infection and arthritis (<10 days), and an asymmetric nonmigratory type of arthritis that usually has a poor response to treatment with aspirin. Affected joints often remain symptomatic for many months despite various nonsteroidal medications. The American Academy of Pediatrics Red Book indicates that some experts recommend penicillin prophylaxis for 1 year to prevent carditis.

Reiter Syndrome

Reiter syndrome (RS) often presents as a clinical triad of conjunctivitis or acute uveitis, urethritis, and arthritis. Reiter syndrome is triggered by specific gastrointestinal (*Salmonella, Shigella, Yersinia,* or *Campylobacter*) and genitourinary *(Chlamydia)* infections. Athletes may develop gastroenteritis from exposure to infected teammates, animals, foods, or beverages in their home environment or during travel. They may acquire a *Chlamydia* genitourinary tract infection through sexual transmission. Genitourinary *Chlamydia* infections are often asymptomatic, but dysuria and urethral or vaginal discharge may be noted.

One to four weeks after any one of these infections, the clinical features of RS may ensue, especially if the youth is male and HLA-B27 positive. In addition to conjunctivitis and urethritis, affected individuals may develop fever, fatigue, aphthous ulcers, and rashes (erythema nodosum, keratoderma blennorrhagicum, circinate balanitis). Musculoskeletal features can include arthritis, especially in the lower extremities; dactylitis; tenosynovitis/tendinitis; and enthesitis. Enthesitis is an inflammation of the tendon, ligament, fascia, or joint capsule as it inserts on bone. It is most common around the knee and foot and has a similar appearance to traction and microtrauma injuries of the apophyses (Osgood-Schlatter disease and Sever's disease). Chronic apophyseal injury may be differentiated from enthesitis by the lack of clinical or laboratory signs of inflammation (morning stiffness or pain, elevated acute phase reactants), arthritis, and/or sacroiliitis. Reiter arthritis is usually self-limited but may evolve into an identifiable chronic spondyloarthropathy (eg, ankylosing spondylitis) with chronic sacroiliitis. Treatment usually includes nonsteroidal (NSAID) medication (especially indomethicin) and intra-articular steroid injections.

Other Acute Conditions

Drug-Induced Rheumatic Diseases   Physicians treating young athletes should identify all medications (sanctioned or not) taken by their young athletes. Individuals on certain medications like isotretinoin, which may be prescribed to athletes with severe acne, can develop side effects, such as arthritis and hyperostosis, and serious complications, such as stroke, seizures, acne fulminans, hepatitis, glomerulonephritis, and systemic vasculitis.

Serum sickness-like disease is a relatively common cause of acute arthritis in children, with an estimated incidence of 4.7/100 000. Affected individuals have acute joint pain that often leads to an inability to walk about 7 to 14 days after exposure to certain agents. Drugs, particularly antibiotics (cefaclor), are usually implicated (**Table 45.2**). The cardinal features of

TABLE 45.2

Common Drugs Associated With Serum Sickness

Commonly Implicated Drugs	Uncommonly Implicated Drugs
Cefaclor	Aspirin
Penicillin	Naproxen
Trimethoprim-sulfamethoxazole	Minocycline
Amoxicillin	Rifampin
	Ciprofloxacin
	Itraconazole
	Carbamazapine
	Phenytoin
	Metronidazole
	Sulfonamides

serum sickness are a pruritic, nonscarring rash (morbilliform, maculopapular, purpuric, urticarial), fever, malaise, and polyarthralgias or polyarthritis. The affected joints rarely exhibit significant swelling and erythema. Many patients with minimal disease do not require treatment other than withdrawing the offending agent. Antihistamines may be sufficient for those with pruritus, mild rash, and low-grade fever; NSAIDs and analgesics are generally effective for arthralgias. Once a serum sickness-like reaction develops, the responsible drug and drugs that are closely related should be avoided.

Patients with hypersensitivity vasculitis may have joint pain and share many overlapping features with serum sickness. Hypersensitivity vasculitis is a small-vessel disease precipitated by an immune response to various exogenous antigens, especially *Streptococcus* and drugs taken 7 to 10 days earlier (**Table 45.3**). The major clinical manifestation is a palpable purpuric or petechial rash, although fever, myalgia, malaise, arthralgia, and arthritis may be present. Renal, cardiorespiratory, gastrointestinal, and nervous system involvement have been reported. The diagnosis is usually made clinically, but eosinophilia, low serum complement levels, and a skin biopsy showing a leukocytoclastic vasculitis are additionally helpful. The discontinuation of the inciting drug should lead to disease resolution within days to a few weeks. Patients with constitutional symptoms, musculoskeletal pain, or arthritis may benefit from NSAIDs while more severe disease may require corticosteroids.

Some medication can cause drug-induced lupus that may lead to arthritis. Diphenylhydantoin, mephenytoin, trimethadione, minocycline, and ethosuximide are most frequently implicated. Individuals with drug-induced lupus can develop fever, rash, myalgias, arthralgias, arthritis, and serositis usually after years of exposure to the drug. Hematologic abnormalities,

TABLE 45.3

Common Drugs Associated With Hypersensitivity Vasculitis

Anti-infective Agents

Penicillin
Tetracycline
Erythromycin
Rifampin
Ciprofloxacin
Trimethoprim-sulfamethoxazole
Ampicillin

NSAIDs

Aspirin
Indomethicin
Ibuprofen
Naproxen

Anticonvulsants

Valproate
Carbamazapine

Cardiovascular Drugs

Atenolol
Captopril
Chlorothiazide
Furosemide
Hydralazine
Spironolactone

Miscellaneous

Allopurinol
Colchicine
Isoniazid
Metformin
Propylthiouracil
Quinidine
Isotretinoin
Vitamin B6

with transient but severe joint pain is a typical musculoskeletal feature and occasionally predates the rash by 1 to 2 days. The detection of perivascular deposits of immunoglobulin (Ig) A on a biopsy of an early skin lesion and/or similar deposits in the mesangium of the kidney confirms the diagnosis. HSP is generally a self-limited disease, although analgesia and NSAIDs may be required for symptom control, and immunosuppressive medications are warranted in severe renal disease.

Benign and Malignant Neoplastic Conditions

Any physician caring for children with musculoskeletal pain should consider the possibility of an underlying benign or malignant tumor of bone, cartilage, bone marrow, fibrous tissue, or soft tissue with metastases to bone.

Benign Painful Tumors of Bone Osteoid osteomas account for 5% of all bone tumors and are most common in males between 10 and 20 years. These benign tumors typically are located in the proximal femur or tibia and posterior elements of the vertebrae. A dull, penetrating ache that is worse at night and responds quickly to NSAIDs is nearly diagnostic. Occasionally there is an adjacent synovial effusion if the tumor resides within the joint capsule. Routine radiographs may be of low diagnostic value, but CT scans are useful. Radiographically, this tumor appears as an oval radiolucent nidus (sometimes with a central nucleus of increased bone density) that is surrounded by sclerotic bone. Some children heal spontaneously and many are asymptomatic on NSAIDs, but intolerance or nonadherence to medication may occur. Some children are also quite debilitated with pain, so surgical excision is generally recommended. This is usually curative as long as the entire lesion is removed. Alternatively, percutaneous thermal ablation may be considered for tumors located in nonoperable locations. Osteoblastomas are larger than osteoid osteomas and are most commonly seen in teenage boys. This painful tumor is found typically in the vertebral arch. Malignant transformation has been reported, hence surgical excision is warranted, but given the location it may be a difficult procedure. Chondromas are composed of mature hyaline cartilage and often present as an asymptomatic mass that becomes painful because of a pathologic fracture. These tumors typically are located in the metaphysis of the small tubular bones in the hands and feet. Surgical excision is not necessary, but follow-up should be provided long-term since there is a possibility of malignant transformation. Periosteal chondromas are much less common. These painful tumors are most commonly located in the proximal humerus and require excision.

kidney disease, and central nervous system involvement are uncommon. The presence of antinuclear antibodies (ANAs) and antihistone antibodies without other autoantibodies strongly suggests this diagnosis. Spontaneous resolution usually occurs 1 to 7 months after discontinuing the offending agent. A short course of NSAIDs and antimalarials can be used if constitutional and musculoskeletal symptoms do not clear rapidly. Corticosteroids are infrequently required.

Henoch-Schönlein Purpura Henoch-Schönlein purpura (HSP) may be confused with hypersensitivity vasculitis since both are types of small-vessel vasculitis with some overlapping clinical features. HSP is suggested by the classic tetrad of purpuric rash, abdominal pain, renal disease, and arthropathy. Periarticular swelling of the ankles and knees

Benign Tumors of Soft Tissue Pigmented villonodular synovitis (PVNS) is a proliferative disorder of the synovium that is rare in children. Patients, usually 20 to 30 years old, most commonly present with swelling, stiffness, and progressive pain in the knee or hip. Both sexes are affected equally. Aspirated synovial fluid is typically serosanguineous. As demonstrated on MRI, this condition is characterized by synovial membrane proliferation leading to the formation of villi and nodules with deposits of intracellular hemosiderin. MRI demonstrates a characteristic lack of signal on both T1 and T2 images that has been attributed to the presence of large amounts of hemosiderin in the synovium. However, the diagnosis should be confirmed by histology because other causes of hemorrhagic and chronic hyperplastic synovitis may appear similarly. PVNS also progressively destroys local cartilage and bone. Surgical excision (complete synovectomy) is indicated.

The synovial hemangioma is an uncommon mass-lesion located most often in the knee. Affected patients have intermittent hemarthroses after minor trauma. Recurrent bleeding into the joint results in chronic inflammatory synovitis and eventual joint damage. MRI demonstrates the extent of the lesion, and surgical excision is indicated. Synovial chondromatosis is an uncommon tumor of the knee. Cartilaginous and osteocartilaginous bodies develop in the synovium, which are released into the intra-articular fluid, resulting in pain, swelling, locking, and giving way of the knee. This may be confused with a meniscal tear. Surgical excision is recommended.

Other Benign Tumors The unicameral bone cyst located in the metaphysis of long bones is most common in boys between 6 and 10 years of age. It is a large lesion that presents asymptomatically or with local swelling, pain, and pathologic fractures. Surgical treatment is indicated if >50% of the diameter of bone is involved. Smaller lesions may be followed by serial radiographs and receive local injection with corticosteroids. Aneurysmal bone cysts are more common in girls during their adolescent years and are commonly located in the metaphysis of long bones or the posterior elements of the spine. Differentiation from unicameral bone cysts is aided by MRI. Treatment may include surgical curettage and local radiation. Patients with eosinophilic granulomas present with local pain and swelling over a solitary mass in the skull, spine, femur, or pelvis. A percutaneous needle biopsy is required to confirm the diagnosis; surgical excision with or without low-dose irradiation is the recommended treatment.

Malignant Bone Tumors Osteogenic sarcomas account for 60% of all bone tumors in children. These occur most commonly during the second decade of life, especially in children with certain underlying acquired or genetic disorders or those who received prior irradiation to that region of bone. This tumor causes localized pain and swelling and signs suggestive of metastatic spread (fever, lymph-adenopathy, hypertrophic osteoarthropathy). Plain radiographs demonstrate a moth-eaten bony lesion with cortical destruction and periosteal elevation. The extent of the lesion can be demonstrated by CT or MRI, and treatment includes surgical resection and chemotherapy.

Ewing sarcoma is the second most common bone tumor in childhood but is the most malignant. It is typically found in the diaphysis of the long bones of Caucasian boys during the second decade of life. Localized pain and swelling are common at presentation. Plain radiographs reveal an aggressive, elongated lytic lesion with roughening of the periosteum resembling onion skin or a sunburst appearance. Surgical resection, irradiation, and chemotherapy are provided in combination for best results.

Metastatic Bone Tumors Neuroblastoma is a tumor of the sympathetic nervous system occurring primarily in young children. This lesion metastasizes early to multiple bony locations (spine, skull, femur, ribs, pelvis), resulting in severe bone pain. Plain radiographs demonstrate lytic lesions arising from the bone marrow, and scintigraphy is the most sensitive method for locating all metastatic sites. Treatment includes surgical removal of the primary tumor in combination with irradiation and chemotherapy.

Leukemia Leukemia is the most common (30%-40%) of all childhood malignancies. Fever, lymphadenopathy, weight loss, hepatosplenomegaly, and petechial rash may not be present immediately. Up to 30% of affected children present with musculoskeletal pain or joint swelling before a definitive diagnosis is made. They typically complain of pain in the metaphyses of long bones. Pain (especially at night) is much more severe than one might expect in children with juvenile arthritis. The complete blood count may be normal initially, but a reduction of 2 cell lines despite elevation of LDH and ESR is suggestive of the diagnosis. The 3 most important factors predicting a diagnosis of leukemia include a history of night pain, a low white count, and a low-normal platelet count. Radiographs and scintigraphy may or may not be helpful, thus bone marrow analysis is essential for diagnosis. Current chemotherapeutic strategies have improved survival to 90% for acute lymphoblastic leukemia.

CHRONIC INFLAMMATORY CONDITIONS

Athletes may also develop chronic joint complaints that are of an inflammatory nature. Thus, physicians should have a good understanding of a variety of chronic rheumatic diseases so that appropriate treatment can be instituted in a timely manner. In general, morning stiffness, gelling (stiffness) after inactivity, improvement of joint symptoms with activity, absence of instability and locking, and extra-articular symptoms help differentiate inflammatory joint pain from pain associated with injury.

Juvenile Idiopathic Arthritis

Juvenile idiopathic arthritis (JIA) (previously called juvenile rheumatoid arthritis) is a common chronic disease of child-hood with a prevalence of approximately 1 in 1000. There are 7 subtypes of JIA (**Table 45.4**), which likely have different pathogenetic mechanisms. JIA occurs in youth younger than 16 years and is more common in girls. It is a clinical diagno-sis defined by the presence of a joint effusion or 2 or more of the following: stress pain, warmth, and limited range of mo-tion for at least 6 weeks. Children may experience joint pain (rarely at rest) or swelling, altered gait, or decreased function. Minor trauma may bring attention to an affected joint, but joint findings following a major traumatic event suggest me-chanical causes. A complete joint and systemic examination is essential for diagnostic purposes, and a pediatric rheuma-tologist should conduct ongoing management.

Constitutional signs and symptoms include anorexia, weight loss, growth failure, and fatigue. Chronic uveitis is a common extra-articular manifestation in some subtypes, es-pecially if ANAs are present. Key musculoskeletal findings in-clude a swollen, warm joint (erythema is unusual) with joint line tenderness and painful (uncommonly severe), limited range of motion. Sometimes these features are subtle and pain may not be a major issue. Even children without joint

---

TABLE 45.4

International League of Associations for Rheumatology (ILAR) Classification Criteria for Juvenile Idiopathic Arthritis (JIA)

Subtypes of JIA (first 6 months of disease)

Systemic onset juvenile arthritis
Oligoarticular juvenile arthritis
   a) Persistent oligoarthritis (remains oligoarthritis)
   b) Extended oligoarthritis (becomes polyarthritis)
Polyarthritis rheumatoid factor–negative
Polyarthritis rheumatoid factor–positive
Psoriatic arthritis
Enthesitis-related arthritis
Other arthritis

Petty RE, Southwood TR, Manners P, et al: International League of Associations for Rheumatology. International League of Associations for Rheumatology classification of juvenile idiopathic arthritis: second revision, Edmonton, 2001. *J Rheumatol.* 2004;2:390-392. Reprinted with permission.

---

pain can develop contractures, regional muscle atrophy, and joint damage. Those with polyarthritis or systemic onset dis-ease may develop micrognathia or cervical spine involvement that may include C1-C2 instability.

Enthesitis-related arthritis, one subtype of JIA, is unique in that it is more common in school-age boys and is frequently associated with the genetic marker HLA-B27. Inflammation of the entheses may be a prominent finding and may be confused with mechanical conditions that re-sult in microinjury to the apophyses. These include Sever's (calcaneus), Osgood-Schlatter (tibial tuberosity), or Sinding-Larsen Johansson disease (inferior pole patella). Plantar fascia pain and pain around the apophyses of the iliac crest and sacroiliac joint can also be seen from repetitive microtrauma. Enthesitis is usually associated with arthritis, and symptoms are more prominent in the morning, which helps to differentiate enthesitis from osteochondroses and traction apophysitis.

Treatment of JIA depends on the subtype and may include nonsteroidal anti-inflammatory drugs, intra-articular steroids, disease-modifying agents (methotrexate, sulfasalazine) and biologic agents (anti-TNF agents), and physiotherapy. Up to 55% of children with JIA continue to be symptomatic into adulthood (depending on the individ-ual subtype), and this may have a major effect on function. However, in many cases, children have better functional out-comes with early recognition and treatment.

Habitual Physical Activity Levels Physical activity is an important component of healthy lifestyles and is paramount for all children, even those with juvenile arthritis. Unfortu-nately, children with JIA may not be as active as their healthy peers for many reasons, including disease symptoms (pain, stiffness, fatigue); treatment-related side effects (nausea, abdominal pain); or concerns of parents, teachers, and physicians that exercise may aggravate their disease. There is scant literature on the activity patterns of children with JIA. Studies combining objective measures of movement with motion sensors and subjective measures of physical activ-ity suggest children with JIA move as much as their peers but report less vigorous activity and lower participation in organized sports. The factors limiting activity are not well defined, but non–disease-related factors such as perceived fitness potential and perceived athletic ability may be important.

Physiologic Fitness (Aerobic and Anaerobic Capacity) Children with JIA can have lower aerobic and an-aerobic fitness than their peers or reference norms. Children with JIA show a reduction in muscle strength that is most pronounced in muscles surrounding inflamed joints (disuse atrophy) and often persists after clinical resolution of inflammation, especially if the disease onset was before 3 years of age. Aerobic fitness results are mixed, but many suggest lower levels in children with JIA. Anemia and muscle atrophy and weakness are likely contributing factors, but the overall deconditioning that accompanies reduced physical activity is the most likely cause. Fitness does not appear to be related to disease activity or function but may correlate with disease duration.

Risks of Exercise　Traditionally, children with arthritis were advised to avoid weight-bearing exercise because this might aggravate joint pain, and swollen and inflamed joints may be more prone to instability and injury. Also, muscle atrophy surrounding active joints and periarticular osteopenia could increase the risk of fracture. Recent reports over the past decade, however, suggest weight-bearing exercise programs can be safe. When advising parents about sport participation, the clinician should note that young children with arthritis may have gross motor delays and lag behind their peers in sport skills development. Children with cervical spine arthritis may be at greater risk for spinal cord injury, especially during collision and contact sports. Children with JIA may develop micrognathia and are at risk for dental injury. Uveitis and its sequelae (visual impairment) may increase the risk of eye injury from local trauma. Children with cardiac involvement (systemic or HLA-B27–associated arthritis) may be at risk for cardiac complications with exercise. Treatment with systemic steroids and methotrexate may be required, which can lead to side effects including infection, osteoporosis, and avascular necrosis. Exercise may need to be modified under these circumstances.

Benefits of Exercise

Physical activity favorably affects children's musculoskeletal health and overall aerobic fitness. There is good evidence that children with JIA can participate in aquatic or land-based exercise programs (biking, elliptical machine) without disease exacerbation. The literature suggests exercise programs lasting a minimum of 6 weeks can lead to improved aerobic fitness; improved muscle strength and function; decreased disease activity; improved self-efficacy, energy level, and quality of life; and decreased pain and medication use with no clear effect on functional status.

Recommendations　Most pediatric rheumatologists encourage their patients to be physically active. Although non–weight-bearing activities (swimming, biking) continue to have the highest participation rates for children with JIA, weight-bearing exercise is critical to the development of optimal bone mineral density. Recent guidelines advise moderate fitness, flexibility, and strengthening exercises. Children with well-controlled disease and adequate

physical capacity can participate in impact activities and competitive contact sports. Children with JIA who have moderate to severe impairment or actively inflamed joints should limit activities according to their pain level. They should be encouraged to participate in physical activities as tolerated and gradually return to activity if a disease flare has caused a disruption of activity. Exercise programs providing individualized training (especially for children with severe joint disease) within a group-exercise format may provide physical and social benefits.

Children with arthritis at C1-C2 should be screened for instability prior to participation in collision or contact sports. If atlantoaxial instability is present, further clinical evaluation to assess the risk of spinal cord injury during sports participation is recommended. Children with jaw involvement should wear appropriately fitted mouth guards during activities with jaw and dental injury risk. Appropriate eye protection is required in JIA patients during activities with ocular injury risk. These guidelines do not differ from guidelines for the general pediatric population. Any patient requiring treatment with systemic steroids and disease-modifying agents requires careful monitoring for drug side effects.

Systemic Lupus Erythematosus

Systemic lupus erythematosus (SLE) is a chronic, episodic, multisystem autoimmune disease characterized by the presence of antinuclear antibodies, especially to native DNA. Girls, especially during the teenage years, are affected more often than boys. Children may present acutely ill, but a history of chronic, intermittent symptoms is more common. Arthritis affects two-thirds of children and commonly involves the small joints of the hands, wrists, elbows, shoulders, knees, and ankles. Joint pain is often significant, but objective findings of warmth and swelling are uncommon. Other musculoskeletal manifestations of SLE include avascular necrosis, osteopenia, pathologic fracture (worse with prolonged systemic steroids), myalgias, and myositis. Extra-articular features may include constitutional symptoms, rash, renal disease, pericarditis/myocarditis, pleuritis, and neurologic involvement. Treatment may involve use of corticosteroids, other immunosuppressant agents (such as methotrexate, azathioprine, and cyclophosphamide), and antimalarials, as well as management of specific organ system disease.

Potential risks of exercise in patients with SLE include osteoporotic fracture, cardiac complications, and flare-up of disease. Individuals with Raynaud syndrome may sustain injury to their digits upon exposure to cold; thus, they should wear layered clothing to keep the body warm.

Direct exposure to the sun may result in disease exacerbation, and sun protection is advised during all outdoor activities. Children receiving immunosuppressive agents are at a risk for serious infections, and those with major organ system disease (CNS, renal) may require careful clinical evaluation before sport participation. Potential benefits of exercise include improved strength and bone mineral density; prevention of significant corticosteroid-related weight gain; and decreased inflammatory-associated dyslipidemia. Graded aerobic physical activity has been shown to be well tolerated without disease exacerbation in adults and to have a positive impact on fatigue, pain, and fitness. Similar studies have yet to be done in children.

Juvenile Dermatomyositis

Juvenile dermatomyositis (JDM) is the most common idiopathic inflammatory myopathy in childhood. It is characterized by progressive proximal muscle weakness and rash (eyelid heliotrope and erythematous papules over the knuckles). Children often have fatigue, malaise, muscle pain, and fever. In the early stages, weakness may be subtle and manifest as decreased exercise tolerance or performance. Later, children may have some difficulty moving from sitting to standing, sitting up from a supine position without rolling over, getting up off the floor, climbing stairs, and doing overhead arm activity. In severe cases, there is gastrointestinal and respiratory muscle involvement. Investigations show elevated muscle enzymes, EMG, MRI, and muscle biopsy changes. Up to 35% have arthritis, which is usually mild. Children with JDM are treated with immunosuppressive agents, physical therapy, and occupational therapy. There is insufficient scientific investigation of the risks and benefits of exercise in this population. Physical activity is generally encouraged to preserve muscle function, but it is probably prudent to avoid vigorous exercise when there is active muscle inflammation. This may result in rhabdomyolysis or increased muscle fatigue and weakness. Children with contracted or inflamed joints may be more prone to injury and those with osteoporosis are at greater risk of fracture. Direct exposure to the sun may cause disease flare; thus, sun protection is recommended during outdoor play. Children receiving immunosuppressive agents who develop infection should be carefully evaluated before they are cleared to participate in sports.

PAIN AMPLIFICATION SYNDROMES

Many cases of severe, chronic musculoskeletal pain in children do not have an identified inflammatory or mechanical cause. Often these individuals have been seen by many physicians and have undergone numerous investigations before the correct diagnosis is made. Up to 8% of all new patients presenting to pediatric rheumatologists in North America have some form of amplified musculoskeletal pain. This condition can affect any ethnic group but is more common in Caucasian girls. It may occur as early as 2 years of age, but most cases begin in late childhood and adolescence. The cause of amplified musculoskeletal pain is not known, but minor trauma, underlying chronic illnesses, and psychological distress have been associated. There is commonly an adult role model for chronic pain or disability, and a distinct enmeshment between the patient and parent (often the mother) may be seen. Amplified musculoskeletal pain may be subdivided into localized and diffuse types.

Localized Amplified Musculoskeletal Pain Syndrome (AMPS)

Many terms have been used to describe this condition, including reflex sympathetic dystrophy (RSD), sympathetic mediated pain syndrome, reflex neurovascular dystrophy (RND), complex regional pain syndrome, and chronic musculoskeletal pain syndrome with or without autonomic dysfunction. Typically, an affected child sustains minor trauma to an extremity (especially lower), which results in pain out of proportion to the injury. The condition presents along a spectrum from isolated localized pain to a totally dysfunctional extremity. Medications that typically relieve pain due to minor trauma are generally not effective in patients with AMPS. Immobilization may help minimize the discomfort initially, but ultimately this tends to make the condition worse.

On physical examination, a number of features help to identify children with AMPS. These include an unwillingness to use the extremity or to bear weight; allodynia (pain generated by stimuli that normally don't cause pain); and autonomic changes such as excessive perspiration, edema, cyanosis, mottling, and coolness of the skin. Patients may be extremely sensitive to pinprick, light touch, or even air blowing on the skin of the affected limb. Importantly, there are no findings on general and neurovascular exam to suggest an underlying causative disease. Additionally, psychological dysfunction is frequently noted as an underlying cause of this condition or as an indicator of the effect AMPS has on the child and family. Psychological findings range from anxiety or poor coping to a borderline personality disturbance. Despite severe pain, the affected child often exhibits an incongruent disposition or *la belle indifference.* Screening bloodwork such as a complete blood count and sedimentation rate is normal. Diagnostic studies are not usually helpful in confirming the diagnosis but may be necessary to rule out other diagnostic possibilities. X-rays may show osteopenia from disuse in children with significant disability. MRI can show regional bone marrow edema, and a 3-phase bone scan may show an increase or decrease in uptake or be completely normal.

There are no well-controlled therapeutic trials demonstrating proven therapies for children with AMPS. However, clinical strategies based on aggressive exercise regimens focused at reversing immobility and increasing function have been shown to be effective. This typically involves exercise rehabilitation as well as a desensitization program (towel and lotion rubs) to relieve allodynia 3 to 5 days per week for about 4 to 6 weeks. Transcutaneous electrical nerve stimulation, sympathetic blocks, and sympathectomy have also been used with variable success. A coordinated team approach with musculoskeletal specialists, allied health personnel, and psychologists is ideal. Progressive muscle relaxation, guided imagery, and cognitive behavioral therapy can help an affected child cope with discomfort. Those with more severe psychological dysfunction may require more psychotherapy or other psychiatric intervention.

The prognosis for children with localized AMPS is much better than for adults. Almost 90% of affected children without autonomic dysfunction are free of pain and fully functional after 5 years. Relapses or transition to another disorder (headaches, conversion, panic attacks, and eating disorders) may occur, but these are far more likely if the child has underlying psychopathology.

Generalized Amplified Musculoskeletal Pain Syndrome (GAMPS)

Generalized amplified musculoskeletal pain syndrome (GAMPS) has been called fibromyalgia and diffuse idiopathic pain syndrome. It begins gradually and can be quite vague in nature and location. Affected individuals often indicate their whole body is painful, which is quite different from localized AMPS. Conversion symptoms may occur, and a number of nonspecific conditions such as headache, abdominal pain, back pain, and sleep disturbances are common. Parents frequently report the child is a perfectionist and aims to please others. Most have specific tender points all over the body. The 1990 American College of Rheumatology criteria for fibromyalgia requires widespread pain above and below the waist for at least 3 months and pain on digital palpation of 11/18 sites using 4 kg of pressure. These fibromyalgia tender point sites include the occiput, lower cervical area, trape-zius, supraspinatus second rib, lateral epicondyle, gluteus medius, greater trochanter, and the medial fat pad of the knees. As in localized AMPS, psychological dysfunction is typical and the affected child appears indifferent. Management involves a combination of education, graduated aerobic exercise, and psychological support. Returning the child to usual activities, including school, is critical. Good sleep hygiene (including low-dose tricyclic antidepressant therapy) is recommended, but the degree to which this is effective is not well known. The prognosis for children with generalized AMPS is better than for similarly affected adults but not as good as for those with localized AMPS, with 50% of patients reaching a pain-free status over 5 years in one cohort. Of note, 90% of these remained in school or were fully employed.

SUMMARY POINTS

- Physicians managing young athletes need to be aware of nontraumatic causes of joint and bone pain, which may include infectious, inflammatory, and oncologic conditions as well as amplified musculoskeletal pain syndromes.

- Nontraumatic inflammatory causes of joint pain and swelling usually have associated morning stiffness and/or soreness.

- Children with neoplastic causes of musculoskeletal discomfort frequently wake at night from severe pain.

- Despite the potential risks facing children with juvenile arthritis and connective tissue diseases who participate in sport, they should be encouraged to be physically active whenever possible because in most instances the benefits will outweigh the risks.

- Children with amplified musculoskeletal pain syndromes have pain out of proportion to the history of injury or physical examination findings. It is important to avoid immobilization of painful extremities or global restrictions of painful activity. Exercise is part of the treatment; hence, they should be encouraged to return to daily activities, including exercise and sport, as soon as possible.

SUGGESTED READING

Bar-Or O. Pathophysiological factors which limit the exercise capacity of the sick child. *Med Sci Sports Exer.* 1986;18(3):276-282.

Bar-Or O, Rowland TW. *Pediatric Exercise Medicine From*

Physiologic Principles to Health Care Application. Champaign, IL: Human Kinetics; 2004.

De Boek H. Osteomyelitis and septic arthritis in children. *Acta Orthop Belg.* 2005;71:505-515.

Dubost JJ, Souteyrand P, Sauvezie B. Drug-induced vasculitides. *Bailliere's Clin Rheumatol.* 1991;5(1):119-138.

Erffmeyer JE. Serum sickness. *Ann Allergy.* 1986;56:105-110.

Goldmuntz EA, White PH. Juvenile idiopathic arthritis: a review for the pediatrician. *Pediatr Rev.* 2006;27:e24-e32.

Jones OY, Spencer CH, Bowyer SL, Dent PB, Gottlieb BS, Rabinovich CE. A multicenter case-control study on predictive factors distinguishing childhood leukemia from juvenile rheumatoid arthritis. *Pediatrics.* 2006;117:840-844.

Kitsoulis P, Mantellos G, Vlychou M. Ostoid osteoma. *Acta Orthop Belg.* 2006;72:119-125.

Klepper SE. Exercise and fitness in children with arthritis: evidence of benefits for exercise and physical activity. *Arthritis Rheum (Arthritis Care Res).* 2003;49(3): 435-443.

Kunnamo I, Kallio P, Pelkonen P, Viander M. Serum-sickness-like disease is a common cause of acute arthritis in children. *Acta Paediatr Scand.* 1986;75:964-969.

Llauger J, Palmer J, Roson N, Bague S, Camins A, Cremades R. Nonseptic monoarthritis: imaging features with clinical and histopathologic correlation. *Radiographics.* 2000;20:S263-S278.

Murray CS, Cohen A, Perkins T, Davidson JE, Sills JA. Morbidity in reflex sympathetic dystrophy. *Arch Dis Child.* March 2000;82(3):231-233.

Pickering LK, Baker CJ, Long SS, McMillan JA, eds. Group A streptococcal infections. In: *Red Book: 2006 Report of the Committee on Infectious Diseases.* 27th ed. Elk Grove Village, IL: American Academy of Pediatrics; 2006:611-620.

Pickering LK, Baker CJ, Long SS, McMillan JA, eds. Lyme disease. In: *Red Book: 2006 Report of the Committee on Infectious Diseases.* 27th ed. Elk Grove Village, IL: American Academy of Pediatrics; 2006:611-620.

Sherry DD. An overview of amplified musculoskeletal pain syndromes. *J Rheumatol Suppl.* 2000;58:44-48.

Tse SML, Laxer RM. Approach to acute limb pain in childhood. *Pediatr Rev.* 2006;27(5):170-180.

Wilder RT. Management of pediatric patients with complex regional pain syndrome. *Clin J Pain.* June 2006;22(5): s443-s448.

CHAPTER 46

Sport-Specific Injury Prevention Strategies

Sally S. Harris, MD, MPH

Steven J. Anderson, MD

This chapter presents preventive strategies for common injuries and provides information to help advise athletes and parents about risks and safety considerations specific to their individual sports. Prompt recognition and treatment of existing injuries in their early or less-severe stages are critical to reducing recurrence and preventing more serious injuries.

General principles of injury prevention are discussed in Chapter 13. Rehabilitation principles and guidelines for safe return to play after an injury are discussed in detail in Chapter 31, "Rehabilitation," and Chapter 14, "Return to Play Decisions."

Injuries and relevant preventive strategies can be generic (ie, pertinent for a variety of sports), sport-specific, or both. The physical demands of many sports are similar and therefore may predispose athletes to similar types of injuries. Other injuries and preventive strategies may be unique to a given sport. For example, athletes who participate in sports involving sustained running (eg, cross-country, track, soccer, and lacrosse) are vulnerable to many of the same overuse injuries of the knees and lower legs. Athletes who participate in sports requiring jumping and hard landings (eg, gymnastics, ice-skating, basketball, volleyball, and jumping events in track) are at higher risk for overuse conditions of the lower extremities, such as stress fractures and anterior knee pain. Athletes who participate in sports requiring repetitive overhead movements of the arms (eg, baseball, volleyball, tennis, and swimming) are at risk for similar overuse injuries to the shoulders. Athletes involved in sports causing repetitive extension of the spine (eg, gymnastics, figure skating, diving, or serving in tennis) are at high risk for pars

interarticularis stress fractures of the lumbar spine. Athletes participating in sports requiring jumping, pivoting, and cutting maneuvers are at high risk of knee ligament sprains.

On the other hand, some injuries tend to be very sport-specific, such as pudendal neuropathy (bicycling), auricular hematoma (wrestling), and stress fractures of the ribs (crew and golf). Preventive strategies may have features in common (eg, core strengthening to prevent back pain, patellofemoral pain, leg pain) and strategies specific to the sport (eg, tilting the bicycle seat forward to prevent compression on the pudendal nerve).

The tables in this chapter provide preventive strategies for injuries that are common to multiple sports as well as preventive strategies for specific sports. Some of the recommendations for injury prevention are based on scientific studies; other recommendations are based on common practice patterns relative to the sport or injury in question. Recommendations to "avoid improper technique" may require more specific guidance from a coach or athletic trainer. Recommendations to "avoid or limit" certain aspects of training are meant to suggest ways to temporarily modify participation to limit exposure and decrease the risk of occurrence, progression, or recurrence of injury. Because poor fitness and deconditioning are general risk factors for injury, it is helpful to recommend some level of safe activity that can be continued during rehabilitation.

In some cases, the recommendations may suggest changes or modifications that appear incompatible with the practice patterns or demands of the sport in question. However, such recommendations are still offered because within a given sport, there may or may not be flexibility in how much training, technique, and/or equipment may be altered in the interest of safety. The ability to modify participation in such a way as to make it safer may be a factor in an athlete's or parent's choice to participate or allow participation in a given sport.

The tables in this chapter do not include all potential injuries or all prevention strategies; nor do they address diagnosis and treatment of specific injuries. The evaluation and treatment of injuries in each anatomic region are discussed in Section 5, "Musculoskeletal Conditions." General information for athletes and parents can be found in the sport-specific patient education handouts and can serve as an adjunct to these tables. **Table 46.1,** "Injury Prevention Guidelines for Common Injuries," addresses common injuries and general preventive strategies that pertain to multiple sports. **Tables 46.2-46.28,** "Injury Prevention Guidelines for Specific Sports," address the most common injuries seen in each sport and provide additional sport-specific preventive strategies.

Table 46.1

Injury Prevention Guidance for COMMON INJURIES

Common Injuries	Prevention Strategies/Comments
General prevention	• Schedule a preparticipation sports examination to address deficits from prior injury, risk factors for future injury, medical conditions that may be affected by participation, and safety recommendations that are specific to the participant, the sport, and/or the environment where the sport is played. • Allow time for general conditioning and sport-specific conditioning before starting practice. • Use well-fitting and well-maintained protective gear. • Fields, surfaces, bases, goals, and equipment related to the sport should be appropriately designed, maintained, and used. • Learn and practice safe techniques for performing the skills that are integral to the sport or activity; enforce safety rules. • Seek medical consultation if symptoms or signs of injury develop, rather than trying to play through pain.
Shoulder overuse injuries • Impingement • Rotator cuff tendonitis	• Allow time to gradually build up to repetitive overhead activity (eg, throwing, tennis, swimming). • Limit activity if pain develops. • Do rotator cuff and scapular strengthening program during preseason; emphasize external rotators and serratus anterior. • Stretch shoulder internal rotators. • Correct forward shoulder (kyphotic) posture by stretching anterior chest wall muscles and strengthening interscapular and spinal extensor muscles.
Finger injuries	• Reduce risk of reinjury by buddy taping. • These injuries are often caused by the ball hitting the end of the finger or the finger getting caught on another player's jersey.

Lumbar injuries
• Muscle strains
• Disk injuries
• Pars interarticularis injuries
  • Pars interarticularis stress fracture (spondylolysis)
  • Pars interarticularis stress reaction
	• Increase flexibility in hamstrings, quadriceps, and hip flexors.
	• Do core strengthening and lumbar stabilization exercises.
	• Use proper technique when lifting.
	• Use caution in sports or training activities that require extreme flexion or extension of the spine.
	• Seek medical evaluation early if symptoms of pain, spasm, restricted mobility, numbness, weakness, or referred pain into lower extremity are present.
	• High-impact activities increase the risk of disk injuries and pars injuries.
	• Risk of disk injuries is increased with activities that require rounding the low back, particularly in combination with lumbar rotation.
	• Risk of pars injury is increased by repetitive lumbar extension and rotation; unilateral low back pain is a warning sign for these conditions.

Muscle strains	• Rehabilitate prior injuries. • Evaluate and treat sources of muscle tightness, including associated lumbar spine disorders, underlying bony pathology, and nutritional and metabolic disorders. • Initiate a stretching program to correct deficits in flexibility. • Perform strengthening to correct deficits from previous injury, correct strength imbalances, and strengthen target muscles at the speed of contraction that occurs in sports.
Knee overuse injuries • Patellofemoral stress syndrome • Patellar tendonitis • Osgood-Schlatter disease	• Gradually build up to activities that involve running, jumping, lunging, or squatting; limit activity if knee pain develops. • Use shoes and/or insoles that provide stability, support, and neutral patellar alignment (eg, arch support for correction of pronation). • Perform a quadriceps/hamstring stretching program. • Strengthen hip abductors and core musculature.

Anterior cruciate ligament (ACL) sprain	• Consider an ACL-injury prevention program:
	  • Preseason conditioning and balance training.
	  • Proper stopping, landing, cutting, and pivoting techniques.
	  • Hamstring strengthening.
	  • No ACL prevention program is 100% effective in preventing all injuries. These programs are options that are still being investigated and refined.

Table 46.1–cont'd

Injury Prevention Guidance for COMMON INJURIES

Common Injuries	Prevention Strategies/Comments
Lower leg overuse injuries • Medial tibial stress syndrome (shin splints) • Achilles tendonitis • Stress fractures of the lower leg and foot	• Gradually build up to activities that involve running, jumping, or high impact. • Limit activity if pain develops. • Consider low-impact cross training to supplement aerobic conditioning (eg, bicycling, stair climber, elliptical trainer, swimming). • Use shoes, insoles, and/or orthotics to provide appropriate support for unstable foot structure, such as pronation, and adequate shock absorption to cushion rigid feet, such as high-arched feet. • Perform Achilles tendon, calf, and hamstring stretching. • Strengthen hip abductors and core musculature. • Recognize and treat prestress fracture conditions (eg, shin splints) before a stress fracture develops. • Seek medical evaluation if persistent bony pain or achiness develops. • Evaluate for female athlete triad.
Ankle sprain	• Initiate a preseason and in-season ankle-strengthening and proprioception program. • Use ankle brace and/or tape for practice and play in running, jumping, and pivoting sports, particularly if there is a history of sprains. • Ensure that previous ankle sprains are completely rehabilitated, because previous sprains are a common cause of future sprains.
Calcaneal apophysitis (Sever's disease)	• Use heel cups in athletic shoes, especially in cleated shoes and shoes that have inadequate heel lift or cushion. • If foot is hyperpronated, use a shoe with good arch support or consider adding an orthotic. • Allow time to gradually build up to running and jumping sports. • Perform Achilles tendon, calf, and hamstring stretching. • If heel pain develops, consider low-impact aerobic cross training such as cycling, swimming, elliptical trainer, stair climber, in-line skating, or rowing.
Eating disorders and/or amenorrhea	• Encourage proper nutritional intake to meet the caloric demands of training and to maintain appropriate body weight. • Ensure adequate calcium and iron intake, particularly in female athletes. • Review menstrual calendar with athlete. • Avoid setting predetermined performance weight goals. • The pressure to be lean can result in unhealthy weight loss practices. • Weight loss can cause injury as a result of the indirect consequences of weight loss (eg, dehydration, electrolyte imbalance, decreased lean body mass, osteopenia).
Dehydration and/or heat illness • Heat cramps • Heat exhaustion • Heat stroke	• Allow 10-14 days for players to acclimate to hot/humid conditions. • Schedule practices at cooler times of day. • Wear appropriate light-colored clothing. • Remove helmet frequently during hot and humid conditions. • Maintain adequate hydration during practice and games; confirm adequacy of hydration by weighing before and after practice. • Allow water breaks every 20 minutes during practice. • Encourage fluid intake even though athlete may not feel thirsty. • Promote rehydration before the next practice. • Encourage the buddy system to allow players to notify coaches if their buddy is not feeling or acting normal.
Sun damage • Sunburn • Skin cancer • Eye damage	• Use sunscreens on exposed areas, even in overcast conditions. • Use lip applications (eg, lip gloss, lip balm) with sunblock. • Wear hats or visors and appropriate light-colored clothing. • Apply aloe for symptom relief from sunburn. • Use complete block to cover any sunburn that has blistered or peeled. • Use sunglasses or goggles to protect eyes from sun exposure.

Table 46.2

Injury Prevention Guidance for BALLET/DANCE

Common Injuries	Prevention Strategies/Comments

Lumbar injuries*
• Muscle strains
• Disk injuries
• Pars interarticularis injuries
  • Pars interarticularis stress fracture (spondylolysis)
  • Pars interarticularis stress reaction
	• Use proper mechanics for male dancers performing lifts of their partner; generate power by bending the knees and avoid rounding or hyperextension of the low back.
	
	• Risk of pars injury is increased as a result of jumps and movements requiring hyperextension of the low back.

Knee overuse injuries* • Patellofemoral pain syndrome • Patellar tendonitis	• Limit grand pliés and jumps if anterior knee pain develops. • Avoid compensating for inadequate hip turnout by excessively turning out the ankle and lower leg. • Supportive shoes and/or orthotics are generally not an option while dancing but may be useful for general activity and nondance conditioning.
Lower leg overuse injuries* • Medial tibial stress syndrome (shin splints) • Achilles tendonitis • Stress fractures of the lower leg and foot	• Supportive shoes and/or orthotics may not be an option while dancing but may be useful during activity that is not performed while wearing a dance shoe.
Ankle sprain*	• Traditional taping or bracing for ankle sprain is too restrictive for dancers to function, so this is not a good prevention strategy.
Anterior ankle overuse conditions • Anterior talar impingement of the ankle	• If anterior ankle pain, swelling, or a pinching sensation develops, minimize activities that involve excessive dorsiflexion of the ankle (eg, plié, preparing to jump, landing from jumps).
Posterior ankle overuse conditions • Posterior talar impingement • Flexor hallucis longus (FHL) tendonitis • Symptomatic os trigonum	• Do not initiate pointe work until the dancer's skills and strength warrant advancement. This can usually be determined by a dance instructor who has experience training professional ballet dancers. • If posterior ankle pain, swelling, or a pinching sensation develops, limit excessive plantar flexion of the ankle, such as being en pointe and relevé. For FHL tendonitis, restrict demi-pointe and pushing off for jumps • Strengthening toe flexors is a common dance practice, but it has not been shown to reduce injuries.
Eating disorders and/or amenorrhea*	• Risk is increased as a result of pressure to maintain an aesthetically appealing, lean body.

* See Table 46.1

Table 46.3

Injury Prevention Guidance for BASEBALL/SOFTBALL

Common Injuries	Prevention Strategies/Comments
Injuries for which protective gear is recommended • Head and eye injuries • Throat injuries • Chest trauma • Scrotal injuries	Use proper protective gear: • Catchers should wear helmets with face guards, throat guards, and chest protectors. Chest trauma can result in a fatal arrhythmia called *commotio cordis*. • Batters should wear batting helmets; face guards or polycarbonate eye protectors attached to batting helmets should be considered. • Boys should wear protective cups. Other preventive measures: • Players should wear shoes with rubber spikes. • Softer low-impact safety balls should be considered for children ages 5-14, particularly children under age 10. • Ensure dugouts and benches include protective fencing. • Eliminate the on-deck circle. • Prohibit headfirst sliding for children under age 10.
Shoulder injuries from throwing* • Impingement • Rotator cuff strain or tendonitis • Labral tears • Stress reaction of the proximal humeral physis (epiphysiolysis)	• See "Elbow injuries" (below).
Elbow injuries • Medial epicondyle pain • Ulnar collateral ligament sprain • Ulnar neuritis • Osteochondritis dissecans	• Initiate preseason throwing program or gradual buildup for throwing and pitching. • General strengthening of other muscle groups that enhance throwing (eg, rotator cuff, scapular stabilizers, legs, hips, trunk). • Monitor the number and types of pitches thrown per game and per week.[†] • Pitches such as curveballs, sliders, and breaking pitches stress the elbow more; young pitchers should master the fastball and changeup before throwing more advanced pitches. • Limit the number of teams an athlete can play on at one time or the number of days the athlete can play or practice per week (5-6 days per week). • Teach the athlete proper throwing mechanics to include the entire kinetic chain. • To avoid elbow and shoulder injuries, teach the athlete to use the whole body, rather than just the arm, to generate power.
Finger injuries*	–

Lumbar injuries*
• Muscle strains
• Disk injuries
• Pars interarticularis injuries
  • Pars interarticularis stress fracture (spondylolysis)
  • Pars interarticularis stress reaction
	• Pars injuries are most common in pitchers as a result of repetitive rotation and extension of the low back.

Patellofemoral stress syndrome in catchers*	• Limit prolonged or repetitive squatting and kneeling. • Catchers should wear knee-saver pads.
Knee sprains, medial collateral ligament sprain	• Use breakways bases. • Teach proper sliding technique.
Ankle sprains*	• Teach proper sliding technique.

* See Table 46.1.
[†]Source: Protecting Young Pitching Arms. The Little League Pitch Count Regulation Guide for Parents, Coaches and League Officials. http://www.littleleague.org/Assets/old_assets/media/Pitch_Count_Publication_2008.pdf

Table 46.4

Injury Prevention Guidance for BASKETBALL/VOLLEYBALL

Common Injuries	Prevention Strategies/Comments
Injuries for which protective gear is recommended • Eye injuries, corneal abrasion • Mouth, facial, and dental injuries	Use proper protective gear, including protective eyewear and mouth guards. • Basketball is the leading cause of mouth, facial, and dental injuries in sports, and the second leading cause of eye injuries.
Shoulder injuries* • Instability/dislocation • Impingement • Rotator cuff strain or tendonitis	• Limit excessive spiking and serving in volleyball to avoid overuse of the shoulder.
Finger injuries*	–

Lumbar injuries*
• Muscle strains
• Disk injuries
• Pars interarticularis injuries
  • Pars interarticularis stress fracture (spondylolysis)
  • Pars interarticularis stress reaction
	• In both basketball and volleyball, risk of pars injury is increased as a result of jumping.
	• In volleyball, risk of pars injury is increased as a result of the lumbar extension and rotation involved in serving and overhead hitting.
	• Limit excessive spiking and serving in volleyball to avoid repetitive hyperextension of the back

Knee overuse injuries* • Patellofemoral stress syndrome • Patellar tendonitis • Osgood-Schlatter disease	• Limit excessive bending (running between and touching lines "liners"), lunging, and defensive stance position.
Anterior cruciate ligament sprain*	–
Lower leg overuse injuries* • Medial tibial stress syndrome (shin splints) • Achilles tendonitis • Stress fractures of the lower leg and foot	• Play on shock-absorbing surfaces. • Wear shoes with appropriate support for lateral movements and shock absorption. • Wear insoles for correction of pronation and arch support. • Perform calf and Achilles tendon stretching.
Ankle sprain*	• Risk is increased as a result of close contact and possibility of stepping on another player's foot. • Ankle braces are often worn for preventive purposes, particularly in athletes with flexible ankles or history of sprains.
Calcaneal apophysitis (Sever's disease)*	–

* See Table 46.1

Table 46.5

Injury Prevention Guidance for BICYCLING

Common Injuries	Prevention Strategies/Comments
General prevention	Ensure proper bike fitting: • *Frame size:* There should be approximately 1-2 inches between the top tube and the rider's crotch when straddling the bike with both feet on the ground. • *Seat height:* When pedaling, the knees should be slightly bent when the foot is all the way down (pedal closest to the ground). • *Seat angle:* The seat is usually level, but it may be tilted slightly back to decrease stress on arms and neck; however, tilting backward may increase pressure on perineum. • *Seat position:* The nose of the saddle should be behind the bottom bracket (the part of the bike that holds the pedal crank in the frame). With the pedals parallel to the ground, the front knee should be directly over the front pedal spindle (middle of the pedal) to prevent knee pain. The distance from the tip of the seat to the handlebars should not be greater than the length of the arm from elbow to fingertips.
Injuries for which protective gear is recommended • Head injuries • Abrasions, contusions, and lacerations • Eye injuries • Toe injuries • Ulnar nerve compression (hand) • Pudendal neuropathy	Use proper protective gear: • Helmet (legally mandatory for children under age 18, but recommended for all). • Low-profile pads for knees, elbows, and wrists for bicycling activities likely to cause frequent falling (mountain biking, BMX). • Protective eyewear to reduce risk of objects flying into the eyes. • Sturdy closed-toe shoes that protect the toes from trauma. • Padded gloves and handlebars. • Padded cycling shorts; avoid seat that is tilted back.
Neck pain (muscular)	Ensure proper bike fitting, particularly distance from seat to handlebars. • Vary position on handlebars and seat frequently. • Limit hyperextension of the neck and rounding of the low back.
Shoulder and arm trauma • acromioclavicular separation • clavicle fracture • Wrist and forearm fracture	Minimize risk of falls and collisions: • Follow the rules of the road. • Ride cautiously and remain in control. • Wear bright-colored clothing to increase visibility.
Lumbar injuries* • Muscle stains • Disk injuries	• See "Neck pain" (above). • Limit rounding of the low back. • Limit cycling uphill with high resistance.
Knee overuse injuries* • Patellofemoral pain syndrome • Iliotibial band syndrome (ITB) • Quadriceps and patellar tendonitis	Ensure proper seat height and position. • A slightly higher seat (straighter knee) can decrease patellofemoral pain. • A slightly lower seat (more bent knee) can decrease iliotibial band tendonitis.
Sun damage* • Sunburn • Skin cancer • Eye damage	–

* See Table 46.1

Table 46.6

Injury Prevention Guidance for BOXING

Common Injuries	Prevention Strategies/Comments
General prevention	• The AAP vigorously opposes boxing as a sport (or any other activity that rewards blows to the head) for any child or adolescent. Encourage athletes to participate in other sports.

Table 46.7

Injury Prevention Guidance for CHEERLEADING

Common Injuries	Prevention Strategies/Comments
Injuries due to falls • Concussion • Neck injuries (sprains and fractures) • Trauma from falls	• Coaches should be experienced in proper technique and safety. • Use mats. • Use spotters. • Follow restrictions from the National Federation of High Schools regarding skills such as basket toss, pyramid heights, and twisting/flipping stunts. • Advance difficulty of stunts gradually as skills and strength warrant. • Have an emergency plan in place. • These injuries occur most commonly in flyers as a result of falling from a height. • Over half of all catastrophic head and neck injuries in female athletes occur in cheerleaders.
Shoulder injuries* • Impingement • Rotator cuff strain or tendonitis	• Use proper lifting technique; keep elbows in front of plane of body, avoid forward bending of back, bend knees, and use legs for power. • These injuries occur most frequently in athletes in base positions (ie, athletes who perform partner lifts or are at the base of pyramids).

Lumbar injuries*
• Muscle strains
• Disk injuries
• Pars interarticularis injuries
  • Pars interarticularis stress fracture (spondylolysis)
  • Pars interarticularis stress reaction
	• Use proper mechanics for performing lifts of partners; generate power by bending the knees, and avoid rounding or hyperextension of the low back.
	• These injuries occur most frequently in athletes in base positions (ie, athletes who perform partner lifts or are at the base of pyramids).

Knee overuse injuries* • Patellofemoral stress syndrome • Patellar tendonitis • Osgood-Schlatter disease	• Limit excessive high impact activities such as jumps, tumbling, and dismounts. • Practice on soft surfaces.
Lower leg overuse injuries* • Medial tibial stress syndrome (shin splints) • Achilles tendonitis • Stress fractures of the lower leg and foot	• See "Knee overuse injuries" above.
Ankle sprains*	–
Eating disorders and/or amenorrhea*	• Risk is increased as a result of pressure to maintain an aesthetically appealing, lean body.

* See Table 46.1

Table 46.8

Injury Prevention Guidance for CREW/ROWING

Common Injuries	Prevention Strategies/Comments
Wrist overuse injuries	• Use proper feathering technique: • Avoid hyperextension of the wrist. • Do scapular stabilization exercises to strengthen shoulder blade muscles. • Consider taping wrists.
• Intersection syndrome	• Intersection syndrome is caused by inflammation on the dorsal radial aspect of the forearm and wrist due to friction where 2 tendons (abductor pollicis longus and extensor pollicis brevis) cross over another set of 2 tendons (extensor carpi radialis longus and brevis). • This injury affects the feathering hand as a result of repetitive extension of the wrist to pull the blade out of the water.
Hand injuries • Calluses/blisters	• Tape hands or use gloves designed for rowing. • Use hand lotion and regularly shave calluses to decrease callous buildup.
Rib pain • Intercostal muscle strain • Stress fractures of the ribs	• Avoid hatchet blades, which increase forces to chest wall. • Avoid improper rowing technique that may predispose the athlete to rib injuries: • Not sitting up enough at the finish. • Pulling into the rib cage too much at the finish. • Reaching too far at the catch (phase of the stroke when the oar enters the water). • Consider switching to rowing on the opposite side of the boat.
Lumbar injuries* • Muscle strains • Disk injuries	• Ensure adequate leg strength and use of legs, rather than back, to generate power during the drive portion of the stroke. • Sit up appropriately at the finish of the stroke. • Avoid excessive rounding of the back. • Ensure proper adjustment of boot rigging. • Use appropriate technique when lifting shells in and out of the water. • Avoid poor technique or excessive resistance while rowing on an ergometer. • Ensure proper technique and resistance for weight training, especially squats.
Knee overuse injuries* • Patellofemoral stress syndrome • Patellar tendonitis • Iliotibial band syndrome	• Limit excessive bend (flexion) of knees and excessive loading at the catch. • Modify the shoes or foot stretcher position to decrease the bend of the knees at the catch. • Avoid improper squatting technique during weight training, such as bending knees too deep, or having feet turned inward or outward.
Lower leg injuries • Track bites (skin irritations such as abrasions, blisters, or bleeding that occur on the back of the calves when the legs hit the slide at the finish of the stroke)	• Tape or cover the affected skin. • Adjust foot stretchers and slide. • Avoid jamming the legs down at the finish.
Eating disorders and/or amenorrhea*	• Set realistic weight goals for athletes participating in weight classes, such as lightweight crew, to prevent acute weight loss and dehydration to meet weight class goal. • Risk is increased as a result of: • Pressure to meet individual weight goals. • Pressure to decrease overall weight of the scull with the rowers inside. • Belief that decreased body fat improves endurance.
Sun damage* • Sunburn • Skin cancer • Eye damage	–

* See Table 46.1

Table. 46.9

Injury Prevention Guidance for CROSS-COUNTRY/TRACK

Common Injuries	Prevention Strategies/Comments
General overuse injuries	• Gradual increase in total weekly mileage by no more than 10% per week at the beginning of the season, and if returning after illness, injury, or other disruption of training. • Limit speed work to 1-2 days per week. • Cross train with aqua jogging, cycling, or elliptical trainer.

Lumbar injuries*
• Muscle strains
• Disk injuries
• Pars interarticularis injuries
  • Pars interarticularis stress fracture (spondylolysis)
  • Pars interarticularis stress reaction
	• Risk of pars injury is increased in track events that involve jumping (eg, hurdles, high jump, long jump, triple jump, pole vault).
	• Risk of pars injury is increased in track events that involve throwing (eg, shot put, discus throw, javelin throw, hammer throw) as a result of the repetitive lumbar extension and rotation used for the throwing motion.

Hip overuse injuries • Iliotibial band syndrome at the hip • Iliac crest apophysitis	• Stretch hip flexors and iliotibial band. • Strengthen hip abductors and external rotators (ie, gluteus medius). • Limit uphill running, sprinting, and hurdles. • These conditions are exacerbated by long strides, which require the leg to extend further behind the plane of the body.
Knee overuse injuries* • Patellofemoral stress syndrome • Patellar tendonitis • Osgood-Schlatter disease	• Run on soft, even surfaces when possible. • Limit hill running.
Iliotibial band syndrome of the knee	• Stretch the iliotibial band • Limit downhill running , which exacerbates this condition
Lower leg overuse injuries* • Medial tibial stress syndrome (shin splints) • Achilles tendonitis • Stress fractures of the lower leg and foot	• Change shoes every 6 months or 300-500 miles. • Run on soft, even surfaces when possible. • Limit hill running.
Ankle sprain*	—
Eating disorders and/or amenorrhea*	• Risk is increased because of the belief that decreased body fat improves endurance.
Iron-deficiency anemia	• Ensure adequate iron intake, particularly in female runners.
Exercise-associated diarrhea (runner's trot)	• Limit fiber intake the 24 hours before competition.

* See Table 46.1

Table 46.10 A

Injury Prevention Guidance for DIVING: SPRINGBOARD AND PLATFORM

Common Mechanisms of Diving Injuries

Injuries from board work (approach, hurdle, jump/takeoff)

- Patellofemoral stress syndrome (PFSS)
- Patellar tendonitis
- Quadriceps tendonitis
- Medial tibial stress syndrome (shin splints)
- Stress fracture of the lower leg and
- Dorsal wrist impingement (from handstand dives)

Injuries from airborne phase of dive

- Lumbar disk (from trunk flexion with dives in pike position or flexion-rotation on front-twisting dives)
- Lumbar facet/pars interarticularis injury (from lumbar hyperextension on back dives or back-twisting dives)

Injuries for hitting board or platform

- Concussion
- Cervical spine/spinal cord
- Laceration/abrasion
- Fracture

Injuries from entering the water

- Fracture (wrist, hand, rib)
- Dislocation (shoulder, elbow)
- Sprain (wrist, thumb, medial collateral ligament of elbow)
- Strain (triceps)
- Tendonitis/dorsal wrist impingement (from repetitive entries)
- Nerve (cervical radiculopathy from cervical disk herniation, transient quadriparesis from cord contusion, stinger [brachial plexus traction], ulnar nerve)
- Stinger
- Contusion (chest, back, legs)
- Pneumothorax/hemopneumothorax
- Tympanic membrane rupture
- Cervical stain, facet injury
- Lumbar injuries (lumbar strain, facet injury, pars interarticularis injury, disk injury)
  - Hyperextension (from underrotating [landing short] on back dive and overrotating [landing long] on front dive)
  - Hyperflexion (from underrotating on front dive and overrotating on back dive)

Injuries from exiting the water

- Dorsal wrist impingement from pushing up to get out of water
- Triceps tendonitis from pushing out of water
- Patellofemoral stress syndrome from ladders/stairs

Injuries from dry land training (eg, weights, trampoline, dry board with landing pit, pike-ups, plyometrics)

- Patellofemoral stress syndrome
- Patellar tendonitis
- Medial tibial stress syndrome (shin splints)
- Lumbar disk (from heavy lifting, pike-ups, spotting belt)

Prevention Strategies/Comments

General prevention: Equipment/facility

- Ensure adequate pool depth for board height.
- Ensure adequate bottom contour (needs to be flat in landing area).
- Ensure adequate clearance of landing area from pool edge, landing areas from other boards/platforms, and other swimmers.
- Ensure adequate design, maintenance of boards, stands, and fulcrums.
- Ensure nonslip surfaces on boards, platforms, ladders, stairs, and decks.

General prevention: Training

- Teach athletes proper techniques for approach, hurdle, and jump.
- Start with feet-first landings; follow skill progressions as outlined by USA Diving (http://usadiving.org/).
- Always swim immediately away from landing area after dive, preferably in a direction away from where other divers may be entering.
- Learn spotting techniques to avoid disorientation during summersault or twisting dives.
- Use proper grab position with arms locked during entry.

General prevention: Medical

- Athletes with active middle ear infection, ruptured tympanic membrane, or vertigo should not dive.
- Triceps weakness from tendonitis, triceps strain, brachial plexus or cervical nerve root irritation can interfere with ability to hold entries and can result in more serious triceps strains, cervical strains, and hand fractures.
- Tight hamstrings may indicate a lumbar spine problem and can contribute to increased lumbar disk compression, particularly during pike dives.
- Unstable ankle, painful knee, or weak hip abductor may interfere with ability to jump or take off straight from the springboard or platform, leading to collisions with other divers and awkward landings in the water.
- Excessive weight loss, eating disorders, and amenorrhea can adversely affect training and lead to injury, including stress fractures.

Table 46.10 B

Injury Prevention Guidance for DIVING: SPRINGBOARD AND PLATFORM

Common Injuries	Prevention Strategies/Comments
Neck conditions • Strain • Facet joint inflammation • Brachial plexus injuries	• Higher risk for 10-m platform divers. • Perform neck-strengthening exercises. • Correct kyphotic posture and forward shoulder position to help maintain more neutral alignment in the cervical spine.
Shoulder injuries* • Instability (subluxation or dislocation) • Impingement • Rotator cuff strain or tendonitis • Labral tears	• Caused by excessive extension of arms behind the plane of the body during entry. • Repetitive forced extension can cause impingement or instability. • Instability with continued impact forces at entry may lead to glenoid labrum tears. • Postural correction to reduce kyphosis and strengthening cuff and scapular stabilizers may reduce impingement.
Elbow injuries • Ulnar neuritis • Medial collateral ligament sprains • Osteochondritis dissecans	• Caused by elbow hyperextension during entry. • Medical instability can contribute to ulnar neuritis. • Repetitive loading of radiocapitellar joint upon entry can cause osteochondritis dissecans; this may also be a carryover from gymnastics, which is a common cause of osteochondritis dissecans.
Wrist/hand injuries • Dorsal wrist impingement	• Caused by hyperextension (dorsiflexion) of the wrist during entry. • Taping or bracing wrist to prevent dorsiflexion and strengthening forearm/wrist may help to prevent injury or reinjury.
Lumbar injuries*	–
• Muscle strains • Disk injuries	• Caused by repetitive flexion of pike and tuck position. • Caused by dry land training and weight lifting. • Dives in tuck position or back dives may be better tolerated.

• Pars interarticularis injuries
  • Pars interarticularis stress reaction
  • Pars interarticularis stress fracture (spondylolysis)
	• Limit repetitive hyperextension of the spine, particularly with back dives or reverse dives.
	• Dives in front tuck or pike position may be better tolerated.

Knee overuse injuries* • Patellofemoral stress syndrome • Patellar tendonitis • Osgood-Schlatter disease	• Repetitive jumping on board and platform, and dry land training lead to overuse anterior knee pain. • Back dives and inward dives cause less stress on the knee and may often be continued if anterior knee pain is present. • Modifying training and optimizing flexibility may reduce injuries. • Supportive shoes and/or orthotics may be helpful for dry land training or for daily activity.
Eating disorders and/or amenorrhea*	• Risk is increased as a result of pressure to maintain an aesthetically appealing, lean body.
Otitis externa (swimmer's ear)	• Dry ears well after participation. • Limit participation if pain or vertigo interferes with balance or spatial awareness.

* See Table 46.1

Table 46.11

Injury Prevention Guidance for EQUESTRIAN/RODEO

Common Injuries	Prevention Strategies/Comments

General prevention to avoid injuries due to falls from the horse
 	
• Head injuries
• Contusions
• Sprains
• Strains
• Fractures
• Dislocations
	Use proper protective gear:
	
	  • Helmets.
	  • Riding boots.
	  • Safety stirrups.
	  • Protective vest.
	Other preventive measures:
	  • Use experienced instructors for novices (most injuries occur in novices).
	  • Teach proper technique and safety standards.
	  • Ensure appropriate matching between rider skill and horse temperament.

Injuries from being kicked by the horse	• Ensure adult supervision. • Avoid startling horse from behind.
Thumb amputation (Rodeo thumb)	• Avoid rope being caught around the thumb and on the horn of the saddle during calf roping.
Lumbar injuries* • Muscle strains • Disk injuries	• Maintain erect riding posture; avoid rounding of low back. • Avoid abnormal or repetitive pelvic motion. • Do hamstring and adductor stretching to avoid contractures that increase stress on the low back.
Ischial bursitis	• Avoid repetitive friction at this point of contact between rider and saddle. • Wear appropriate riding clothes and use a saddle.
Hip adductor strain or contracture	• Perform adductor stretching and strengthening program.

* See Table 46.1

Table 46.12

Injury Prevention Guidance for FIELD HOCKEY

Common Injuries	Prevention Strategies/Comments

Injuries due to being struck by stick or ball
 	
• Head and facial trauma
 	
• Eye trauma (infrequent but serious)
• Hand finger fractures and contusions
• Shin injuries
	• Enforce rules preventing dangerous use of stick and ball.
	Use proper protective gear:
	  • Helmet with face mask for goalies.
	  • Mouth guards.
	  • Consider protective eyewear.
	  • Consider protective gloves.
	  • Shin guards.

Lumbar injuries*
 	
• Muscle strains
• Disk injuries
 	
• Pars interarticularis injuries
  • Pars interarticularis stress fracture (spondylolysis)
  • Pars interarticularis stress reaction
	• Risk of disk injuries is increased as a result of movements requiring bending forward and rotation.
	• Limit excessive lumbar flexion with rotation when bending forward to hit the ball.
	• Risk of pars injuries is increased as a result of repetitive rotation when hitting the ball.

Knee overuse injuries* • Patellofemoral stress syndrome • Patellar tendonitis • Osgood-Schlatter disease	–
Lower leg overuse injuries* • Medial tibial stress syndrome (shin splints) • Achilles tendonitis • Stress fractures of the lower leg and foot	–
Ankle sprain*	–

* See Table 46.1

Table 46.13

Injury Prevention Guidance for FIGURE SKATING

Common Injuries	Prevention Strategies/Comments

Injuries due to falls
 	
• Lacerations
• Contusions to elbow, knees, hips, and tailbone
• Forearm and wrist fractures
	Use appropriate protective gear (especially for novices or while learning risky skills):
	
	  • Wrist guards.
	  • Elbow pads.
	  • Knee pads.
	  • Buttocks pads.
	
	Learn how to fall correctly:
	
	  • Learn the safety roll.
	  • Preferably land on the fleshy parts of the body (hips and shoulders).
	  • Avoid falling on outstretched arm; bend elbow if falling on arm.
	  • Keep your head up; if falling backward, tuck chin into chest.
	
	General prevention of falls:
	
	  • Avoid skating with hands in pockets.
	  • Avoid doing tricks and moves beyond skill level or training.
	  • Maintain appropriate sharpness of skate blades (overly sharp blades stick, and dull blades skid).
	  • Check that the screws that fasten the blade to the skate are tight to prevent the blade from falling off while skating.
	• Pair skaters and ice dancers are at higher risk of falls as a result of height of throws and lifts of the female skater by the male skater, and as a result of skaters moving close together at high speeds.

Concussions/head injuries	• See "General prevention of falls" (above). • Helmets are not required but should be encouraged, especially for children during recreational ice skating, particular at indoor skating rinks. • Head injury risk is higher than for skateboarders, roller skaters, and in-line skaters, for whom helmets are recommended or required.
Shoulder strains*	• Use proper lifting mechanics for male pair skaters and ice dancers lifting their partners; keep elbows in front of plane of body, avoid forward bending of back, bend knees, and use legs for power. • Perform shoulder-strengthening program.

Lumbar injuries*
 	
• Muscle strains
• Disk injuries
• Pars interarticularis injuries
  • Pars interarticularis stress fracture (spondylolysis)
  • Pars interarticularis stress reaction
	• Limit hard landings and jumps.
	• Male pair skaters should use proper mechanics when performing partner lifts: generate power by bending the knees and avoid rounding or hyperextension of the low back.
	• Limit repetitive hyperextension of the spine, which contributes to pars injuries.
	• Female pair skaters are more susceptible to spondylolysis because of the need for holding the free leg very high in the air much of the time, which increases extension of the lumbar spine.

Iliac crest apophysitis	• Limit excessive jumping, especially triple jumps. • Maintain adequate flexibility and strength of hip girdle muscles, particularly hip flexors and adductors. • Perform iliotibial band stretching.
Knee overuse injuries* • Patellofemoral stress syndrome • Patellar tendonitis • Osgood-Schlatter disease	• Limit jumps and high-impact off-ice training.
Medial tibial stress syndrome (shin splints)*	• Wear orthotics or modify boots to correct pronation. • Ensure proper blade placement to prevent skates from leaning inward. • Pad medial boot top to relieve pressure.
Stress fractures of the lower leg and foot*	• Wear orthotics or modify boots to correct pronation if stress fracture of medial tibia or medial foot is present. • Limit excessive jumping and high-impact activities, particularly during off-ice practice.

* See Table 46.1.

Table 46.13–cont'd

Injury Prevention Guidance for FIGURE SKATING

Common Injuries	Prevention Strategies/Comments
Lower leg injuries to skin • Skin irritation or thickening where the top of the boot hits the posterior ankle or lower leg during plantar flexion	• Wear padding and silicon sleeves, such as Bunga Pads. • Modify skates to include a dance back (soft, closed-cell foam material to replace a portion of the posterior-superior upper).
Achilles tendonitis*	• Limit excessive jumping, particularly during off-ice practice. • Avoid overly stiff boots, which increase eccentric load on the back of the leg. • Modify the boot to decrease pressure of boot top against the Achilles tendon.
Ankle • Sprains*	• Ensure that boots have enough upper support and have not worn out. • Use caution during off-ice training, when ankle injuries occur more frequently. • Maintain strong peroneal muscles; they may weaken as a result of time spent in a stiff boot. • Ankle braces do not fit inside ice-skating boots and are not a good preventive strategy.
• Malleolar bursitis (inflammation and swelling over the medial malleolus of the ankle) due to the pressure of the skating boots, often caused by pronation, particularly in persons with flat feet	• Stretch out boots at the sides. • Protect the ankles with silicone sleeves, such as Bunga Pads. • Use donut-shaped padding around the medial malleolus, not directly over it, to decrease pressure. • Use orthotics or modify boots to correct pronation.
• Tenosynovitis of the anterior tibialis or extensor hallucis tendon at the anterior ankle	• Wear more flexible boots. • Use silicone sleeves, such as Bunga Pads.
• "Lace bites" (caused by upper two laces crossing in boots that are too stiff); can progress to cysts and tendonitis	• Pad the tongue of the boot. • Add midline lace hooks or alternate lacing to keep tongue in neutral or slightly medial position or to avoid lateral migration of the tongue. • Rebuild boot tongue of aging skates.
Heel • Retrocalcaneal bursitis (Haglund's deformity) • "Pump bump"	• Select a boot that is narrow enough in the heel to prevent excessive movement of the heel. • Change fit of boot by using padding to narrow the heel.
Foot overuse conditions • Metatarsal stress fractures • Navicular stress fractures • Metatarsalgia • Sesamoiditis	• Metatarsal pads or bars under the forefoot may be used to redistribute the pressure of impact. • Wear orthotics. • Limit excessive jumping, particularly during off-ice practice.
Foot injuries to skin • Foot bunions, calluses, and blisters (at base of fifth metatarsal, tarsal navicular, or toes)	• Use properly fitting skates and avoid lacing too tightly. • Modify skates or use donut padding for blisters and calluses. • Shave down calluses.
Eating disorders and/or amenorrhea*	• Risk is increased as a result of pressure to maintain an aesthetically appealing, lean body.

* See Table 46.1

Table 46.14

Injury Prevention Guidance for FOOTBALL

Common Injuries	Prevention Strategies/Comments
Injuries for which protective gear is recommended • Head injuries/facial injuries	Wear proper protective gear: • Helmet. • Face mask. • Mouth guard. Ensure helmet fits properly: • Eyebrows should be 1-1.5 inches below the helmet's front rim. • The back of the helmet should cover the occiput. • The player's ear openings should be in the center of the helmet's ear openings. • Jaw pads should be snug against athlete's jaw. • The chin strap should be centered over the chin and tightened to prevent movement of the helmet. • Helmet padding and chin strap should be tight enough to prevent any rotation of the helmet on the head. • Face mask should be attached to helmet. Additional protection can be provided by a clear Plexiglas shield. • Mouth guard should be in place.
• Contusions to knee, thigh, iliac crest (hip pointer), tail bone, ribs, shoulder	• To prevent contusions, wear properly fitting football pants incorporating knee pads, thigh pads, and girdle that includes hip pads and tailbone pads. • Wear shoulder pads. • Wear additional pads available for hand, forearm, and ribs.
• Testicular injuries	• Wear a protective cup.

• Shoulder injuries
  • Shoulder separation (acromioclavicular joint sprain)
  • Dislocation
	• Ensure shoulder pads that are large enough to extend $3/4$ to 1 inch beyond the acromioclavicular joint.
	• Shoulder harness that restricts abduction is available for athletes with prior subluxation or dislocation.

Concussion	• Ensure that helmet, face mask, and mouth guard are worn. • Educate coaches on signs and symptoms of concussions to decrease chance of secondary injury, second-impact syndrome, or postconcussion syndrome. • Insist on medical clearance to return to play after any concussion. • Continued play for athletes with multiple concussions may not be advisable even if they appear to have recovered.
Neck strain or fracture • Brachial plexopathy (stinger or burner)	• Ensure proper tackling technique: instruct athlete to keep head up. • Initiate neck- and shoulder-strengthening program. • Consider cervical roll to prevent recurrent injuries.

Lumbar injuries*
• Muscle strains
• Disk injuries
• Pars interarticularis injuries
  • Pars interarticularis stress fracture (spondylolysis)
  • Pars interarticularis stress reaction
	• Use caution with drills that involve repetitive lumbar hyperextension, such as a blocking sled, which contributes to pars injuries.

* See Table 46.1

Table 46.14–cont'd

Injury Prevention Guidance for FOOTBALL

Common Injuries	Prevention Strategies/Comments
Muscle strains* • Hamstring • Quadriceps • Calf	• Perform preseason conditioning to strengthen hamstring and reduce discrepancies between hamstring and quadriceps strength. • Correct deficits in flexibility before sprinting or practicing at full speed. • Restore flexibility and strength if muscle tightness develops or a mild strain occurs.
Knee ligament injuries*	• Prophylactic knee braces are often recommended and used. • Efficacy for anterior cruciate ligament injury prevention has not been demonstrated.
Lower leg overuse injuries* • Medial tibial stress syndrome (shin splints) • Achilles tendonitis • Stress fractures of the lower leg and foot	–
Ankle sprains*	• Prophylactic taping or bracing is commonly recommended, but its efficacy has not been proven.
First metacarpophalangeal joint sprain (turf toe)	• Earlier return to play after injury may be helped by taping or inserting a stiff plate in the shoe.
Dehydration and/or heat illness* • Heat cramps • Heat exhaustion • Heatstroke	• Risk is increased as a result of wearing helmets and multiple layers of clothing and padding. • Increase salt in the diet 24 hours before and then during games for players with history of cramping. • Remove helmet frequently during hot and humid conditions.

* See Table 46.1

Table 46.15

Injury Prevention Guidance for GOLF

Common Injuries	Prevention Strategies/Comments
General prevention	• Use appropriate equipment: a golf professional can help the athlete identify clubs that are appropriate length, weight, grip size, and shaft stiffness on the basis of the size, strength, swing speed, and skill level of the player. • Ensure the athlete learns proper golf swing technique by taking lessons or other form of professional instruction. • Warm up by stretching back and shoulder muscles, swinging 2 clubs or a heavy club back and forth, and, if possible, hitting practice shots on the driving range before playing. • Exercise to improve overall flexibility and strength, particularly in rotational planes of motion. • Maintain adequate distance from other golfers to avoid injuries from getting hit by the golf club or ball. • Be aware of golfers playing other holes: yell "fore" if a shot is heading in the direction of other players, and duck for cover if another player yells "fore."
Shoulder overuse injuries* • Impingement • Rotator cuff tendonitis (more frequent in the leading arm)	• Use caution when lifting golf bag or carrying golf bag on one shoulder. It is preferable to carry golf bag over both shoulders.

* See Table 46.1

Table 46.15—cont'd

Injury Prevention Guidance for GOLF

Common Injuries	Prevention Strategies/Comments
Elbow overuse injuries • Medial epicondylitis (golfer's elbow) • Lateral epicondylitis	• Avoid overswinging with the dominant arm (right arm in right-handed golfer); it can lead to medial epicondylitis of the dominant arm. • Overswinging with the lead arm or hitting shots "fat" can cause lateral epicondylitis of the nondominant arm. • Perform forearm stretching and strengthening exercises, and warm up before play.
Wrist injuries • Tendonitis • Carpal tunnel syndrome • Wrist dorsal impaction syndrome • Ligament sprains • Traumatic arthritis	• Perform exercises to establish full motion in wrist and to strengthen hand, wrist, and forearm. • If wrist pain or stiffness is present, limit extra practice swings and swings through heavy material (eg, rough, sand).
Stress fracture of ribs	• Avoid general overuse by increasing practice and playing time gradually. • Use proper swing biomechanics. • This injury is most common in novices. • This injury involves the posterior lateral portion of the fourth to seventh ribs on the side of the nondominant arm.
Lumbar injuries* • Muscle stains • Disk injuries	• Warm up and stretch before playing; consider strengthening exercises for core musculature, including exercises for abdominal obliques. • Limit full swings and carrying golf bag if symptoms of back pain develop; seek medical evaluation if back pain persists or starts interfering with daily activity. • Lift and carry golf bag following the rules of good mechanics. Use a double-strapped bag to distribute the weight evenly and to allow an upright posture while walking.
Knee overuse injuries* • Patellofemoral stress syndrome	• Limit squatting while lining up putts and picking up balls. • Limit walking on hills. • Hitting balls on driving range and putting is less aggravating for this condition than walking and playing over greater distances on the course.
Meniscal tears of the knee	• Limit repetitive squatting, twisting, and walking on uneven surfaces. • No exercises can clearly help with prevention of a meniscal tear; however, avoiding attempts to push through symptoms of a small meniscus tear (ie, swelling, stiffness, catching) may prevent a small meniscus tear from becoming a bigger tear or requiring surgery.
Sun damage* • Sunburn • Skin cancer • Eye damage	—
Lightning strikes	• Adhere to warnings issued by weather service or golf course officials. • Avoid standing in the middle of a fairway, near isolated trees, or by metal poles during storms. • Stand apart from other golfers rather than in a group. • Lie down in a sand trap and wait for the storm to pass if a designated shelter or car is not available.

* See Table 46.1

Table 46.16

Injury Prevention Guidance for GYMNASTICS

Common Injuries	Prevention Strategies/Comments
General prevention	• Use well-trained coaches experienced in proper technique and safety. • Ensure appropriate spotting. • Advance difficulty of routines gradually as skills and strength warrant. • Have an emergency plan in place.
Shoulder injuries* • Shoulder instability • Impingement • Rotator cuff strain or tendonitis	—
Elbow conditions • Osteochondritis dissecans • Olecranon apophysitis	• Limit upper extremity weight bearing and impact.
Wrist overuse injuries • Dorsal wrist impingement or capsulitis • Radial epiphysitis (stress reaction of the distal radial physis)	• Tape wrists or use wrist braces, such as "Tiger Paws." • Limit upper extremity weight bearing and impact.
Torn skin on hands (rips)	• Use chalk and leather grips to decrease friction. • Use hand lotion and regularly shave calluses to decrease callous buildup.

Lumbar injuries*
• Muscle strains
• Disk injuries
• Pars interarticularis injuries
  • Pars interarticularis stress fracture (spondylolysis)
  • Pars interarticularis stress reaction
	• Limit tumbling and dismounts to decrease high-impact activities.
	• Limit excessive lumbar flexion, which contributes to disk injuries.
	• Limit dismounts in position of lumbar extension, which contributes to pars injuries.
	• Limit skills requiring extreme lumbar extension, such as back walkovers and back handsprings, which contribute to pars injuries.

Knee overuse injuries* • Patellofemoral stress syndrome • Patellar tendonitis • Osgood-Schlatter disease	• Practice tumbling and dismounts on soft surfaces such as mats, tumble track, and trampoline.
Anterior cruciate ligament injuries*	• Teach stopping and landing techniques for dismounts and floor exercises.
Lower leg overuse injuries* • Medial tibial stress syndrome (shin splints) • Achilles' tendonitis • Stress fractures of the lower leg and foot	• See "Knee overuse injuries" (above). • Limit tumbling and dismounts to decrease high-impact activities. • Risk is increased as a result of high-impact activities performed barefoot, without the cushioning and support provided by athletic shoes.
Ankle sprains*	—
Calcaneal apophysitis (Sever's disease)*	• Use ankle brace that incorporates heel cushioning ("Cheetah") or silicone heel cups in an ankle brace.
Eating disorders and/or amenorrhea*	• Risk is increased as a result of pressure to maintain an aesthetically appealing, lean body.

* See Table 46.1

Table 46.17

Injury Prevention Guidance for ICE HOCKEY/ROLLER HOCKEY

Common Injuries	Prevention Strategies/Comments
Injuries for which protective gear is recommended • Facial injuries • Mouth injuries • Scrotal injuries • Elbow injuries • Knee injuries • Shoulder injuries • Neck injuries • Kidney injuries • Hand and wrist injuries • Hip and thigh injuries • Head injuries	Use appropriate protective gear: • Full cage helmet with strap around the chin. • Mouth guard. • Protective cup. • Elbow pads. • Knee pads. • Shoulder pads. • Neck guard. • Kidney pads. • Padded hockey gloves. • Hip/thigh pads. • Helmet. Other preventive measures: • Enforce safety rules. • Ensure the net slides out of holes when athlete strikes the pipe. • Enforce rules that limit contact in certain age groups, such as not allowing checking for children under age 15.
Injuries to goalies	Use specialized protective equipment for goalies: • More substantial helmet and mask, and padding. • Skates with longer blades for stability. • Reinforcement along the inner foot of the skates for protection from pucks and skates.
Concussions	• Use full cage helmet with strap around chin. • Teach athlete how to strike the boards at an angle with the head up when a collision cannot be avoided. • Avoid overly aggressive or dangerous play. • Educate coaches on signs and symptoms of concussions to decrease chance of secondary injury, second-impact syndrome, or postconcussion syndrome.
Shoulder injuries • Shoulder separation (acromioclavicular joint sprain) • Dislocation (glenohumeral)	• Perform upper-body strengthening program focusing on shoulder strengthening and stabilization. • Wear shoulder pads. • Enforce rules that limit contact in certain age groups, such as not allowing checking for children under age 15.
Lumbar injuries* • Muscle strains • Disk injuries	• Limit rounding of the back while bending forward to hit the puck.
Groin strains	• Perform proper warm-up and stretching.
Knee sprains • Medial collateral ligament sprain	• Enforce rules that limit contact in certain age groups, such as not allowing checking for children under age 15.
Skin infections from gear contaminated with bacteria or fungus	Wash or disinfect hockey gear in direct contact with skin: • Most equipment can be washed in a commercial washing machine. • Disinfect helmets and face masks with antibacterial wipes. • Spray the inside of leather gloves with spray cleaner. • Special dry-cleaning machines can disinfect entire bags of gear. • Dry all damp equipment before repacking in hockey bag.
Dehydration*	• Encourage hydration even though athlete may not feel thirsty or hot. • Risk is increased as a result of wearing helmets and many layers of clothing and padding.
Hypothermia/frostbite	• Change to dry clothing when clothing is wet. • Avoid tight-fitting skates. • Dress in underlayers of wicking, fast-drying fabrics (eg, wool, polypropylene).
Exercise-induced asthma	• Risk is increased with exposure to cold, dry air. • Use baseline asthma medications and use an additional inhaler treatment before exercise sessions.

* See Table 46.1

Table 46.18

Injury Prevention Guidance for LACROSSE

Common Injuries	Prevention Strategies/Comments
Injuries for which protective gear is recommended	Use appropriate protective gear
	• Proper athletic gear for male athletes (required): • Helmet with face mask.
• Head injuries • Facial injuries • Eye injuries	

• Mouth injuries
• Wrist/hand injuries
• Scrotal injuries
• Shoulder and elbow injuries
	• Mouth guard.
	• Gloves.
	• Protective cup.
	• Shoulder pads.
	• Elbow pads.
	• Proper athletic gear for female athletes (required):
	  • Eye goggles.
	  • Mouth guard.
	  • Gloves.
	• Optional gear for female athletes:
	  • Soft helmet made of foam-type material.
	  • Nose guard.
	• Additional gear for goalkeepers (males and females):
	  • Helmet with face mask.
	  • Separate throat protector.
	  • Padded gloves.
	  • Chest protector.
	  • Mouth guard.
	  • Padding on shins and thighs (required for high school level and below).
	  • Padding on arms and shoulders (optional).

Lumbar injuries*
• Muscle strains
• Disk injuries
• Pars interarticularis injuries
  • Pars interarticularis stress fracture (spondylolysis)
  • Pars interarticularis stress reaction
	• Risk of pars injury is increased as a result of repetitive rotation when using the lacrosse stick to pass the ball.

Knee sprain	• Enforce rules to prevent overly aggressive or dangerous play.
Lower leg overuse injuries* • Medial tibial stress syndrome (shin splints) • Achilles tendonitis • Stress fractures of the lower leg and foot	–

* See Table 46.1

Table 46.19

Injury Prevention Guidance for MARATHON AND TRIATHALON

Common Injuries	Prevention Strategies/Comments
Overuse injuries* • Medial tibial stress syndrome (shin splints) • Stress fractures of the lower leg and foot • Patellofemoral stress syndrome • Rotator cuff strain or tendonitis • Iliotibial band syndrome	• See Cross-country, Bicycling, and Swimming prevention strategies. • Increase training distance by no more than 10% per week. • Gradually increase in training distance by no more than 10% per week when initiating training and if returning after illness, injury, or other disruption of training. • Encourage participation in youth age categories with shorter distances, and discourage participation in full-length marathons and triathlons.
Eating disorders and/or amenorrhea*	• Risk is increased because of the belief that decreased body fat improves endurance.
Iron-deficiency anemia	• Ensure adequate iron intake, particularly in female runners.
Hyponatremia	• Educate marathon runners about proper hydration with water and sports drinks; avoid overhydration.
Hypothermia and hyperthermia	• Enforce weather-related guidelines. • Use wet suits and hoods for open-water swims.
Burnout	• See "Overuse injuries" (above)
Sun damage* • Sunburn • Skin cancer • Eye damage	–

* See Table 46.1

Table 46.20

Injury Prevention Guidance for MARTIAL ARTS

Common Injuries	Prevention Strategies/Comments

Injuries for which protective gear is recommended
• Rib fracture
• Shin contusion
• Mouth and dental injuries
• Head injuries
• Hand injuries
	Use proper protective gear:
	  • Chest protection.
	  • Shin guards.
	  • Mouth guards.
	  • Protective headgear, when applicable (see below).
	  • Gloves.

Concussion	• Wear protective headgear, when the rules allow, for sparring or for activities with risk of falling, such as high jumps or flying kicks. • Teach proper technique. • Discourage contact to the head. • Educate coaches on signs and symptoms of concussions to decrease chance of secondary injury, second-impact syndrome, or postconcussion syndrome.
Knee sprain	• Enforce safety rules. • Teach proper kicking and punching techniques.
Renal contusion	
Hand and foot trauma	
Ankle sprain*	• Risk is increased as a result of lack of supportive shoe wear.

* See Table 46.1

Table 46.21

Injury Prevention Guidance for RACQUET SPORTS (TENNIS, RACQUETBALL, SQUASH, PADDLE TENNIS)

Common Injuries	Prevention Strategies/Comments
Eye injuries (due to being struck by ball or racquet)	• Wear protective eyewear, particularly for racquetball and squash.
Shoulder overuse injuries* • Impingement • Rotator cuff strain or tendonitis	• Limit excessive serving or overheads.
Elbow overuse injuries	• Teach proper stroke mechanics. • Ensure proper fitting of racquet grip and appropriate string tension: • Avoid grips that are too large. • Avoid racquets that are too heavy. • Use larger racquet head. • Decrease string tension. • Use racquets that decrease impact and vibration.
• Medial epicondylitis/apophysitis	• This injury is often the result of introducing a new service motion or topspin; introduce these changes gradually.
• Lateral epicondylitis	• This injury is often due to incorrect technique while hitting backhand. • Lateral epicondylitis is not common in children and adolescents; it should raise concern for other pathology, such as osteochondritis dissecans.
Wrist tendonitis	• Avoid poor stroke mechanics: • Failure to fully extend the elbow on ground strokes. • Bending the wrist on ground strokes. • Hitting the ball too late. • Serving behind one's head. • Ensure proper fitting of racquet grip and strings. • Extensor carpi ulnaris tendonitis is common as a result of repetitive wrist rotation.
Fracture of the hook of the hamate of the hand	• Avoid pressure of racquet handle over volar ulnar aspect of the wrist.
Ulnar neuropathy affecting fourth and fifth fingers	• Avoid excessive pressure of the grip against the hypothenar eminence of the hand.
Digital nerve palsy of fingers	• Avoid excessive compression of grip against hand.
Lumbar injuries* • Muscle strains • Disk injuries	• Risk of disk injuries is increased as a result of movements requiring bending forward and rotation.
• Pars interarticularis injuries • Pars interarticularis stress fracture (spondylolysis) • Pars interarticularis stress reaction	• Risk of pars injury is increased as a result of repetitive lumbar extension and rotation required for serving and hitting overheads.
Knee overuse injuries* • Patellofemoral stress syndrome • Patellar tendonitis • Osgood-Schlatter disease	–
Lower leg overuse injuries* • Medial tibial stress syndrome (shin splints) • Achilles tendonitis • Stress fractures of the lower leg and foot	• Avoid sudden changes from soft to hard surfaces. • Avoid sudden increases in hours of playing.
Ankle sprains*	• Clear away extra balls to avoid stepping on them.
Dehydration and/or heat illness* • Heat cramps • Heat exhaustion • Heat stroke	• Increase salt in the diet 24 hours before matches for players with a history of cramping.
Sun damage* • Sunburn • Skin cancer • Eye damage	–

* See Table 46.1

Table 46.22

Injury Prevention Guidance for SKATEBOARDING/IN-LINE SKATING

Common Injuries	Prevention Strategies/Comments
General prevention	Skate safely in appropriate environments:
	• For in-line skaters and skateboarders:
	• Skate under control and within capabilities in a safe environment.
	• Skate on smooth pavement in areas closed off from traffic.
	• Do not skate on wet, oily, or irregular surfaces.
	• Avoid tricks and moves beyond the athlete's skill level or training.
	• Avoid skating with hands in pockets.
	• Do not use headphones while skating.
	• "Skitching a ride" (holding onto the side or rear of a moving vehicle while riding a skateboard or in-line skates) should never be done.
	• For in-line skaters:
	• Novice in-line skaters should learn at an indoor skating rink.
	• For skateboarders:
	• Novice skateboarders should be particularly cautious.
	• One-third of skateboard injuries occur within the first week.
	• The injury rate for skateboarding is twice as high as for in-line skating.
	• Avoid homemade skateboard ramps.
	• Skate parks are associated with higher severity of fractures, particularly ramps and bars.
	• Never put more than one person on a skateboard.
	• Children under age 5 should not ride skateboards; children ages 6-10 should be closely supervised.
	Use appropriate equipment:
	• For in-line skaters and skateboarders:
	• Ensure that wheels are worn down symmetrically and turn freely.
	• Replace worn wheels and check for cracks, nicks, or debris.
	• For in-line skaters:
	• Use properly fitting skates.
	• Novice in-line skaters should wear 3- or 4- wheeled skates; 5-wheeled skates are for high-performance distance or competitive skaters.
	• Maintain brake pads on in-line skates.
	• For skateboarders:
	• Wear closed, slip-resistant shoes.
	• Novice skateboarders should use skateboards with shorter decks.
	Learn how to fall correctly:
	• Preferably land on the fleshy parts of the body (thighs/hips and arms/shoulders).
	• Avoid falling on an outstretched arm; bend elbow if falling on arm.
	• Keep head up while falling.
	• If falling backward, tuck chin into chest.

Injuries for which protective gear is recommended
• Head injuries
• Wrist/hand/forearm fractures
• Knee abrasions/contusions
• Elbow injuries
	Use proper protective gear
	  • Helmets (mandatory in some states for children under age 18).
	  • Wrist guards.
	  • Knee pads.
	  • Elbow pads.

Ankle injuries (skateboarders)*	• See "General prevention" (above).

* See Table 46.1

Table 46.23

Injury Prevention Guidance for SKIING (DOWNHILL AND CROSS-COUNTRY)/SNOWBOARDING

Common Injuries	Prevention Strategies/Comments
General prevention	• Ski under control and within capabilities. • Do not ski alone. • Use devices to prevent runaway equipment. • Teach athlete how and when to fall (see below).
Injuries for which protective gear is recommended • Concussions/head injuries	Use proper protective gear: • Ski helmet.
Shoulder injuries • Shoulder separation (acromioclavicular joint sprain) • Dislocation (glenohumeral)	• Avoid falling directly on the side of the shoulder. • Do not drag poles to stop or slow falls; this can cause the arms to be pulled behind the plane of the body and increase the risk of shoulder dislocation.
Ulnar collateral ligament sprain of thumb (skier's thumb)	• Avoid falling on the hand while still gripping ski pole.
Splenic injuries (snowboarding)	• Avoid skiing or snowboarding if athlete has any underlying condition associated with splenic enlargement, such as infectious mononucleosis. • This injury occurs most often from falling onto the edge of a snowboard.

Knee ligament injuries (particularly skiing)
• Anterior cruciate ligament sprain
• Medial collateral ligament sprain
	• Ensure proper fit of equipment and adjustment of bindings that allow for appropriate release.
	• Teach athlete how to stop after a fall.
	• Teach athlete how and when to fall:
	  • Avoid trying to sit down when out of control.
	  • Avoid attempting to recover when off balance or falling.
	  • Avoid falling backward on the tail of the skis; fall to side or along the fall line.
	  • Avoid position of "phantom foot"; this occurs when the skier is off balance and falling backward with weight on the inside edge of the downhill ski and uphill ski is in the air.
	  • Avoid landing from a jump with extended knees or with the weight primarily on the back of the skis.
	  • Try to lift ski tips out from under snow.

Medial tibial stress syndrome (cross-country)*	–
Achilles tendonitis (cross-country)*	–
Ankle fracture • Lateral process of talus (snowboarder's fracture)	• Beginners should wear soft-shell boots.
Hypothermia/frostbite	• Limit exposure to extreme temperatures. • Wear layered, sweat-wicking clothing. • Wear appropriate foot, hand, and head wear.
Altitude syndrome • Acute mountain sickness • High-altitude pulmonary edema • High-altitude cerebral edema	• Allow time for acclimatization to altitude with gradual ascent. • Maintain proper hydration. • Avoid use of alcohol, caffeine, and sedatives.
Sun damage* • Sunburn • Skin cancer • Eye damage	• Sun damage to skin and eyes is increased as a result of the sun's reflection off the snow and increased exposure to ultraviolet light at high altitude.

* See Table 46.1

Table 46.24

Injury Prevention Guidance for SOCCER

Common Injuries	Prevention Strategies/Comments
Injuries for which protective gear is recommended: • Eye injuries • Facial, mouth, and dental injuries • Shin injuries	Use proper preventive gear: • Consider wearing protective eyewear; eye injuries in soccer are rare but are often severe. • Use mouth guard; soccer is the second leading cause of facial, mouth, and dental injuries in sports. • Wear shin guards.
Neck strain	• Teach proper heading technique with an appropriate-sized ball. • Perform neck-strengthening exercises to protect neck during heading. • Discourage heading in children younger than 10 because most younger children lack adequate neck strength and coordination to head the ball safely and correctly.
Concussion	• Educate coaches on signs and symptoms of concussions to decrease chance of secondary injury, second-impact syndrome, or postconcussion syndrome. • Teach proper heading technique with an appropriate-sized ball for age. • Minimize heading near goalposts (which is a common cause of concussion). • Ensure goalposts are anchored into the ground. • Minimize heading from behind (ie, heading the ball backward, when the player cannot see if another player is directly behind, thus increasing the risk of collision of the heads of the 2 players). • Discourage excessive heading drills. • Minimize heading in children less than 10 because younger children lack adequate neck strength and coordination to head the ball safely and correctly; the risk of permanent cognitive impairment has not been determined.

Lumbar injuries*
• Muscle strains
• Disk injuries
• Pars interarticularis injuries
  • Pars interarticularis stress fracture (spondylolysis)
  • Pars interarticularis stress reaction
	• Risk of pars injury is increased as a result of repetitive kicking, which causes lumbar extension and rotation.

Groin strains and pelvic ring avulsion fractures	• Perform hip flexor, adductor, and hamstring stretching, particularly during growth spurts.
Knee ligament injuries (especially anterior cruciate ligament tears)*	• Enforce rules to prevent overly aggressive or dangerous play, particularly fouling from behind.
Lower leg overuse injuries* • Medial tibial stress syndrome (shin splints) • Achilles' tendonitis • Stress fractures of the lower leg and foot	• Use correct type of running shoe when not doing soccer-specific drills. • Run on soft, even surfaces when cross training. • Insoles for arch support and correction of pronation are particularly beneficial in soccer shoes, which typically have little support.
Tibial shaft fracture	• Use shin guards. • Enforce rules to prevent overly aggressive or dangerous play.
Ankle sprain*	–
Calcaneal apophysitis (Sever's disease)*	• This condition is particularly common in soccer as a result of cleated shoes with little heel cushioning; consider switching to a uncleated turf shoe.
Turf toe (1st Metacarpophalangeal joint sprain)	• To prevent reinjury, tape or insert a stiff plate in the shoe.

* See Table 46.1

Table 46.25

Injury Prevention Guidance for SWIMMING

Common Injuries	Prevention Strategies/Comments
Shoulder overuse injuries* • Impingement • Rotator cuff strain or tendonitis • Labral tears	Teach proper stoke technique: • Ensure adequate rotation of the shoulders and trunk and avoid swimming flat on the water. • Avoid pulling with a straight arm, too much adduction during the pull (pulling across the midline of the body), and excessive internal rotation of the arm. • Strokes that place the most stress on the shoulder are butterfly, followed by freestyle, backstroke, and breaststroke. • Hand paddles and pull buoys increase stress on the shoulders.
Medial knee pain • Medial collateral ligament sprain • Patellofemoral dysfunction • Medial plica syndrome	• Limit time performing breaststroke kick and ensure proper technique.
Skin rashes and eye irritation	• Check pool water for excessive chemicals and chlorine. • Wear swimming goggles.
Sun damage* • Sunburn • Skin cancer • Eye damage	• Wear swimming caps. • Wear sun-protective water shirts.
Hypothermia	• Wear a wet suit and hood for open-water swims in cold water.

* See Table 46.1

Table 46.26

Injury Prevention Guidance for WATER POLO

Common Injuries	Prevention Strategies/Comments
Injuries for which protective equipment is recommended • Ear injuries • Mouth injuries • Eye injuries	Use proper protective gear: • Polo caps with ear guards.
Neck pain	• Water polo players swim with their heads above the water and looking forward, known as the heads-up crawl. This is more stressful on the neck and shoulder than the traditional crawl stroke. • Neck injuries can occur as a result of direct contact.
Shoulder injuries • Instability • Impingement • Rotator cuff strain or tendonitis • Labral tears	• Limit use of devices that increase stress on the shoulders, such as hand paddles and pull buoys. • Limit excessive throwing. • See "Neck pain" above
Quadriceps contusion	• Enforce rules and regulations.
Concussions (usually from head hit by another player's elbow)	
Nasal fracture	
Knee injuries • Medial knee pain (from eggbeater kick) • Medial collateral ligament sprain • Patellofemoral stress syndrome* • Medial plica syndrome	• Limit excessive eggbeater kicking. • Stress can be taken off the knees by sculling more to tread water and modifying the eggbeater kick to a more narrow or bicycle-type kick.
Scratches, abrasions, and lacerations; corneal abrasion	• Keep fingernails and toenails trimmed. • Officials should inspect nails before competitions for proper trimming.
Skin rashes/eye irritation	• Persons in charge of pool maintenance should check pool water for excessive chemicals and chlorine.
Sun damage* • Sunburn • Skin cancer • Eye damage	–

* See Table 46.1

Table 46.27

Injury Prevention Guidance for WRESTLING

Common Injuries	Prevention Strategies/Comments
Auricular hematoma (cauliflower ear)	• Use properly fitting headgear with ear protectors. • Perform prompt aspiration and compression of blood in auricle to prevent cartilage deformity (cauliflower ear).
Brachial plexopathy	• Perform neck-strengthening exercises.
Shoulder injuries • Shoulder separation (acromioclavicular sprain) • Shoulder dislocation (glenohumeral) • Clavicle fracture	• Initiate an upper-body strengthening program focusing on shoulder strengthening and stabilization.
Elbow injuries • Medial collateral ligament strains • Elbow dislocation • Olecranon bursitis	• Avoid elbow hyperextension. • Avoid hard falls directly on the elbow.
Lumbar injuries* • Muscle stains • Disk injuries	• Risk is increased as a result of positions requiring rounding of the back under load.
Knee injuries • Meniscal tear • Anterior cruciate ligament sprain • Medial collateral ligament sprain • Patellar dislocations • Prepatellar bursitis	• Teach proper technique. • Enforce safety rules.
Dermatologic infection • Herpesvirus (herpes gladiatorum) • Impetigo • Methicillin-resistant *Staphylococcus aureus* • Tinea corporis	• Educate athletes to have skin lesions evaluated early. • Perform skin checks before practices and matches. • Ensure mats are cleaned daily with commercial antibacterial solutions. • Educate athletes to shower after practice and matches, and not to share towels.
Disordered eating • Excessive weight loss • Dehydration	• Encourage proper nutritional intake to meet the caloric demands of training and to maintain appropriate body weight, usually at least 2000 kcal per day. • Enforce minimum weight-class rules to prevent acute weight loss and dehydration. • Maintain body fat of at least 7% for males and 12% for females wrestling at the high school level. • Restrict weight loss to no more than 1.5% of body weight per week. • Avoid use of rubber suits, steam baths or saunas, prolonged fasting, fluid restriction, vomiting, drugs, laxatives, diuretics, diet pills, stimulants, ergogenic aids, and supplements. • Measure weight before and after wrestling, and replace each pound lost with 16 ounces of fluid.

* See Table 46.1

APPENDIX

Council on Sports Medicine and Fitness: Policy Statements

All policy statements from the American Academy of Pediatrics automatically expire 5 years after publication unless reaffirmed, revised, or retired at or before that time.

STATEMENTS PUBLISHED

Active Healthy Living: Prevention of Childhood Obesity Through Increased Physical Activity
Pediatrics Vol. 117, No. 5, May 2006
http://aappolicy.aappublications.org/cgi/reprint/pediatrics;
117/5/1834.pdf

Athletic Participation by Children and Adolescents Who Have Systemic Hypertension
Pediatrics Vol. 99, No. 4, April 1997
Reaffirmed January 2009
http://aappolicy.aappublications.org/cgi/reprint/pediatrics;
99/4/637.pdf

Climatic Heat Stress and the Exercising Child and Adolescent
Pediatrics Vol. 106, No. 1, July 2000
Reaffirmed September 2007
http://aappolicy.aappublications.org/cgi/reprint/pediatrics;
106/1/158.pdf

Human Immunodeficiency Virus and Other Blood-Borne Viral Pathogens in the Athletic Setting
Pediatrics Vol. 104, No. 6, December 1999
Reaffirmed May 2009
http://aappolicy.aappublications.org/cgi/reprint/pediatrics;
104/6/1400.pdf

In-Line Skating Injuries in Children and Adolescents
Reaffirmed May 2009
Pediatrics Vol. 101, No. 4, April 1998
http://aappolicy.aappublications.org/cgi/reprint/pediatrics;
101/4/720.pdf

Intensive Training and Sports Specialization in Young Athletes
Pediatrics Vol. 106, No. 1, July 2000
Reaffirmed May 2006
http://aappolicy.aappublications.org/cgi/reprint/pediatrics;
106/1/154.pdf

Medical Concerns in the Female Athlete
Pediatrics Vol. 106, No. 3, September 2000
Reaffirmed August 2008
http://aappolicy.aappublications.org/cgi/reprint/pediatrics;
106/3/610.pdf

Medical Conditions Affecting Sports Participation
Pediatrics Vol. 121, No. 4, April 2008
http://aappolicy.aappublications.org/cgi/reprint/pediatrics;
121/4/841.pdf

Organized Sports for Children and Preadolescents
Pediatrics Vol. 107, No. 6, June 2001
Reaffirmed September 2007
http://aappolicy.aappublications.org/cgi/reprint/pediatrics;
107/6/1459.pdf

Overuse Injuries, Overtraining, and Burnout in Children and Adolescent Athletes
Pediatrics Vol. 119, No. 6, June 2007
http://aappolicy.aappublications.org/cgi/reprint/pediatrics;
119/6/1242.pdf

Promotion of Healthy Weight-Control Practices in Young Athletes
Pediatrics Vol. 116, No. 6, December 2005
http://aappolicy.aappublications.org/cgi/reprint/pediatrics;
116/6/1557.pdf

Protective Eyewear for Young Athletes

Pediatrics Vol. 113, No. 3, March 2004

Reaffirmed August 2008

http://aappolicy.aappublications.org/cgi/reprint/pediatrics;
113/3/619.pdf

Risk of Injury from Baseball and Softball in Children

Pediatrics Vol. 107, No. 4, April 2001

Reaffirmed May 2006

http://aappolicy.aappublications.org/cgi/reprint/pediatrics;
107/4/782.pdf

Safety in Youth Ice Hockey: The Effects of Body Checking

Pediatrics Vol. 105, No. 3, March 2000

Reaffirmed September 2007

http://aappolicy.aappublications.org/cgi/reprint/pediatrics;
105/3/657.pdf

Strength Training by Children and Adolescents

Pediatrics Vol. 121, No. 4, April 2008

http://aappolicy.aappublications.org/cgi/reprint/pediatrics;
121/4/835.pdf

Technical Report: Knee Brace Use in the Young Athlete

Pediatrics Vol. 108, No. 2, August 2001

Reaffirmed May 2007

http://aappolicy.aappublications.org/cgi/reprint/pediatrics;
108/2/503.pdf

Trampolines at Home, School, and Recreational Centers

Pediatrics Vol. 103, No. 5, May 1999

Reaffirmed May 2006

http://aappolicy.aappublications.org/cgi/reprint/pediatrics;
103/5/1053.pdf

Use of Performance-Enhancing Substances

Pediatrics Vol. 115, No. 4, April 2005

Reaffirmed August 2008

http://aappolicy.aappublications.org/cgi/reprint/pediatrics;
115/4/1103.pdf

Active Healthy Living: Prevention of Childhood Obesity Through Increased Physical Activity

Organizational Principles to Guide and Define the Child Health Care System and/or Improve the Health of All Children

Council on Sports Medicine and Fitness and Council on School Health

ABSTRACT

The current epidemic of inactivity and the associated epidemic of obesity are being driven by multiple factors (societal, technologic, industrial, commercial, financial) and must be addressed likewise on several fronts. Foremost among these are the expansion of school physical education, dissuading children from pursuing sedentary activities, providing suitable role models for physical activity, and making activity-promoting changes in the environment. This statement outlines ways that pediatric health care providers and public health officials can encourage, monitor, and advocate for increased physical activity for children and teenagers.

INTRODUCTION

IN 1997, THE World Health Organization declared obesity a global epidemic with major health implications.[1] According to the 1999–2000 National Health and Nutrition Examination Survey (www.cdc.gov/nchs/nhanes.htm), the prevalence of overweight or obesity in children and youth in the United States is over 15%, a value that has tripled since the 1960s.[2] The health implications of this epidemic are profound. Insulin resistance, type 2 diabetes mellitus, hypertension, obstructive sleep apnea, nonalcoholic steatohepatitis, poor self-esteem, and a lower health-related quality of life are among the comorbidities seen more commonly in affected children and youth than in their unaffected counterparts.[3-7] In addition, up to 80% of obese youth continue this trend into adulthood.[8,9] Adult obesity is associated with higher rates of hypertension, dyslipidemia, and insulin resistance, which are risk factors for coronary artery disease, the leading cause of death in North America.[10]

Assessment of Overweight

Ideally, methods of measuring body fat should be accurate, inexpensive, and easy to use; have small measurement error; and be well documented with published reference values. Direct measures of body composition, such as underwater weighing, magnetic resonance imaging, computed axial tomography, and dual-energy radiograph absorptiometry, provide an estimate of total body fat mass. These techniques, however, are used mainly in tertiary care centers for research purposes. Anthropometric measures of relative fatness may be inexpensive and easy to use but rely on the skill of the measurer, and their relative accuracy must be validated against a "gold-standard" measure of adiposity. Such indirect methods of

www.pediatrics.org/cgi/doi/10.1542/peds.2006-0472

doi:10.1542/peds.2006-0472

All policy statements from the American Academy of Pediatrics automatically expire 5 years after publication unless reaffirmed, revised, or retired at or before that time.

Key Words
healthy living, physical activity, obesity, overweight, advocacy, children, youth

Abbreviations
PE—physical education
AAP—American Academy of Pediatrics

PEDIATRICS (ISSN Numbers: Print, 0031-4005; Online, 1098-4275). Copyright © 2006 by the American Academy of Pediatrics

estimating body composition include measuring weight and weight for height, body mass index (BMI), waist circumference, skinfold thickness, and ponderal index.[11] Of these, perhaps the most convenient is BMI, which can be calculated according to the following formulas (www.cdc.gov/growthcharts):

$$BMI = weight\ (kg)/(height)\ (m^2)\ or$$

$$BMI = weight\ (kg)/height\ (cm)/height\ (cm) \times 10\,000$$

$$BMI = weight\ (lb)/height\ (in)/height\ (in) \times 703$$

BMI varies with age and gender. It typically increases during the first months of life, decreases after the first year, and increases again around 6 years of age.[11] A specific BMI value, therefore, should be evaluated against age- and gender-specific reference values. In the United States, such reference charts based on early 1970s survey data of children 2 to 20 years of age are readily available for clinical use.[12] Children and youth with a BMI greater than the 95th percentile are classified as overweight or obese, and those between the 85th and 95th percentiles are designated at risk of overweight.[13] Although BMI tends to underestimate overweight in tall individuals and overestimate overweight in short individuals and those with high lean body mass (ie, athletes), it generally correlates well with more precise measures of adiposity in individuals with BMI in the 95th percentile or greater.[14]

Factors Contributing to Obesity

Some children have medical conditions associated with obesity and/or require pharmacologic treatments resulting in significant weight gain. Others (1%–2% of obese children) have underlying genetic conditions such as Down, Prader-Willi, or Bardet-Biedle syndrome, which can be associated with obesity. Rarely, single-gene disorders, including congenital leptin deficiency and defects in the melanocortin 4 receptor, cause morbid childhood obesity.

Observations in twin, sibling, and family studies suggest that children are more likely to be overweight if relatives are similarly affected and that heritability may play a role in as many as 25% to 85% of cases. However, to suggest that only genetic factors have caused the recent global epidemic of childhood obesity would not be realistic. It is more likely that most of the world's population carries a combination of genes that may have evolved to cope with food scarcity. In obesogenic environments in which calorie-dense foods are readily available and low-energy expenditure is commonplace, this genetic predisposition would be maladaptive and could lead to an obese population.[11]

Nutritional factors contributing to the increase in obesity rates include, in no particular order, (1) insufficient infant breastfeeding, (2) a reduction in cereal fiber, fruit,

and vegetable intake by children and youth, and (3) the excessive consumption of oversized fast foods and soda, which are encouraged by fast-food advertising during children's television programming and a greater availability of fast foods and sugar-containing beverages in school vending machines.[15,16] Although nutritional issues have a significant role to play, this statement focuses on factors associated with decreased energy expenditure, namely excessive sedentary behaviors and lack of adequate physical activity.

Children and youth are more sedentary than ever with the widespread availability of television, videos, computers, and video games. Data from the 1988–1994 National Health and Nutrition Examination Survey indicated that 26% of American children (up to 33% of Mexican American and 43% of non-Hispanic black children) watched at least 4 hours of television per day, and these children were less likely to participate in vigorous physical activity. They also had greater BMIs and skinfold measurements than those who watched <2 hours of television per day.[17]

Not only are the rates of sedentary activities rising, but participation in physical activity is not optimal. In a 2002 Youth Media Campaign Longitudinal Survey, 4500 children 9 to 13 years of age and their parents were polled about physical activity levels outside of school hours. The report indicated that 61.5% of 9- to 13-year-olds did not participate in any organized physical activities and 22.6% did not partake in nonorganized physical activity during nonschool hours.[18]

Youth at Risk of Decreased Physical Activity

Particular individuals at increased risk of having low levels of physical activity have been identified and include children who are from ethnic minorities (especially girls) in the preadolescent/adolescent age groups, children living in poverty, children with disabilities, children residing in apartments or public housing, and children living in neighborhoods where outdoor physical activity is restricted by climate, safety concerns, or lack of facilities.[19,20] According to the Centers for Disease Control and Prevention (www.cdc.gov/nccdphp/sgr/adoles.htm), inactivity is twice as common among females (14%) as males (7%) and among black females (21%) as white females (12%). In a meta-analysis that evaluated physical activity and cardiorespiratory fitness, 6- to 7-year-olds were more active in moderate to vigorous physical activity (46 minutes/day) compared with 10- to 16-year-olds (16–45 minutes/day). Boys were approximately 20% more active than girls, and mean activity levels decreased with age by 2.7% per year in boys compared with 7.4% per year in girls.[21] Many reasons are stated for the general lack of physical activity among children and youth. These reasons include inactive role models (eg, parents and other caregivers), competing demands/time pressures, unsafe environments, lack of recreation facilities or insufficient funds to begin recreation programs, and inadequate access to quality daily physical education (PE).

Physical Activity in Schools

Children and youth spend most of their waking hours at school, so the availability of regular physical activity in that setting is critical. Although the *Healthy People 2010* report recommends increasing the amount of daily PE for all students in a larger proportion of US schools, such changes do not seem to be forthcoming.[19] In 2000, a school health policies and program study[22] looked at a nationally representative sample of private and public schools and found that only 8% of American elementary schools, 6.4% of middle schools, and 5.8% of high schools with existing PE requirements provided daily PE classes for all grades for the entire year. In addition, although approximately 80% of states have policies calling for students to participate in PE in all schools, 40% of elementary schools, 52% of middle schools, and 60% of high schools allow exemption from PE classes, particularly for students with permanent physical disabilities and those having religious reasons.[22] The National Association of State Boards of Education recommends 150 minutes per week of PE for elementary students and 225 minutes per week for middle and high school students.[23] Unfortunately, these requirements are not being implemented. In a study of 814 third-grade students from 10 different US data-collection sites, the mean duration of PE was 33 minutes twice a week, with only 25 minutes per week at a moderate to vigorous intensity level.[24] In addition, 1991–2003 Youth Risk Behavior Surveillance data showed that although the percentage of high school students enrolled in PE class remained constant (48.9%–55.7%), the percentage of students with daily PE attendance decreased from 41.6% in 1991 to 25.4% in 1995 and remained stable thereafter (25.4%–28.4%).[25]

Management of the Obese Child

The successful treatment of obesity in the pediatric age group has been somewhat obscure to date. Studies have shown that younger children seem to respond better to treatment than adolescents and adults.[11,26] Reasons given for this include greater motivation, more influence of the family on behavioral change, and the ability to take advantage of longitudinal growth, which allows children to "grow into their weight." Treatment programs that include nutritional intervention in combination with exercise have higher success rates than diet modification alone. Indeed, a research program that included dietary modification, exercise, and family-based behavioral modification demonstrated enhanced weight loss and better maintenance of lost weight over 5 years.[27] Successful activity-related interventions include a reduction in sedentary behavior and an increase in energy expenditure. Improvements in BMI have been shown to occur

when television viewing is restricted.[28] In this regard, the American Academy of Pediatrics (AAP) recommends no more than 2 hours of quality television programming per day for children older than 2 years.[29] Lifestyle-related physical activity, as opposed to calisthenics or programmed aerobic exercise, seems to be more important for sustained weight loss.[30] Such treatment programs should be individually tailored to each child, and their success should be measured not just in terms of weight loss but also in terms of the effects of the programs on associated morbidities.

Health Benefits of Physical Activity

Regular physical activity is important in weight reduction and improving insulin sensitivity in youth with type 2 diabetes.[31] Aerobic exercise has been shown in a prospective randomized, controlled study of 64 children (9–11 years old) with hypertension to reduce systolic and diastolic blood pressure over 8 months.[32] Resistance training (eg, weight lifting) after aerobic exercise seems to prevent the return of blood pressure to preintervention levels in hypertensive adolescents.[33] Weight loss through moderate aerobic exercise has been shown to reduce the hyperinsulinemia, hepatomegaly, and liver enzyme elevation seen in patients with steatohepatitis.[6,34] Regular physical activity is also beneficial psychologically for all youth regardless of weight. It is associated with an increase in self-esteem and self-concept and a decrease in anxiety and depression.[35]

Prevention of Overweight in Children and Youth

Given the challenges of reversing existing obesity in the pediatric population, preventive tactics are likely to be the key to success. Unfortunately, controlled prevention trials have been somewhat disappointing to date. In a systematic Cochrane Database review,[36] 3 of 4 long-term studies combining dietary education with physical activity showed no difference in overweight, and 1 long-term physical activity intervention study showed a slight reduction in overweight. However, the randomized control design may not be ideal for the study of most health-promotion interventions. This is because these are typically population-based programs, which tend to be complex, are delivered over long periods of time, and present some difficulties in controlling all variables.[11] Solution-oriented research, which evaluates promising interventions, often in a quasi-experimental manner, may be more appropriate in the long run.[37] It is unlikely, however, that any single strategy will be sufficient to reverse current trends in pediatric obesity. Success is more likely to be achieved by the implementation of sustainable, economically viable, culturally acceptable active-living policies that can be integrated into multiple sectors of society.

Increasing Physical Activity Levels in Children and Youth

Physical activity needs to be promoted at home, in the community, and at school, but school is perhaps the most encompassing way for all children to benefit. As of June 2005, there is a new opportunity for pediatricians to get involved with school districts. Section 204 of the Child Nutrition and WIC [Supplemental Nutrition Program for Women, Infants, and Children] Reauthorization Act of 2004 (Public Law 108–265) requires that every school receiving funding through the National School Lunch and/or Breakfast Program develop a local wellness policy that promotes the health of students, with a particular emphasis on addressing the problem of childhood obesity. By the 2006–2007 school year, each school or school district is required to set goals for healthy nutrition, physical activity, and other strategies to promote student wellness. Parents, students, school personnel, and members of the community are required to be involved in the policy development. Pediatricians can take advantage of this requirement to get involved. In light of the school wellness policy, many schools are looking to modify their present PE programs to improve their physical activity standards.

In past years, PE classes used calisthenics and sport-specific skill acquisition to promote fitness. This approach did not meet the needs of all students, such as those with obesity or physical disabilities. PE curricula and instruction should emphasize the knowledge, attitudes, and motor and behavioral skills required to adopt and maintain lifelong habits of physical activity.[38] Cross-sectional school-based studies have shown modest correlation between physical activity and lower BMI, although long-term follow-up data are lacking. In an observational study of 9751 kindergarten students, an increase in PE instruction time was associated with a significant reduction in BMI among overweight girls.[39] Project SPARK (Sports, Play, and Active Recreation for Kids Curriculum) looked at increasing physical activity through modified PE and classroom-based teaching on health and skill fitness. Physical activity levels increased during PE classes, and fitness levels in girls improved as a result.[40] It is interesting to note that, despite a significant increase in PE class time, there was no interference with academic attainment, and some achievement test results improved. A recent review of the literature suggests that school-based physical activity programs may modestly enhance academic performance in the short-term, but additional research is required to establish any long-term improvements. There does not seem to be sufficient evidence to suggest that daily physical activity detracts from academic success.[41]

An increase in school PE participation alone is not likely to be sufficient to reverse the childhood obesity epidemic. A 2-year study of elementary students showed that those who had enhanced physical activity education as well as modified PE classes to increase lifestyle aerobic activity increased their physical activity inside the classroom, but lower levels were noted outside the classroom in their leisure time, and no improvements on fitness testing or body fat percentage were seen.[42] The PLAY (Promoting Lifestyle Activity for Youth) program, which encourages the accumulation of 30 to 60 minutes of moderate to vigorous physical activity daily beyond school time and during regular school hours outside of PE classes, has been shown to increase the physical activity levels of children, especially girls.[43] Children can increase their physical activity levels in many other ways during school and nonschool hours, including active transportation, unorganized outdoor free play, personal fitness and recreational activities, and organized sports. Parents of children in organized sports should be encouraged to stimulate their children to be physically active on days when they are not participating in these sports and not rely solely on the sports to provide all their away-from-school physical activity. This should include participation in physical activities with the entire family. Communities designed with green spaces and biking trails help provide families the means to enjoy such active lifestyles.

During late childhood and adolescence, strength training may be additionally beneficial. Youth taking part in this type of exercise may gain strength, improve sport performance, and derive long-term health benefits.[44] Obese children often prefer strength training because it does not require agility or aerobic ability, and the benefits become apparent within as little as 2 to 3 weeks. Because of their added body mass, overweight participants also tend to be stronger than their peers, giving them a relative psychological advantage. Recent studies have shown that obese students are more compliant and increase their free fat mass when weight training is added to aerobic exercise or a standardized energy-reduction diet.[45,46]

Recommended physical activity levels for children and youth vary somewhat in different countries. The Centers for Disease Control and Prevention and the United Kingdom Health Education Authority recommend that children and youth accumulate at least 60 minutes daily of moderate to vigorous physical activity in a variety of enjoyable individual and group activities.[47,48] Health Canada guidelines recommend increasing physical activity above the current level by at least 30 minutes (10 minutes vigorous) and reducing sedentary activity by the same amount per day. Each month, physical activity should be increased and sedentary behavior should be decreased by 15 minutes until at least 90 minutes more active time and 90 minutes less inactive time are accumulated (www.paguide.com). The Canadian Paediatric Society has endorsed these recommendations and emphasizes a wide variety of activities as part of recreation, transportation, chores, work, and planned exercise to encourage lifestyle changes that may last a lifetime.[49]

Age-Appropriate Recommendations for Physical Activity

Clinicians should encourage parents to limit sedentary activity and make physical activity and sport recommendations to parents and caregivers that are consistent with the developmental level of the child.[50] The following are guidelines from the AAP for different age groups.

Infants and Toddlers

There is insufficient evidence to recommend exercise programs or classes for infants and toddlers as a means of promoting increased physical activity or preventing obesity in later years. The AAP has recommended that children younger than 2 years not watch any television. The AAP suggests that parents be encouraged to provide a safe, nurturing, and minimally structured play environment for their infant.[51] Infants and toddlers should also be allowed to develop enjoyment of outdoor physical activity and unstructured exploration under the supervision of a responsible adult caregiver. Such activities include walking in the neighborhood, unorganized free play outdoors, and walking through a park or zoo.

Preschool-Aged Children (4–6 Years)

Free play should be encouraged with emphasis on fun, playfulness, exploration, and experimentation while being mindful of safety and proper supervision. Preschool-aged children should take part in unorganized play, preferably on flat surfaces with few variables and instruction limited to a show-and-tell format. Appropriate activities might include running, swimming, tumbling, throwing, and catching. Preschoolers should also begin walking tolerable distances with family members. In addition, parents should reduce sedentary transportation by car and stroller and, as applies to all age groups, limit screen time to <2 hours per day.

Elementary School-Aged Children (6–9 Years)

In this age group, children improve their motor skills, visual tracking, and balance. Parents should continue to encourage free play involving more sophisticated movement patterns with emphasis on fundamental skill acquisition. These children should be encouraged to walk, dance, or jump rope and may enjoy playing miniature golf. There is little difference between the sexes in weight, height, endurance, and motor skill development at this age; thus, co-ed participation is not contraindicated. Organized sports (soccer, baseball) may be initiated, but they should have flexible rules and short instruction time, allow free time in practices, and focus on enjoyment rather than competition. These children have a limited ability to learn team strategy.

Middle School-Aged Children (10–12 Years)

Preferred physical activities that focus on enjoyment with family members and friends should be encouraged as with previous groups. Emphasis on skill development and increasing focus on tactics and strategy as well as factors promoting continued participation are needed. Fully developed visual tracking, balance, and motor skills are typical in late childhood. Middle school–aged children are better able to process verbal instruction and integrate information from multiple sources so that participation in complex sports (football, basketball, ice hockey) is more feasible. Puberty may begin at different rates, making some individuals bigger and stronger than others. Basing placement in contact and collision sports on maturity rather than chronologic age may result in less risk of injury and enhanced chance of success, especially for those at lower Tanner stages. Weight training may be initiated, provided that the program is well supervised, that small free weights are used with high repetitions (15–20), that proper technique is demonstrated, and that shorter sets using heavier weights and maximum lifts (squat lifts, clean and jerk, dead lifts) are avoided.[44]

Adolescents

Adolescents are highly social and influenced by their peers. Identifying activities that are of interest to the adolescent, especially those that are fun and include friends, is crucial for long-term participation. Physical activities may include personal fitness preferences (eg, dance, yoga, running), active transportation (walking, cycling), household chores, and competitive and noncompetitive sports. Ideally, enrollment in competitive contact and collision sports should be based on size and ability instead of chronologic age. Weight training may continue, and as the individual reaches physical maturity (Tanner stage 5), longer sets using heavier weights and fewer repetitions may be safely pursued while continuing to stress the importance of proper technique.

Office-Based Physical Activity Assessment

An accurate assessment of an individual child's physical activity level by history or questionnaire is difficult and fraught with methodologic problems. It may be easier for parents to recall the number of times per week their child plays outside for at least 30 minutes than to estimate the average daily minutes spent in physical activity. In addition, asking parents about the number of hours per day their child spends in front of a television, video game, or computer screen may be simpler to quantify and track than time spent in active play. Pedometers may also be helpful, because they provide a simple and more objective method of measuring activity, are inexpensive, and have a "gadget appeal" among youngsters. It has been recommend that adults accumulate 10 000 steps per day to follow a healthy lifestyle.[52] Requirements are less clearly defined in children, but guidelines range from 11 000 to 12 000 steps per day for girls and 13 000 to 15 000 steps per day for boys.[53,54]

CONCLUSIONS

The prevalence of pediatric obesity has reached epidemic proportions. It is unlikely that the medical profession alone will be able to solve this serious health problem. The promotion of decreased caloric intake and increased energy expenditure will need to take place within all aspects of society. Among the most difficult but most important challenges for society are making exercise alternatives as attractive, exciting, and enjoyable as video games for children, convincing school boards that PE and other school-based physical activity opportunities are as important to long-term productivity as are academics, changing both supplier and consumer attitudes about food selection and portion sizes, and reengineering living environments to promote physical activity.

RECOMMENDATIONS

Research has shown the importance of social, physical, and cultural environments in determining the extent to which people are able to be active in all facets of daily life, including work, education, family life, and leisure.[55] Creating active school communities is an ideal way to ensure that children and youth adopt active, healthy lifestyles. These communities require a collaborative framework between families, schools, community recreation leaders, and health care professionals. Physicians can be instrumental in the development of active school communities by advocating for policy changes at the community, state, and national levels that support healthy nutrition, reducing sedentary time, and increasing physical activity levels while providing education and health supervision about regular physical activity and reduced sedentary time to families in their practices.

ADVOCACY

In addition to promoting healthy nutrition recommendations suggested by the AAP Committee on Nutrition, physicians and health care professionals and their national organizations should advocate for:

- Social marketing that promotes increased physical activity.

- The appropriate allocation of funding for quality research in the prevention of childhood obesity.

- The development and implementation of a school wellness counsel on which local physician representation is encouraged.

- A school curriculum that teaches children and youth the health benefits of regular physical activity.

- Comprehensive community sport and recreation programs that allow for community and school facilities to be open after hours and make physical activities available to all children and youth at reasonable costs; access to recreation facilities should be equally available to both sexes.

- The reinstatement of compulsory, quality, daily PE classes in all schools (kindergarten through grade 12) taught by qualified, trained educators. The curricula should emphasize enjoyable participation in physical activity that helps students develop the knowledge, attitudes, motor skills, behavioral skills, and confidence required to adopt and maintain healthy active lifestyles. These classes should allow participation by all children regardless of ability, illness, injury, and developmental disability, including those with obesity and those who are disinterested in traditional competitive team sports. Commitment of adequate resources for program funding, trained PE personnel, safe equipment, and facilities is also recommended.

- The provision of a variety of physical activity opportunities in addition to PE, including the protection of children's recess time and the requirement of extracurricular physical activity programs and nonstructured physical activity before, during, and after school hours, that address the needs and interests of all students.

- The reduction of environmental barriers to an active lifestyle through the construction of safe recreational facilities, parks, playgrounds, bicycle paths, sidewalks, and crosswalks.

PROMOTING A HEALTHY LIFESTYLE

Physicians and health care professionals should promote active healthy living within each family unit by:

- Serving as role models through the adoption of an active lifestyle.

- Inquiring about nutritional intake, calculating and plotting BMI, identifying obesity-related comorbidities, and promoting healthy eating as suggested by the AAP Committee on Nutrition.

- Documenting the number of hours per day spent on sedentary activities and limiting screen (television, video game, and computer) time according to AAP guidelines.

- Determining physical activity levels of the child and family members at regular health care visits.

- Tabulating the amount of physical activity the child or youth does each day at home, school, or child care as part of transportation, work, recreation, and unorganized sports, which should include determining the actual minutes of PE and recess-related physical activity achieved at school each week. In addition, the number of times per week spent in outdoor play for at least 30 minutes and/or the number of daily steps achieved (monitored by using a pedometer) should be documented. Specific involvement in organized sports and dance also should be noted.

- Encouraging children and adolescents to be physically active for at least 60 minutes per day, which does not need to be acquired in a continuous fashion but rather may be accumulated by using smaller increments. Events should be of moderate intensity and include a wide variety of activities as part of sports, recreation, transportation, chores, work, planned exercise, and school-based PE classes. These activities should be primarily unstructured and fun if they are to achieve best compliance.

- Identifying any barriers the child, youth, or parent might have against increasing physical activity, which might include lack of time, competing interests, perceived lack of motor skills, and fear of injury on the part of the child. Parents might be additionally concerned about financial and safety issues. Efforts must then be made to work with the family to educate them regarding the importance of lifelong physical activity and to identify potential strategies to overcome some of their barriers.

- Recommending that parents become good role models by increasing their own level of physical activity. Parents should also incorporate physical activities that family members of all ages and abilities can do together. They should encourage children to play outside as much as possible. Safety should be promoted by the use of appropriate protective equipment (bicycle helmets, life jackets, etc).

- Advising parents to support their children and youth in developmentally and age-appropriate sports and recreational activities. The child's favorite types of physical activity should be a priority. These might best occur in the school setting during extracurricular activities, in which parents/grandparents can take part as leaders and coaches.

- Suggesting that overweight children partake in activities that take advantage of their tall stature and muscle strength, such as water-based sports and strength training, rather than those that require weight bearing (eg, jumping, jogging).

- Recommending that parents of overweight children and youth play a supporting, accepting, and encouraging role in returning them to healthier lifestyles to increase self-esteem.

- Encouraging youth to promote physical activities for their peers and become role models and leaders for younger students.

REFERENCES

1. World Health Organization. *Obesity: Preventing and Managing the Global Epidemic. Report of a WHO Consultation on Obesity, 3–5 June 1997, Geneva.* Geneva, Switzerland: World Health Organization; 2001. WHO/NUT/NCD 98.1
2. Ogden CL, Carroll MD, Flegal KM. Epidemiologic trends in overweight and obesity. *Endocrinol Metab Clin North Am.* 2003; 32:741–760, vii

3. Rosenbloom AL. Increasing incidence of type 2 diabetes in children and adolescents: treatment considerations. *Paediatr Drugs*. 2002;4:209–221

4. Sorof JM, Lai D, Turner J, Poffenbarger T, Portman RJ. Overweight, ethnicity, and the prevalence of hypertension in school-aged children. *Pediatrics*. 2004;113:475–482

5. Wing YK, Hui SH, Pak WM, et al. A controlled study of sleep related disordered breathing in obese children. *Arch Dis Child*. 2003;88:1043–1047

6. Rashid M, Roberts EA. Nonalcoholic steatohepatitis in children. *J Pediatr Gastroenterol Nutr*. 2000;30:48–53

7. Schwimmer JB, Burwinkle TM, Varni JW. Health-related quality of life of severely obese children and adolescents. *JAMA*. 2003;289:1813–1819

8. Whitaker RC, Wright JA, Pepe MS, Seidel KD, Dietz WH. Predicting obesity in young adulthood from childhood and parental obesity. *N Engl J Med*. 1997;337:869–873

9. Guo SS, Chumlea WC. Tracking of body mass index in children in relation to overweight in adulthood. *Am J Clin Nutr*. 1999;70(1 pt 2):145S–148S

10. Belay B, Belamarich P, Racine AD. Pediatric precursors of adult atherosclerosis. *Pediatr Rev*. 2004;25:4–16

11. Lobstein T, Baur L, Uauy R. Obesity in children and young people: a crisis in public health. *Obesity Rev*. 2004;5(suppl 1):4–104

12. Kuczmarski RJ, Ogden CL, Grummer-Strawn LM, et al. CDC growth charts: United States. *Adv Data*. 2000;(314):1–28

13. Himes JH, Dietz WH. Guidelines for overweight in adolescent preventive services: recommendations from an expert committee. The Expert Committee on Clinical Guidelines for Overweight in Adolescent Preventive Services. *Am J Clin Nutr*. 1994;59:307–316

14. Sardinha LB, Going SB, Teixeira PJ, Lohman TG. Receiver operating characteristic analysis of body mass index, triceps skinfold thickness, and arm girth for obesity screening in children and adolescents. *Am J Clin Nutr*. 1999;70:1090–1095

15. Krebs NF, Jacobson MS; American Academy of Pediatrics, Committee on Nutrition. Prevention of pediatric overweight and obesity. *Pediatrics*. 2003;112:424–430

16. American Academy of Pediatrics, Committee on School Health. Soft drinks in schools. *Pediatrics*. 2004;113:152–154

17. Andersen RE, Crespo CJ, Bartlett SJ, Cheskin LJ, Pratt M. Relationship of physical activity and television watching with body weight and level of fatness among children: results from the Third National Health and Nutrition Examination Survey. *JAMA*. 1998;279:938–942

18. Centers for Disease Control and Prevention. Physical activity levels among children aged 9–13 years: United States, 2002. *MMWR Morb Mortal Wkly Rep*. 2003;52:785–788

19. US Department of Health and Human Services. *Healthy People 2010: Understanding and Improving Health*. 2nd ed. Washington, DC: US Department of Health and Human Services; 2001

20. Raine KD. *Overweights and Obesity in Canada: A Population Health Perspective*. Ottawa, Ontario, Canada: Canadian Institute for Health Information; 2004. Available at: http://secure.cihi.ca/cihiweb/products/CPHIOverweightandObesityAugust2004_e.pdf. Accessed March 30, 2005

21. Sallis JF. Epidemiology of physical activity and fitness in children and adolescents. *Crit Rev Food Sci Nutr*. 1993;33:403–408

22. Burgeson CR, Wechsler H, Brener ND, Young JC, Spain CG. Physical education and activity: results from the School Health Policies and Programs Study 2000. *J Sch Health*. 2001;71:279–293

23. National Association of State Boards of Education. *Fit, Healthy, and Ready to Learn: A School Health Policy Guide*. Alexandria, VA: National Association of State Boards of Education; 2000

24. Nader PR. Frequency and intensity of activity of third-grade children in physical education. National Institute of Child Health and Human Development Study of Early Child Care and Youth Development Network. *Arch Pediatr Adolesc Med*. 2003;157:185–190

25. Grunbaum JA, Kann L, Kinchen S, et al. Youth risk behavior surveillance: United States, 2003 [published corrections appear in *MMWR Morb Mortal Wkly Rep*. 2004;53(24):536 and *MMWR Morb Mortal Wkly Rep*. 2005;54(24):608]. *MMWR Surveill Summ*. 2004;53(2):1–96

26. Summerbell CD, Ashton V, Campbell KJ, Edmonds L, Kelly S, Waters E. Interventions for treating obesity in children. *Cochrane Database Syst Rev*. 2003;(3):CD001872

27. Epstein LH. Methodological issues and ten-year outcomes for obese children. *Ann N Y Acad Sci*. 1993;699:237–249

28. Robinson TN. Reducing children's television viewing to prevent obesity: a randomized controlled trial. *JAMA*. 1999;282:1561–1567

29. American Academy of Pediatrics, Committee on Public Education. Children, adolescents, and television. *Pediatrics*. 2001;107:423–426

30. Epstein LH, Wing RR, Koeske R, Valoski A. A comparison of lifestyle exercise, aerobic exercise, and calisthenics on weight loss in obese children. *Behav Ther*. 1985;16:345–356

31. American Diabetes Association. Type 2 diabetes in children and adolescents. *Pediatrics*. 2000;105:671–680

32. Hansen HS, Froberg K, Hyldebrandt N, Nielsen JR. A controlled study of eight months of physical training and reduction of blood pressure in children: the Odense schoolchild study. *BMJ*. 1991;303:682–685

33. Hagberg JM, Ehsani AA, Goldring D, Hernandez A, Sinacore DR, Holloszy JO. Effect of weight training on blood pressure and hemodynamics in hypertensive adolescents. *J Pediatr*. 1984;104:147–151

34. Roberts EA. Nonalcoholic steatohepatitis in children. *Curr Gastroenterol Rep*. 2003;5:253–259

35. Calfas KJ, Taylor WC. Effects of physical activity on psychological variables in adolescents. *Pediatr Exerc Sci*. 1994;6:406–423

36. Campbell K, Waters E, O'Meara S, Kelly S, Summerbell C. Interventions for preventing obesity in children. *Cochrane Database Syst Rev*. 2002;(2):CD001871

37. Robinson TN, Sirard JR. Preventing childhood obesity: a solution-oriented research paradigm. *Am J Prev Med*. 2005;28(2 suppl 2):194–201

38. Centers for Disease Control and Prevention. Youth risk behavior surveillance: National College Health Risk Behavior Survey—United States, 1995. *MMWR CDC Surveill Summ*. 1997;46(6):1–56

39. Datar A, Sturm R. Physical education in elementary school and body mass index: evidence from the Early Childhood Longitudinal Study. *Am J Public Health*. 2004;94:1501–1506

40. Sallis JF, McKenzie TL, Kolody B, Lewis M, Marshall S, Rosengard P. Effects of health-related physical education on academic achievement: project SPARK. *Res Q Exerc Sport*. 1999;70:127–134

41. Taras H. Physical activity and student performance at school. *J Sch Health*. 2005;75:214–218

42. Donnelly JE, Jacobsen DJ, Whatley JE, et al. Nutrition and physical activity program to attenuate obesity and promote physical and metabolic fitness in elementary school children. *Obes Res*. 1996;4:229–243

43. Pangrazi RP, Beighle A, Vehige T, Vack C. Impact of Promoting Lifestyle Activity for Youth (PLAY) on children's physical activity. *J Sch Health*. 2003;73:317–321

44. Bernhardt DT, Gomez J, Johnson MD, et al. Strength training by children and adolescents. *Pediatrics*. 2001;107:1470–1472

45. Sothern MS, Loftin JM, Udall JN, et al. Safety, feasibility, and

efficacy of a resistance training program in preadolescent obese children. *Am J Med Sci.* 2000;319:370–375

46. Schwingshandl J, Sudi K, Eibl B, Wallner S, Borkenstein M. Effect of an individualised training programme during weight reduction on body composition: a randomised trial. *Arch Dis Child.* 1999;81:426–428

47. Strong WB, Malina RM, Blimkie CJ, et al. Evidence based physical activity for school-age youth. *J Pediatr.* 2005;146:732–737

48. Biddle S, Sallis J, Cavill N. Policy framework for young people and health-enhancing physical activity. In: Biddle S, Sallis J, Cavill N, eds. *Young and Active: Young People and Physical Activity.* London, England: Health Education Authority; 1998:3–16

49. Canadian Paediatric Society, Healthy Active Living Committee. Healthy active living for children and youth. *Paediatr Child Health.* 2002;7:339–345

50. Harris SS. Readiness to participate in sports. In: Sullivan JA, Anderson SJ, eds. *Care of the Young Athlete.* Rosemont, IL:

American Academy of Orthopaedic Surgeons/American Academy of Pediatrics; 2000:19–24

51. American Academy of Pediatrics, Committee on Sports Medicine and Fitness. Infant exercise programs. *Pediatrics.* 1988;82:800

52. Hatano Y. Use of the pedometer for promoting daily walking exercise. *Int Council Health Phys Ed Rec.* 1993;29:4–8

53. Vincent SD, Pangrazi RP. An examination of the activity patterns of elementary school children. *Pediatr Exerc Sci.* 2002;14:432–441

54. Tudor-Locke C, Pangrazi RP, Corbin CB, et al. BMI-referenced standards for recommended pedometer-determined steps/day in children. *Prev Med.* 2004;38:857–864

55. Health Canada, Population and Public Health Branch, Policy Directorate. *The Population Health Template: Key Elements and Actions That Define a Population Health Approach.* Ottawa, Ontario, Canada: Health Canada; 2001

AMERICAN ACADEMY OF PEDIATRICS

Committee on Sports Medicine and Fitness

Athletic Participation by Children and Adolescents Who Have Systemic Hypertension

ABSTRACT. Children and adolescents who have systemic hypertension may be at risk for complications when exercise causes their blood pressures to rise even higher. The purpose of this statement is to make recommendations concerning the athletic participation of individuals with hypertension using the 26th Bethesda Conference on heart disease and athletic participation and of the Second Task Force on Blood Pressure Control in Children as a basis.

Hypertension is the most common cardiovascular condition seen in people who engage in competitive athletics.[1] Recently, the National Institutes of Health convened the 26th Bethesda Conference to make recommendations concerning the participation of athletes who have heart disease. One of the panels considered hypertension.[1] In 1987, the Second Task Force on Blood Pressure Control in Children also briefly addressed exercise for hypertensive youth.[2] This policy statement summarizes the recommendations of these two groups of experts and makes these guidelines more available to pediatricians.

Table 1 presents the classification of hypertension of the Second Task Force[2] and includes some values from the 26th Bethesda Conference.[1] All values given in the table apply to patients who are not taking antihypertensive drugs and who are not acutely ill. When the systolic and diastolic blood pressures fall into different categories, the higher category should be selected to classify the patient's blood pressure status.

Care must be taken to obtain reliable blood pressure recordings.[1,2] Some athletes have exceedingly large biceps or triceps, and others have long extremities. The width of the blood pressure bladder must be adequate to cover at least 66%[1] or 75%[2] of the individual's upper arm measured between the top of the shoulder and the olecranon and should be of adequate length to encircle the arm completely,[2] which may require the use of a thigh cuff. The athlete should be seated, at rest, and the arm should be supported at heart level.[2] Only after several elevated readings are obtained on separate occasions should the diagnosis of systemic hypertension be made. Further details concerning the measurement of blood pressure are available.[1,2]

Once the diagnosis of systemic hypertension is confirmed, an evaluation including a history, thorough physical examination, and appropriate laboratory testing should be performed, as outlined in the report of the Second Task Force on Blood Pressure Control in Children.[2]

Reports of cerebrovascular accidents during maximal exercise have raised concerns that the rise in blood pressure accompanying strenuous activity may cause harm.[1] The following guidelines recommend temporary restriction for those athletes who have severe hypertension, but the available data do not indicate that strenuous dynamic exercise places these athletes at risk of acute complications of hypertension during exercise or of worsening of their baseline blood pressure values.[1] In dynamic exercise, intramuscular force is not greatly increased as muscles lengthen and contract and joints move through their range of motion. There is a sizable increase in systolic blood pressure, a moderate increase in mean arterial pressure, and a fall in diastolic pressure and total peripheral resistance. In static exercise, relatively large intramuscular forces develop without much change in muscle length or joint motion. Systolic, mean arterial, and diastolic blood pressures rise significantly, and total peripheral resistance remains essentially unchanged. It is the acute increase in diastolic pressure that particularly concerns the experts, as well as the possible increases in muscle mass that may elevate resting blood pressure. Although the limited evidence shows no greater risk with highly static exercise[1] (Table 2), experts are more cautious about allowing athletes with severe hypertension to participate in this type of activity.

Most physical activities and sports have both static and dynamic components. Guidelines for restricting participation should be based on the cardiovascular demands of the activity and the demands of the practice, training, and/or preparation for that activity.

The experts from the 26th Bethesda Conference[1] and those from the Second Task Force on Blood Pressure Control in Children[2] agree on temporary restriction of athletes who have severe hypertension. However, the definition of severe hypertension of the 26th Bethesda Conference is more liberal for youth greater than 12 years old than is that of the Second Task Force (Table 1, last column). We recommend the use of the values of the Second Task Force because this group of experts was more pediatric oriented. Since the Second Task Force did not define severe hypertension in youth older than 18 years,

TABLE 1. Classification of Hypertension[2]

Age, y	High Normal, mm Hg*	Significant Hypertension, mm Hg†	Severe Hypertension, mm Hg‡
6–9			
Systolic	111–121	122–129	>129 (129)§
Diastolic	70–77	70–85	>85 (84)
10–12			
Systolic	117–125	126–133	>133 (134)
Diastolic	75–81	82–89	>89 (89)
13–15			
Systolic	124–135	136–143	>143 (149)
Diastolic	77–85	86–91	>91 (94)
16–18			
Systolic	127–141	142–149	>149 (159)
Diastolic	80–91	92–97	>97 (99)
>18			
Systolic	Not given	[140–179]‖	> (179)
Diastolic		[90–109]	> (109)

* 90th to 94th percentile for age, boys and girls combined.[2]
† 95th to 98th percentile for age, boys and girls combined.[2]
‡ 99th percentile for age, boys and girls combined.[2]
§ The values in parentheses are those used for the classification of severe hypertension by the 26th Bethesda Conference on cardiovascular disease and athletic participation.[1] See text for explanation.
‖ Because the Second Task Force did not discuss youth older than 18 years, the values in brackets are those for mild and moderate hypertension given by the 26th Bethesda Conference.[1]

only the values of the 26th Bethesda Conference are given for this age group (Table 1).

RECOMMENDATIONS

The American Academy of Pediatrics recommends:

1. The presence of significant (Table 1) hypertension in the absence of target organ damage or concomitant heart disease should not limit a person's eligibility for competitive athletics. Athletes with significant hypertension should have their blood pressure measured regularly (every 2 months at the physician's office) to monitor the impact of exercise on blood pressure.
2. Youth who have severe (Table 1) hypertension need to be restricted from competitive sports and highly static (isometric) activities (Table 2) until their hypertension is under adequate control and they have no evidence of target organ damage. Since cardiovascular conditioning may be less strenuous than competitive athletics, complete restriction of exercise may not be necessary for those with severe hypertension.
3. When hypertension and other cardiovascular diseases coexist, eligibility for participation in competitive athletics is usually based on the type and severity of the other cardiovascular disease.[1]
4. The young athlete with hypertension, regardless of the degree of severity, should be strongly encouraged to adopt healthy lifestyle behaviors, including the avoidance of exogenous androgens, growth hormone, drugs of abuse (especially cocaine), alcohol, use of tobacco (by all routes), and high sodium intake.[1] In addition, the athlete

TABLE 2. Sports That Have a High Static Component*

Low Dynamic	Moderate Dynamic	High Dynamic
Bobsledding	Body building	Boxing†
Field events (throwing)	Downhill skiing	Canoeing/kayaking
Gymnastics	Wrestling	Cycling
Karate/judo		Decathlon
Luge		Rowing
Sailing		Speeding skating
Rock climbing		
Waterskiing		
Weight lifting		
Windsurfing		

* Adapted from Mitchell et al[3] with permission.
† The American Academy of Pediatrics recommends that youth not participate in boxing.

should be advised that the use of diuretic drugs and β blockers has been prohibited by some athletic governing bodies. In these instances, other types of medication may need to be considered.

ADDENDUM

An update to the 1987 Task Force report on high blood pressure[2] has recently appeared (*Pediatrics.* 1996;98:649–658). It provides new data on the 90th and 95th percentile values for blood pressure categorized by age, sex, and height and mentions new information on the diagnosis, treatment, and prevention of hypertension in youth. It does not address sports participation for hypertensive patients other than to say that hypertension is "usually not" a contraindication. Members of the working group that developed the update indicate that the 1987 report's recommendations concerning severe hypertension still stand (Stephen R. Daniels, Jennifer M. H. Logie, personal communication).

COMMITTEE ON SPORTS MEDICINE AND FITNESS, 1995 TO 1996
William L. Risser, MD, PhD, Chair
Steven J. Anderson, MD
Stephen P. Bolduc, MD
Elizabeth Coryllos, MD
Bernard Griesemer, MD
Larry McLain, MD
Suzanne M. Tanner, MD

LIAISON REPRESENTATIVES
Kathryn Keely, MD
    Canadian Paediatric Society
Richard Malacrea, ATC
    National Athletic Trainers Association
Judith C. Young, PhD
    National Association for Sport and
    Physical Education

AAP SECTION LIAISONS
Reginald L. Washington, MD
    Section on Cardiology
Frederick E. Reed, MD
    Section on Orthopaedics

REFERENCES

1. Kaplan NM, Deveraux RB, Miller HS Jr. Task Force 4: systemic hypertension. *J Am Coll Cardiol.* 1994;24:885–888
2. American Academy of Pediatrics, Task Force on Blood Pressure Control in Children. Report of the Second Task Force on Blood Pressure Control in Children—1987. *Pediatrics.* 1987;79:1–25
3. Mitchell JH, Haskell WL, Raven PB. Classification of sports. *J Am Coll Cardiol.* 1994;24:864–866

AMERICAN ACADEMY OF PEDIATRICS

Committee on Sports Medicine and Fitness

Climatic Heat Stress and the Exercising Child and Adolescent

ABSTRACT. For morphologic and physiologic reasons, exercising children do not adapt as effectively as adults when exposed to a high climatic heat stress. This may affect their performance and well-being, as well as increase the risk for heat-related illness. This policy statement summarizes approaches for the prevention of the detrimental effects of children's activity in hot or humid climates, including the prevention of exercise-induced dehydration.

Heat-induced illness is preventable. Physicians, teachers, coaches, and parents need to be aware of the potential hazards of high-intensity exercise in hot or humid climates and to take measures to prevent heat-related illness in children and adolescents.

Exercising children do not adapt to extremes of temperature as effectively as adults when exposed to a high climatic heat stress.[1] The adaptation of adolescents falls in between. The reasons for these differences include:

1. Children have a greater surface area-to-body mass ratio than adults, which causes a greater heat gain from the environment on a hot day and a greater heat loss to the environment on a cold day.
2. Children produce more metabolic heat per mass unit than adults during physical activities that include walking or running.[2]
3. Sweating capacity is considerably lower in children than in adults,[1,3,4] which reduces the ability of children to dissipate body heat by evaporation.

Exercising children are able to dissipate heat effectively in a neutral or mildly warm climate. However, when air temperature exceeds 35°C (95°F), they have a lower exercise tolerance than do adults. The higher the air temperature, the greater the effect on the child.[4-7] It is important to emphasize that humidity is a major component of heat stress, sometimes even more important than air temperature.

On transition to a warmer climate, exercising persons must allow time to become acclimatized. Intense and prolonged exercise undertaken before acclimatization may be detrimental to the child's physical performance and well-being and may lead to heat-related illness, including heat exhaustion or fatal heat stroke.[8] The rate of acclimatization for children is slower than that of adults.[9] A child will need

as many as 8 to 10 exposures (30 to 45 minutes each) to the new climate to acclimatize sufficiently. Such exposures can be taken at a rate of one per day or one every other day.

Children frequently do not feel the need to drink enough to replenish fluid loss during prolonged exercise. This may lead to severe dehydration.[10,11] Children with mental retardation are at special risk for not recognizing the need to replace the fluid loss. A major consequence of dehydration is an excessive increase in core body temperature. Thus, the dehydrated child is more prone to heat-related illness than the fully hydrated child.[12,13] For a given level of hypohydration, children are subject to a greater increase in core body temperature than are adults.[10] Although water is an easily available drink, a flavored beverage may be preferable because the child may drink more of it.[14,15] Another important way to enhance thirst is by adding sodium chloride (approximately 15 to 20 mmol/L, or 1 g per 2 pints) to the flavored solution. This has been shown to increase voluntary drinking by 90%, compared with unflavored water.[15] The above concentration is found in commercially available sports drinks. Salt tablets should be avoided, because of their high content of sodium chloride.

The likelihood of heat intolerance increases with conditions that are associated with excessive fluid loss (febrile state, gastrointestinal infection, diabetes insipidus, diabetes mellitus), suboptimal sweating (spina bifida, sweating insufficiency syndrome), excessive sweating (selected cyanotic congenital heart defects), diminished thirst (cystic fibrosis),[11,12] inadequate drinking (mental retardation, young children who may not comprehend the importance of drinking), abnormal hypothalamic thermoregulatory function (anorexia nervosa, advanced undernutrition, prior heat-related illness), and obesity.[7,8]

Proper health habits can be learned by children and adolescents. Athletes who may be exposed to hot climates should follow proper guidelines for heat acclimatization, fluid intake, appropriate clothing, and adjustment of activity according to ambient temperature and humidity. High humidity levels, even when air temperature is not excessive, result in high heat stress.

Based on this information, the American Academy of Pediatrics recommends the following for children and adolescents:

1. The intensity of activities that last 15 minutes or more should be reduced whenever relative humidity, solar radiation, and air temperature are above critical levels. For specific recommenda-

TABLE 1. Restraints on Activities at Different Levels of Heat Stress*

WBGT		Restraints on Activities
°C	°F	
<24	<75	All activities allowed, but be alert for prodromes of heat-related illness in prolonged events
24.0–25.9	75.0–78.6	Longer rest periods in the shade; enforce drinking every 15 minutes
26–29	79–84	Stop activity of unacclimatized persons and other persons with high risk; limit activities of all others (disallow long-distance races, cut down further duration of other activities)
>29	>85	Cancel all athletic activities

* From the American Academy of Pediatrics, Committee on Sports Medicine and Fitness.[16] WBGT is *not* air temperature. It indicates wet bulb globe temperature, an index of climatic heat stress that can be measured on the field by the use of a psychrometer. This apparatus, available commercially, is composed of 3 thermometers. One (wet bulb [WB]) has a wet wick around it to monitor humidity. Another is inside a hollow black ball (globe [G]) to monitor radiation. The third is a simple thermometer (temperature [T]) to measure air temperature. The heat stress index is calculated as WBGT = 0.7 WB temp + 0.2 G temp + 0.1 T temp.
It is noteworthy that 70% of the stress is due to humidity, 20% to radiation, and only 10% to air temperature.

tions, see Table 1. One way of increasing rest periods on a hot day is to substitute players frequently.

2. At the beginning of a strenuous exercise program or after traveling to a warmer climate, the intensity and duration of exercise should be limited initially and then gradually increased during a period of 10 to 14 days to accomplish acclimatization to the heat. When such a period is not available, the length of time for participants during practice and competition should be curtailed.

3. Before prolonged physical activity, the child should be well-hydrated. During the activity, periodic drinking should be enforced (eg, each 20 minutes 150 mL [5 oz] of cold tap water or a flavored salted beverage for a child weighing 40 kg (88 lbs) and 250 mL [9 oz] for an adolescent weighing 60 kg (132 lbs)), even if the child does not feel thirsty. Weighing before and after a training session can verify hydration status if the child is weighed wearing little or no clothing.

4. Clothing should be light-colored and lightweight and limited to one layer of absorbent material to facilitate evaporation of sweat. Sweat-saturated garments should be replaced by dry garments. Rubberized sweat suits should never be used to produce loss of weight.

COMMITTEE ON SPORTS MEDICINE AND FITNESS, 1999–2000
Steven J. Anderson, MD, Chairperson
Bernard A. Griesemer, MD
Miriam D. Johnson, MD
Thomas J. Martin, MD
Larry G. McLain, MD
Thomas W. Rowland, MD
Eric Small, MD

LIAISON REPRESENTATIVES
Claire LeBlanc, MD
  Canadian Paediatric Society
Robert Malina, PhD
  Institute for the Study of Youth Sports
Carl Krein, ATc, PT
  National Athletic Trainers Association
Judith C. Young, PhD
  National Association for Sport and Physical Education

SECTION LIAISONS
Frederick E. Reed, MD
  Section on Orthopaedics
Reginald L. Washington, MD
  Section on Cardiology

CONSULTANT
Oded Bar-Or, MD

STAFF
Heather Newland

REFERENCES

1. Bar-Or O. Temperature regulation during exercise in children and adolescents. In: Gisolfi C, Lamb DR, eds. *Perspectives in Exercise Sciences and Sports Medicine, II. Youth, Exercise and Sport.* Indianapolis, IN: Benchmark Press; 1989:335–367

2. Astrand PO. *Experimental Studies of Physical Working Capacity in Relation to Sex and Age.* Copenhagen, Denmark: Munksgaard; 1952

3. Haymes EM, McCormick RJ, Buskirk ER. Heat tolerance of exercising lean and obese prepubertal boys. *J Appl Physiol.* 1975;39:457–461

4. Drinkwater BL, Kupprat IC, Denton JE, et al. Response of prepubertal girls and college women to work in the heat. *J Appl Physiol.* 1977;43:1046–1053

5. Drinkwater BL, Horvath SM. Heat tolerance and aging. *Med Sci Sports Exerc.* 1979;11:49–55

6. Wagner JA, Robinson S, Tzankoff SP, et al. Heat tolerance and acclimatization to work in the heat in relation to age. *J Appl Physiol.* 1972;33:616–622

7. Haymes EM, Buskirk ER, Hodgson JL, et al. Heat tolerance of exercising lean and heavy prepubertal girls. *J Appl Physiol.* 1974;36:566–571

8. Fox EL, Mathews DK, Kaufman WS, et al. Effects of football equipment on thermal balance and energy cost during exercise. *Res Q.* 1966;37:332–339

9. Inbar O. *Acclimatization to Dry and Hot Environment in Young Adults and Children 8–10 Years Old.* New York, NY: Columbia University; 1978. Dissertation

10. Bar-Or O, Dotan R, Inbar O, et al. Voluntary hypohydration in 10- to 12-year-old boys. *J Appl Physiol.* 1980;48:104–108

11. Bar-Or O, Blimkie CJ, Hay JA, et al. Voluntary dehydration and heat tolerance in patients with cystic fibrosis. *Lancet.* 1992;339:696–699

12. Danks DM, Webb DW, Allen J. Heat illness in infants and young children: a study of 47 cases. *Br Med J.* 1962;2:287–293

13. Taj-Eldin S, Falaki N. Heat illness in infants and small children in desert climates. *J Trop Med Hyg.* 1968;71:100–104

14. Meyer F, Bar-Or O, Salsberg A, et al. Hypohydration during exercise in children: effect on thirst, drink preference, and rehydration. *Int J Sport Nutr.* 1994;4:22–35

15. Wilk B, Bar-Or O. Effect of drinking flavor and NaCl on voluntary drinking and rehydration in boys exercising in the heat. *J Appl Physiol.* 1996;80:1112–1117

16. American Academy of Pediatrics, Committee on Sports Medicine and Fitness. *Sports Medicine: Health Care for Young Athletes.* 2nd ed. Elk Grove Village, IL: American Academy of Pediatrics; 1991:98

AMERICAN ACADEMY OF PEDIATRICS

Committee on Sports Medicine and Fitness

Human Immunodeficiency Virus and Other Blood–borne Viral Pathogens in the Athletic Setting

ABSTRACT. Because athletes and the staff of athletic programs can be exposed to blood during athletic activity, they have a very small risk of becoming infected with human immunodeficiency virus, hepatitis B virus, or hepatitis C virus. This statement, which updates a previous position statement of the American Academy of Pediatrics,[1] discusses sports participation for athletes infected with these pathogens and the precautions needed to reduce the risk of infection to others in the athletic setting. Each of the recommendations in this statement is dependent upon and intended to be considered with reference to the other recommendations in this statement and not in isolation.

ABBREVIATIONS. HIV, human immunodeficiency virus; HBV, hepatitis B virus; HCV, hepatitis C virus; CI, 95% confidence interval; AAP, American Academy of Pediatrics; OSHA, Occupational Safety and Health Administration.

During sports participation, the blood of an athlete who is infected with human immunodeficiency virus (HIV), hepatitis B virus (HBV), or hepatitis C virus (HCV) may occasionally contaminate the skin or mucous membranes of other athletes or the staff of athletic programs. Common sense suggests that this likelihood is greatest in contact sports, but transmission can potentially occur indirectly or in noncontact sports. Even in contact sports, the very limited available data indicate that bleeding wounds are not necessarily common.[2]

HIV INFECTION

The risk of HIV infection via skin or mucous membrane exposure to blood or other infectious bodily fluids during sports participation is very low. The most relevant research has been conducted with health care workers, for whom the risk from skin or mucous membrane exposure is less than the risk from parenteral exposure, which is .2% to .3% per exposure (95% confidence interval [CI], .1%–.5%).[3] The risk from exposure to mucous membranes or damaged skin determined from pooling 6 prospective studies was 1 infection in 1007 exposures, or .1% (95% CI, .01%–.5%). Such transmission appears to require, in addition to a portal of entry, prolonged

exposure to large quantities of blood.[3] Transmission through intact skin has not been documented: no HIV infections occurred after 2712 such exposures in 1 large prospective study (95% CI, 0%–.1%).[3] Transmission of HIV in sports has not been documented. One unsubstantiated report describes possible transmission during a collision between professional soccer players.[4]

HBV INFECTION

The HBV is more easily transmitted via exposure to infected blood than is HIV.[3] In 2 studies of health care professionals who had percutaneous exposure to HBV-infected blood, the risk of infection was 27% and 45%; approximately 25% of cases were symptomatic. The risk of infection was greater if the blood was positive for HBV e antigen. The health care workers received immune serum globulin, and so some of them were protected from infection.[5,6] Transmission of infection by contamination of mucous membranes or broken skin with infected blood has been documented, but the magnitude of risk has not been quantified.[3]

Although transmission of HBV is apparently rare in sports, 2 reports document such transmission. An asymptomatic high school sumo wrestler who had a chronic infection transmitted HBV to other members of his team.[7] An epidemic of HBV infection occurred through unknown means among Swedish athletes participating in track finding (orienteering).[8] The epidemiologists concluded that the most likely route of infection was the use of water contaminated with infected blood to clean wounds caused by branches and thorns.

An effective way of preventing HBV transmission in the athletic setting is through immunization of athletes. The American Academy of Pediatrics (AAP) recommends that all children and adolescents be immunized.[9] Clinicians and the staff of athletic programs should aggressively promote immunization.

HCV INFECTION

Although the transmission risks of HCV infection are not completely understood, the risk of infection from percutaneous exposure to infected blood is estimated to be 10 times greater than that of HIV but lower than that of HBV.[3] Transmission via contamination of mucous membranes or broken skin also probably has a risk intermediate between that for blood infected with HIV and HBV.[3]

SUMMARY

Because of the very low probability of transmission of their infection to other athletes, athletes infected with HIV, HBV, or HCV should be allowed to participate in all sports.

CONFIDENTIALITY AND OTHER LEGAL ISSUES

Confidentiality about an athlete's infection with a blood–borne pathogen is necessary to prevent exclusion of the athlete from sports because of inappropriate fear among others in the program. Except for the reporting required by law, the patient (and parent or guardian if the patient is a minor) must give informed consent for clinicians to share information about these medical conditions with a school or sports organization. Testing of athletes for these viral infections is not indicated. Infected athletes should be told that they have a very small risk of infecting other competitors. This risk, although unknown for any sport, is probably greatest in wrestling and boxing. Infected athletes can be encouraged not to participate in these activities or in others in which contamination of skin or mucous membranes with blood is relatively likely. This may also be protective for infected athletes themselves, reducing their possible exposure to blood–borne pathogens other than the one(s) with which they are infected.

The AAP opposes boxing as a sport for youth. Pediatricians should counsel athletes not to participate in this sport, whatever their infection status.

Athletic programs should inform athletes and parents that athletes have a very small but finite risk of contracting a blood–borne infection from another athlete. This is part of the duty to warn about risks of participation that is the responsibility of all athletic programs.

Pediatricians can avoid reporting the presence of infections with blood–borne pathogens by making it clear on the preparticipation form or elsewhere that they support the AAP policy, "Human Immunodeficiency Virus and Other Blood–borne Pathogens in the Athletic Setting," and that the AAP policy acknowledges that the physician should respect the right of infected athletes to confidentiality.

The US Supreme Court has not ruled specifically on the legality of excluding from competition an athlete who has a chronic infection with a blood–borne viral pathogen but has held that a person infected with a contagious disease may be handicapped and therefore entitled to protection from unlawful discrimination. On the basis of this authority, when considering whether an athlete infected with a blood–borne viral pathogen can be excluded from competition, an inquiry would have to be made "based on reasonable medical judgements given the state of medical knowledge" into whether the athlete poses a significant risk of communicating the disease to others in the competition that cannot be eliminated by reasonable accommodation.[10,11]

PREVENTION OF INFECTION

Strict safety precautions are particularly important for those persons in athletic programs who provide first aid and have repeated exposure to blood or other bodily fluids visibly contaminated with blood. Specific precautions are discussed in Recommendation 10 below. Other discussions of safety precautions appropriate for sports programs, with some additional information, are available elsewhere.[10,12–14]

EDUCATION OF ATHLETES

Coaches, athletic trainers, and health care professionals can expand discussions about the risks of transmission of blood–borne viral pathogens during sports participation to teach athletes about how these pathogens are transmitted and how to prevent infection.

RECOMMENDATIONS

1. Athletes infected with HIV, HBV, or HCV should be allowed to participate in all competitive sports.
2. The physician should respect the right of infected athletes to confidentiality. This includes not disclosing the patient's infection status to other participants or the staff of athletic programs.
3. Athletes should not be tested for blood–borne pathogens because they are sports participants.
4. Pediatricians are encouraged to counsel athletes who are infected with HIV, HBV, or HCV that they have a very small risk of infecting other competitors. Infected athletes can consider choosing a sport in which this risk is apparently relatively low. This may be protective for other participants and for infected athletes themselves, reducing their possible exposure to blood–borne pathogens other than the one(s) with which they are infected. Wrestling and boxing, a sport opposed by the AAP, probably have the greatest potential for contamination of injured skin by blood.
5. Athletic programs should inform athletes and their parents that the program is operating under the policies in Recommendations 1 through 3 and that the athletes have a very small risk of becoming infected with a blood–borne pathogen.
6. Clinicians and the staff of athletic programs should aggressively promote HBV immunization among athletes and among coaches, athletic trainers, equipment handlers, laundry personnel, and any other persons at risk of exposure to athletes' blood as an occupational hazard. All athletes should, if possible, receive HBV immunization; >95% of those who receive this immunization will be protected against infection.[9]
7. Each coach and athletic trainer must receive training in first aid and emergency care and in the prevention of transmission of blood–borne pathogens in the athletic setting. These staff members can then help to implement recommendations made here.
8. Coaches and members of the health care team should educate athletes about the precautions described in these recommendations and about the greater risks of transmission of HIV and other blood–borne pathogens through sexual ac-

tivity and needle sharing during the use of illicit drugs, including anabolic steroids. Athletes should be told not to share personal items, such as razors, toothbrushes, and nail clippers that might be contaminated with blood.

9. In some states, depending on state law, schools may need to comply with Occupational Safety and Health Administration (OSHA) regulations[13] for the prevention of transmission of blood–borne pathogens. The athletic program must determine what rules apply. Compliance with OSHA regulations is a reasonable and recommended precaution even if this is not specifically required by the state.

10. The following precautions should be adopted in sports with direct body contact and other sports in which an athlete's blood or other bodily fluids visibly tinged with blood may contaminate the skin or mucous membranes of other participants or staff members of the athletic program. Even if these precautions are adopted, the risk that a participant or staff member may become infected with a blood–borne pathogen in the athletic setting will not be entirely eliminated.

- Athletes must cover existing cuts, abrasions, wounds, or other areas of broken skin with an occlusive dressing before and during participation. Caregivers should cover their own damaged skin to prevent transmission of infection to or from an injured athlete.
- Disposable, water-impervious vinyl or latex gloves should be worn to avoid contact with blood or other bodily fluids visibly tinged with blood and any object such as equipment, bandages, or uniforms contaminated with these fluids. Hands should be cleaned with soap and water or an alcohol-based antiseptic handwash as soon as possible after gloves are removed.
- Athletes with active bleeding should be removed from competition as soon as possible and the bleeding stopped. Wounds should be cleaned with soap and water. Skin antiseptics may be used if soap and water are not available. Wounds must be covered with an occlusive dressing that remains intact during further play before athletes return to competition.
- Athletes should be advised to report injuries and wounds in a timely fashion before or during competition.
- Minor cuts or abrasions that are not bleeding do not require interruption of play but can be cleaned and covered during scheduled breaks. During these breaks, if an athlete's equipment or uniform fabric is wet with blood, the equipment should be cleaned and disinfected (see below), or the uniform should be replaced.
- Equipment and playing areas contaminated with blood must be cleaned until all visible blood is gone and then disinfected with an appropriate germicide such as a freshly-made bleach solution containing 1 part bleach in 10 parts of water. The decontaminated equipment or area should be in contact with the

bleach solution for at least 30 seconds. The area may be wiped with a disposable cloth after the minimum contact time or be allowed to air dry.[9]

- Emergency care must not be delayed because gloves or other protective equipment is not available. If the caregiver does not have the appropriate protective equipment, a towel may be used to cover the wound until an off-the-field location is reached where gloves can be used during more definitive treatment.
- Breathing (Ambu) bags and oral airways should be available for giving resuscitation. Mouth-to-mouth resuscitation is recommended only if this equipment is not available.[12]
- Equipment handlers, laundry personnel, and janitorial staff must be trained in proper procedures for handling washable or disposable materials contaminated with blood.[9, 12]

Committee on Sports Medicine and Fitness, 1999–2000
Steven J. Anderson, MD, Chairperson
Bernard A. Griesemer, MD
Miriam D. Johnson, MD
Thomas J. Martin, MD
Larry G. McLain, MD
Thomas W. Rowland, MD
Eric Small, MD

Liaison Representatives
Claire LeBlanc, MD
  Canadian Paediatric Society
Carl Krein, AT, PT
  National Athletic Trainers Association
Robert Malina, PhD
  Institute for the Study of Youth Sports
Judith C. Young, PhD
  National Association for Sport and Physical Education

Section Liaisons
Frederick E. Reed, MD
  Section on Orthopaedics
Reginald L. Washington, MD
  Section on Cardiology

Consultant
William L. Risser, MD, PhD

REFERENCES

1. American Academy of Pediatrics. Human immunodeficiency virus [acquired immunodeficiency syndrome (AIDS) virus] in the athletic setting. *Pediatrics.* 1991;88:640–641
2. Brown LS Jr, Drotman P, Chu A, Brown CLJ, Knowlan D. Bleeding injuries in professional football: estimating the risk for HIV transmission. *Ann Intern Med.* 1995;122:271–274
3. Gerberding JL. Management of occupational exposures to blood-borne viruses. *N Engl J Med.* 1995;332:444–451
4. Torre D, Sampietro C, Ferraro G, Zeroli C, Speranza F. Transmission of HIV-1 infection via sports injury. *Lancet.* 1990;335:1105
5. Seeff LB, Wright EC, Zimmerman HJ, et al. Type B hepatitis after needle-stick exposure: prevention with hepatitis B immune globulin, final report of the Veterans Administration cooperative study. *Ann Intern Med.* 1978;88:285–293
6. Grady, GF, Lee VA, Prince AM, et al. Hepatitis B immune globulin for accidental exposures among medical personnel: final report of a multicenter controlled trial. *J Infect Dis.* 1978;138:625–638
7. Kashiwagi S, Hayashi J, Ikematsu H, et al. An outbreak of hepatitis B in members of a high school sumo wrestling club. *JAMA.* 1982;248:213–214
8. Ringertz O, Zetterberg B. Serum hepatitis among Swedish track finders:

an epidemiologic study. *N Engl J Med.* 1967;276:540–546

9. American Academy of Pediatrics. In: Pickering LK, ed. *2000 Red Book. Report of the Committee on Infectious Diseases.* 25th ed, Elk Grove Village, IL: American Academy of Pediatrics. In press

10. American Medical Society for Sports Medicine and the American Academy of Sports Medicine. Human immunodeficiency virus and other blood-borne pathogens in sports. *Clin J Sport Med.* 1995;5:199–204

11. Mitten MJ. Athletic participation with a contagious blood-borne disease. *Clin J Sport Med.* 1995;5:153–154

12. Centers for Disease Control and Prevention. Guidelines for prevention of transmission of human immunodeficiency virus and hepatitis B virus to health-care and public-safety workers. *MMWR Morb Mortal Wkly Rep.* 1989;38:1–37

13. American Academy of Pediatrics. *OSHA. Materials to Assist the Pediatric Office in Implementing the Bloodborne Pathogen, Hazard Communication, and Other OSHA Standards.* 2nd ed. Elk Grove Village, IL: American Academy of Pediatrics; 1994

14. Mast EE, Goodman RA, Bond WW, Favero MS, Drotman DP. Transmission of blood-borne pathogens during sports: risk and prevention. *Ann Intern Med.* 1995;122:283–285

AMERICAN ACADEMY OF PEDIATRICS

Committee on Injury and Poison Prevention and Committee on Sports Medicine and Fitness

In-line Skating Injuries in Children and Adolescents

ABSTRACT. In-line skating has become one of the fastest-growing recreational sports in the United States. Recent studies emphasize the value of protective gear in reducing the incidence of injuries. Recommendations are provided for parents and pediatricians, with special emphasis on the novice or inexperienced skater.

Since its introduction in 1980, in-line skating has become one of the fastest growing recreational sports for children and teenagers in the United States. An estimated 17.7 million people younger than 18 years participated in this sport in 1996, a 24% increase over the previous year.[1] The sport offers the benefits of aerobic fitness,[2] independent transportation for younger children, the opportunity to play roller hockey or cross-train for other sports, and venues for competition in artistic, speed skating, and endurance events. Entry-level skates now cost less than $20 per pair, a 10-fold decrease in the past decade. The low cost and multiple benefits of participation have allowed the sport to thrive beyond the limits of a "fad," as evidenced by the existence of a professional roller hockey league, in-line speed skating competition at the Pan American Games, trick-skating competition at the Entertainment and Sports Programming Network (ESPN) Extreme Games, several periodicals for enthusiasts, an international skaters association, a formal training program for instructors,[3] and summer training camps.

As the sport has grown, so has the number of participants injured. In 1996, an estimated 76 000 children and teenagers younger than 21 years were injured sufficiently while in-line skating to require emergency department care, compared with about 415 000 bicyclists. The most common reasons cited for injuries during in-line skating were losing one's balance because of a road defect or debris, being unable to stop, out-of-control speeding, or doing a trick.[4] In one study, novice skaters incurred 14% of all injuries requiring treatment.[4] The wrist is the most common site of injury (37% of all injuries), and two thirds of wrist injuries are fractures. Few skaters die. Of a total of 36 who died since 1992, the US Consumer Product Safety Commission Clearinghouse reported that 31 had collided with a motor vehicle.

Wearing proper gear is essential for safe skating. This includes a helmet, wrist guards, knee pads, and elbow pads. Wrist guards are designed to prevent

wrist injuries by preventing sudden extreme hyperextension, absorbing some shock of impact, dissipating kinetic forces by forward sliding on their hard volar plates, and preventing local gravel burns. A helmet, elbow pads, and knee pads are recommended for shock absorption.[5–9] Recent research[4] has evaluated the effectiveness of such gear and indicates that wearing wrist guards could reduce the number of wrist injuries by 87%, wearing elbow pads could reduce the number of elbow injuries by 82%, and wearing knee pads could reduce the number of knee injuries by 32%. Although in this study the number of in-line skaters who sustained a head injury was not sufficient to determine the degree of protection afforded by helmets, others[10] have reported that a bicycle helmet or similar approved sports helmet[11] is strongly protective against the occurrence of a head injury to bicyclists in the same physical environment to which a skater is exposed. Helmet use by child and adolescent skaters is required by law in New York and Oregon. Skaters who participate in roller hockey or perform tricks should wear heavy-duty protective gear, including well-constructed wrist guards, knee pads, elbow pads, and a full-head helmet that covers the ears.

"Truck-surfing" or "skitching" refers to skating behind or alongside a vehicle while the skater holds on to the vehicle. This enables a skater to travel at the same velocity as the vehicle. However, it can be very dangerous because the skater cannot slow down fast enough to prevent colliding with the vehicle or being thrown into oncoming traffic or the roadbed if the vehicle suddenly slows, stops, or turns. If the skater falls, his or her enhanced momentum will likely result in a greater force of impact, and consequently, a more severe injury. Several deaths have been caused by skitching.

The design of the skates should match the ability of the skater. Three- or four-wheeled skates are suitable for novice- or intermediate-level skaters, depending on the child's foot size. Five-wheeled skates are high-performance, extremely low-friction skates that should be used only by competitive or long-distance skaters. Skates should fit snugly to allow good, responsive control. Skates, whether rented or owned, should be well maintained: the brake pads should not be worn down, the wheels should be worn symmetrically and turn freely. Skates with expandable shells or interchangeable liners are now available to accommodate the child's growing foot.

Skating skill is not acquired easily or quickly. Good balance and speed control are essential skills to learn. In the past, children acquired skating skills on traditional "quad" skates, rather than in-line skates, but that pattern appears to be changing. The age at which children are ready to use in-line skates safely is not known with certainty because a combination of factors are involved: physical factors (foot size and body strength); skill factors (general athletic ability and large-muscle coordination); and behavioral factors (vigilance in watching the surface for debris and defects, sufficient attention to traffic, judgment). Although most 7- and 8-year-olds can acquire the skills needed to in-line skate, some children may acquire these skills earlier or later. Judgment and ability to avoid obstacles, including bicyclists, pedestrians, and other skaters, are needed. Training may help the novice learn the sport; more than 2000 certified instructors now teach in the United States.

With either type of skate, the novice should preferably learn indoors at a skating rink, where surface conditions, speed, and lighting are controlled without the presence of motor vehicle traffic or other obstacles. Novices particularly need a flat, smooth surface free of debris.

Once a skater can control speed and direction on an indoor rink, he or she is ready to skate on a path or open lot. Hills (even small ones) should be avoided at first. The path selected should be isolated from motor vehicle, bicycle, and pedestrian traffic to the greatest extent possible until the skater is competent enough to avoid such obstacles. Separate trails are advisable where possible. Trail designs have been published, including recommendations for design speed, surface composition, drainage, trail width, and sight distances.[8] Trails should be kept free of sand, dirt, leaves, and twigs, which can become trapped between the wheels and cause a sudden change in velocity with loss of balance. Good drainage is needed so that puddles do not form—water changes the coefficient of friction and results in a sudden change in velocity. Trails should also flatten for at least 30 ft before intersections.[8]

RECOMMENDATIONS

The American Academy of Pediatrics recommends that pediatricians provide the following advice to patients and families concerned with this activity:

1. Parents need to understand both the benefits and risks of in-line skating. Children and their parents should appreciate that injuries are particularly common in novice skaters, roller hockey players, and those performing tricks.
2. Full protective gear needs to be used at all times, including a helmet, wrist guards, knee pads, and elbow pads. The helmet should be certified by the American National Standards Institute (ANSI), the American Society for Testing and Materials (ASTM), the Snell Memorial Foundation, or the Consumer Product Safety Commission. Skaters performing tricks need special heavy-duty protective gear.
3. If skating takes place on the streets, pediatricians should strongly encourage parents, children, and adolescents to use streets that are blocked off or closed to through traffic (eg, dead-end streets or cul-de-sacs).

4. Special attention should be paid to the needs of novice skaters to avoid injuries. They should skate on an indoor or outdoor rink, rather than on a path or street. Inexperienced children should not attempt to do tricks.
5. "Truck-surfing" or "skitching" should be prohibited for all skaters under any circumstance.
6. The type and fit of the skates should be carefully considered when they are purchased or rented and should be appropriate for the child's size, ability, and purpose.
7. Skaters should vigilantly watch for road debris and defects, which may precipitate a loss of balance. They should be trained to react appropriately to these and other rapidly occurring and unpredictable circumstances by learning to stop quickly and fall safely and by avoiding traffic. Instruction in skating by a teacher certified by the International In-Line Skating Association is recommended.
8. Children with large-muscle motor skill or balance problems and those with any uncorrected hearing or vision deficit should skate only in a protected environment. Appropriate areas include a skating rink or outdoor area where the skater is either alone or where no motor vehicle or bicycle traffic occurs and where all other skaters and pedestrians travel in same direction.
9. State legislation that requires helmet use while skating should be encouraged.

COMMITTEE ON INJURY AND POISON PREVENTION, 1997 TO 1998
Murray L. Katcher, MD, PhD, Chairperson
Phyllis Agran, MD, MPH
Danielle Laraque, MD
Susan H. Pollack, MD
Barbara L. Smith, MD
Gary A. Smith, MD, DrPh
Howard R. Spivak, MD
Susan B. Tully, MD

LIAISON REPRESENTATIVES
Ruth A. Brenner, MD
    National Institute of Child Health and Human Development
Stephanie Bryn, MPH
    Maternal and Child Health Bureau
William P. Tully, MD
    Pediatric Orthopaedic Society of North America
Cheryl Neverman
    US Dept of Transportation
Richard A. Schieber, MD, MPH
    Centers for Disease Control and Prevention
Richard Stanwick, MD
    Canadian Paediatric Society
Deborah Tinsworth
    US Consumer Product Safety Commission

SECTION LIAISONS
Marilyn Bull, MD, MPH
    Section on Injury and Poison Prevention
Victor Garcia, MD
    Section on Surgery

COMMITTEE ON SPORTS MEDICINE AND FITNESS, 1997 TO 1998
Steven J. Anderson, MD, Chairperson
Stephen P. Bolduc, MD

Bernard Griesemer, MD
Miriam D. Johnson, MD
Larry G. McLain, MD
Thomas W. Rowland, MD
Eric Small, MD

LIAISON REPRESENTATIVES
Kathryn Keely, MD
   Canadian Paediatric Society
Richard Malacrea, ATC
   National Athletic Trainers Association
Judith C. Young, PhD
   National Association for Sport and Physical
   Education

SECTION LIAISONS
Reginald L. Washington, MD
   Section on Cardiology
Frederick E. Reed, MD
   Section on Orthopaedics

REFERENCES

1. American Sports Data, Inc. *American Sports Analysis: Summary Report.* Hartsdale, NY: American Sports Data, Inc; 1996

2. Snyder AC, O'Hagan KP, Clifford PS, Hoffman MD, Foster C. Exercise responses to in-line skating: comparisons to running and cycling. *Int J Sports Med.* 1993;14:38–42

3. International In-Line Skating Association. *Level I Certified Instructor Manual.* Minneapolis, MN: International In-line Skating Association; 1993

4. Schieber R, Branche-Dorsey CM, Ryan GW, Rutherford GW, Stevens JA, O'Neil J. Risk factors for injuries from in-line skating and the effectiveness of safety gear. *N Engl J Med.* 1996;335:1630–1635

5. Schieber RA, Branche-Dorsey CM, Ryan GW. Comparison of in-line skating injuries with roller-skating and skateboarding injuries. *JAMA.* 1994;271:1856–1858

6. Calle SC. In-line skating injuries, 1987 through 1992. *Am J Public Health.* 1994;84:675

7. Heller D. Rollerblading injuries. *Hazard.* 1993;15:11–13

8. International In-line Skating Association. *Guidelines for Establishing In-line Skate Trails in Parks and Recreational Areas.* Minneapolis, MN: International In-line Skating Association; 1992

9. US Consumer Product Safety Commission. *Safety Commission Warns About Hazards With In-line Roller Skates: Safety Alert.* Bethesda, MD: US Consumer Product Safety Commission; August 1991

10. Sacks JJ, Holmgreen P, Smith SM, Sosin DM. Bicycle-associated head injuries and deaths in the United States from 1984 through 1988: how many are preventable? *JAMA.* 1991;266:3016–3018

11. Centers for Disease Control and Prevention. Injury-control recommendations: bicycle helmets. *MMWR.* 1995;44(RR-1):1–17

AMERICAN ACADEMY OF PEDIATRICS

Committee on Sports Medicine and Fitness

Intensive Training and Sports Specialization in Young Athletes

ABSTRACT. Children involved in sports should be encouraged to participate in a variety of different activities and develop a wide range of skills. Young athletes who specialize in just one sport may be denied the benefits of varied activity while facing additional physical, physiologic, and psychologic demands from intense training and competition.

This statement reviews the potential risks of high-intensity training and sports specialization in young athletes. Pediatricians who recognize these risks can have a key role in monitoring the health of these young athletes and helping reduce risks associated with high-level sports participation.

There appear to be increasing numbers of children who specialize in a sport at an early age, train year-round for a sport, and/or compete on an "elite" level. Media coverage of national and international competition in sports such as gymnastics, figure skating, swimming, diving, and tennis has focused attention on a number of very talented but very young competitors. The successes of young athletes can serve as a powerful inducement for others to follow. Most Olympic sports have selection processes that attempt to identify future champions and initiate specialized training—often before the prospect finishes elementary school. The lure of a college scholarship or a professional career can also motivate athletes (and their parents) to commit to specialized training regimens at an early age. The low probability of reaching these lofty goals does not appear to discourage many aspirants.

To be competitive at a high level requires training regimens for children that could be considered extreme even for adults. The ever-increasing requirements for success creates a constant pressure for athletes to train longer, harder, more intelligently, and, in some cases, at an earlier age. The unending efforts to outdo predecessors and outperform contemporaries are the nature of competitive sports. The necessary commitment and intensity of training raises concerns about the sensibility and safety of high-level athletics for any young person.

Adverse consequences from intense training and competition have been reported in the lay and medical literature.[1,2] Many pediatricians can cite examples of undesirable outcomes from sports participation involving patients in their own practices. Unfortunately, anecdotal reports and case studies are insuf-

ficient grounds for drawing conclusions about the safety of intense training or high-level competition.

The short-term and long-term health consequences of such training in young athletes need to be further investigated. Physical, physiologic, and psychologic tolerances to stress in children have been studied in laboratory settings and can be defined by observing the threshold for injury in clinical settings. Unfortunately, this information is difficult to directly apply to the specific clinical scenarios of concern to the pediatrician. Studying the risks of "specialized," "intensely trained," or "elite" athletes is hampered by the lack of clear definitions of these at-risk populations. Even if a study group could be defined, the level of variation between sports, individuals, and training regimens creates further methodologic challenges for investigators.

Despite recognized inadequacies of current information, pediatricians can still help safeguard their young athletic patients by being aware of potential problems associated with intense training. Because pediatricians serve as the primary medical contact for most young athletes, they may have the best opportunity to recognize, treat, and monitor injuries or illnesses resulting from strenuous training. To respond to parental concerns and to more effectively monitor the child athlete engaged in intensive training, increased awareness of the following issues is suggested.

CARDIAC

Child athletes have superior cardiac functional capacity compared with nonathletes. Nonetheless, there is some cause for caution. Data obtained from studies using animals and humans indicate that myocardial function can be depressed, at least transiently, after intense exercise. Echocardiographic studies have indicated a transient decrease in left ventricular contractility after extremes of athletic competition (ie, 24-hour ultramarathon runs).[3]

A limited number of studies have failed to identify an adverse effect of intense endurance training on the heart of the child athlete. In these investigations, no differences in resting echocardiograms or electrocardiograms have been observed between trained prepubertal runners and nonathletes.[4,5] Rost studied a group of young swimmers longitudinally with echocardiograms over a 10-year period. Cardiac volume and chamber size exceeded those of nonathletic children.[6] The effects of sustained submaximal exercise on cardiac function are similar in children and adults.[7] Evaluation of cardiac function before and immediately after a 4-km road race by echocardiograms in run-trained boys ages 9 to 14 years showed no evidence of change in left ventricular contractility.[8]

Based on these limited data, currently there is no indication that intense athletic training of the child athlete results in injury to the heart. However, closer study of the cardiac characteristics of children training at elite levels is necessary before this conclusion can be verified. Careful assessment of cardiovascular status (heart murmurs, abnormal rhythms) remains important in ongoing medical care of the child athlete.

MUSCULOSKELETAL INJURY AND GROWTH

With low or absent physical activity, muscle tissue becomes atrophic, and bone mineral content decreases. An increase in physical activity stimulates musculoskeletal growth and repetitive stress can stimulate positive adaptive responses in musculoskeletal structures. However, excessive stress or overload can lead to tissue breakdown and injury. To realize maximum gains, athletes must correctly identify and train just below the threshold for injury.

Overuse injuries (tendinitis, apophysitis, stress fractures) can be consequences of excessive sports training in child and adult athletes. Certain aspects of the growing athlete may predispose the child and adolescent to repetitive stress injuries such as traction apophysitis (Osgood-Schlatter disease, Sever disease, medial epicondylitis [Little League elbow]), injuries to developing joint surfaces (osteochondritis dissecans), and/or injuries to the immature spine (spondylolysis, spondylolisthesis, vertebral apophysitis).[9]

Because of the potential for long-term growth disturbances, injuries to epiphyseal growth centers are a particular concern for young athletes. Because the physeal plate may be weaker than surrounding ligamentous structures, external stress may disrupt a growth plate rather than damaging a ligament or related soft-tissue structure. Physeal fractures can result in growth arrest or deformity of long bones. Fortunately, there is no evidence that epiphyseal fractures or growth complications caused by epiphyseal injuries are seen disproportionately in children who participate in organized sports or higher levels of competition.

The long-term effects of repetitive microtrauma to the epiphysis is still under investigation. Damage to the distal radial epiphysis with subsequent alterations in radial-ulnar growth has been described in highly competitive gymnasts.[10] Epiphyseal injuries to the long bones of prepubertal children involved in distance running and other weight-bearing sports (that might potentially affect development of stature) have not been described. Similarly, cross-sectional and longitudinal studies describing growth in child athletes indicate that size and rate of growth of athletes are not negatively influenced by intensive training and competition.[11] Short stature in gymnasts has been considered most likely a consequence of genetic and physique preselection rather than a result of training, although some have concluded that training

starting before and maintained throughout puberty can alter growth rates.[12]

NUTRITION

Proper nutrition is critical for both good health and optimal sports performance. For child athletes, an adequate diet is critical because nutritional needs are increased by both training and the growth process. Young athletes and their parents are frequently unaware of the appropriate components of a training diet. The following 4 areas are of particular concern.

Total Caloric Intake

Athletic training creates a need for increased caloric intake, and requirements relative to body size are higher in growing children and adolescents than at any other time in life. In child athletes, the energy intake must be increased beyond the needs of training to maintain adequate growth. Children who engage in sports in which slenderness is considered important for optimizing performance (ie, gymnastics, ballet dancing) may be at risk for compromising their growth. A risk for pathologic eating behaviors also may be increased in children participating in sports where leanness is rewarded.

Balanced Diet

Balance, moderation, and a variety of food choices should be promoted. The Food Guide Pyramid can be used to plan a diet that is balanced and provides sufficient nutrients and calories for both growth and training needs. Athletes who focus on particular dietary constituents (such as carbohydrates) at the expense of a well-rounded diet may potentially compromise their performance as well as their health.

Iron

The body's requirement for iron is greater during the growing years than at any other time in life. Adequate iron stores are important to the athlete to provide adequate oxygen transport (hemoglobin), muscle aerobic metabolism (Krebs' cycle enzymes), and cognitive function. However, athletes often avoid eating red meat and other iron-containing foods. Moreover, sports training itself may increase body iron losses.

Calcium

Inadequate calcium intake is common in athletes, presumably because of their concern about the fat content in dairy foods. Normal bone growth, and possibly, prevention and healing of stress fractures, are contingent on sufficient dietary calcium.

SEXUAL MATURATION

Athletic girls tends to experience menarche at a later age than nonathletic girls, leading to concern that intensive sports training might delay sexual maturation. The average age of menarche in healthy North American girls is 12.3 to 12.8 years, while that of athletes in a wide variety of sports is typically 1 to 2 years later. Undernutrition, training stress, and low levels of body fat have been hypothesized to account for this delay. Alternatively, it is possible that the later age of menarche in athletes simply reflects a preselection phenomenon.[13] Girls who have narrow hips, slender physiques, long legs, and low levels of body fat—advantageous characteristics in many girls' sports—are more likely to experience later menarche regardless of sports participation.

Secondary amenorrhea, or cessation of menstrual cycles after menarche, can occur as a result of intense athletic training. Prolonged amenorrhea may cause diminished bone mass from the associated decrease in estrogen secretion, augmenting the risk for stress fractures and the potential for osteoporosis in adulthood. Efforts to improve nutrition or diminish training volume in these girls may permit resumption of menses and diminish these risks.

Studies of males have indicated no evidence of an adverse effect on sexual maturation related to sports training. Progression of Tanner stages of pubertal development has not been observed to be retarded in athletic compared with nonathletic adolescents.[11]

PSYCHOSOCIAL DEVELOPMENT

Considerable research has addressed anxiety and stress that affect children who engage in competitive sports but little data exist about the effects of more intense or sustained training on young athletes. Anecdotal reports suggest risks of "burnout" from physical and emotional stress, missed social and educational opportunities, and disruptions of family life. Unrealistic parental expectations and/or exploitation of young athletes for extrinsic gain can contribute to negative psychological consequences for elite young athletes. Survey studies suggest, however, that while such adverse effects occur, they are experienced by only a small minority of intensely training athletes.[13] Most athletes find elite-level competition to be a positive experience.

Research supports the recommendation that child athletes avoid early sports specialization. Those who participate in a variety of sports and specialize only after reaching the age of puberty tend to be more consistent performers, have fewer injuries, and adhere to sports play longer than those who specialize early.[15]

HEAT STRESS

Child athletes differ from adults in their thermoregulatory responses to exercise in the heat.[16] They sweat less, create more heat per body mass, and acclimatize slower to warm environments. As a result, child athletes may be more at risk for heat-related injuries in hot, humid conditions. It is particularly critical that coaches, parents, and young athletes are aware of signs of heat injury. They also should be aware that limiting sports play and training in hot, humid conditions and ensuring adequate fluid intake can prevent heat injury.

RECOMMENDATIONS

Although many concerns surround intense sports competition in children, little scientific information is available to support or refute these risks. Nonetheless, it is important to make efforts to assist young athletes in avoiding potential risks from early excessive training and competition. The following guidelines are suggested keeping in mind 1) the importance of assuring safe and healthy sports play for children, 2) the need to provide practical and realistic guidelines, and 3) the limited research basis for making such recommendations.

1. Children are encouraged to participate in sports at a level consistent with their abilities and interests. Pushing children beyond these limits is discouraged as is specialization in a single sport before adolescence.
2. Pediatricians should work with parents to ensure that the child athlete is being coached by persons who are knowledgeable about proper training techniques, equipment, and the unique physical, physiologic, and emotional characteristics of young competitors.
3. In the absence of prospective markers of excessive physical stress, physicians and coaches should strive for early recognition and prevention and treatment of overuse injuries (tendinitis, apophysitis, stress fractures, "shin splints"). Child athletes should never be encouraged to "work through" such injuries. Treatment recommendations for overuse injuries that include only "rest" or cessation of the sport are unlikely to be followed by the committed child athlete and are unlikely to adequately address the risk of further injury.
4. The conditions of child athletes involved in intense training should be monitored regularly by a pediatrician. Attention should be focused on serial measurements of body composition, weight, and stature; cardiovascular findings; sexual maturation; and evidence of emotional stress. The pediatrician should be alert for signs and symptoms of overtraining, including decline in performance, weight loss, anorexia, and sleep disturbances.
5. The intensely trained, specialized child athlete needs ongoing assessment of nutritional intake, with particular attention to total calories, a balanced diet, and intake of iron and calcium. Serial measurements of body weight are particularly important in ensuring the adequacy of caloric intake and early identification of pathologic eating behaviors.
6. The child athlete, family, and coach should be educated by the pediatrician about the risks of heat injury and strategies for prevention.

COMMITTEE ON SPORTS MEDICINE AND FITNESS, 1999–2000
Steven J. Anderson, MD, Chairperson
Bernard A. Griesemer, MD
Miriam D. Johnson, MD
Thomas J. Martin, MD
Larry G. McLain, MD
Thomas W. Rowland, MD
Eric Small, MD

LIAISON REPRESENTATIVES
Claire LeBlanc, MD
  Canadian Paediatric Society
Robert Malina, PhD
  Institute for the Study of Youth Sports

Carl Krein, ATc, PT
  National Athletic Trainers Association
Judith C. Young, PhD
  National Association for Sport and Physical
  Education

SECTION LIAISONS
Frederick E. Reed, MD
  Section on Orthopaedics
Reginald L. Washington, MD
  Section on Cardiology

CONSULTANT
Oded Bar-Or, MD

STAFF
Heather Newland

REFERENCES

1. Ryan J. *Little Girls in Pretty Boxes: The Making and Breaking of Elite Gymnasts and Figure Skaters.* New York, NY: Warner Books; 1996
2. Tofler IR, Stryer BK, Micheli LJ, Herman LR. Physical and emotional problems of elite female gymnasts. *N Engl J Med.* 1996;25:335:281–283
3. Niemela KO, Palatski IJ, Ikaheimo MJ, Takkunen JT, Vuori JJ. Evidence of impaired left ventricular performance after an uninterrupted competitive 24-hour run. *Circulation.* 1984;70:350–356
4. Rowland TW, Delaney BC, Siconolfi SF. "Athlete's heart" in prepubertal children. *Pediatrics.* 1987;79:800–804
5. Rowland TW, Unnithan VB, McFarlane NG, Gibson NG, Paton JY. Clinical manifestations of the "athlete's heart" in prepubertal male runners. *Int J Sports Med.* 1994;15:515–519
6. Rost R. *Athletics and the Heart.* Chicago, IL: Yearbook Medical Publishers; 1987
7. Rowland TW, Rimany TA. Physiological responses to prolonged exercise in premenarcheal and adult females. *Pediatr Exerc Science.* 1995;7: 183–191
8. Rowland TW, Goff D, Popowski B, DeLuca P. Cardiac effects of a competitive road race in trained child runners. *Pediatrics.* 1997;100(3). URL: http://www.pediatrics.org/cgi/content/full/100/3/e2
9. Micheli LJ. Overuse injuries in children's sports: the growth factor. *Orthop Clin North Am.* 1983;14:337–349
10. Caine DJ. Growth plate injury and bone growth: an update. *Pediatr Exerc Science.* 1990;2:209–229
11. Malina RM. Physical growth and biological maturation of young athletes. *Exerc Sports Sci Rev.* 1994;22:389–434
12. Thientz GE, Howald H, Weiss V, Sizonenko PC. Evidence for a reduction of growth potential in adolescent female gymnasts. *J Pediatr.* 1993; 122:306–313
13. Malina RM. Menarche in athletes: a synthesis and hypothesis. *Ann Hum Biol.* 1983;10:1–24
14. Donnelly P. Problems associated with youth involvement in high-performance sport. In: Cahill BR, Pearl AJ. *Intensive Participation in Children's Sports.* Champaign, IL: Human Kinetics Publishers; 1993: 95–126
15. Bompa T. *From Childhood to Champion Athlete.* Toronto, Canada: Veritas Publishing, Inc; 1995
16. Bar-Or O. *Pediatric Sports Medicine for the Practitioner.* New York, NY: Springer-Verlag; 1983

AMERICAN ACADEMY OF PEDIATRICS

Committee on Sports Medicine and Fitness

Medical Concerns in the Female Athlete

ABSTRACT. Female children and adolescents who participate regularly in sports may develop certain medical conditions, including disordered eating, menstrual dysfunction, and decreased bone mineral density. The pediatrician can play an important role in monitoring the health of young female athletes. This revised policy statement provides updated and expanded information for pediatricians on these health concerns as well as recommendations for evaluation, treatment, and ongoing assessments of female athletes.

ABBREVIATIONS. BMD, bone mineral density; LH, luteinizing hormone.

Exercise is good for female children and adolescents. Special medical concerns should be considered, however, when caring for young female athletes. Athletes can develop abnormal eating patterns (termed disordered eating), which can be associated with menstrual dysfunction (amenorrhea or oligomenorrhea) and subsequent decreased bone mineral density (BMD), or osteoporosis. These 3 conditions—disordered eating, amenorrhea, and osteoporosis—often occur together and have been termed the female athlete triad.[1] Although these conditions may also be seen in the nonathlete, this statement will concentrate on the physically active and athletic female.

DISORDERED EATING

Some physically active females, particularly adolescents, may develop an energy deficit when the energy (calories) they expend exceeds their energy (calorie) intake.[2] This deficit may be unintentional, resulting from inadequate replenishment of the caloric (energy) demands of training, or may be intentional—a conscious attempt to lose weight or body fat in the interest of improved appearance or athletic performance. These athletes often restrict food intake but may develop other disordered eating behaviors, such as binge eating and/or purging by vomiting or use of laxatives, diuretics, and diet pills. Compulsive exercise, defined as excessive exercise in addition to a normal training regimen, is another form of "purging," or energy expenditure often overlooked in athletes. The spectrum of disordered eating behaviors ranges from mild—slight restriction of food intake or occasional binge eating and purging—to severe—significant restriction of food intake, as in anorexia

nervosa, or regular binge eating and purging, as in bulimia nervosa.[3] Disordered eating may result in adverse health consequences, with the risk of morbidity and mortality increasing as the severity of the behavior increases.

Disordered eating behavior has been reported in young female athletes and dancers.[4–6] One study of young elite swimmers revealed that 60.5% of average-weight girls and 17.9% of underweight girls were trying to lose weight. Most of the girls were trying to lose weight by decreasing their food intake[7]; however, 12.7% were vomiting, 2.5% were using laxatives, and 1.5% were using diuretics.[7] Disordered eating can be seen in athletes participating in all sports. Sports that may place athletes at higher risk for the development of these behaviors include those in which leanness is emphasized (eg, gymnastics, ballet dancing, diving, and figure skating) or perceived to optimize performance (eg, long-distance running and cross-country skiing) and those that use weight classification (eg, martial arts and rowing).[3] A variety of factors may contribute to the development of disordered eating patterns in the young athlete, including pressure to optimize performance or meet inappropriate weight or body fat goals, social factors (eg, idealization of thinness in Western cultures), psychological factors (eg, poor coping skills, unhealthy family dynamics, and low self-esteem), and personality traits (eg, perfectionism, compulsiveness, and high achievement expectations).[3]

Disordered eating behaviors may impair athletic performance and increase risk of injury. Decreased energy (caloric) intake and fluid and electrolyte imbalance can result in decreased endurance, strength, reaction time, speed, and ability to concentrate. Because the body initially adapts to these changes, a decrease in performance may not be seen for some time, and athletes may falsely believe disordered eating practices are harmless. To the contrary, food restriction and purging can result not only in menstrual dysfunction and potentially irreversible bone loss but also in psychological and other medical complications, including depression, fluid and electrolyte imbalance, and changes in the cardiovascular, endocrine, gastrointestinal, and thermoregulatory systems.[8,9] Some of these complications are potentially fatal.

MENSTRUAL DYSFUNCTION

Menstrual dysfunction in athletes may include primary amenorrhea, secondary amenorrhea, oligomenorrhea, and luteal phase deficiency.[10–12]

An adolescent is considered to have delayed pu-

PEDIATRICS (ISSN 0031 4005). Copyright © 2000 by the American Academy of Pediatrics.

berty when breast development has not begun by 13.3 years of age.[13] Because sports involvement or poor nutrition may be associated with a delay in development, evaluation might be postponed until 14 years of age, as determined by clinical judgment. Primary amenorrhea is defined as the absence of menses by age 16 years. If menses have not occurred within 4.5 years after the onset of breast development, evaluation should be considered. Secondary amenorrhea is typically defined as the absence of at least 3 to 6 consecutive menstrual cycles in a female who has begun menstruating. Oligomenorrhea refers to menstrual periods that occur at intervals longer than every 35 days.[11,12,14] Although adolescents may have irregular periods or amenorrhea for 3 to 6 months in the first several years after menarche, the cessation of menses for longer than 3 months after regular cycles have begun or persistent oligomenorrhea is considered abnormal.[15]

Menstrual dysfunction is more common in athletes than in the general population. Athletes and dancers who begin training before menarche occurs may experience a later menarche and have an increased incidence of menstrual dysfunction when compared with girls who begin training after menarche occurs.[16–19] The prevalence of secondary amenorrhea in adult athletes ranges from 3.4% to 66% (depending on the sport studied and the criteria used to define amenorrhea),[10–12] compared with 2% to 5% of women in the general population.[12] The prevalence of secondary amenorrhea in the young athlete is unknown.

Luteinizing hormone (LH) pulsatility and, therefore, normal menstrual function are dependent on energy availability (dietary energy intake minus energy expenditure from exercise).[20] Low energy availability causes a hypometabolic state characterized by a variety of substrate and hormonal alterations, including hypoglycemia, hypoinsulinemia, hypothyroidemia, hypercortisolemia, and the suppression of the 24-hour mean and amplitude of the diurnal rhythm of leptin.[2,20–23] Amenorrheic and regularly menstruating athletes display reduced LH pulse frequencies[24] and similarly low 24-hour mean leptin levels.[25] However, amenorrheic athletes are distinctive in having a more extreme suppression and disorganization of LH pulsatility[24] and a complete suppression of the amplitude of the diurnal rhythm of leptin.[25] It is not known whether a particular threshold of energy availability is required to maintain normal reproductive function or whether the macronutrient composition of the diet is important.

Menstrual dysfunction may lead to decreased BMD. Other long-term consequences of a chronically estrogen-depleted state in young women are unknown at this time.

DECREASED BONE MINERAL DENSITY

Hypoestrogenism associated with amenorrhea may predispose to osteoporosis.[26,27] Osteoporosis is defined as premature bone loss and/or inadequate bone formation resulting in low bone mass and microarchitectural deterioration.[1] Adequate levels of estrogen slow bone resorption and improve or maintain bone mass.[28,29] The prevalence of osteoporosis in adult and adolescent women is unknown.[1] Studies of adult female athletes have shown that premature osteoporosis may occur as a result of amenorrhea and oligomenorrhea and may be partially irreversible despite resumption of menses, estrogen replacement, or calcium supplementation.[27,30,31] Amenorrheic adolescents, both athletes and nonathletes, have been found to have lower BMD than eumenorrheic adolescents.[28,32–34] This may be attributable to decreased bone accretion as well as increased bone loss.[35] An overall increase in BMD is demonstrated throughout adolescence. However, the amenorrheic teenager remains osteopenic in comparison with regularly menstruating teenagers.[28,32–35]

High-intensity exercise in some sports for many years may actually increase BMD in specific skeletal sites despite amenorrhea. Elite adolescent ice skaters and gymnasts have been found to have increased BMD in the lower skeleton, compared with controls, despite menstrual dysfunction.[29,36,37]

Girls who begin menarche at a later age and have a lower weight during adolescence have been found to have the lowest BMD when compared with their peers.[34,35] An increased incidence of stress fracture in dancers has been associated with older age at menarche.[38] Weight gain and the resumption of menses result in increased BMD.[33,35] Estrogen replacement therapy may decrease bone loss and potentially increase BMD in the adolescent with secondary amenorrhea.[28,35,39]

CLINICAL EVALUATION

The physical examination that precedes participation in sports is an ideal opportunity to screen for problems of disordered eating, menstrual dysfunction, and decreased BMD.[40] Signs of disordered eating may be recognized by parents, coaches, athletic trainers, teammates, or school nurses and brought to the physician's attention. If an athlete shows signs of disordered eating behavior, further evaluation by the physician, a nutritionist, and a mental health professional may be necessary.[3]

The diagnosis of primary amenorrhea or secondary amenorrhea in an athlete first requires a full evaluation to rule out pregnancy and underlying pathologic conditions. Pathologic conditions that may cause menstrual dysfunction include pituitary tumors (especially prolactinomas), thyroid dysfunction, polycystic ovary disease, premature ovarian failure, and other chronic illnesses.[10]

Evaluation of amenorrhea includes a complete physical examination and pelvic examination when indicated. A pregnancy test is usually indicated. Laboratory studies may include measurement of thyroid-stimulating hormone, prolactin, and follicle-stimulating hormone (FSH). If the athlete shows signs of androgen excess (eg, hirsutism, acne) or if the pelvic examination reveals polycystic ovaries, a determination of levels of LH, testosterone, dehydroepiandrosterone sulfate (DHEA-S), and 17-hydroxyprogesterone may need to be done. A progesterone challenge may help determine if the patient is hypoestrogenemic.[10,15] The possible use of anabolic steroids should also be considered.

In the athlete who has been amenorrheic, a study to evaluate BMD may be helpful.[29]

TREATMENT

The female athlete who has restrictive eating patterns because she is unaware of her energy needs may require only nutritional counseling. The female athlete who purposefully engages in disordered eating behaviors is often best treated using a multidisciplinary team approach: with a physician who monitors her medical status and ability to participate safely in sports, a nutritionist who provides appropriate nutritional guidance, and a mental health professional who addresses any psychological issues.[3]

Increased dietary energy intake or decreased energy expenditure (exercise) usually results in the development or resumption of menses and ovulation in adolescent girls and women with exercise-associated amenorrhea.[29,31] Daily requirements for calories, carbohydrates, and protein are greater in athletes than in more sedentary women and girls,[41] and diet should be changed accordingly. The recommended daily dietary allowance of calcium for adolescents is 1200 mg. Amenorrheic athletes should be encouraged to increase their calcium intake to at least 1500 mg daily. If intake of dietary sources of calcium is inadequate, calcium supplements may be recommended. If estrogen levels are deficient, the efficacy of calcium supplementation in improving bone mass may be impaired.[10,29,42]

In adolescents and young women with hypothalamic amenorrhea, estrogen-progesterone supplementation may help maintain bone density, protect the endometrium, and promote regular menses at predictable times.[10,28,35] The criteria for initiating estrogen replacement therapy and the optimal dosing schedule have not been determined. The minimum daily estrogen dose that has been shown to prevent bone loss in postmenopausal women is 0.625 mg of conjugated estrogens[43]; this dose, however, has not been shown to increase BMD in young women with hypothalamic amenorrhea.[28] Supplementation with a low-dose oral contraceptive (<50 μg of estrogen per day) is a readily available source of estrogen and may be associated with an increase in total body BMD.[39]

RECOMMENDATIONS

1. Exercise and sports participation should be promoted in girls and adolescents for health benefits and enjoyment.
2. Dietary practices; exercise intensity, duration, and frequency; and menstrual history need to be reviewed during evaluations that precede participation in sports or other medical encounters in which related problems may present.
3. Amenorrhea should not be considered a normal response to exercise. Exercise-associated amenorrhea or amenorrhea attributable to decreased energy availability should be considered a diagnosis of exclusion. A complete medical evaluation is required for any adolescent with primary or secondary amenorrhea or persistent oligomenorrhea.
4. Disordered eating should be considered in adolescents with amenorrhea. Treatment often requires a team of health care professionals, including a physician, nutritionist, and mental health professional, all experienced in the treatment of eating disorders, in addition to cooperation by coaches, parents, and teammates.
5. Education and counseling should be provided to athletes, parents, and coaches regarding disordered eating, menstrual dysfunction, decreased bone mineralization, and adequate energy (calorie) and nutrient intake to meet energy expenditure and maintain normal growth and development.
6. When athletes and coaches want to know what weight and amount of body fat are best for a given athlete, it is preferable to establish a range of values rather than specific values. It is difficult and potentially dangerous to define an ideal level of weight and/or body fat for each sport or individual participant. Weight is not an accurate estimate of fitness or fatness, and when weight is lost, muscle and fat are lost.
7. An adolescent with menstrual dysfunction attributed to exercise should be encouraged to increase her energy (caloric) intake and modify excessive exercise activity. If an athlete's weight is low, she may be required to gain weight before resuming athletic activity.
8. Estrogen-progesterone supplementation may be considered in the mature amenorrheic athlete.
9. Measurement of BMD may be considered as a tool when making treatment decisions for the amenorrheic athlete.

Committee on Sports Medicine and Fitness, 1999–2000
Steven J. Anderson, MD, Chairperson
Bernard A. Griesemer, MD
Miriam D. Johnson, MD
Thomas J. Martin, MD
Larry G. McLain, MD
Thomas W. Rowland, MD
Eric Small, MD

Liaisons
Claire LeBlanc, MD
  Canadian Paediatric Society
Carl Krein, AT, PT
  National Athletic Trainers Association
Judith C. Young, PhD
  National Association for Sport and Physical Education
Robert Malina, PhD
  Institute for the Study of Youth Sports

Section Liaisons
Frederick E. Reed, MD
  Section on Orthopaedics
Reginald L. Washington, MD
  Section on Cardiology

Consultants
Oded Bar-Or, MD
Anne Loucks, PhD
Suzanne Tanner, MD

STAFF

Heather Newland

REFERENCES

1. Yeager KK, Agostini R, Nattiv A, Drinkwater B. The female athlete triad: disordered eating, amenorrhea, osteoporosis. *Med Sci Sports Exerc.* 1993;25:775–777

2. Loucks AB, Heath EM. Induction of low-T_3 syndrome in exercising women occurs at a threshold of energy availability. *Am J Physiol.* 1994; 266:R817–R823

3. Johnson MD. Disordered eating in active and athletic women. *Clin Sports Med.* 1994;13:355–369

4. Benson J, Gillien DM, Bourdet K, Loosli AR. Inadequate nutrition and chronic calorie restriction in adolescent ballerinas. *Phys Sportsmed.* 1985; 13:79–90

5. Loosli AR, Benson J, Gillien DM, Bourdet K. Nutrition habits and knowledge in competitive adolescent female gymnasts. *Phys Sportsmed.* 1986;14:118–130

6. Rosen LW, McKeag DB, Hough DO, Curley V. Pathogenic weight-control behavior in female athletes. *Phys Sportsmed.* 1986;14:79–84

7. Dummer GM, Rosen LW, Heusner WW, Roberts PJ, Counsilman JE. Pathogenic weight-control behaviors of young competitive swimmers. *Phys Sportsmed.* 1987;5:22–27

8. Palla B, Litt IF. Medical complications of eating disorders in adolescents. *Pediatrics.* 1988;81:613–623

9. Ratnasuriya RH, Eisler I, Szmuckler GI, Russell GF. Anorexia nervosa: outcome and prognostic factors after 20 years. *Br J Psychiatry.* 1991;158: 495–502

10. Shangold M, Rebar RW, Wentz AC, Schiff I. Evaluation and management of menstrual dysfunction in athletes. *JAMA.* 1990;263:1665–1669

11. Loucks AB. Effects of exercise training on the menstrual cycle: existence and mechanisms. *Med Sci Sports Exerc.* 1990;22:275–280

12. Loucks AB, Horvath SM. Athletic amenorrhea: a review. *Med Sci Sports Exerc.* 1985;17:56–72

13. Sperling MA, ed. *Pediatric Endocrinology.* Philadelphia, PA: WB Saunders; 1996

14. Sperhoff L, Glass RH, Kase NG. Amenorrhea. In: *Clinical Gynecologic Endocrinology and Infertility.* 5th ed. Philadelphia, PA: Williams & Wilkins; 1994:401–456

15. Emans SJ, Goldstein DP. *Pediatric and Adolescent Gynecology.* 3rd ed. Boston, MA: Little, Brown, and Co; 1990

16. Frisch RE, Gotz-Welbergen AV, McArthur JW, et al. Delayed menarche and amenorrhea of college athletes in relation to age of onset of training. *JAMA.* 1981;246:1559–1563

17. Warren MP. The effects of exercise on pubertal progression and reproductive function in girls. *J Clin Endocrinol Metab.* 1980;51:1150–1157

18. Malina RM. Menarche in athletes: a synthesis and hypothesis. *Ann Hum Biol.* 1983;10:1–24

19. Malina RM. Physical activity, sport, social status and Darwinian fitness. In: Strickland SS, Shetty PS, eds. *Human Biology and Social Inequality.* Cambridge, England: Cambridge University Press; 1998:165–192

20. Loucks AB, Verdun M, Heath EM. Low energy availability, not stress of exercise alters LH pulsatility in exercising women. *J Appl Physiol.* 1998; 84:37–46

21. Loucks AB, Callister R. Induction and prevention of low-T_3 syndrome in exercising women. *Am J Physiol.* 1993;264:R924–R930

22. Loucks AB, Heath EM. Dietary restriction reduces luteinizing hormone (LH) pulse frequency during waking hours and increases LH pulse amplitude during sleep in young menstruating women. *J Clin Endocrinol Metab.* 1994;78:910–915

23. Laughlin GA, Yen SS. Nutritional and endocrine-metabolic aberrations in amenorrheic athletes. *J Clin Endocrinol Metab.* 1996;81:4301–4309

24. Loucks AB, Mortola JF, Girton L, Yen SS. Alterations in the hypotha-lamic-pituitary-ovarian and hypothalamic-pituitary-adrenal axes in athletic women. *J Clin Endocrinol Metab.* 1989;68:402–411

25. Laughlin GA, Yen SS. Hypoleptinemia in women athletes: absence of a diurnal rhythm with amenorrhea. *J Clin Endocrinol Metabol.* 1997;82: 318–321

26. Cann CE, Genant HK, Ettinger B, Gordon GS. Spinal mineral loss in oophorectomized women: determination by quantitative computed tomography. *JAMA.* 1980;244:2056–2059

27. Cann CE, Martin MC, Genant HK, Jaffe RB. Decreased spinal mineral content in amenorrheic women. *JAMA.* 1984;251:626–629

28. Emans SJ, Grace E, Hoffer FA, Gundberg C, Ravnikar V, Woods ER. Estrogen deficiency in adolescents and young adults: impact on bone mineral content and effects of estrogen replacement therapy. *Obstet Gynecol.* 1990;76:585–592

29. Snow-Harter CM. Bone health and prevention of osteoporosis in active and athletic women. *Clin Sports Med.* 1994;13:389–404

30. Drinkwater BL, Bruemner B, Chesnut CH. Menstrual history as a determinant of current bone density in young athletes. *JAMA.* 1990;263: 545–548

31. Drinkwater BL, Nilson K, Ott S, Chestnut CH. Bone mineral density after resumption of menses in amenorrheic athletes. *JAMA.* 1986;256: 380–382

32. Bachrach LK, Guido D, Katzman D, Litt IF, Marcus R. Decreased bone density in adolescent girls with anorexia nervosa. *Pediatrics.* 1990;86: 440–447

33. Dhuper S, Warren MP, Brooks-Gunn J, Fox R. Effects of hormonal status on bone density in adolescent girls. *J Clin Endocrinol Metab.* 1990;71: 1983–1088

34. White CM, Hergenroeder AC, Klish WJ. Bone mineral density in 15 to 21 year old eumenorrheic and amenorrheic subjects. *Am J Dis Child.* 1992;146:31–35

35. Bachrach LK, Katzman DK, Litt IF, Guido D, Marcus R. Recovery from osteopenia in adolescent girls with anorexia nervosa. *J Clin Endocrinol Metab.* 1991;72:602–606

36. Robinson T, Snow-Harter C, Gillis D, Shaw J. Bone mineral density and menstrual cycle status in competitive female runners and gymnasts. *Med Sci Sports Exerc.* 1993;25:549. Abstract

37. Slemenda CW, Johnston CC. High intensity activities in young women: site specific bone mass effects among female figure skaters. *Bone Miner.* 1993;20:125–132

38. Warren MP, Brooks-Gunn J, Hamilton LH, Warren LF, Hamilton WG. Scoliosis and fractures in young ballet dancers: relation to delayed menarche and secondary amenorrhea. *N Engl J Med.* 1986;314:1348–1353

39. Hergenroeder AC, Smith EO, Shypailo R, Jones LA, Klish WJ, Ellis K. Bone mineral changes in young women with hypothalamic amenorrhea treated with oral contraceptives, medroxyprogesterone, or placebo over 12 months. *Am J Obstet Gynecol.* 1997;176:1017–1025

40. Johnson MD. Tailoring the preparticipation exam to female athletes. *Phys Sportsmed.* 1992;20:60–72

41. Steen SN. Nutritional concerns of athletes who must reduce body weight. *Sports Science Exchange, Nutrition.* Oct 1989;2(20)

42. Drinkwater BL, Chesnut CH. Site specific skeletal response to increased calcium in amenorrheic athletes. *Med Sci Sports Exerc.* 1992;24:545

43. Lindsay R, Hart DM, Clark DM. The minimum effective dose of estrogen for prevention of postmenopausal bone loss. *Obstet Gynecol.* 1984; 63:759–763

Medical Conditions Affecting Sports Participation

Guidance for the Clinician in Rendering Pediatric Care

Stephen G. Rice, MD, PhD, MPH, and the Council on Sports Medicine and Fitness

ABSTRACT

Children and adolescents with medical conditions present special issues with respect to participation in athletic activities. The pediatrician can play an important role in determining whether a child with a health condition should participate in certain sports by assessing the child's health status, suggesting appropriate equipment or modifications of sports to decrease the risk of injury, and educating the athlete, parent(s) or guardian, and coach regarding the risks of injury as they relate to the child's condition. This report updates a previous policy statement and provides information for pediatricians on sports participation for children and adolescents with medical conditions.

www.pediatrics.org/cgi/doi/10.1542/peds.2008-0080

doi:10.1542/peds.2008-0080

All clinical reports from the American Academy of Pediatrics automatically expire 5 years after publication unless reaffirmed, revised, or retired at or before that time.

The guidance in this report does not indicate an exclusive course of treatment or serve as a standard of medical care. Variations, taking into account individual circumstances, may be appropriate.

Key Words
youth, athletes, risk of injury, contact and collision sports, prevention management, strenuousness, safety

PEDIATRICS (ISSN Numbers: Print, 0031-4005; Online, 1098-4275). Copyright © 2008 by the American Academy of Pediatrics

In 2001, the American Academy of Pediatrics published an analysis of medical conditions affecting sports participation.[1] This updated report replaces the 2001 policy statement and provides additions and changes to increase the accuracy and completeness of the information.

Health care professionals must determine whether a child with a health condition should participate in a particular sport. One way of determining this is by estimating the relative risk of an acute injury to the athlete by categorizing sports as contact, limited-contact, or noncontact sports (Table 1). This categorization may subdivide contact sports into collision and contact sports; although there may be no clear dividing line between the 2, collision implies greater injury risk. In collision sports (eg, boxing, ice hockey, football, lacrosse, and rodeo), athletes purposely hit or collide with each other or with inanimate objects (including the ground) with great force. In contact sports (eg, basketball and soccer), athletes routinely make contact with each other or with inanimate objects but usually with less force than in collision sports. In limited-contact sports (eg, softball and squash), contact with other athletes or with inanimate objects is infrequent or inadvertent. However, some limited-contact sports (eg, skateboarding) can be as dangerous as collision or contact sports. Even in noncontact sports (eg, power lifting), in which contact is rare and unexpected, serious injuries can occur.

Overuse injuries are related not to contact or collision but to repetitive microtrauma; furthermore, overuse injuries generally are not acute. For these reasons, the categorization of sports in Table 1 insufficiently reflects the relative risks of injury. However, the categorization indicates the comparative likelihood that participation in different sports will result in acute traumatic injuries from blows to the body.

For most chronic health conditions, current evidence supports and encourages the participation of children and adolescents in most athletic activities. However, the medical conditions listed in Table 2 have been assessed to determine whether participation would create an increased risk of injury or affect the child's medical condition adversely. These guidelines can be valuable when a physician examines an athlete who has one of the listed problems. Decisions about sports participation are often complex, and the usefulness of Table 2 is limited by the frequency with which it recommends individual assessment when a "qualified yes" or a "qualified no" appears.

The physician's clinical judgment is essential in the application of these recommendations to a specific patient. This judgment is enhanced by consideration of the available published information on the risks of participation, the risk of acquiring a disease as a result of participation in the sport, and the severity of that disease. Other variables to consider include (1) the advice of knowledgeable experts, (2) the current health status of the athlete, (3) the sport in which the athlete participates, (4) the position played, (5) the level of competition, (6) the maturity of the competitor, (7) the relative size of the athlete (for collision/contact sports), (8) the availability of effective protective equipment that is acceptable to the athlete and/or sport governing body, (9) the availability and efficacy of treatment, (10) whether treatment (eg, rehabilitation of an injury) has been completed, (11) whether the sport can be modified to allow safer participation, and (12) the ability of the athlete's parent(s) or guardian and coach to understand and

TABLE 1   Classification of Sports According to Contact

Contact	Limited-Contact	Noncontact
Basketball	Adventure racing[a]	Badminton
Boxing[b]	Baseball	Bodybuilding[c]
Cheerleading	Bicycling	Bowling
Diving	Canoeing or kayaking (white water)	Canoeing or kayaking (flat water)
Extreme sports[d]	Fencing	Crew or rowing
Field hockey	Field events	Curling
Football, tackle	High jump	Dance
Gymnastics	Pole vault	Field events
Ice hockey[e]	Floor hockey	Discus
Lacrosse	Football, flag or touch	Javelin
Martial arts[f]	Handball	Shot-put
Rodeo	Horseback riding	Golf
Rugby	Martial arts[f]	Orienteering[g]
Skiing, downhill	Racquetball	Power lifting[c]
Ski jumping	Skating	Race walking
Snowboarding	Ice	Riflery
Soccer	In-line	Rope jumping
Team handball	Roller	Running
Ultimate Frisbee	Skiing	Sailing
Water polo	Cross-country	Scuba diving
Wrestling	Water	Swimming
	Skateboarding	Table tennis
	Softball	Tennis
	Squash	Track
	Volleyball	
	Weight lifting	
	Windsurfing or surfing	

[a] Adventure racing has been added since the previous statement was published and is defined as a combination of 2 or more disciplines, including orienteering and navigation, cross-country running, mountain biking, paddling, and climbing and rope skills.[1]

[b] The American Academy of Pediatrics opposes participation in boxing for children, adolescents, and young adults.[2]

[c] The American Academy of Pediatrics recommends limiting bodybuilding and power lifting until the adolescent achieves sexual maturity rating 5 (Tanner stage V).

[d] Extreme sports has been added since the previous statement was published.

[e] The American Academy of Pediatrics recommends limiting the amount of body checking allowed for hockey players 15 years and younger, to reduce injuries.

[f] Martial arts can be subclassified as judo, jujitsu, karate, kung fu, and tae kwon do; some forms are contact sports and others are limited-contact sports.

[g] Orienteering is a race (contest) in which competitors use a map and a compass to find their way through unfamiliar territory.

to accept the risks involved in participation. Potential dangers of associated training activities that lead to repetitive and/or excessive overload also should be considered.

Unfortunately, adequate data on the risks of a particular sport for athletes with medical problems often are limited or lacking, and an estimate of risk becomes a necessary part of the decision-making process. If primary care physicians are uncertain or uncomfortable with the evaluation and/or the decision-making process, they should seek the counsel of a sports medicine specialist or a specialist in the specific area of medical concern. If the physician thinks that restriction from a sport is necessary for a particular patient, then he or she should counsel the athlete and family about safe alternative activities.

Physicians making decisions about sports participation for athletes with cardiovascular disease (Table 2) are strongly encouraged to consider consulting a cardiologist and to review carefully recommendations from the 36th Bethesda Conference.[12] The complexities and nuances of cardiovascular disease make it difficult to provide important detailed information in a single table.

An athlete's underlying cardiac pathologic condition and the stress that a sport places on that condition are the 2 primary factors determining the risk of participating in that sport. A strenuous sport can place dynamic (volume) and static (pressure) demands on the cardiovascular system. These demands vary not only with activities of the sport but also with factors such as the associated training activities and the environment, as well as the level of emotional arousal and fitness of the competitors. Figure 1 lists sports according to their dynamic and static demands, as classified by cardiopulmonary experts of the 36th Bethesda Conference.[12]

New recommendations on sports participation for athletes with hypertension (Table 2) are available.[10,12] The latest blood pressure tables provide the 50th, 90th, 95th, and 99th percentiles based on age, gender, and height.[10] The blood pressure reading must be at least 5 mm Hg above the 99th percentile before any exclusion from sports is indicated.[10] Periodic monitoring of resting (preexercise) blood pressure levels is preferred for readings above the 90th percentile. A more-complete evaluation is performed for sustained blood pressure readings above the 95th percentile.[10,12]

In earlier legal decisions, athletes have been permitted to participate in sports despite known medical risks and against medical advice, usually in cases involving missing or nonfunctioning paired organs. In recent years, however, courts have been reluctant to permit athletes to participate in competitive athletics contrary to the team physician's medical recommendation. When an athlete's family seeks to disregard such medical advice against participation, the physician should ask all parents or guardians to sign a written informed consent statement indicating that they have been advised of the potential dangers of participation and that they understand these dangers. The physician should document, with the athlete's signature, that the child or adolescent athlete also understands the risks of participation. To ensure that parents or guardians truly understand the risks and dangers of participation against medical advice, it is recommended that these adults write the statement in their own words and handwriting.[59–62]

Additional information on the effects of medical problems on the risk of injury during sports participation is available in *Care of the Young Athlete* by the American Academy of Orthopaedic Surgeons and the American Academy of Pediatrics[63] and *Preparticipation Physical Evaluation, Third Edition,* by the American Academy of Family Physicians, American Academy of Pediatrics, American College of Sports Medicine, American Medical Society for Sports Medicine, American Orthopaedic Society for Sports Medicine, and American Osteopathic Academy of Sports Medicine.[7] In addition, other American Academy of Pediatrics policy statements include relevant material.[64–67]

TABLE 2   **Medical Conditions and Sports Participation**

Condition	May Participate
Atlantoaxial instability (instability of the joint between cervical vertebrae 1 and 2)	Qualified yes
Explanation: Athlete (particularly if he or she has Down syndrome or juvenile rheumatoid arthritis with cervical involvement) needs evaluation to assess the risk of spinal cord injury during sports participation, especially when using a trampoline.[4–7]	
Bleeding disorder	Qualified yes
Explanation: Athlete needs evaluation.[8,9]	
Cardiovascular disease	
Carditis (inflammation of the heart)	No
Explanation: Carditis may result in sudden death with exertion.	
Hypertension (high blood pressure)	Qualified yes
Explanation: Those with hypertension >5 mm Hg above the 99th percentile for age, gender, and height should avoid heavy weightlifting and power lifting, bodybuilding, and high-static component sports (Fig 1). Those with sustained hypertension (>95th percentile for age, gender, and height) need evaluation.[10–12] The National High Blood Pressure Education Program Working Group report defined prehypertension and stage 1 and stage 2 hypertension in children and adolescents younger than 18 years of age.[10]	
Congenital heart disease (structural heart defects present at birth)	Qualified yes
Explanation: Consultation with a cardiologist is recommended. Those who have mild forms may participate fully in most cases; those who have moderate or severe forms or who have undergone surgery need evaluation. The 36th Bethesda Conference[12] defined mild, moderate, and severe disease for common cardiac lesions.	
Dysrhythmia (irregular heart rhythm)	Qualified yes
Long-QT syndrome	
Malignant ventricular arrhythmias	
Symptomatic Wolff-Parkinson-White syndrome	
Advanced heart block	
Family history of sudden death or previous sudden cardiac event	
Implantation of a cardioverter-defibrillator	
Explanation: Consultation with a cardiologist is advised. Those with symptoms (chest pain, syncope, near-syncope, dizziness, shortness of breath, or other symptoms of possible dysrhythmia) or evidence of mitral regurgitation on physical examination need evaluation. All others may participate fully.[13–15]	
Heart murmur	Qualified yes
Explanation: If the murmur is innocent (does not indicate heart disease), full participation is permitted. Otherwise, athlete needs evaluation (see structural heart disease, especially hypertrophic cardiomyopathy and mitral valve prolapse).	
Structural/acquired heart disease	
Hypertrophic cardiomyopathy	Qualified no
Coronary artery anomalies	Qualified no
Arrhythmogenic right ventricular cardiomyopathy	Qualified no
Acute rheumatic fever with carditis	Qualified no
Ehlers-Danlos syndrome, vascular form	Qualified no
Marfan syndrome	Qualified yes
Mitral valve prolapse	Qualified yes
Anthracycline use	Qualified yes
Explanation: Consultation with a cardiologist is recommended. The 36th Bethesda Conference provided detailed recommendations.[12,13,15–18] Most of these conditions carry a significant risk of sudden cardiac death associated with intense physical exercise. Hypertrophic cardiomyopathy requires thorough and repeated evaluations, because disease may change manifestations during later adolescence.[12,13,17] Marfan syndrome with an aortic aneurysm also can cause sudden death during intense physical exercise.[18] Athlete who has ever received chemotherapy with anthracyclines may be at increased risk of cardiac problems because of the cardiotoxic effects of the medications, and resistance training in this population should be approached with caution; strength training that avoids isometric contractions may be permitted.[19,20] Athlete needs evaluation.	
Vasculitis/vascular disease	Qualified yes
Kawasaki disease (coronary artery vasculitis)	
Pulmonary hypertension	
Explanation: Consultation with a cardiologist is recommended. Athlete needs individual evaluation to assess risk on the basis of disease activity, pathologic changes, and medical regimen.[21]	
Cerebral palsy	Qualified yes
Explanation: Athlete needs evaluation to assess functional capacity to perform sports-specific activity.	
Diabetes mellitus	Yes
Explanation: All sports can be played with proper attention and appropriate adjustments to diet (particularly carbohydrate intake), blood glucose concentrations, hydration, and insulin therapy. Blood glucose concentrations should be monitored before exercise, every 30 min during continuous exercise, 15 min after completion of exercise, and at bedtime.	
Diarrhea, infectious	Qualified no
Explanation: Unless symptoms are mild and athlete is fully hydrated, no participation is permitted, because diarrhea may increase risk of dehydration and heat illness (see fever).	
Eating disorders	Qualified yes
Explanation: Athlete with an eating disorder needs medical and psychiatric assessment before participation.	
Eyes	Qualified yes
Functionally 1-eyed athlete	
Loss of an eye	
Detached retina or family history of retinal detachment at young age	
High myopia	
Connective tissue disorder, such as Marfan or Stickler syndrome	
Previous intraocular eye surgery or serious eye injury	

TABLE 2	Continued

Condition	May Participate
Explanation: A functionally 1-eyed athlete is defined as having best-corrected visual acuity worse than 20/40 in the poorer-seeing eye. Such an athlete would suffer significant disability if the better eye were seriously injured, as would an athlete with loss of an eye. Specifically, boxing and full-contact martial arts are not recommended for functionally 1-eyed athletes, because eye protection is impractical and/or not permitted. Some athletes who previously underwent intraocular eye surgery or had a serious eye injury may have increased risk of injury because of weakened eye tissue. Availability of eye guards approved by the American Society for Testing and Materials and other protective equipment may allow participation in most sports, but this must be judged on an individual basis.[22,23]	
Conjunctivitis, infectious	Qualified no
Explanation: Athlete with active infectious conjunctivitis should be excluded from swimming.	
Fever	No
Explanation: Elevated core temperature may be indicative of a pathologic medical condition (infection or disease) that is often manifest by increased resting metabolism and heart rate. Accordingly, during athlete's usual exercise regimen, the presence of fever can result in greater heat storage, decreased heat tolerance, increased risk of heat illness, increased cardiopulmonary effort, reduced maximal exercise capacity, and increased risk of hypotension because of altered vascular tone and dehydration. On rare occasions, fever may accompany myocarditis or other conditions that may make usual exercise dangerous.	
Gastrointestinal	Qualified yes
Malabsorption syndromes (celiac disease or cystic fibrosis)	
Explanation: Athlete needs individual assessment for general malnutrition or specific deficits resulting in coagulation or other defects; with appropriate treatment, these deficits can be treated adequately to permit normal activities.	
Short-bowel syndrome or other disorders requiring specialized nutritional support, including parenteral or enteral nutrition	
Explanation: Athlete needs individual assessment for collision, contact, or limited-contact sports. Presence of central or peripheral, indwelling, venous catheter may require special considerations for activities and emergency preparedness for unexpected trauma to the device(s).	
Heat illness, history of	Qualified yes
Explanation: Because of the likelihood of recurrence, athlete needs individual assessment to determine the presence of predisposing conditions and behaviors and to develop a prevention strategy that includes sufficient acclimatization (to the environment and to exercise intensity and duration), conditioning, hydration, and salt intake, as well as other effective measures to improve heat tolerance and to reduce heat injury risk (such as protective equipment and uniform configurations).[24,25]	
Hepatitis, infectious (primarily hepatitis C)	Yes
Explanation: All athletes should receive hepatitis B vaccination before participation. Because of the apparent minimal risk to others, all sports may be played as athlete's state of health allows. For all athletes, skin lesions should be covered properly, and athletic personnel should use universal precautions when handling blood or body fluids with visible blood.[26]	
HIV infection	Yes
Explanation: Because of the apparent minimal risk to others, all sports may be played as athlete's state of health allows (especially if viral load is undetectable or very low). For all athletes, skin lesions should be covered properly, and athletic personnel should use universal precautions when handling blood or body fluids with visible blood.[26] However, certain sports (such as wrestling and boxing) may create a situation that favors viral transmission (likely bleeding plus skin breaks). If viral load is detectable, then athletes should be advised to avoid such high-contact sports.	
Kidney, absence of one	Qualified yes
Explanation: Athlete needs individual assessment for contact, collision, and limited-contact sports. Protective equipment may reduce risk of injury to the remaining kidney sufficiently to allow participation in most sports, providing such equipment remains in place during activity.[22]	
Liver, enlarged	Qualified yes
Explanation: If the liver is acutely enlarged, then participation should be avoided because of risk of rupture. If the liver is chronically enlarged, then individual assessment is needed before collision, contact, or limited-contact sports are played. Patients with chronic liver disease may have changes in liver function that affect stamina, mental status, coagulation, or nutritional status.	
Malignant neoplasm	Qualified yes
Explanation: Athlete needs individual assessment.[27]	
Musculoskeletal disorders	Qualified yes
Explanation: Athlete needs individual assessment.	
Neurologic disorders	
History of serious head or spine trauma or abnormality, including craniotomy, epidural bleeding, subdural hematoma, intracerebral hemorrhage, second-impact syndrome, vascular malformation, and neck fracture.[4,5,28–30]	Qualified yes
Explanation: Athlete needs individual assessment for collision, contact, or limited-contact sports.	
History of simple concussion (mild traumatic brain injury), multiple simple concussions, and/or complex concussion	Qualified yes
Explanation: Athlete needs individual assessment. Research supports a conservative approach to concussion management, including no athletic participation while symptomatic or when deficits in judgment or cognition are detected, followed by graduated return to full activity.[28–32]	
Myopathies	Qualified yes
Explanation: Athlete needs individual assessment.	
Recurrent headaches	Yes
Explanation: Athlete needs individual assessment.[33]	
Recurrent plexopathy (burner or stinger) and cervical cord neuropraxia with persistent defects	Qualified yes
Explanation: Athlete needs individual assessment for collision, contact, or limited-contact sports; regaining normal strength is important benchmark for return to play.[34,35]	
Seizure disorder, well controlled	Yes
Explanation: Risk of seizure during participation is minimal.[36]	
Seizure disorder, poorly controlled	Qualified yes
Explanation: Athlete needs individual assessment for collision, contact, or limited-contact sports. The following noncontact sports should be avoided: archery, riflery, swimming, weightlifting, power lifting, strength training, and sports involving heights. In these sports, occurrence of a seizure during activity may pose a risk to self or others.[36]	

TABLE 2   Continued

Condition	May Participate
Obesity	Yes
Explanation: Because of the increased risk of heat illness and cardiovascular strain, obese athlete particularly needs careful acclimatization (to the environment and to exercise intensity and duration), sufficient hydration, and potential activity and recovery modifications during competition and training.[37]	
Organ transplant recipient (and those taking immunosuppressive medications)	Qualified yes
Explanation: Athlete needs individual assessment for contact, collision, and limited-contact sports. In addition to potential risk of infections, some medications (eg, prednisone) may increase tendency for bruising.	
Ovary, absence of one	Yes
Explanation: Risk of severe injury to remaining ovary is minimal.	
Pregnancy/postpartum	Qualified yes
Explanation: Athlete needs individual assessment. As pregnancy progresses, modifications to usual exercise routines will become necessary. Activities with high risk of falling or abdominal trauma should be avoided. Scuba diving and activities posing risk of altitude sickness should also be avoided during pregnancy. After the birth, physiological and morphologic changes of pregnancy take 4 to 6 weeks to return to baseline.[38,39]	
Respiratory conditions	
Pulmonary compromise, including cystic fibrosis	Qualified yes
Explanation: Athlete needs individual assessment but, generally, all sports may be played if oxygenation remains satisfactory during graded exercise test. Athletes with cystic fibrosis need acclimatization and good hydration to reduce risk of heat illness.	
Asthma	Yes
Explanation: With proper medication and education, only athletes with severe asthma need to modify their participation. For those using inhalers, recommend having a written action plan and using a peak flowmeter daily.[40–43] Athletes with asthma may encounter risks when scuba diving.	
Acute upper respiratory infection	Qualified yes
Explanation: Upper respiratory obstruction may affect pulmonary function. Athlete needs individual assessment for all except mild disease (see fever).	
Rheumatologic diseases	Qualified yes
Juvenile rheumatoid arthritis	
Explanation: Athletes with systemic or polyarticular juvenile rheumatoid arthritis and history of cervical spine involvement need radiographs of vertebrae C1 and C2 to assess risk of spinal cord injury. Athletes with systemic or HLA-B27-associated arthritis require cardiovascular assessment for possible cardiac complications during exercise. For those with micrognathia (open bite and exposed teeth), mouth guards are helpful. If uveitis is present, risk of eye damage from trauma is increased; ophthalmologic assessment is recommended. If visually impaired, guidelines for functionally 1-eyed athletes should be followed.[44]	
Juvenile dermatomyositis, idiopathic myositis	
Systemic lupus erythematosis	
Raynaud phenomenon	
Explanation: Athlete with juvenile dermatomyositis or systemic lupus erythematosis with cardiac involvement requires cardiology assessment before participation. Athletes receiving systemic corticosteroid therapy are at higher risk of osteoporotic fractures and avascular necrosis, which should be assessed before clearance; those receiving immunosuppressive medications are at higher risk of serious infection. Sports activities should be avoided when myositis is active. Rhabdomyolysis during intensive exercise may cause renal injury in athletes with idiopathic myositis and other myopathies. Because of photosensitivity with juvenile dermatomyositis and systemic lupus erythematosis, sun protection is necessary during outdoor activities. With Raynaud phenomenon, exposure to the cold presents risk to hands and feet.[45–48]	
Sickle cell disease	Qualified yes
Explanation: Athlete needs individual assessment. In general, if illness status permits, all sports may be played; however, any sport or activity that entails overexertion, overheating, dehydration, or chilling should be avoided. Participation at high altitude, especially when not acclimatized, also poses risk of sickle cell crisis.	
Sickle cell trait	Yes
Explanation: Athletes with sickle cell trait generally do not have increased risk of sudden death or other medical problems during athletic participation under normal environmental conditions. However, when high exertional activity is performed under extreme conditions of heat and humidity or increased altitude, such catastrophic complications have occurred rarely.[8,49–52] Athletes with sickle cell trait, like all athletes, should be progressively acclimatized to the environment and to the intensity and duration of activities and should be sufficiently hydrated to reduce the risk of exertional heat illness and/or rhabdomyolysis.[25] According to National Institutes of Health management guidelines, sickle cell trait is not a contraindication to participation in competitive athletics, and there is no requirement for screening before participation.[53] More research is needed to assess fully potential risks and benefits of screening athletes for sickle cell trait.	
Skin infections, including herpes simplex, molluscum contagiosum, verrucae (warts), staphylococcal and streptococcal infections (furuncles [boils], carbuncles, impetigo, methicillin-resistant *Staphylococcus aureus* [cellulitis and/or abscesses]), scabies, and tinea	Qualified yes
Explanation: During contagious periods, participation in gymnastics or cheerleading with mats, martial arts, wrestling, or other collision, contact, or limited-contact sports is not allowed.[54–57]	
Spleen, enlarged	Qualified yes
Explanation: If the spleen is acutely enlarged, then participation should be avoided because of risk of rupture. If the spleen is chronically enlarged, then individual assessment is needed before collision, contact, or limited-contact sports are played.	
Testicle, undescended or absence of one	Yes
Explanation: Certain sports may require a protective cup.[22]	

This table is designed for use by medical and nonmedical personnel. "Needs evaluation" means that a physician with appropriate knowledge and experience should assess the safety of a given sport for an athlete with the listed medical condition. Unless otherwise noted, this need for special consideration is because of variability in the severity of the disease, the risk of injury for the specific sports listed in Table 1, or both.

INCREASING DYNAMIC COMPONENT →

INCREASING STATIC COMPONENT ↑	A. Low (< 40% Max O_2)	B. Moderate (40-70% Max O_2)	C. High (> 70% Max O_2)
III. High (>50% MVC)	**IIIA (Moderate)** Bobsledding/luge[a,b] Field events (throwing) Gymnastics[a,b] Martial arts[a] Sailing Sport climbing Water skiing[a,b] Weight lifting[a,b] Windsurfing[a,b]	**IIIB (High Moderate)** Body building[a,b] Downhill skiing[a,b] Skateboarding[a,b] Snowboarding[a,b] Wrestling[a]	**IIIC (High)** Boxing[a,c] Canoeing/kayaking Cycling[a,b] Decathlon Rowing Speed-skating[a,b] Triathlon[a,b]
II. Moderate (20-50% MVC)	**IIA (Low Moderate)** Archery Auto racing[a,b] Diving[a,b] Equestrian[a,b] Motorcycling[a,b]	**IIB (Moderate)** American football[a] Field events (jumping) Figure skating[a] Rodeoing[a,b] Rugby[a] Running (sprint) Surfing[a,b] Synchronized swimming[b]	**IIC (High Moderate)** Basketball[a] Ice hockey[a] Cross-country skiing (skating technique) Lacrosse[a] Running (middle distance) Swimming Team handball
I. Low (< 20% MVC)	**IA (Low)** Billiards Bowling Cricket[d] Curling Golf Riflery	**IB (Low Moderate)** Baseball/softball[a] Fencing Table tennis Volleyball	**IC (Moderate)** Badminton Cross-country skiing (classic technique) Field hockey[a] Orienteering Race walking Racquetball/squash Running (long distance) Soccer[a] Tennis

FIGURE 1
Classification of sports according to cardiovascular demands (based on combined static and dynamic components).[12] This classification is based on peak static and dynamic components achieved during competition. It should be noted, however, that the higher values may be reached during training. The increasing dynamic component is defined in terms of the estimated percentage of maximal oxygen uptake (Max O_2) achieved and results in increasing cardiac output. The increasing static component is related to the estimated percentage of maximal voluntary contraction (MVC) reached and results in increasing blood pressure load. Activities with the lowest total cardiovascular demands (cardiac output and blood pressure) are shown in box IA, and those with the highest demands are shown in box IIIC. Boxes IIA and IB depict activities with low/moderate total cardiovascular demands, boxes IIIA, IIB, and IC depict activities with moderate total cardiovascular demands, and boxes IIIB and IIC depict high/moderate total cardiovascular demands. These categories progress diagonally across the graph from lower left to upper right. [a] Danger of bodily collision. [b] Increased risk if syncope occurs. [c] Participation is not recommended by the American Academy of Pediatrics.[2] [d] The American Academy of Pediatrics classifies cricket in the IB box (low static component and moderate dynamic component).[58] (Reproduced with permission from Mitchell JH, Haskell W, Snell P, Van Camp SP. 36th Bethesda Conference. Task force 8: classification of sports. *J Am Coll Cardiol.* 2005;45(8):1364–1367.)

COUNCIL ON SPORTS MEDICINE AND FITNESS, EXECUTIVE COMMITTEE, 2006–2007

Eric W. Small, MD, Chairperson
Teri M. McCambridge, MD, Chairperson-elect
Holly Benjamin, MD
David T. Bernhardt, MD
Joel S. Brenner, MD, MPH
Charles Cappetta, MD
Joseph A. Congeni, MD
Andrew J. Gregory, MD
Bernard A. Griesemer, MD
Frederick E. Reed, MD
Stephen G. Rice, MD, PhD, MPH

PAST MEMBERS

Jorge E. Gomez, MD
Douglas B. Gregory, MD
Paul R. Stricker, MD

LIAISONS

Claire Marie Ann LeBlanc, MD
  Canadian Paediatric Society
James Raynor, MS, ATC
  National Athletic Trainers Association

CONSULTANT

Michael F. Bergeron, PhD

STAFF

Anjie Emanuel, MPH
Jeanne Lindros, MPH

REFERENCES

1. American Academy of Pediatrics, Committee on Sports Medicine and Fitness. Medical conditions affecting sports participation. *Pediatrics.* 2001;107(5):1205–1209
2. American Academy of Pediatrics, Committee on Sports Medicine and Fitness. Participation in boxing by children, adolescents, and young adults. *Pediatrics.* 1997;99(1):134–135
3. American Academy of Pediatrics, Committee on Sports Medicine and Fitness. Safety in youth ice hockey: the effects of body checking. *Pediatrics.* 2000;105(3):657–658
4. American Academy of Pediatrics, Committee on Injury and Poison Prevention, Committee on Sports Medicine and Fitness.

Trampolines at home, school, and recreational centers. *Pediatrics.* 1999;103(5):1053–1056

5. Maranich AM, Hamele M, Fairchok MP. Atlanto-axial subluxation: a newly reported trampolining injury. *Clin Pediatr (Phila).* 2006;45(5):468–470

6. American Academy of Pediatrics, Committee on Sports Medicine and Fitness. Atlanto-axial instability in Down syndrome: subject review. *Pediatrics.* 1995;96(1):151–154

7. American Academy of Family Physicians, American Academy of Pediatrics, American College of Sports Medicine, American Medical Society for Sports Medicine, American Orthopaedic Society for Sports Medicine, American Osteopathic Academy of Sports Medicine. *Preparticipation Physical Evaluation.* 3rd ed. New York, NY: McGraw-Hill; 2004

8. Mercer KW, Densmore JJ. Hematologic disorders in the athlete. *Clin Sports Med.* 2005;24(3):599–621

9. National Hemophilia Foundation. *Playing It Safe: Bleeding Disorders, Sports and Exercise.* New York, NY: National Hemophilia Foundation; 2005

10. National High Blood Pressure Education Program Working Group on High Blood Pressure in Children and Adolescents. The fourth report on the diagnosis, evaluation, and treatment of high blood pressure in children and adolescents. *Pediatrics.* 2004;114(2 suppl):555–576

11. American Academy of Pediatrics, Committee on Sports Medicine and Fitness. Athletic participation by children and adolescents who have systemic hypertension. *Pediatrics.* 1997;99(4):637–638

12. American College of Cardiology Foundation. 36th Bethesda Conference: eligibility recommendations for competitive athletes with cardiovascular abnormalities. *J Am Coll Cardiol.* 2005; 45(8):1313–1375

13. Maron BJ, Thompson PD, Ackerman MJ, et al. Recommendations and considerations related to preparticipation screening for cardiovascular abnormalities in competitive athletes: 2007 update: a scientific statement from the American Heart Association Council on Nutrition, Physical Activity and Metabolism: endorsed by the American College of Cardiology Foundation. *Circulation.* 2007;115(12):1643–1655

14. American Academy of Pediatrics, Committee on Sports Medicine and Fitness. Cardiac dysrhythmias and sports. *Pediatrics.* 1995;95(5):786–788

15. Freed LA, Levy D, Levine RA, et al. Prevalence and clinical outcome of mitral-valve prolapse. *N Engl J Med.* 1999;341(1): 1–7

16. Maron BJ. Sudden death in young athletes. *N Engl J Med.* 2003;349(11):1064–1075

17. Maron BJ. Hypertrophic cardiomyopathy: a systematic review. *JAMA.* 2002;287(10):1308–1320

18. Pyeritz RE. The Marfan syndrome. *Annu Rev Med.* 2000;51: 481–510

19. American Academy of Pediatrics, Council on Sports Medicine and Fitness. Strength training by children and adolescents. *Pediatrics.* 2008;121(4):835–840

20. Steinherz L, Steinherz P, Tan C, et al. Cardiac toxicity 4 to 20 years after completing anthracycline therapy. *JAMA.* 1991; 266(12):1672–1677

21. Newburger JW, Takahashi M, Gerber MA, et al. Diagnosis, treatment, and long-term management of Kawasaki disease: a statement for health professionals from the Committee on Rheumatic Fever, Endocarditis, and Kawasaki Disease, Council on Cardiovascular Disease in the Young, American Heart Association. *Pediatrics.* 2004;114(6):1708–1733

22. Gomez JE. Paired organ loss. In: Delee JC, Drez D Jr, Miller MD, eds. *Delee and Drez's Orthopaedic Sports Medicine: Principles and Practice.* 2nd ed. Philadelphia, PA: Saunders; 2003:264–271

23. American Academy of Pediatrics, Committee on Sports Medi-cine and Fitness. Protective eyewear for young athletes. *Pediatrics.* 2004;113(3):619–622

24. American Academy of Pediatrics, Committee on Sports Medicine and Fitness. Climatic heat stress and the exercising child and adolescent. *Pediatrics.* 2000;106(1):158–159

25. Bergeron MF, McKeag DB, Casa DJ, et al. Youth football: heat stress and injury risk. *Med Sci Sports Exerc.* 2005;37(8): 1421–1430

26. American Academy of Pediatrics, Committee on Sports Medicine and Fitness. Human immunodeficiency virus and other blood-borne viral pathogens in the athletic setting. *Pediatrics.* 1999;104(6):1400–1403

27. Dickerman JD. The late effects of childhood cancer therapy. *Pediatrics.* 2007;119(3):554–568

28. Wojtys EM, Hovda D, Landry G, et al. Current concepts: concussion in sports. *Am J Sports Med.* 1999;27(5):676–687

29. McCrory P, Johnston K, Meeuwisse W, et al. Summary and agreement statement of the 2nd International Conference on Concussion in Sport, Prague 2004. *Clin J Sport Med.* 2005;15(2): 48–55

30. Aubry M, Cantu R, Dvorak J, et al. Summary and agreement statement of the 1st International Symposium on Concussion in Sport, Vienna 2001. *Clin J Sport Med.* 2002;12(1):6–11

31. Herring SA, Bergfeld JA, Boland A, et al. Concussion (mild traumatic brain injury) and the team physician: a consensus statement. *Med Sci Sports Exerc.* 2006;38(2):395–399

32. Guskiewicz KM, Bruce SL, Cantu RC, et al. National Athletic Trainers' Association position statement: management of sport-related concussion. *J Athl Train.* 2004;39(3):280–297

33. Lewis DW, Ashwal S, Dahl G, et al. Practice parameter: evaluation of children and adolescents with recurrent headaches: report of the Quality Standards Subcommittee of the American Academy of Neurology and the Practice Committee of the Child Neurology Society. *Neurology.* 2002;59(4):490–498

34. Castro FP Jr. Stingers, cervical cord neuropraxia, and stenosis. *Clin Sports Med.* 2003;22(3):483–492

35. Weinberg J, Rokito S, Silber JS. Etiology, treatment, and prevention of athletic "stingers." *Clin Sports Med.* 2003;22(3): 493–500, viii

36. Hirtz D, Berg A, Bettis D, et al. Practice parameter: treatment of the child with a first unprovoked seizure: report of the Quality Standards Subcommittee of the American Academy of Neurology and the Practice Committee of the Child Neurology Society. *Neurology.* 2003;60(2):166–175

37. American Academy of Pediatrics, Council on Sports Medicine and Fitness and Council on School Health. Active healthy living: prevention of childhood obesity through increased physical activity. *Pediatrics.* 2006;117(5):1834–1842

38. American College of Obstetricians and Gynecologists, Committee on Obstetric Practice. ACOG committee opinion: exercise during pregnancy and the postpartum period. *Obstet Gynecol.* 2002;99(1):171–173

39. Morales M, Dumps P, Extermann P. Pregnancy and scuba diving: what precautions? [in French]. *J Gynecol Obstet Biol Reprod (Paris).* 1999;28(2):118–123

40. National Heart, Lung, and Blood Institute. *National Asthma Education and Prevention Program Expert Panel Report 3: Guidelines for the Diagnosis and Management of Asthma: Full Report.* Bethesda, MD: National Institutes of Health; 2007. Available at: www.nhlbi.nih.gov/guidelines/asthma/asthupdt.htm. Accessed October 2, 2007

41. American College of Allergy, Asthma, and Immunology. *Asthma Disease Management Resource Manual.* Arlington Heights, IL: American College of Allergy, Asthma, and Immunology. Available at: www.acaai.org/Member/Practice_Resources/manual.htm. Accessed November 17, 2006

42. Storms WW. Review of exercise-induced asthma. *Med Sci Sports Exerc.* 2003;35(9):1464–1470

43. Holzer K, Brukner P. Screening of athletes for exercise-induced bronchospasm. *Clin J Sport Med.* 2004;14(3):134–138

44. Giannini MJ, Protas EJ. Exercise response in children with and without juvenile rheumatoid arthritis: a case-comparison study. *Phys Ther.* 1992;72(5):365–372

45. Tench C, Bentley D, Vleck V, McCurdie I, White P, D'Cruz D. Aerobic fitness, fatigue, and physical disability in systemic lupus erythematosis. *J Rheumatol.* 2002;29(3):474–481

46. Carvalho MR, Sato EI, Tebexreni AS, Heidecher RT, Schenckman S, Neto TL. Effects of supervised cardiovascular training program on exercise tolerance, aerobic capacity, and quality of life in patients with systemic lupus erythematosis. *Arthritis Rheum.* 2005;53(6):838–844

47. Hicks JE, Drinkard B, Summers RM, Rider LG. Decreased aerobic capacity in children with juvenile dermatomyositis. *Arthritis Rheum.* 2002;47(2):118–123

48. Clarkson PM, Kearns AK, Rouzier P, Rubin R, Thompson PD. Serum creatine kinase levels and renal function measures in exertional muscle damage. *Med Sci Sports Exerc.* 2006;38(4):623–627

49. Pretzlaff RK. Death of an adolescent athlete with sickle cell trait caused by exertional heat stroke. *Pediatr Crit Care Med.* 2002;3(3):308–310

50. Kark J. *Sickle Cell Trait.* Washington, DC: Howard University School of Medicine; 2000. Available at: http://sickle.bwh.harvard.edu/sickle_trait.html. Accessed November 17, 2006

51. Kerle KK, Nishimura KD. Exertional collapse and sudden death associated with sickle cell trait. *Am Fam Physician.* 1996;54(1):237–240

52. Bergeron MF, Cannon JG, Hall EL, Kutlar A. Erythrocyte sickling during exercise and thermal stress. *Clin J Sport Med.* 2004;14(6):354–356

53. National Heart, Lung, and Blood Institute. *The Management of Sickle Cell Disease.* 4th ed. Bethesda, MD: National Institutes of Health; 2002:15–18. NIH publication 02-2117

54. Mast EE, Goodman RA. Prevention of infectious disease transmission in sports. *Sports Med.* 1997;24(1):1–7

55. Sevier TL. Infectious disease in athletes. *Med Clin North Am.* 1994;78(2):389–412

56. Centers for Disease Control and Prevention. Methicillin-resistant *Staphylococcus aureus* infections among competitive sports participants: Colorado, Indiana, Pennsylvania, and Los Angeles County, 2000–2003. *MMWR Morb Mortal Wkly Rep.* 2003;52(33):793–795. Available at: www.cdc.gov/mmwr/preview/mmwrhtml/mm5233a4.htm. Accessed November 17, 2006

57. Centers for Disease Control and Prevention. Community-associated MRSA information for clinicians. Available at: www.cdc.gov/ncidod/dhqp/ar_mrsa_ca_clinicians.html. Accessed November 17, 2006

58. American Academy of Pediatrics. General physical activities defined by level of intensity. Available at: www.aap.org/sections/seniormembers/docs/Fit-ActvsIntensity.pdf. Accessed October 2, 2007

59. Baxter JS. Legal aspects of sports medicine. In: Garrick JG, ed. *Orthopaedic Knowledge Update: Sports Medicine 3.* Rosemont, IL: American Academy of Orthopaedic Surgeons; 2004:397–402

60. Mitten MJ. When is disqualification from sports justified? Medical judgment vs patients' rights. *Phys Sports Med.* 1996;24(10):75–78

61. Mitten MJ. Emerging legal issues in sports medicine: a synthesis, summary, and analysis. *St John's Law Rev.* 2002;76(1):5–86

62. Mitten MJ. Legal issues affecting medical clearance to resume play after mild brain injury. *Clin J Sport Med.* 2001;11(3):199–202

63. Sullivan JA, Anderson SJ, eds. *Care of the Young Athlete.* Elk Grove Village, IL: American Academy of Pediatrics; 2000

64. Washington RL, Bernhardt DT, Gomez J, et al. Organized sports for children and preadolescents. *Pediatrics.* 2001;107(6):1459–1462

65. American Academy of Pediatrics, Committee on Sports Medicine and Fitness. Risk of injury from baseball and softball in children. *Pediatrics.* 2001;107(4):782–784

66. American Academy of Pediatrics, Committee on Sports Medicine and Fitness. Intensive training and sports specialization in young athletes. *Pediatrics.* 2000;106(1):154–157

67. American Academy of Pediatrics, Committee on Sports Medicine and Fitness. Promotion of healthy weight-control practices in young athletes. *Pediatrics.* 2005;116(6):1557–1564

ADDITIONAL RESOURCE

Brenner JS, American Academy of Pediatrics, Council on Sports Medicine and Fitness. Overuse injuries, overtraining, and burnout in athletes. *Pediatrics.* 2007;119(6):1232–1241

AMERICAN ACADEMY OF PEDIATRICS

Committee on Sports Medicine and Fitness and Committee on School Health

Organized Sports for Children and Preadolescents

ABSTRACT. Participation in organized sports provides an opportunity for young people to increase their physical activity and develop physical and social skills. However, when the demands and expectations of organized sports exceed the maturation and readiness of the participant, the positive aspects of participation can be negated. The nature of parental or adult involvement can also influence the degree to which participation in organized sports is a positive experience for preadolescents. This updates a previous policy statement on athletics for preadolescents and incorporates guidelines for sports participation for preschool children. Recommendations are offered on how pediatricians can help determine a child's readiness to participate, how risks can be minimized, and how child-oriented goals can be maximized.

INTRODUCTION

Participation in organized sports can have physical and social benefits for children. However, the younger the participant, the greater the concern about safety and benefits. The involvement of preadolescents in organized sports is a relatively recent phenomenon. In the early 20th century, physical activity was a more regular part of life for the average child. Sports and games provided an additional outlet for physical activity and were characterized by play that was generally spontaneous, unstructured, and without adult involvement. Participation in such sports and games allowed for development of motor skills, social interaction, creativity, and enjoyment for participants.

During the latter part of the 20th century, "free play" or unstructured games primarily gave way to organized sports. The starting age for organized sports programs has also evolved to the point that infant and preschool training programs are now available for many sports. Organization of sports has potential benefits of coaching, supervision, safety rules, and proper equipment but can also create demands and expectations that exceed the readiness and capabilities of young participants. Organization can also shift the focus to goals that are not necessarily child oriented. Clearly, the nature of the organization can determine if it has a positive or negative influence.

This statement is an update to a previous policy statement on athletics for preadolescents[1] and incorporates guidelines for sports participation for preschool children.[2] Recommendations are made on

how pediatricians can help determine a child's readiness to participate in organized sports, how risks can be minimized, and how child-oriented goals can be maximized.

ORGANIZED SPORTS PROGRAMS: LIMITATIONS AND RISKS

The effects of organized sports participation on growth and maturation have come under question, as have the effects of growth and maturation on the ability to participate in sports. Because children are beginning to train and compete at earlier ages, there is increasing concern about potential negative effects on growth and maturation. Reports of gymnasts and divers with short stature or ballet dancers with lean body types or late menarche have contributed to such concerns. Despite such reports, it is unclear if these characteristics were a result of intensive training or other factors, such as dietary practices, psychological and emotional stress, or selection bias for the sport.[3]

The effects of immaturity on sports participation are more obvious. When the demands of a sport exceed a child's cognitive and physical development, the child may develop feelings of failure and frustration. Even with coaches available to teach rules and skills of a sport, children may not be ready to learn or understand what is being taught. Furthermore, many coaches are not equipped to deal with the needs or abilities of children. Basic motor skills, such as throwing, catching, kicking, and hitting a ball, do not develop sooner simply as a result of introducing them to children at an earlier age.[4] Teaching or expecting these skills to develop before children are developmentally ready is more likely to cause frustration than long-term success in the sport.[5] Because most youth sports coaches are volunteers with little or no formal training in child development, they cannot be expected to correctly match demands of a sport with a child's readiness to participate. Educational programs are available for youth sports coaches, but most coaches do not participate. Nonetheless, coaches may still try to teach what often cannot be learned and blame resulting failures on shortcomings of athletes or themselves.

Parental or adult supervision of children's activity is usually considered to be desirable. However, in organized sports, inappropriate or overzealous parental or adult influences can have negative effects. Adults' involvement in children's sports activities may bring goals or outcome measures that are not oriented toward young participants. Tournaments, all-star teams, most valuable player awards, trophies, and awards banquets are by-products of adult influences. Despite good intentions, increased involvement of adults does not necessarily enhance the child athlete's enjoyment. The familiar image of a parent imploring their 5-year-old to "catch the ball," "kick the ball," or "run faster" is a reminder of how adult encouragement can have discouraging effects.

ORGANIZED SPORTS PROGRAMS: BENEFITS

In contrast to unstructured or free play, participation in organized sports provides a greater opportunity to develop rules specifically designed for health and safety. Organization can allow for the establishment of developmentally sound criteria for determining readiness to play. Organization can also allow for a fair process in choosing teams,[6] matching competitors,[7] and enforcing rules. Rules specifically targeted at younger athletes can reduce injuries. Recommendations have been made to limit dangerous practices, such as headfirst sliding in baseball[8] and body checking in hockey.[9] Safety accommodations associated with organized youth sports can also include smaller playing fields, shorter contest times, pitch counts for Little League pitchers, softer baseballs, matching opponents by weight in youth football, and adjusting play for extreme climatic conditions.[10] The availability of qualified coaches in organized sports can be a key factor in providing safety and a positive experience.

In this regard, the effects of organization provide positive environments for young participants. Unfortunately, not all youth sports participants have access to all known safety measures. Furthermore, a great deal remains to be learned about safety in youth sports. Additional resources are needed to study injury prevention and ensure that all participants will benefit from existing safety measures. The prospects for additional development and implementation of safety measures are far greater for organized sports than for unstructured free play.

Despite many potential benefits of organization, there is no consensus as to the overall value of organized sports for preadolescents. A return to the days of free play has been suggested as one means to eliminate negative aspects of organized sports. Unfortunately, the days when children had the time, opportunity, or inclination to play in neighborhoods or local parks have passed. Today, there are more demands on a young person's time, more options for free time, diminished requirements for regular physical activity, and fewer opportunities for free play. School-based physical education programs have also been reduced throughout the years and can no longer be relied on to provide adequate levels of healthy activity.[11]

Regular physical activity can help reduce the risk of many adult health problems, including diabetes, obesity, and heart disease.[12] However, with less time dedicated to free play and school physical education programs, the result may be lower activity levels and lower levels of fitness for children. There is a greater need to protect opportunities for structured and unstructured physical activity for children. Organized sports may not provide all physical activity needs but can be a viable means to increase activity levels in children and, hopefully, lead to the adoption of active lifestyles as adults.

Organized Sports Programs: Optimizing the Benefit-to-Risk Ratio

If organized sports are going to be safe, healthy, and beneficial for children and preadolescents, there must be reasonable goals for participation and appropriate strategies to attain these goals. Reasonable goals for children and preadolescents participating in organized sports include acquisition of basic motor skills, increasing physical activity levels, learning social skills necessary to work as a team, learning good sportsmanship, and having fun.[13]

Organized sports sessions should be tailored to match the developmental level of participants. Most preschool children have short attention spans and are easily distracted; therefore, exercise sessions should be short and emphasize playfulness, experimentation, and exploration of a wide variety of movement experiences. A reasonable format would consist of no longer than 15 to 20 minutes of structured activity combined with 30 minutes of free play. Concentration will be maximized if instructional sessions take place in a setting with minimal distraction. Instructing younger children using a show-and-tell format with physical demonstration may be more effective than with verbal instruction.

For children and preadolescents, factors such as fun, success, variety, freedom, family participation, peer support, and enthusiastic leadership encourage and maintain participation, whereas others such as failure, embarrassment, competition, boredom, regimentation, and injuries discourage subsequent participation.[14]

Pediatricians, as experts in child development, can help parents and coaches determine readiness of a child to participate in organized sports. Readiness is often defined relative to the demands of the sport. Because different sports and even the same sport may vary widely with respect to demands and expectations, pediatricians must understand these demands to help determine if they are appropriate for the physical and cognitive maturation of participants. Preparticipation examinations are typically not mandated until junior high and high school. However, annual examinations for younger children afford an opportunity to promote physical activity and address issues of readiness as they apply to organized sports.

Pediatricians can further advocate safe sports participation by promoting better education and training of youth sports coaches. Standards for coaching competency are available, and certification for youth sports coaches should address these competencies.[15] In addition, pediatricians can work with sports administrators and coaches within their community to share relevant information on child development, injury assessment, first aid, and injury prevention. Pediatricians can also take an active role in developing safety programs while ensuring that existing safety measures are observed. A pediatrician may be one of the few adults who can objectively determine when pressures and expectations of organized sports become excessive for any individual or group. Finally, pediatricians can serve as role models for appropriate sideline behavior and can help parents and other adults remember the reasons children want to participate.

SUMMARY AND RECOMMENDATIONS

Organized sports for children and preadolescents provide an opportunity for increased physical activity and an opportunity to learn sports and team skills in an environment where risks of participation can potentially be controlled. Unfortunately, when demands and expectations of the sport exceed the maturation or readiness of the participant, benefits of participation are offset. The shift from child-oriented goals to adult-oriented goals can further negate positive aspects of organized sports.

To optimize the safety and benefits of organized sports for children and preadolescents and to preserve this valuable opportunity for young people to increase their physical activity levels, the American Academy of Pediatrics recommends the following:

1. Organized sports programs for preadolescents should complement, not replace, the regular physical activity that is a part of free play, child-organized games, recreational sports, and physical education programs in the schools. Regular physical activity should be encouraged for all children whether they participate in organized sports or not.
2. Pediatricians are encouraged to help assess developmental readiness and medical suitability for children and preadolescents to participate in organized sports and assist in matching a child's physical, social, and cognitive maturity with appropriate sports activities.
3. Pediatricians can take an active role in youth sports organizations by educating coaches about developmental and safety issues, monitoring the health and safety of children involved in organized sports, and advising committees on rules and safety.
4. Pediatricians are encouraged to take an active role in identifying and preserving goals of sports that best serve young athletes.
5. Additional research and resources are needed to:
   a. determine the optimal time for children to begin participating in organized sports;
   b. identify safe and effective training strategies for growing and developing athletes;
   c. educate youth sports coaches about unique needs and characteristics of young athletes; and
   d. develop effective injury prevention strategies.

COMMITTEE ON SPORTS MEDICINE AND FITNESS, 2000–2001
Reginald L. Washington, MD, Chairperson
David T. Bernhardt, MD
Jorge Gomez, MD
Miriam D. Johnson, MD
Thomas J. Martin, MD

Thomas W. Rowland, MD
Eric Small, MD

LIAISONS
Claire LeBlanc, MD
  Canadian Pediatric Society
Carl Krein, AT, PT
  National Athletic Trainers Association
Robert Malina, PhD
  Institute for the Study of Youth Sports
Judith C. Young, PhD
  National Association for Sport and Physical Education

SECTION LIAISON
Frederick E. Reed, MD
  Section on Orthopaedics

CONSULTANTS
Steven Anderson, MD
Stephen Bolduc, MD
Oded Bar-Or, MD

STAFF
Heather Newland

COMMITTEE ON SCHOOL HEALTH, 2000–2001
Howard L. Taras, MD, Chairperson
David A. Cimino, MD
Jane W. McGrath, MD
Robert D. Murray, MD
Wayne A. Yankus, MD
Thomas L. Young, MD

LIAISONS
Missy Fleming, PhD
  American Medical Association
Maureen Glendon, RNCS, MSN, CRNP
  National Association of Pediatric Nurse Practitioners
Lois Harrison-Jones, EdD
  American Association of School Administrators
Jerald L. Newberry, MEd, Executive Director
  National Education Association, Health Information Network
Evan Pattishall III, MD
  American School Health Association
Mary Vernon, MD, MPH
  Centers for Disease Control and Prevention
Linda Wolfe, RN, BSN, MEd, CSN
  National Association of School Nurses

STAFF
Su Li, MPA

REFERENCES

1. American Academy of Pediatrics, Committee on Sports Medicine and Fitness. Organized athletics for preadolescent children. *Pediatrics.* 1989; 84:583
2. American Academy of Pediatrics, Committee on Sports Medicine and Fitness. Fitness, activity, and sports participation in the preschool child. *Pediatrics.* 1992;90:1002–1004
3. Malina RM. Physical growth and biological maturation of young athletes. *Exerc Sports Sci Rev.* 1994;22:389–433
4. Branta C, Haubenstricker J, Seefeldt V. Age changes in motor skills during childhood and adolescence. *Exerc Sports Sci Rev.* 1984;12:467–520
5. Stryer B, Toffler IR, Lapchick R. A developmental overview of child and youth sports in society. *Child Adolesc Psychiatr Clin North Am.* 1998;7: 697–724
6. Kamm RL. A developmental and psychoeducational approach to reducing conflict and abuse in Little League and youth sports. *Child Adolesc Psychiatr Clin North Am.* 1998;7:891–918

7. Roemmich JN, Rogol A. Physiology of growth and development: its relationship to performance in the young athlete. *Clin Sports Med.* 1995;14:483–503

8. American Academy of Pediatrics, Committee on Sports Medicine and Fitness. Risk of injury from baseball and softball in children. *Pediatrics.* 2000;107:782–784

9. American Academy of Pediatrics, Committee on Sports Medicine and Fitness. Safety in youth ice hockey: the effects of body checking. *Pediatrics.* 2000;105:657–658

10. American Academy of Pediatrics, Committee on Sports Medicine and Fitness. Climatic heat stress and the exercising child. *Pediatrics.* 2000; 106:158–159

11. American Academy of Pediatrics, Committee on Sports Medicine and Fitness. Physical fitness and the schools. *Pediatrics.* 2000;105:1156–1157

12. US Department of Health and Human Services. *Physical Activity and Health: A Report of the Surgeon General.* Atlanta, GA: Centers for Disease Control and Prevention; 1996

13. Martens R, Seefeldt V, eds. *Guidelines for Children's Sports.* Reston, VA: National Association for Sport and Physical Education; 1979:1–47

14. Rowland TW. Clinical approaches to the sedentary child. In: *Exercise and Children's Health.* Champaign, IL: Human Kinetics Books; 1990:259–274

15. National Association for Sport and Physical Education. *National Standards for Athletic Coaches: Quality Coaches, Quality Sports.* Dubuque, IA: Kendall/Hunt Publishing Co; 1995:1–124

Overuse Injuries, Overtraining, and Burnout in Child and Adolescent Athletes

Guidance for the Clinician in Rendering Pediatric Care

Joel S. Brenner, MD, MPH, and the Council on Sports Medicine and Fitness

ABSTRACT

Overuse is one of the most common etiologic factors that lead to injuries in the pediatric and adolescent athlete. As more children are becoming involved in organized and recreational athletics, the incidence of overuse injuries is increasing. Many children are participating in sports year-round and sometimes on multiple teams simultaneously. This overtraining can lead to burnout, which may have a detrimental effect on the child participating in sports as a lifelong healthy activity. One contributing factor to overtraining may be parental pressure to compete and succeed. The purpose of this clinical report is to assist pediatricians in identifying and counseling at-risk children and their families. This report supports the American Academy of Pediatrics policy statement on intensive training and sport specialization.

INTRODUCTION

Overuse injuries, overtraining, and burnout among child and adolescent athletes are a growing problem in the United States. Although inactivity and obesity are on the rise, the number of children and adolescents who participate in organized or recreational athletics has grown considerably over the past 2 decades. It is estimated that 30 to 45 million youth 6 to 18 years of age participate in some form of athletics. Sports participation is more accessible to all youth, from recreational play and school activities, to highly organized and competitive traveling teams, to pre-Olympic training opportunities. The variety of available, organized sporting activities has also grown from the typical American favorites, such as football, baseball, and soccer, to include lacrosse, field hockey, rugby, cheerleading, and dance, each with its own list of sports medicine concerns. This report will assist the clinician managing young athletes by first defining the medical, psychological, and developmental concerns of intensive, focused athletic participation. In addition, it will highlight specific overtraining issues such as participation in endurance events, weekend athletic tournaments, year-round training on multiple teams, and the multisport athlete. This clinical report should be used in conjunction with the American Academy of Pediatrics policy statement on intensive training and sports specialization in young athletes.[1] There is currently a very small body of scientific evidence pertaining to these issues. Therefore, some of the recommendations are based on committee opinion and/or expertise.

www.pediatrics.org/cgi/doi/10.1542/peds.2007-0887

doi:10.1542/peds.2007-0887

All clinical reports from the American Academy of Pediatrics automatically expire 5 years after publication unless reaffirmed, revised, or retired at or before that time.

The guidance in this report does not indicate an exclusive course of treatment or serve as a standard of medical care. Variations, taking into account individual circumstances, may be appropriate.

Key Words
overuse, injuries, overtraining, burnout, athlete

PEDIATRICS (ISSN Numbers: Print, 0031-4005; Online, 1098-4275). Copyright © 2007 by the American Academy of Pediatrics

Overuse Injuries

An overuse injury is microtraumatic damage to a bone, muscle, or tendon that has been subjected to repetitive stress without sufficient time to heal or undergo the natural reparative process. Overuse injuries can be classified into 4 stages: (1) pain in the affected area after physical activity; (2) pain during the activity, without restricting performance; (3) pain during the activity that restricts performance; and (4) chronic, unremitting pain even at rest.[2] The incidence of overuse injuries in the young athlete has paralleled the growth of youth participation in sports. Up to 50% of all injuries seen in pediatric sports medicine are related to overuse.[3]

The risks of overuse are more serious in the pediatric/adolescent athlete for several reasons. The growing bones of the young athlete cannot handle as much stress as the mature bones of adults.[4,5] For example, a young baseball pitcher who has not yet learned proper throwing mechanics (ie, recruiting the entire kinetic chain—from foot to hand—instead of just the arm) is at risk of traction apophysitis of the medial elbow. A young gymnast who performs repetitive hyperextension activities may develop spondylolysis (ie, a stress fracture of the spine), which is an injury particular to the pediatric age group. In addition, young swimmers may not recognize signs of rotator cuff tendonitis, because they may be unable to cognitively connect vague symptoms, such as fatigue or poor performance, as a sign of injury. Identifying youth at risk of overuse injuries is the first step to prevention. Guidelines for parents, coaches, and athletes need to be developed to provide opportunities for education, injury reduction, and early recognition of overuse injuries.

Overtraining

A question often asked of the practitioner who cares for young athletes is, "How much athletic training is too much?" There are no scientifically determined guidelines to help define how much exercise is healthy and beneficial to the young athlete compared with what might be harmful and represent overtraining. However, injuries tend to be more common during peak growth velocity, and some are more likely to occur if underlying biomechanical problems are present.

A sound training regimen is essential, recognizing that although repetition is important, it may induce harm. Sport-specific drills that use a variety of modalities, such as water running for the track athlete on alternate days, may provide similar fitness benefits with less stress to the body. The American Academy of Pediatrics Council on Sports Medicine and Fitness recommends limiting 1 sporting activity to a maximum of 5 days per week with at least 1 day off from any organized physical activity. In addition, athletes should have at least 2 to 3 months off per year from their particular sport during which they can let injuries heal, refresh the

mind, and work on strength, conditioning, and proprioception in hopes of reducing injury risk. In addition to overuse injuries, if the body is not given sufficient time to regenerate and refresh, the youth may be at risk of "burnout."

"Burnout" or Overtraining Syndrome

Burnout, or overtraining syndrome, has been well described in the literature for adult athletes, but little is found regarding its applicability in youth. The overtraining syndrome can be defined as a "series of psychological, physiologic, and hormonal changes that result in decreased sports performance."[6] Common manifestations may include chronic muscle or joint pain, personality changes, elevated resting heart rate, and decreased sports performance.[6,7] The pediatric athlete may also have fatigue, lack of enthusiasm about practice or competition, or difficulty with successfully completing usual routines. Burnout should be recognized as a serious sequela of overtraining syndrome. Prevention of burnout should be addressed by encouraging the athlete to become well rounded and well versed in a variety of activities rather than 1 particular sport. The following guidelines are suggested to prevent overtraining/burnout:

1. Keep workouts interesting, with age-appropriate games and training, to keep practice fun.

2. Take time off from organized or structured sports participation 1 to 2 days per week to allow the body to rest or participate in other activities.

3. Permit longer scheduled breaks from training and competition every 2 to 3 months while focusing on other activities and cross-training to prevent loss of skill or level of conditioning.

4. Focus on wellness and teaching athletes to be in tune with their bodies for cues to slow down or alter their training methods.[6]

Endurance Events

Endurance athletic events (triathlons, marathons, and half-marathons) are becoming more popular in the United States, and legitimate concerns have been raised for the safety of youth participating in these events. The American Academy of Pediatrics has stated that triathlons for children and adolescents are reasonably safe as long as the events are modified to be age appropriate.[8] Specifically, such events should be of shorter duration/length, and careful attention should be given to safety and environmental conditions.[8,9] Children and adolescents must be properly trained to avoid hypothermia or hyperthermia, overtraining, overuse injuries, and burnout.

Recent concerns regarding the participation of children in marathon running has led to different opinions being expressed in the literature.[10–12] There is, at present, no scientific evidence that supports or refutes the safety of children who participate in marathons. There are no recorded data on injuries sustained by children who run marathons. Marathon training requires a gradual increase in total weekly mileage, which may be less than or equal to the total weekly distance that is generally logged by high school cross-country teams (35–40 miles). Regardless, a clearly devised weekly plan, ensuring that safe running conditions are in place, and the provision of proper education on endurance activities (including environmental conditions and appropriate hydration) should all be part of the training process. A critical environmental safety concern is the ambient temperature and relative humidity, because a child is less able than an adult to handle heat stress.[13] Weather-related guidelines have been set for all marathons, and these guidelines should be strictly enforced by the medical director for all youth endurance events.[14] Ultimately, there is no reason to disallow participation of a young athlete in a properly run marathon as long as the athlete enjoys the activity and is asymptomatic.[15]

Weekend Athletic Tournaments

Weekend-long sports tournaments for soccer, baseball, or tennis are common across the country. Often, these athletes are actively participating at least 6 hours each day in their sport and are exposed to the associated weather elements for an additional 2 to 3 hours. The risks associated with these events include heat-related illness, nutritional deficiencies, overuse injuries (eg, pitching in multiple games over a 48-hour span), and burnout from having a lack of "free time." Research examining the possibility of fatigue contributing to an increased injury risk in the tournament situation does not exist, but the general overtraining-prevention guidelines outlined earlier should also apply.

Year-Round Training on Multiple Teams

Single-sport, year-round training and competition is becoming more common for children and adolescents. A focus on participating in 1 sport, or single-sport specialization, to improve, advance, and compete at the highest level may drive youth to participate for long hours daily on 1 or more teams at a time. This is common in soccer, baseball, and gymnastics. The motivation behind this overinvolvement may be induced by the child or parent. As more young athletes are becoming professionals at a younger age, there is more pressure to grab a piece of the "professional pie," to obtain a college scholarship, or to make the Olympic team. Most young athletes and their parents fail to realize that, depending on the sport, only 0.2% to 0.5% of high school athletes ever make it to the professional level.[16] Yet, youth continue to specialize in 1 sport while participating on multiple teams and risk overuse and/or burnout if there is no break from athletics during the year. Young athletes who participate in a variety of sports have fewer injuries and play sports longer than those who specialize before puberty.[1]

Multisport Athlete

Well-rounded, multisport athletes have the highest potential to achieve the goal of lifelong fitness and enjoyment of physical activity while avoiding some of the pitfalls of overuse, overtraining, and burnout provided that they participate in moderation and are in tune with their bodies for signs of overuse or fatigue. Many youth will play multiple sports throughout the year either simultaneously or during different seasons. They may do this because they enjoy multiple sports or because their coach or parent pushes them to participate in other sports to condition them for their primary sport or in hopes of being noticed by college or professional scouts. There may be additional pressures from other coaches who wish to better their team by calling on well-rounded athletes from other sports. Multisport athletes are at risk of overuse injuries if they do not get sufficient rest between daily activities or if they do not get a break between seasons. Multisport athletes who participate in 2 or more sports for which the major emphasis is the same body part (eg, swimmers and baseball pitchers) are at higher risk of overuse injuries than are those who participate in sports that have a different emphasis (eg, track and golf).

What Is the Goal of the Athlete?

The ultimate goal of youth participation in sports should be to promote lifelong physical activity, recreation, and skills of healthy competition that can be used in all facets of future endeavors. As providers of care for youth, it is important to obtain a physical activity history (type of activity, frequency, duration) and take the opportunity to promote healthy participation and preventive care measures. Education of parents, athletes, and coaches must be part of the plan to promote fun, skill development, and success for each individual athlete. Skilled young athletes must be mentored carefully to prevent overparticipation, which may affect them physically as well as psychologically. The parent or pediatrician may wonder how hard a child should be pushed to train and compete. Ultimately, it is important for the practitioner to discuss the underlying motivation for sport participation with the athlete, the parent, and, possibly, the coach. Unfortunately, too often the goal is skewed toward adult (parent/coach) goals either implicitly or explicitly. The parent often hopes the child will get a scholarship, become a professional athlete, or fulfill the parents' unfulfilled childhood dreams. It is best to identify and focus on the child's motivation and goals to provide guidance.

GUIDANCE FOR THE CLINICIAN

1. Encourage athletes to strive to have at least 1 to 2 days off per week from competitive athletics, sport-specific training, and competitive practice (scrimmage) to allow them to recover both physically and psychologically.

2. Advise athletes that the weekly training time, number of repetitions, or total distance should not increase by more than 10% each week (eg, increase total running mileage by 2 miles if currently running a total of 20 miles per week).

3. Encourage the athlete to take at least 2 to 3 months away from a specific sport during the year.

4. Emphasize that the focus of sports participation should be on fun, skill acquisition, safety, and sportsmanship.

5. Encourage the athlete to participate on only 1 team during a season. If the athlete is also a member of a traveling or select team, then that participation time should be incorporated into the aforementioned guidelines.

6. If the athlete complains of nonspecific muscle or joint problems, fatigue, or poor academic performance, be alert for possible burnout. Questions pertaining to sport motivation may be appropriate.

7. Advocate for the development of a medical advisory board for weekend athletic tournaments to educate athletes about heat or cold illness, overparticipation, associated overuse injuries, and/or burnout.

8. Encourage the development of educational opportunities for athletes, parents, and coaches to provide information about appropriate nutrition and fluids, sport safety, and the avoidance of overtraining to achieve optimal performance and good health.

9. Convey a special caution to parents with younger athletes who participate in multigame tournaments in short periods of time.

COUNCIL ON SPORTS MEDICINE AND FITNESS, 2005–2006

Eric W. Small, MD, Chairperson
David T. Bernhardt, MD
Joel S. Brenner, MD, MPH
Joseph A. Congeni, MD
Jorge E. Gomez, MD
Andrew J. M. Gregory, MD
Douglas B. Gregory, MD
Teri M. McCambridge, MD
Frederick E. Reed, MD
Stephen G. Rice, MD, PhD, MPH

Paul R. Stricker, MD
Bernard A. Griesemer, MD

LIAISONS

Claire M. A. Le Blanc, MD
 Canadian Paediatric Society
James Raynor, MS, ATC
 National Athletic Trainers Association

STAFF

Jeanne Lindros, MPH
Anjie Emanuel, MPH

REFERENCES

1. American Academy of Pediatrics, Committee of Sports Medicine and Fitness. Intensive training and sports specialization in young athletes. *Pediatrics*. 2000;106:154–157
2. Mellion MB, Walsh WM, Madden C, Putukian M, Shelton GL. *Team Physician's Handbook*. 3rd ed. Philadelphia, PA: Hanley & Belfus Inc; 2002
3. Dalton SE. Overuse injuries in adolescent athletes. *Sports Med*. 1992;13:58–70
4. Maffulli N, Chan D, Aldridge M. Overuse injuries of the olecranon in young gymnasts. *J Bone Joint Surg Br*. 1992;74: 305–308
5. Carter SR, Aldridge MJ, Fitzgerald R, Davies AM. Stress changes of the wrist in adolescent gymnasts. *Br J Radiol*. 1988; 61:109–112
6. Small E. Chronic musculoskeletal pain in young athletes. *Pediatr Clin North Am*. 2002;49:655–662
7. Budgett R. Fatigue and underperformance in athletes: the overtraining syndrome. *Br J Sports Med*. 1998;32:107–110
8. American Academy of Pediatrics, Committee of Sports Medicine and Fitness. Triathlon participation by children and adolescents. *Pediatrics*. 1996;98:511–512
9. USA Triathlon. Juniors. Available at: www.usatriathlon.org/AthleteFocus/Junior.aspx. Accessed March 30, 2006
10. Rice SG, Waniewski S; American Academy of Pediatrics, Committee on Sports Medicine and Fitness; International Marathon Medical Directors Association. Children and marathoning: how young is too young? *Clin J Sport Med*. 2003;13:369–373
11. Roberts W. Children and running: at what distance safe? *Clin J Sport Med*. 2005;15:109–110
12. Mohtadi N. Children and marathoning. *Clin J Sport Med*. 2005; 15:110
13. American Academy of Pediatrics, Committee of Sports Medicine and Fitness. Climatic heat stress and the exercising child and adolescent. *Pediatrics*. 2000;106:158–159
14. Armstrong L, Epstein Y, Greenleaf L. American College of Sports Medicine position stand: heat and cold illnesses during distance running. *Med Sci Sports Exerc*. 1996;28:i–x
15. American Academy of Pediatrics, Committee on Sports Medicine and Fitness. Risks in distance running for children. *Pediatrics*. 1990;86:799–800
16. National Collegiate Athletic Association. Fact sheet. Available at: www.ncaa.org/about/fact_sheet.pdf. Accessed March 30, 2006

AMERICAN ACADEMY OF PEDIATRICS

POLICY STATEMENT
Organizational Principles to Guide and Define the Child Health Care System and/or Improve the Health of All Children

Committee on Sports Medicine and Fitness

Promotion of Healthy Weight-Control Practices in Young Athletes

ABSTRACT. Children and adolescents are often involved in sports in which weight loss or weight gain is perceived as an advantage. This policy statement describes unhealthy weight-control practices that may be harmful to the health and/or performance of athletes. Healthy methods of weight loss and weight gain are discussed, and physicians are given resources and recommendations that can be used to counsel athletes, parents, coaches, and school administrators in discouraging inappropriate weight-control behaviors and encouraging healthy methods of weight gain or loss, when needed. *Pediatrics* 2005;116:1557–1564; *athlete, weight gain, weight loss, wrestling, eating disorders.*

ABBREVIATION. NWCA, National Wrestling Coaches' Association.

INTRODUCTION

With the growth and advancement of youth sports, children and adolescents are becoming more involved in sports in which weight control is perceived to be advantageous for the individual and/or team. Bodybuilding, cheerleading, dancing, distance running, cross-country skiing, diving, figure skating, gymnastics, martial arts, rowing, swimming, weight-class football, and wrestling all emphasize thinness, leanness, and/or competing at the lowest possible weight. Other sports, such as football, rugby, basketball, and power lifting emphasize gaining weight by increasing lean muscle mass. In their attempt to lose weight and body fat or gain weight and muscle mass, some athletes resort to unhealthy weight-control practices,[1–5] which can potentially be harmful to their performance and/or their health. Pediatricians need to be able to recognize the young athlete who is at risk of developing unsafe weight-control practices and provide the athlete, family members, coaches, athletic trainers, and athletic directors with accurate information about healthy weight-control practices.

WEIGHT LOSS

Many athletes attempt to lose weight or body fat, hoping to improve performance, improve appearance, or meet weight expectations. Practices that are used to reduce weight include food restriction, vomiting, overexercising, diet-pill use, inappropriate use of prescribed stimulants or insulin, nicotine use, and

voluntary dehydration (Table 1). Voluntary dehydration practices include fluid restriction, spitting, and the use of laxatives and diuretics, rubber suits, steam baths, and saunas. Weight loss becomes a problem when nutritional needs are not met or adequate hydration is not maintained.

Athletes may practice weight-control methods during the sports season only or year-round. These practices can impair athletic performance and increase injury risk. They also may result in medical complications including delayed physical maturation; oligomenorrhea and amenorrhea in female athletes; development of eating disorders; potential permanent growth impairment; an increased incidence of infectious diseases; changes in the cardiovascular, endocrine, gastrointestinal, renal and thermoregulatory systems; and depression.[1,4,6–9]

Dehydration

Hypohydration and dehydration are used by athletes in weight-sensitive sports in an attempt to lose weight or appear more lean and, thus, obtain a perceived advantage. Because the body does not store fluid or electrolytes before exercise, it is predisposed to dehydration.[10] The extent of the dehydration is determined by sweat loss and the inability or refusal to replace those losses with oral fluids.[11] On the basis of studies in adults, weight loss by dehydration results in suboptimal performance because of impaired strength, reaction time, endurance, and electrolyte imbalance and acidosis. It also may result in temporary learning deficits,[4,12–14] inability to concentrate, lethargy, mood swings, and changes in cognitive state.[15–20]

Hypohydration affects prolonged aerobic exercise more than it affects short, high-intensity anaerobic exercise.[10,21] In adults, a decrease in performance is seen when hypohydration is 2% or more (Table 2). Two to 3% hypohydration results in decreased reflex activity, maximal oxygen uptake, physical work capacity, and muscle endurance and impaired temperature regulation.[22] With additional hypohydration,

TABLE 1. Definition of Hydration

Euhydration: a normal state of body-water content
Dehydration: the process of incurring water deficit
Hypohydration: the extent (or level) of this deficit (usually described as percent of initial body weight)
Voluntary dehydration: purposeful restriction of fluids or use of measures to dehydrate oneself, often to produce weight loss

doi:10.1542/peds.2005-2314
PEDIATRICS (ISSN 0031 4005). Copyright © 2005 by the American Academy of Pediatrics.

TABLE 2.   Effects of Various Levels of Hypohydration

Adults
  2–3% hypohydration
    Decreases reflex activity
    Maximal oxygen uptake decreases by 10%[22]
    Physical work capacity decreases by 22%[22]
    Muscle strength decreases
    Muscle endurance decreases
    Impairment in temperature regulation
  4–6% hypohydration
    Maximal oxygen uptake decreases by 27%[22]
    Physical work capacity decreases by 48%[22]
    Muscle strength decreases more
    Endurance time is reduced
    Severe impairment in temperature regulation
    Headaches, difficulty with concentration, impatience,
      sleepiness
  >8% hypohydration
    Heat cramps
    Heat exhaustion
    Heat stroke
Children
  1% hypohydration
    Reduces aerobic performance[25]
    Increases core temperature[26]
  No studies in children for higher levels of hypohydration
    exist

these parameters decrease even more,[22] and additional symptoms including reduced muscle strength, headache, difficulty concentrating, impatience, and sleepiness occur.[23] Dehydration retards the acclimation process and affects thermoregulation during exercise. The thermoregulatory effect of dehydration intensifies when athletes exercise. For every 1% hypohydration in adults, there is an associated increase of 0.1 to 0.4°C in body temperature.[23,24] When hypohydration exceeds 8%, heat cramps occur, followed by heat exhaustion and heat stroke (body temperature of more than 40.5°C or 105°F). These are serious, life-threatening events.

In children, 1% hypohydration is enough to induce a reduction in aerobic performance.[25] For ethical reasons, studies have not been performed in young children with greater levels of hypohydration. A study with 10- to 12-year-old boys who exercised intermittently in the heat suggested that the increase in their core temperature, at any level of hypohydration, was greater than in adults.[26]

Children have the following characteristics that are similar to adults:

1. Involuntary dehydration can occur with prolonged exercise even if the child is given fluids ad libitum.[11,26,27] This occurs principally when the fluids are unflavored.[28,29]
2. Dehydration causes greater body heat storage (excessive increase in core body temperature),[21,30] decreases blood volume, and results in reduced exercise tolerance,[28] increasing the risk of heat-related illness.[21,30–34]
3. Heat acclimation and training result in an increased sweating rate, which may provide heat dissipation by evaporation but also produces greater fluid loss.[28]
4. The likelihood of heat intolerance increases with conditions that are associated with excessive fluid loss (febrile state, gastrointestinal infection, diabe-

tes insipidus, and diabetes mellitus), suboptimal sweating (spina bifida, sweating-insufficiency syndromes), excessive sweating (selective cyanotic congenital heart disease), abnormal sweating (cystic fibrosis), inadequate drinking (people with mental retardation and young children), abnormal hypothalamic thermoregulatory functions (anorexia nervosa, advanced undernutrition, previous heat-related illness), and obesity.[30,35,36]

Children have certain characteristics that, when compared with adults, predispose them to dehydration and heat illness, including the following:

1. Children produce more heat relative to body mass for the same exercise.[21,30,33]
2. Children have lower cardiac output for any given metabolic level.[30,33]
3. Children have higher thresholds before beginning to sweat.[34,35,37]
4. Sweating capacity is considerably lower in children,[30] reducing their ability to dissipate body heat by evaporation.[30,34,35,37]
5. Children become slightly more dehydrated with lower climatic and metabolic heat stress.
6. Children have a greater ratio of body surface area to body mass, which causes them to absorb heat more quickly when the ambient temperature exceeds skin temperature. Thus, a high level of solar radiation can be more detrimental to children.[28,30]
7. Children's ability to maintain thermohomeostasis during prolonged running in very hot or very cold environments is less efficient.[30,34,38]
8. Children are less efficient in dissipating heat in very hot environments.[11]
9. Children take longer to acclimate to hot, humid environments (2 weeks versus 1 week),[11,30] which increases their risk of heat-related disorders.[38,39]
10. Core body temperature increases more in children for the same level of hypohydration.[11,26]
11. Recent studies indicate that children's thirst is inadequate and that they become dehydrated easier (O. Bar-Or, MD, McMaster University and Chedoke Hospital, Hamilton, Ontario, Canada, verbal communication, October 1, 2003).

Children have a few characteristics that are beneficial in protecting them from dehydration in comparison with adults, including the following:

1. Children have shorter performance times in hot environments, and when exercising at the same intensity as adults. With shorter performance times, children are less likely to dehydrate themselves.[11,30]
2. Sodium and chloride concentrations in the sweat of prepubescent children are lower than those of pubescent children, who in turn have lower sodium losses than adults.[11]
3. Children's sweat rates are reduced, resulting in less sodium and chloride loss.

Dehydration over several days may be cumulative when the athlete who is dehydrated does not sufficiently replace the fluid loss. An athlete may develop 2% to 3% hypohydration one day, not fully rehydrate overnight, and then on subsequent days dehydrate further by repeating the previous day's experience. This process leads to progressive dehydration, to the extent that the athlete becomes 5% to 8% hypohydrated. The greater the body-fluid deficit, the longer it takes to restore this deficit completely.[23] Replacement of intracellular fluids, when dehydration has occurred over 2 or 3 days, requires 48 hours.[40]

When children are given plain water, they will not replace their fluid losses completely. However, when children are given flavored drinks such as grape-, tropical-, or orange-flavored water, voluntary drinking increases by 44.5%,[28,41] a sufficient amount to replace their fluid losses completely.[11,28–30,32] When 6% carbohydrate and 18 mmol/L of sodium are added to flavored water, voluntary drinking is increased by an additional 45.5%.[28–30,41]

Prevention and Treatment of Dehydration

Sweat rates vary among athletes; therefore, one must consider each athlete individually and rely on previous experience with a particular athlete to estimate how much fluid he or she will require.[42]

Fluid ingested before, during, and after exercise reduces dehydration, core temperature, heart rate, and cardiac strain[6]; it maintains skin blood flow and increases exercise performance.[43,44] Thirst is a late indicator of dehydration in adolescents and adults; therefore, efforts must be made to maintain euhydration. The best way to assess hypohydration is to weigh the athlete before and after exercise. The amount of weight lost should be replaced with an equal volume of fluids before the next exercise session. The fluid should contain carbohydrates to replenish glycogen stores as well as sodium chloride.[11,21,45] The concentration of sodium in sports drinks is lower than the sodium concentration in the sweat of both adults and children.[41] Even if children drink enough sports drinks to maintain euhydration, their total body sodium would be decreased and their total sodium loss would not be replaced.[45] If this is repeated over several days and the sodium is not replaced in food or drink, symptomatic hyponatremia may develop.[45]

Food Restrictions/Binge-Purge Behavior

The most common way for athletes to attempt weight loss is by restricting food intake. They may develop other disordered eating behaviors such as purging, with or without bingeing, to decrease total energy (caloric) intake. Compulsive exercise or excessive exercise in addition to the normal training regimen also would be considered a form of purging. The spectrum of these disordered eating behaviors ranges from mild to severe, with the risk of development of an eating disorder and the associated morbidity and mortality increasing as the severity of the behavior increases.[46]

Disordered eating behaviors are prevalent in male and female athletes. Ten to 15% of high school boys who participate in "weight-sensitive sports" practice unhealthy weight-loss behaviors.[1,4,47] Numerous studies have reported these practices in wrestlers, with 1 study revealing that 80% of wrestlers lost weight for the wrestling season.[48] Eleven percent of wrestlers were found to have an eating disorder in 1 study,[49] and as many as 45% of wrestlers were found to be at risk of developing an eating disorder in other studies.[4,19,47]

Many studies have revealed an increased incidence of disordered eating behavior (food restriction, vomiting, laxative and diuretic use) in female athletes involved in weight-sensitive sports such as figure skating, gymnastics, diving, long-distance running, rowing, and swimming.[2,5,46] One study of young swimmers reported that 60% of average-weight girls and 18% of underweight girls were trying to lose weight.[50] Most of these swimmers were restricting food intake to lose weight; however, 15% were vomiting or using laxatives or diuretics. In the female athlete, decreased energy availability (calculated as dietary energy intake minus exercise energy expenditure) can lead to menstrual dysfunction, which can result in potential bone mineral density loss. This has been termed the "female athlete triad" (decreased energy availability or disordered eating, menstrual dysfunction, and bone mineral density loss).[3,51] All female athletes with oligomenorrhea or amenorrhea should be evaluated thoroughly to determine the underlying etiology. If low energy availability is the cause, the athlete should be counseled on increasing energy intake enough to resume normal menses.[3,51] If an eating disorder is suspected, referral to a multidisciplinary team of experts in this field is appropriate.

Healthy Weight Loss

Athletes usually require a greater energy (caloric) intake than do nonathletes.[21] The actual energy intake (number of calories) needed depends on the athlete's body composition, weight, height, age, stage of growth, and level of fitness as well as the intensity, frequency, and duration of exercise activity.[52] Athletes need to eat enough to cover the energy costs of daily living, growth, building and repairing muscle tissue, and participating in sport.[53] Athletes who want to lose weight should be counseled on the harmful effects of unhealthy weight-loss practices and inappropriate weight loss. They need to be informed that weight is not an accurate indicator of body fat or lean muscle mass and that body composition measurements can be much more helpful.[54]

Studies have shown that physique does not markedly influence performance except at the extreme ranges (ie, significant endomorphy or ectomorphy).[55] An excessive amount of body fat interferes with acclimation to heat and can decrease speed, endurance, and work efficiency.[4,56] Therefore, weight loss may be beneficial when it is achieved by healthy means and involves losing excess fat without reducing lean muscle mass or causing dehydration.[4] When weight is lost too rapidly or by significant reduction in energy (caloric) intake, lean muscle mass will be lost, which can affect performance negatively.[57]

Weight loss, when necessary, should be gradual

and should not exceed 1.5% of the total body weight, or 1 to 2 lb, each week.[52,56–59] Weight loss beyond these guidelines results in the breakdown and metabolism of muscle, making an athlete weaker.[52,56–60] To lose 1 lb of fat in 1 week, one must expend 14 700 kJ (3500 kcal) more than one consumes.[60] The ideal way to do this is to consume 7350 kJ (1750 kcal) fewer per week and expend 7350 kJ (1750 kcal) more per week by exercising.[56,60] An appropriate diet for most athletes consists of a minimum of 8400 kJ (2000 kcal) each day. Approximately 55% to 65% of the daily energy (caloric) intake should be from carbohydrates, 15% to 20% should be from protein, and 20% to 30% should be from fat.[52,57] The diet should be well balanced, consisting of foods from all groups of the food pyramid. When possible, the athlete should be counseled by a registered dietitian who has experience working with athletes and their families. Sports and Cardiovascular Nutritionists (SCAN), a practice group of the American Dietetic Association, can provide names of registered dietitians with expertise in nutrition and exercise (see www.eatright-.org, or call 800-877-1600, extension 5000).

Once weight has been lost and the desired weight is obtained, that weight should be maintained. Studies have shown that athletes who maintain their desired weight have higher resting metabolic rates than do athletes who are "cyclic" weight losers (177.2 vs 154.6 kJ/m² per hour, respectively).[61] They also have higher resting energy expenditures (7702.8 vs 6631.8 kJ/day, respectively) and oxygen consumption (266.5 vs 230.4 mL/minute, respectively).[61] Therefore, athletes who maintain a constant weight can eat more calories than the "cyclic" weight losers and maintain the same weight.[61]

With the exception of sports that require mandatory weigh-ins, coaches of most sports should not discuss weight or weight loss with an athlete. Many coaches inappropriately focus on weight instead of body composition and performance, and most coaches do not have an adequate nutritional background to counsel an athlete about weight loss. In addition, when a coach mentions weight loss to an athlete, that athlete is much more likely to begin harmful practices of weight control rather than consult with the appropriate professionals. Any weight loss desired by an athlete should be discussed with a health care professional, a registered dietitian, an athletic trainer (when appropriate), and the family. Athletes involved in sports that require mandatory weigh-ins should be discouraged from using harmful weight-loss practices and should be encouraged to compete at a weight that is appropriate for their age, height, physique, and stage of growth and development. Weigh-ins should take place in such a manner as to encourage good hydration and competing at a healthy weight. It has been determined that the safest and fairest procedure for wrestlers, to ensure that they are well hydrated at all times, is to have mat-side weigh-ins immediately before their matches.[62] This procedure ensures that competing wrestlers will be at or near the same weight during the match. A wrestler is prevented from dehydrating and weighing in at one weight, and then rehydrating and wrestling at a significantly higher weight while his or her opponent weighs in at his or her natural weight and wrestles at that weight. Mat-side weigh-ins would prevent wrestlers from competing when they are weak from dehydration and prevent the temptation of dehydrating themselves to the degree that is life threatening.

Weight and Body-Composition Measurement

An athlete's weight should typically fall between the 25th and 75th percentiles of weight for height for age (by National Center for Health Statistics guidelines),[63] although some athletes weigh more because of increased muscle mass. The use of body mass index (BMI) in athletes is not recommended; however, if used, most athletes should be between the 50th and 75th percentile for BMI.[64] BMI is a measure of one's weight relative to height and has been used as a fairly reliable indicator of total body fat (obesity) in adults. In 2000, the Centers for Disease Control and Prevention published guidelines for BMI in children and adolescents 2 years and older to aid in diagnoses of overweight and underweight.[64] BMI is not a perfect indicator of body fatness and may falsely classify some children, particularly adolescents, who are of normal fatness as being overweight.[65] Because weight and height velocities do not coincide exactly during the growth spurt and individual patterns of growth vary during this time, care must be taken to avoid a false diagnosis of overweight during puberty.[65] BMI also can be falsely elevated in an athlete or nonathlete with a muscular build as well as in someone who has a high torso-to-leg ratio.[65] Therefore, body-composition measurements (body fat and lean muscle mass), in addition to height-for-weight for age measurements, may be more useful in determining the physical status of an athlete.[54,57]

Anthropometric measurements can be performed to estimate lean muscle mass. For most well-nourished athletes, lean muscle mass should be greater than the 25th percentile.[57] Many methods are available to determine body fat.[4] The most precise method is underwater weighing; however, the equipment for underwater weighing is expensive and of limited availability. Other commonly used methods include skinfold-thickness measurements, air displacement, bioelectrical impedance measurements, girth measurements, and computerized calipers.[4,58] Skinfold measurements are easily performed by someone with experience using high-quality calipers (approximately $200). When performed in the correct manner, published reports on skinfold calibration show an error margin of ±3%.[66] Skinfold measurements can be taken from 3, 4, or 5 sites (right biceps, right triceps, right subscapular, right suprailiac, and right abdominal sites [regardless of whether the athlete is right-handed or left-handed, measurements are always performed on the right side]). The more sites used, the more accurate the results are. Instructions on how to perform skinfold measurements are available.[58,59]

No optimal values for body composition have been established for any sport. The association between performance and body composition must be individualized for each athlete. A specific percentage of body fat should never be recommended for an individual athlete, but rather a range that is realistic and appropriate.[67] The body fat of "reference adolescents" ranges from 12.7% to 17.2% for males and 21.5% to 25.4% for females.[68] "Low fat" is considered to be 10% to 13% for males and 17% to 20% for females. "Very low fat" is considered to be 7% to 10% for males and 14% to 17% for females.[69,70] Adolescent females who are meeting their energy (caloric) needs will be eumenorrheic.[51]

WEIGHT GAIN

Sports such as football, rugby, basketball, power lifting, and bodybuilding often motivate athletes to gain weight. If weight is gained improperly, it will lead to excess fat, resulting in decreased speed, endurance, and agility and poor acclimation to heat. Overweight athletes, later in life, are at an increased risk of hypercholesterolemia, gall bladder disease, cardiovascular disease, hypertension, and type 2 diabetes mellitus. Often, athletes use supplements (which may be of unproven value and potentially harmful) or anabolic compounds (which are harmful to athletes' health) to gain weight instead of evaluating their nutritional and training programs.

Before trying to change body composition, athletes must understand potential genetic limitations.[71] Athletes with a solid body build (mesomorphy) can expect to gain more weight than athletes with a slender body build (ectomorphy). Inadequate energy intake is often the limiting factor for athletes trying to increase muscle mass. They may overestimate the protein requirements and underestimate the need for carbohydrates.[71]

Healthy Weight Gain

The rate and amount of weight gained and specific muscles developed are determined by an athlete's genetic predisposition, training program, diet, and motivation.[71] To build 1 lb of muscle in 1 week, one must (1) consume 8400 to 10 500 kJ (2000–2500 kcal) more than one expends, (2) consume 1.5 to 1.75 g of protein per kg of body weight per day, and (3) participate in strength training. Consuming 1.5 to 1.75 g of protein per kg of body weight per day rarely is a problem; the average American diet contains 2 to 3 times that amount of protein.[56] If the athlete has not gained the desired weight despite an appropriate training program, adequate rest, and a nutritionally sound diet, it is appropriate to make a recommendation that he or she increase dietary fat.[71] Studies of elite athletes report dietary fat intakes ranging from 29% to 41% in males and 29% to 34% in females.[71] Increased energy (caloric) intake should always be combined with strength training to induce muscle growth and, therefore, increase muscle mass. Gains in muscle hypertrophy are best achieved by performing multiple sets of weight lifting with a relatively high number of repetitions (8–15 repetitions per set).[72] Young athletes should lift lighter weights with an increased number of repetitions under the supervision of a trained adult.[72] Weight gain needs to be gradual, because a gain in excess of 1.5% of body weight per week may result in unwanted fat.[56,60]

RECOMMENDATIONS

1. Physicians who care for young athletes should have knowledge of healthy weight-gain and weight-loss methods. They should understand minimal recommended weight, normal growth curves, and body composition measurements and be willing to educate athletes, families, coaches, athletic trainers, school administrators, and state and national organizations when appropriate. Physicians should understand that all athletes are unique and each athlete must be evaluated individually.

2. All physical examinations of young athletes should include a weight history and a history of eating patterns, hydration practices, eating disorders, heat illness, and other factors that may influence heat illness or weight control.

3. Physicians should be able to recognize early signs and symptoms of an eating disorder and obtain appropriate medical, psychological, and nutritional consultation for young athletes with these symptoms.

4. Nutritional needs for growth and development must be placed above athletic considerations. Fluid or food deprivation should never be allowed. There is no substitute for a healthy diet consisting of a variety of foods from all food groups with enough energy (calories) to support growth, daily physical activities, and sports activities. Daily caloric intake for most athletes should consist of a minimum of 8400 kJ (2000 kcal). Athletes need to consume enough fluids to maintain euhydration. Physicians should engage the services of a registered dietitian familiar with athletes to help with weight-control issues.

5. In sports for which weigh-ins are required, athletes' weight and body composition should be assessed once or twice per year. The most important assessment is obtained before the beginning of the sport season. This should include a determination of body fat and minimal allowable weight when the athlete is adequately hydrated (the National Wrestling Coaches' Association [NWCA] Internet Weight Classification Program is available at www.nwcaonline.com[58] or by calling 717-653-8009 [see Fig 1 and Appendix]). Weigh-ins for competition should be performed immediately before competition.[62] Athletes should be permitted to compete in championship tournaments only at the weight class in which they have competed for most other athletic events that year.[58,59,62]

6. Male high school athletes should not have less than 7% body fat. This minimal allowable body fat may be too low for some athletes and result in suboptimal performance. Female athletes should consume enough energy (calories) and nutrients to meet their energy requirements and experience normal menses. There are no recommendations on body-fat percentages in female athletes.

Obtain urine specific gravity (by refractometer or urometer)

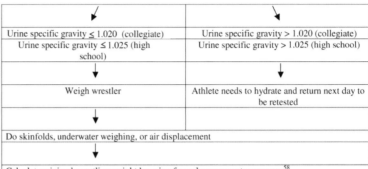

Urine specific gravity ≤ 1.020 (collegiate)	Urine specific gravity > 1.020 (collegiate)
Urine specific gravity ≤ 1.025 (high school)	Urine specific gravity > 1.025 (high school)
Weigh wrestler	Athlete needs to hydrate and return next day to be retested
Do skinfolds, underwater weighing, or air displacement	

Calculate minimal wrestling weight by using formula or computer program[58]

The minimal wrestling weight is calculated using the following formula[58]:

(1) body density = [1.0982 – (sum of the skinfolds × 0.000815)] + [(sum of the skinfolds)^2 × 0.00000084]

(2) % body fat = [(4.57/body density) – 4.142] × 100

(3) fat weight = (body weight) × (% body fat/100)

(4) fat freeweight = (body weight) – (fat weight)

(5) minimal wrestling weight = fat freeweight/0.93 (for high school wrestlers) minimal wrestling weight = fat freeweight/0.95 (for collegiate wrestlers)

Fig 1. Calculating minimal wrestling weight.

Alternatively, the skinfold measurements may be entered into the NWCA Internet weight certification program at www.nwcacalculator.com/certification.

The minimal wrestling weight is calculated for the minimal allowable percent of body fat. As defined by the NWCA, the minimal allowable percent body fat is 7% for male high school wrestlers and 12% for female high school wrestlers. The National Collegiate Athletic Association (NCAA) has determined the minimal allowable percent body fat to be 5% for male collegiate wrestlers. The wrestler may not be able to attain these levels of body fat without resorting to unhealthy weight-control practices. He or she will often perform better at a higher percent body fat than the calculated minimal allowable body fat. Female wrestlers should not permit their weight or percent body fat to be below that level at which they have normal monthly menstrual periods.

7. A program for the purpose of gaining or losing weight should (a) be started early to permit a gradual weight gain or loss over a realistic time period, (b) permit a change of 1.5% or less of one's body weight per week, (c) permit the loss of weight to be fat loss and the gain of weight to be muscle mass, (d) be coupled with an appropriate training program (both strength and conditioning), and (e) incorporate a well-balanced diet with adequate energy (calories), carbohydrates, protein, and fat. After athletes obtain their desired weight, they should be encouraged to maintain a constant weight and avoid fluctuations of weight. A weight-loss plan for athletic purposes should never be instituted before the 9th grade.

8. Any athlete who loses a significant amount of fluid during sports participation should weigh in before and after practices, games, meets, and competitions. Each pound of weight loss should be replaced with 1 pt of fluid containing carbohydrates and electrolytes before the next practice or competition. Fluids should be available, and the drinking of such should be encouraged at all practices and competitions.

9. Weight loss accomplished by overexercising; using rubber suits, steam baths, or saunas; prolonged fasting; fluid reduction; vomiting; or using anorexic drugs, laxatives, diuretics, diet pills, insulin, stimulants, nutritional supplements, or other legal or illegal drugs and/or nicotine should be prohibited at all ages.[73,74]

10. Athletes who need to gain weight should consult their physician for resources on healthy weight gain and referral to a registered dietitian. They should be discouraged from gaining excessive weight, which may impair performance, increase the likelihood of heat illness, and increase the risk of developing complications from obesity.

11. Ergogenic aids and nontherapeutic use of supplements for weight management should be prohibited.[73,74]

12. Young athletes should be involved in a total athletic program that includes acquisition of athletic skills and improvement in speed, flexibility, strength, and physical conditioning while maintaining good nutrition and normal hydration. This should be done under the supervision of a coach who stresses a positive attitude, character building, teamwork, and safety.[75]

APPENDIX: CALCULATING MINIMAL WRESTLING WEIGHT

Calculation of a minimal safe wrestling weight using body-fat measurements was first performed in high school athletes.[18,76–80] In 1998, the National Collegiate Athletic Association[59] and the NWCA[58] incorporated this technique into a mandatory program designed to establish the minimal safe wrestling weight for collegiate wrestlers.[58] This program includes hydration testing, body-composition assessment, calculation of a lowest allowable weight class for each wrestler, development of a weight-loss plan for each wrestler (if appropriate), and a nutrition education program specific to wrestling. The wrestler's minimal wrestling weight is established by determining percent body fat when the wrestler is adequately hydrated (urine specific gravity of 1.020 or less for college wrestlers and 1.025 or less for high school wrestlers). If the wrestler is not well hydrated, the body-fat calculations will result in a low and unsafe minimum weight recommendation.[81] The National Federation of High Schools medical advisory committee has recommended that high school wrestling programs adopt the program of the NWCA by the 2004–2005 academic year.[4]

In establishing minimal weight, skinfold calipers (Lange skinfold calipers; Beta Technology Corp, Cambridge, MD), bioimpedance (Tanita, Arlington Heights, IL), air displacement (Bod Pod; Life Measurement, Inc, Concord, CA), and hydrostatic weighing are the only methods currently approved for body-composition measurements.[58,59] The NWCA formula requires skinfold measurements to be taken at the right triceps, right subscapular, and right abdominal sites (regardless of whether the athlete is right-handed or left-handed, measurements are always performed on the right side).[58]

COMMITTEE ON SPORTS MEDICINE AND FITNESS,
2003–2004
Reginald L. Washington, MD, Chairperson
David T. Bernhardt, MD
Joel S. Brenner, MD, MPH
Jorge Gomez, MD
*Thomas J. Martin, MD
Frederick E. Reed, MD
Stephen G. Rice, MD, PhD, MPH

LIAISONS
Carl Krein, AT, PT
    National Athletic Trainers Association
Claire LeBlanc, MD
    Canadian Paediatric Society
Judith C. Young, PhD
    National Association for Sport and Physical
    Education

CONTRIBUTORS
Oded Bar-Or, MD
*Miriam D. Johnson, MD

STAFF
Jeanne Christensen Lindros, MPH

*Lead authors

REFERENCES

1. Ashley CD, Smith JF, Robinson JB, Richardson MT. Disordered eating in female collegiate athletes and collegiate females in an advanced program of study: a preliminary investigation. *Int J Sport Nutr.* 1996;6: 391–401
2. Brownell KD, Rodin J. Prevalence of eating disorders in athletes. In: Brownell KD, Rodin J, Wilmore JH, eds. *Eating, Body Weight and Performance in Athletes: Disorders of Modern Society.* Philadelphia, PA: Lea & Febiger; 1992:128–145
3. Nattiv A, Loucks AB, Manore MM, Sanborn CF, Sundgot-Borgen J, Warren MP. American College of Sports Medicine position stand: the female athlete triad. *Med Sci Sports Exerc.* 2006; in press
4. Perriello VA Jr. Aiming for healthy weight in wrestlers and other athletes. *Contemp Pediatr.* 2001;18:55–74
5. Rosen LW, McKeag DB, Hough DO, et al. Pathogenic weight-control behavior in female athletes. *Phys Sportsmed.* 1986;14:79–86
6. Montain S, Coyle EF. Influence of the timing of fluid ingestion on temperature regulation during exercise. *J Appl Physiol.* 1993;75:688–695
7. Palla B, Litt IF. Medical complications of eating disorders in adolescents. *Pediatrics.* 1988;81:613–623
8. Ratnasuriya RH, Eisler I, Szmuckler GI, Russell GF. Anorexia nervosa: outcome and prognostic factors after 20 years. *Br J Psychiatry.* 1991;158: 495–502
9. American Psychiatric Association. Practice guideline for the treatment of patients with eating disorders (revision). *Am J Psychiatry.* 2000;157(1 suppl):1–39
10. Gisolfi CV, Duchman SM. Guidelines for optimal replacement beverages for different athletic events. *Med Sci Sports Exerc.* 1992;24:679–687
11. Meyer F, Bar-Or O. Fluid and electrolyte loss during exercise: the paediatric angle. *Sports Med.* 1994;18:4–9
12. Choma CW, Sforzo GA, Keller BA. Impact of rapid weight loss on cognitive function in collegiate wrestlers. *Med Sci Sports Exerc.* 1998;30: 746–749
13. Conners CK, Blouin AG. Nutritional effects on behavior of children. *J Psychiatr Res.* 1982;17:193–201
14. Defeo PV, Gallai V, Mazzotta G, et al. Modest decrements in plasma glucose concentrations cause early impairment in cognitive function and later activation of glucose counterregulation in the absence of hypoglycemic symptoms in normal man. *J Clin Invest.* 1988;82: 436–444
15. Horswill CA, Hickner RC, Scott JR, Costill DL, Gould D. Weight loss, dietary carbohydrate modifications, and high intensity, physical performance. *Med Sci Sports Exerc.* 1990;22:470–476
16. Lakin JA, Steen SN, Oppliger RA. Eating behaviors, weight loss methods, and nutritional practices among high school wrestlers. *J Community Health Nurs.* 1990;7:223–234
17. Morgan BL. Nutritional requirements for normative development of the brain and behavior. *Ann N Y Acad Sci.* 1990;602:127–132
18. Oppliger Ra, Landry GL, Foster SW, Lambrecht AC. Wisconsin minimum weight program reduces weight-cutting practices of high school wrestlers. *Clin J Sport Med.* 1998;8:26–31
19. Steen SN, Brownell KD. Patterns of weight loss and regain in wrestlers: has the tradition changed? *Med Sci Sports Exerc.* 1990;22:762–768
20. Cain K, Oakhill JV, Barnes MA, Bryant PE. Comprehension skill, inference-making ability, and their relation to knowledge. *Mem Cognit.* 2001; 29:850–859
21. Bar-Or O. *Nutrition for Child and Adolescent Athletes.* Chicago, IL: Sports Science Center, Gatorade Sports Science Institute; 2000:13:1–4. Available at: www.gssiweb.com/reflib/refs/235/sse77.cfm?pid-38. Accessed August 19, 2004
22. Craig EN, Cummings EG. Dehydration and muscular work. *J Appl Physiol.* 1966;21:670–674
23. Greenleaf JE. Problem: thirst, drinking behavior, and involuntary dehydration. *Med Sci Sports Exerc.* 1992;24:645–656
24. Sawka MN. Physiological consequences of hypohydration: exercise performance and thermoregulation. *Med Sci Sports Exerc.* 1992;24:657–670
25. Wilk B, Yuxiu H, Bar-Or O. Effect of body hypohydration on aerobic performance of boys who exercise in the heat [abstract]. *Med Sci Sports Exerc.* 2002;34(5 suppl):S48
26. Bar-Or O, Dotan R, Inbar O, Rotshtein A, Zonder H. Voluntary hypohydration in 10- to 12-year-old boys. *J Appl Physiol.* 1980;48:104–108
27. Bar-Or O, Blimkie CJ, Hay JA, MacDougall JD, Ward DS, Wilson WM. Voluntary dehydration and heat intolerance in cystic fibrosis. *Lancet.* 1992;339:696–699
28. Rivera-Brown AM, Gutierrez R, Guterrez JC, Frontera WR, Bar-Or O. Drink composition, voluntary drinking, and fluid balance in exercising, trained, heat-acclimatized boys. *J Appl Physiol.* 1999;86:78–84
29. Wilk B, Bar-Or O. Effect of drink flavor and NaCl on voluntary drinking and rehydration in boys exercising in the heat. *J Appl Physiol.* 1996;80: 1112–1117
30. American Academy of Pediatrics, Committee on Sports Medicine and Fitness. Climatic heat stress and the exercising child and adolescent. *Pediatrics.* 2000;106:158–159
31. Danks DM, Webb DW, Allen J. Heat illness in infants and young children: a study of 47 cases. *Br Med J.* 1962;2(5300):287–293
32. Taj-Eldin S, Falaki N. Heat illness in infants and small children in desert climates. *J Trop Med Hyg.* 1968;71:100–104

33. Astrand PO. *Experimental Studies of Physical Working Capacity in Relation to Sex and Age*. Copenhagen, Denmark: Munksgaard; 1952

34. Bar-Or O. Temperature regulation during exercise in children and adolescence. In: Gisolfi CV, Lamb DR, eds. *Perspectives in Exercise Sciences and Sports Medicine II: Youth, Exercise and Sport*. Indianapolis, IN: Benchmark Press; 1989:335–367

35. Haymes EM, McCormick RJ, Buskirk ER. Heat tolerance of exercising lean and obese prepubertal boys. *J Appl Physiol*. 1975;39:457–461

36. Fox EL, Mathews DK, Kaufman WS, Bowers RW. Effect of football equipment on thermal balance and energy cost during exercise. *Res Q*. 1966;37:332–339

37. Drinwater BL, Horvath SM. Heat tolerance and aging. *Med Sci Sports Exerc*. 1979;11:49–55

38. Bar-Or O. *Pediatric Sports Medicine for the Practitioner: From Physiologic Principles to Clinical Applications*. New York, NY: Springer; 1983

39. Inbar O. *Acclimatization to Dry and Hot Environment in Young Adults and Children 8–10 Years Old* [dissertation]. New York, NY: Columbia University; 1978

40. Costill DL. Water and electrolyte requirements during exercise. *Clin Sports Med*. 1984;3:639–648

41. Meyer F, Bar-Or O, Salsberg A, Passe D. Hypohydration during exercise in children: effect on thirst, drink preferences, and rehydration. *Int J Sport Nutr*. 1994;4:22–35

42. Sparling PB, Millard-Stafford M. Keeping sports participants safe in hot weather. *Phys Sportsmed*. 1999;27:27–34

43. Below PR, Mora-Rodriquez R, Gonzlez-Alonzo J, Coyle EF. Fluid and carbohydrate ingestion independently improve performance during 1 h of intense exercise. *Med Sci Sports Exerc*. 1995;27:200–210

44. Hargreaves M, Dillo P, Angus D, Febbraio M. Effect of fluid ingestion on muscle metabolism during prolonged exercise. *J Appl Physiol*. 1996; 80:363–366

45. Meyer F, Bar-Or O, MacDougall D, Heigenhauser GJ. Sweat electrolyte loss during exercise in the heat: effect of gender and maturation. *Med Sci Sports Exerc*. 1992;24:776–781

46. Johnson MD. Disordered eating in active and athletic women. *Clin Sports Med*. 1994;13:355–369

47. Perriollo VA Jr, Almquist J, Conkwright D Jr, et al. Health and weight control management among wrestlers: a proposed program for high school athletes. *Va Med Q*. 1995;122:179

48. Weissenger E, Housh TJ, Johnson GO, Evans SA. Weight loss behavior in high school wrestling: wrestler and parent perceptions. *Pediatr Exerc Sci*. 1991;3:64–73

49. Garner DM, Rosen LW, Barry D. Eating disorders among athletes: research and recommendations. *Child Adolesc Psychiatr Clin N Am*. 1998; 7:839–857, x

50. Dummer GM, Rosen LW, Huesner WW, Roberts PJ, Counsilman JE. Pathogenic weight-control behaviors of young competitive swimmers. *Phys Sportsmed*. 1987;15:75–86

51. American Academy of Pediatrics, Committee on Sports Medicine and Fitness. Medical concerns in the female athlete. *Pediatrics*. 2000;106: 610–613

52. Steen SN, Berning JR. Sound nutrition for the athlete. In: Brownell KD, Rodin J, Wilmore JH, eds. *Eating, Body Weight, and Performance in Athletes: Disorders of Modern Society*. Philadelphia, PA: Lea & Febiger. 1992;293–314

53. Manore MM. Nutritional needs of the female athlete. *Clin Sports Med*. 1999;18:549–563

54. Wilmore JH. Body weight and body composition. In: Brownell KD, Rodin J, Wilmore JH, eds. *Eating, Body Weight, and Performance in Athletes: Disorders of Modern Society*. Philadelphia, PA: Lea & Febiger. 1992;77–93

55. Malina RM. Physique and body composition: effects on performance and effects of training, semistarvation, and overtraining. In: Brownell KD, Rodin J, Wilmore JH, eds. *Eating, Body Weight, and Performance in Athletes: Disorders of Modern Society*. Philadelphia, PA: Lea & Febiger. 1992;94–111

56. Smith NJ, Roberts BW. *Food for Sport*. Palo Alto, CA: Bull Publishing; 1976

57. American Academy of Pediatrics, Committee on Nutrition. Sports nutrition. In: Kleinman RE, ed. *Pediatric Nutrition Handbook*. 5th ed. Elk Grove Village, IL: American Academy of Pediatrics; 2004:155–166

58. National Wrestling Coaches Association. *The National Wrestling Coaches Association's Wrestling Weight Certification Program Handbook*. Manheim, PA: National Wrestling Coaches Association; 2003:1–31

59. National Collegiate Athletic Association, Wrestling Committee. Appendix H: weight certification procedures. In: *2004 NCAA Wrestling Rules and Interpretations*. Indianapolis, IN: National Collegiate Athletic Association; 2003:WA-27–WA-32

60. Smith NJ. Gaining and losing weight in athletics. *JAMA*. 1976;236: 149–151

61. Steen SN, Oppliger RA, Brownell KD. Metabolic effects of repeated weight loss and regain in adolescent wrestlers. *JAMA*. 1988;260:47–50

62. Oppliger RA, Case HS, Horswill CA, Landry GL, Shelter AC. American College of Sports Medicine position stand: weight loss in wrestlers. *Med Sci Sports Exerc*. 1996;28:ix–xii

63. Hamill PVV, Johnston FE, Lemeshow S. Height and weight of youth 12–17 years: United States. *Vital Health Stat 1*. 1973;11(124):1–81

64. National Heart, Lung, and Blood Institute. Calculate your body mass index. Available at: www.nhlbisupport.com/bmi/bmicalc.htm. Accessed September 26, 2005

65. Roberts SB, Dallal GE. The new childhood growth charts. *Nutr Rev*. 2001;59:31–36

66. Kuta JM, Clark RR, Webber LM, Ward A. Inter and intra tester reliability of skinfold measurements in high school wrestlers [abstract]. *Med Sci Sports Exerc*. 1990;22(2 suppl):S110

67. Sanborn CF, Horea M, Siemers BJ, Dieringer KI. Disordered eating and the female athlete triad. *Clin Sports Med*. 2000;19:199–213

68. Haschke F. Body composition during adolescence. In: Klish WJ, Kretchmer N, eds. *Body Composition Measurements in Infants and Children: Report of the 98th Ross Conference on Pediatric Research*. Columbus, OH: Ross Laboratories; 1989:76–83

69. Getchell B, Anderson W. *Being Fit: A Personal Guide*. New York, NY: John Wiley & Sons; 1982

70. Clark N. *Nancy Clark's Sports Nutrition Guidebook*. Champaign, IL: Leisure Press; 1990

71. Grandjean A. Nutritional requirements to increase lean mass. *Clin Sports Med*. 1999;18:623–632

72. Bernhardt DT, Gomez J, Johnson MD, et al. Strength training by children and adolescents. *Pediatrics*. 2001;107:1470–1472

73. Gomez J; American Academy of Pediatrics, Committee on Sports Medicine and Fitness. Use of performance-enhancing substances. *Pediatrics*. 2005;115:1103–1106

74. National Collegiate Athletic Association. *2004 NCAA Wrestling Rules and Interpretations*. Indianapolis, IN: National Collegiate Athletic Association; 2003:WR-28, WA-10

75. American Academy of Pediatrics, Committee on Sports Medicine and Fitness, Committee on School Health. Organized sports for children and preadolescents. *Pediatrics*. 2001;107:1459–1462

76. Oppliger RA, Harms RD, Herrmann DE, Streich CM, Clark RR. The Wisconsin wrestling minimum weight project: a model for weight control among high school wrestlers. *Med Sci Sports Exerc*. 1995;27: 1220–1224

77. Thorland WG, Tipton CM, Lohman TG. Midwest wrestling study: prediction of minimal weight for high school wrestlers. *Med Sci Sports Exerc*. 1991;23:1102–1110

78. Perriello VA Jr, Benjamin JT, Dickens MD, et al. New medical standards for Virginia's high school athletes. *Va Med*. 1989;116:359–367

79. Tcheng T, Tinton CM. Iowa wrestling study: anthropometric measurements and the prediction of a "minimal" body weight for high school wrestlers. *Med Sci Sports*. 1973;5:1–10

80. Tinton CM, Tcheng T, Zambaski EJ. Iowa wrestling study: weight classification systems. *Med Sci Sports*. 1976;8:101–104

81. Roberts, WO. Certifying wrestlers' minimum weight: a new requirement. *Phys Sportsmed*. 1998;26:79–81

All policy statements from the American Academy of Pediatrics automatically expire 5 years after publication unless reaffirmed, revised, or retired at or before that time.

AMERICAN ACADEMY OF PEDIATRICS

Committee on Sports Medicine and Fitness

AMERICAN ACADEMY OF OPHTHALMOLOGY

Eye Health and Public Information Task Force

POLICY STATEMENT
Organizational Principles to Guide and Define the Child Health Care System and/or Improve the Health of All Children

Protective Eyewear for Young Athletes

ABSTRACT. The American Academy of Pediatrics and American Academy of Ophthalmology strongly recommend protective eyewear for all participants in sports in which there is risk of eye injury. Protective eyewear should be mandatory for athletes who are functionally 1-eyed and for athletes whose ophthalmologists recommend eye protection after eye surgery or trauma.

ABBREVIATIONS. ASTM, American Society for Testing and Materials; ANSI, American National Standards Institute; CSA, Canadian Standards Association; HECC, Hockey Equipment Certification Council.

BACKGROUND

More than 42 000 sports and recreation-related eye injuries were reported in 2000.[1] Seventy-two percent of the injuries occurred in individuals younger than 25 years, 43% occurred in individuals younger than 15 years, and 8% occurred in children younger than 5 years.[1] Children and adolescents may be particularly susceptible to injuries because of their aggressive play, athletic maturity,[2–4] and poor supervision in some recreational situations.

The sports highlighted in this statement were chosen on the basis of their popularity and/or the high incidence of eye injuries in that sport. Participation rates and information on the severity of the injuries are unavailable; therefore, the relative risk of significant injuries cannot be determined for various sports. Baseball and basketball are associated with the most eye injuries in athletes 5 to 24 years old.[1]

The eye-injury risk of a sport is proportional to the chance of the eye being impacted with sufficient energy to cause injury. The risk is not correlated with the classification of sports into collision, contact, and noncontact categories. Instead, the risk of eye injury to the unprotected player is roughly categorized as high risk, moderate risk, low risk, and eye safe. The sports included in each of these categories are listed in Table 1.

EVALUATION

All athletes and their parents should be made aware of the risks associated with participation in

sports and the availability of a variety of certified sports eye protectors. Although eye protectors cannot eliminate the risk of injury, appropriate eye protectors have been found to reduce the risk of significant eye injury by at least 90% when fitted properly.[4–6] It would be ideal if all children and adolescents wore appropriate eye protection for all eye-risk sports and recreational activities.

Physicians should strongly recommend that athletes who are functionally 1-eyed wear appropriate eye protection during all sports, recreational, and work-related activities. Functionally 1-eyed athletes are those who have a best corrected visual acuity of worse than 20/40 in the poorer-seeing eye.[1,4,7] If the better eye is injured, functionally 1-eyed athletes may be handicapped severely and unable to obtain a driver's license in many states.[8]

Athletes who have had eye surgery or trauma to the eye may have weakened eye tissue that is more susceptible to injury.[9] These athletes may need additional eye protection or may need to be restricted from certain sports; they should be evaluated and counseled by an ophthalmologist before sports participation.

PROTECTIVE EYEWEAR OPTIONS

Eye protection and different brands of sports goggles vary significantly in both the way they fit and their capacity to protect the eye from injury. An experienced ophthalmologist, optometrist, optician, physician, or athletic trainer can help an athlete select appropriate protective gear that fits well and provides the maximum amount of protection. Sports programs should assist indigent athletes in evaluating and obtaining protective eyewear.

There are 4 basic types of eyewear. The 2 types that are satisfactory for eye-injury risk sports include:

1. Safety sports eyewear that conforms to the requirements of the American Society for Testing and Materials (ASTM) standard F803 for selected sports (racket sports, baseball fielders, basketball, women's lacrosse, and field hockey).[10]
2. Sports eyewear that is attached to a helmet or for sports in which ASTM standard F803 eyewear is inadequate. Those for which there are standard

TABLE 1.   Categories of Sports Eye-Injury Risk to the Unprotected Player*

High Risk	Moderate Risk	Low Risk	Eye Safe
Small, fast projectiles	Tennis	Swimming	Track and field†
Air rifle	Badminton	Diving	Gymnastics
BB gun	Soccer	Skiing (snow and water)	
Paintball	Volleyball	Noncontact martial arts	
Hard projectiles, "sticks," close contact	Water polo	Wrestling	
Basketball	Football	Bicycling	
Baseball/softball	Fishing		
Cricket	Golf		
Lacrosse (men's and women's)			
Hockey (field and ice)			
Squash			
Racquetball			
Fencing			
Intentional injury			
Boxing			
Full-contact martial arts			

* Vinger PF. A practical guide for sports eye protection. *Phys Sports Med.* 2000;28(6). Available at: http://www.physsportsmed.com/
issues/2000/06_00/vinger.htm
† Javelin and discus have a small but definite potential for injury. However, good field supervision can reduce the extremely low risk of
injury to near-negligible.

specifications include youth baseball batters and base runners (ASTM standard F910), paintball (ASTM standard 1776), skiing (ASTM standard 659), and ice hockey (ASTM standard F513).[10] Other protectors with specific standards are available for football and men's lacrosse.

The 2 types of eyewear that are not satisfactory for eye-injury risk sports include:

1. Streetwear (fashion) spectacles that conform to the requirements of American National Standards Institute (ANSI) standard Z80.3.[11]
2. Safety eyewear that conforms to the requirements of ANSI standard Z87.1,[12] which is mandated by the Occupational Safety and Health Administration for industrial and educational safety eyewear.

Prescription or nonprescription (plano) lenses may be fabricated from any of several types of clear material, including polycarbonate. Polycarbonate is the most shatter-resistant clear lens material and should be used for all safety eyewear.[13]

PROTECTIVE EYEWEAR CERTIFICATION

Protectors that have been tested to an appropriate standard by an independent testing laboratory are often certified and should afford reasonable protection. The Protective Eyewear Certification Council has begun certifying protectors that comply with ASTM standard F803 (racket sports, basketball, baseball, women's lacrosse, and field hockey), ASTM standard F1776 (paintball), and ASTM standard F910 (youth baseball batters and base runners) standards.[10] The Canadian Standards Association (CSA) certifies products that comply with the Canadian racket-sport standard, which is similar to the ASTM standard.[10] The Hockey Equipment Certification Council (HECC) certifies ice hockey equipment including helmets and face shields. The National Operating Committee on Standards in Athletic Equipment certifies baseball and football helmets as well as the face protectors for men's lacrosse and football.

For those sports with certified protectors, it is recommended that products bearing the Protective Eyewear Certification Council, CSA, HECC, or National Operating Committee on Standards for Athletic Equipment seals be used when available.

RECOMMENDATIONS

1. All youths involved in organized sports should be encouraged to wear appropriate eye protection.
2. The recommended sports-protective eyewear as listed in Table 2 should be prescribed. Proper fit is essential. Because some children have narrow facial features, they may be unable to wear even the smallest sports goggles. These children may be fitted with 3-mm polycarbonate lenses in ANSI standard Z87.1 frames designed for children.[12] The parents should be informed that this protection is not optimal, and the choice of eye-safe sports should be discussed.
3. Because contact lenses offer no protection, it is strongly recommended that athletes who wear contact lenses also wear the appropriate eye protection listed in Table 2.
4. An athlete who requires prescription spectacles has 3 options for eye protection: a) polycarbonate lenses in a sports frame that passes ASTM standard F803 for the specific sport; b) contact lenses plus an appropriate protector listed in Table 2; or c) an over-the-glasses eyeguard that conforms to the specifications of ASTM standard F803 for sports in which an ASTM standard F803 protector is sufficient.[10]
5. All functionally 1-eyed athletes should wear appropriate eye protection for all sports.
6. Functionally 1-eyed athletes and those who have had an eye injury or surgery must not participate in boxing or full-contact martial arts. (Eye protection is not practical in boxing or wrestling and is not allowed in full-contact martial arts.) Wrestling has a low incidence of eye injury. Although no standards exist, eye protectors that are firmly

TABLE 2.   Recommended Eye Protectors for Selected Sports

Sport	Minimal Eye Protector	Comment
Baseball/softball (youth batter and base runner)	ASTM standard F910	Face guard attached to helmet
Baseball/softball (fielder)	ASTM standard F803 for baseball	ASTM specifies age ranges
Basketball	ASTM standard F803 for basketball	ASTM specifies age ranges
Bicycling	Helmet plus streetwear/fashion eyewear	
Boxing	None available; not permitted in the sport	Contraindicated for functionally 1-eyed athletes
Fencing	Protector with neck bib	
Field hockey (men and women)	ASTM standard F803 for women's lacrosse (goalie: full face mask)	Protectors that pass for women's lacrosse also pass for field hockey
Football	Polycarbonate eye shield attached to helmet-mounted wire face mask	
Full-contact martial arts	None available; not permitted in the sport	Contraindicated for functionally 1-eyed athletes
Ice hockey	ASTM standard F513 face mask on helmet (goaltenders: ASTM standard F1587)	HECC OR CSA certified Full-face shield
Lacrosse (men)	Face mask attached to lacrosse helmet	
Lacrosse (women)	ASTM standard F803 for women's lacrosse	Should have option to wear helmet
Paintball	ASTM standard F1776 for paintball	
Racquet sports (badminton, tennis, paddle tennis, handball, squash, and racquetball)	ASTM standard F803 for selected sport	
Soccer	ASTM standard F803 for selected sport	
Street hockey	ASTM standard 513 face mask on helmet	Must be HECC or CSA certified
Track and field	Streetwear with polycarbonate lenses/fashion eyewear*	
Water polo/swimming	Swim goggles with polycarbonate lenses	
Wrestling	No standard available	Custom protective eyewear can be made

* Eyewear that passes ASTM standard F803 is safer than streetwear eyewear for all sports activities with impact potential.

fixed to the head have been custom made. The wrestler who has a custom-made eye protector must be aware that the protector design may be insufficient to prevent injury.

7. For sports in which a face mask or helmet with an eye protector or shield must be worn, it is strongly recommended that functionally 1-eyed athletes also wear sports goggles that conform to the requirements of ASTM standard F803 (for any selected sport).[10] This is to maintain some level of protection if the face guard is elevated or removed, such as for hockey or football players on the bench. The helmet must fit properly and have a chinstrap for optimal protection.

8. Athletes should replace sports eye protectors that are damaged or yellowed with age, because they may have become weakened and are, therefore, no longer protective.

COMMITTEE ON SPORTS MEDICINE AND FITNESS, 2003–2004
Reginald L. Washington, MD, Chairperson
David T. Bernhardt, MD
Joel S. Brenner, MD, MPH
Jorge Gomez, MD
Thomas J. Martin, MD
Frederick E. Reed, MD
Stephen G. Rice, MD, PhD, MPH

LIAISONS
Carl Krein, AT, PT
    National Athletic Trainers Association
Claire LeBlanc, MD
    Canadian Paediatric Society

Judith C. Young, PhD
    National Association for Sport and Physical Education

STAFF
Jeanne Christensen Lindros, MPH

EYE HEALTH AND PUBLIC INFORMATION TASK FORCE, 2003–2004
M. Bowes Hamill, MD, Chairperson
Stuart R. Dankner, MD
Roberto Diaz-Rohena, MD
James Garrity, MD
Ana Huaman, MD
Henry Jampel, MD
Terri D. Pickering, MD
Tamara Vrabec, MD

SECRETARIAT
Paul Sternberg, Jr, MD

STAFF
Peggy Kraus
Georgia Alward
Annamarie Harris

REFERENCES

1. US Consumer Product Safety Commission. *Sports and Recreational Eye Injuries.* Washington, DC: US Consumer Product Safety Commission; 2000
2. Nelson LB, Wilson TW, Jeffers JB. Eye injuries in childhood: demography, etiology, and prevention. *Pediatrics.* 1989;84:438–441
3. Grin TR, Nelson LB, Jeffers JB. Eye injuries in childhood. *Pediatrics.* 1987;80:13–17
4. Jeffers JB. An on-going tragedy: pediatric sports-related eye injuries. *Semin Ophthalmol.* 1990;5:216–223
5. Larrison WI, Hersh PS, Kunzweiler T, Shingleton BJ. Sports-related ocular trauma. *Ophthalmology.* 1990;97:1265–1269

6. Strahlman E, Sommer A. The epidemiology of sports-related ocular trauma. *Int Ophthalmol Clin.* 1988;28:199–202

7. Wichmann S, Martin DR. Single-organ patients: balancing sports with safety. *Phys Sportsmed.* 1992;20:176–182

8. Federal Highway Administration. *Manual on Uniform Traffic Control Devices for Streets and Highways.* Washington, DC: US Department of Transportation; 1988

9. Vinger PF. The eye and sports medicine. In: Duane TD, Tasman W, Jaeger EA, eds. *Duane's Clinical Ophthalmology.* Vol 5. Philadelphia, PA: JB Lippincott; 1994:1–103

10. American Society for Testing and Materials. *Annual Book of ASTM Standards: Vol 15.07. Sports Equipment; Safety and Traction for Footwear; Amusement Rides; Consumer Products.* West Conshohocken, PA: American Society for Testing and Materials; 2003

11. American National Standards Institute. Ophthalmics—Nonprescription Sunglasses and Fashion Eyewear—Requirements. Washington, DC: American National Standards Institute; 2001

12. American National Standards Institute. Occupational and Educational Personal Eye and Face Protection Devices. Washington, DC: American National Standards Institute; 2003

13. Vinger PF, Parver L, Alfaro D III, Woods T, Abrams BS. Shatter resistance of spectacle lenses. *JAMA.* 1997;277:142–144

All policy statements from the American Academy of Pediatrics automatically expire 5 years after publication unless reaffirmed, revised, or retired at or before that time.

RESOURCES

American Academy of Ophthalmology, Communications Department, PO Box 7424, San Francisco, CA 94120-7424.

Prevent Blindness America (formerly National Society to Prevent Blindness), 500 E. Remington Rd, Schaumburg, IL 60173.

AMERICAN ACADEMY OF PEDIATRICS

Committee on Sports Medicine and Fitness

Risk of Injury From Baseball and Softball in Children

ABSTRACT. This statement updates the 1994 American Academy of Pediatrics policy statement on baseball and softball injuries in children. Current studies on acute, overuse, and catastrophic injuries are reviewed with emphasis on the causes and mechanisms of injury. This information serves as a basis for recommending safe training practices and the appropriate use of protective equipment.

ABBREVIATION. NOCSAE, National Operating Committee on Standards for Athletic Equipment.

INTRODUCTION

Baseball is one of the most popular sports in the United States, with an estimated 4.8 million children 5 to 14 years of age participating annually in organized and recreational baseball and softball. Highly publicized catastrophic impact injuries from contact with a ball or a bat frequently raise safety concerns. These injuries, as well as ongoing concerns about shoulder and elbow injuries, provide the impetus for this review of the safety of baseball for 5- to 14-year-old participants. The discussion focuses principally on baseball, but softball is considered in accord with the availability of relevant literature. This statement mainly concerns injuries during practices and games in organized settings. Players and bystanders also can be injured in casual play.

INJURY OVERVIEW

The overall incidence of injury in baseball ranges between 2% and 8% of participants per year. Among children 5 to 14 years of age, an estimated 162 000 baseball, softball, and tee-ball injuries were treated in emergency departments in 1995. The number of injuries generally increased with age, with a peak incidence at 12 years. Of the injuries, 26% were fractures, and 37% were contusions and abrasions. The remainder were strains, sprains, concussions, internal injuries, and dental injuries.[1] The potential for catastrophic injury resulting from direct contact with a bat, baseball, or softball exists. Deaths have occurred from impact to the head resulting in intracranial bleeding and from blunt chest impact, probably causing ventricular fibrillation or asystole (commotio cordis).[1] Children 5 to 15 years of age seem to be uniquely vulnerable to blunt chest impact because

their thoraces may be more elastic and more easily compressed.[2] Statistics compiled by the US Consumer Product Safety Commission[1] indicate that there were 88 baseball-related deaths to children in this age group between 1973 and 1995, an average of about 4 per year. This average has not changed since 1973. Of these, 43% were from direct-ball impact with the chest (commotio cordis); 24% were from direct-ball contact with the head; 15% were from impacts from bats; 10% were from direct contact with a ball impacting the neck, ears, or throat; and in 8%, the mechanism of injury was unknown.

Direct contact by the ball is the most frequent cause of death and serious injury in baseball. Preventive measures to protect young players from direct ball contact include the use of batting helmets and face protectors while at bat and on base, the use of special equipment for the catcher (helmet, mask, chest, and neck protectors), the elimination of the on-deck circle, and protective screening of dugouts and benches.

OVERUSE INJURIES

The term "Little League elbow" refers to medial elbow pain attributable to throwing by skeletally immature athletes. Pitchers are most likely to be affected by this condition, but it can occur in other positions associated with frequent and forceful throwing. The throwing motion creates traction forces on the medial portion of the elbow and compression forces on the lateral portion of the elbow. The medial traction forces can cause separation or avulsion of the apophysis from the medial epicondyle of the humerus and overuse injury to the common flexor tendon. The compression forces laterally can cause collapse and deformity of the distal humerus, also known as osteochondritis dissecans of the capitulum of the humerus. Early recognition of the symptoms is important to avoid chronic elbow pain, instability, and arthritis.

In response to concerns about Little League elbow and shoulder, many youth leagues have attempted to limit the stress placed on the pitching arms of youth. For example, Little League Baseball Incorporated limits pitchers to a maximum of 6 innings per week and requires mandatory rest periods between pitching appearances.[3] The number of pitches thrown per outing should be recorded for all young pitchers. Recommendations include limiting the number of pitches to 200 per week, or 90 pitches per outing.[4] A preseason conditioning program that includes strengthening the rotator cuff and the shoulder-stabilizing muscles also may help reduce

PEDIATRICS (ISSN 0031 4005). Copyright © 2001 by the American Academy of Pediatrics.

throwing injuries. Instruction on proper pitching mechanics is another way to prevent serious overuse throwing injuries.[5] Finally, allowing time during the early part of the season to gradually increase the amount and intensity of throwing may allow young arms a better opportunity to adapt to the stresses of throwing.

EQUIPMENT

Modifications in the hardness and compressibility of softballs and baseballs have been developed for use by children of different ages with the intent of reducing the force of impact while maintaining performance characteristics. The National Operating Committee on Standards for Athletic Equipment (NOCSAE) has developed standards for these softer baseballs.[6] An expert review indicated that softer balls that meet the NOCSAE standard are less likely to result in serious head injury or commotio cordis attributable to ball impact.[1]

Chest protectors for batters are a relatively new product. They are produced in 2 styles: a small 6 × 6-in polyethylene square intended to protect the heart from ball impact; and a high-density plastic and foam vest intended to protect the rib cage and the heart and other vital organs. Expert review of the available scientific literature indicated that the way in which baseball impact causes death is unknown at the present. Therefore, the effect of any equipment on the risk of chest impact death remains undetermined.[2]

Concern has been raised about injuries to the eye.[7–9] Baseball is the leading cause of sports-related eye injuries in children, and the highest incidence occurs in children 5 to 14 years of age. Approximately one third of baseball-related eye injuries result from being struck by a pitched ball. As a result, for this age group, Prevent Blindness America has recommended the use of batting helmets with polycarbonate face guards that meet standard F910 of the American Society for Testing and Materials.[10] These cover the lower part of the face from the tip of the nose to below the chin. They also protect against injuries to the teeth and facial bones. Functionally one-eyed athletes (best corrected vision in the worst eye of less than 20/50) must use these face guards. They also must protect their eye when fielding by using polycarbonate sports goggles. Eye protection also may be particularly important for young athletes who have undergone eye surgery or experienced a serious eye injury.

DEVELOPMENTAL CONSIDERATIONS

Compared with older players, children younger than 10 years often have less coordination, slower reaction times, a reduced ability to pitch accurately, and a greater fear of being struck by the ball. Some developmentally appropriate rule modifications therefore are advisable for this age group, including the use of an adult pitcher, a pitching machine, or a batting tee. The avoidance of head-first sliding and the use of softer balls should be considered. For children younger than 10 years, there have been anecdotal reports of rare but serious cervical spine injuries occurring when a player slides head-first, hitting an opponent with the top of the helmet. This injury is similar to that caused by spearing (using the head as the lead object) in football. Such sliding should be banned for players younger than 10 years.

Much of the injury research has concerned baseball and is not differentiated between baseball and softball. Injury risks seem to be similar in softball. Therefore, the same recommendations for injury prevention in baseball apply to softball except for limitations on pitching.

RECOMMENDATIONS

The American Academy of Pediatrics recommends the following:

1. Baseball and softball for children 5 through 14 years of age should be acknowledged by pediatricians as relatively safe sports. Catastrophic and chronically disabling injuries are rare; the frequency of injuries does not seem to have increased during the past 2 decades.
2. Preventive measures should be used to protect young baseball pitchers from throwing injuries. These measures include a restriction on the number of pitches thrown in organized and informal settings and instruction in proper training, conditioning, and throwing mechanics. Parents, coaches, and players should be educated about the early warning signs of an overuse injury and encouraged to seek timely and appropriate treatment if evidence of an injury develops.
3. Serious and potentially catastrophic baseball injuries can be minimized by the proper use of available safety equipment. This includes the use of approved batting helmets; helmets, masks, and chest and neck protectors for all catchers; and rubber spikes. Protective fencing of dugouts and benches and the use of break-away bases also are recommended, as is the elimination of the on-deck circle. Protective equipment should always be properly fitted and well maintained. These preventive measures should be used in games and practices and in organized and informal participation.
4. Baseball and softball players should be encouraged to wear polycarbonate eye protectors on their batting helmets to reduce the risk of eye injury. These eye protectors should be required for functionally one-eyed athletes (best corrected vision in the worst eye of less than 20/50) and for athletes who have undergone eye surgery or experienced severe eye injuries if their ophthalmologists judge them to be at an increased risk for eye injuries. These athletes also should protect their eyes when fielding by using polycarbonate sports goggles.
5. Consideration should be given to using low-impact NOCSAE-approved baseballs and softballs for children 5 to 14 years of age. Particularly, children younger than 10 years should be encouraged to use the lowest impact NOCSAE-approved balls.

6. Developmentally appropriate rule modifications, such as the avoidance of head-first sliding, should be implemented for children younger than 10 years.

7. Because current data are limited, the routine use of chest protectors is not recommended for baseball players other than catchers.

8. Surveillance of baseball and softball injuries should be continued. Studies should continue to determine the effectiveness of low-impact balls for reducing serious impact injuries. Research should be continued to develop other new, improved, and efficacious safety equipment.

COMMITTEE ON SPORTS MEDICINE AND FITNESS, 2000–2001
Reginald L. Washington, MD, Chairperson
David T. Bernhardt, MD
Jorge Gomez, MD
Miriam D. Johnson, MD
Thomas J. Martin, MD
Thomas W. Rowland, MD
Eric Small, MD

LIAISON REPRESENTATIVES
Claire LeBlanc, MD
    Canadian Paediatric Society
Carl Krein, AT, PT
    National Athletic Trainers Association
Judith C. Young, PhD
    National Association for Sport and Physical Education

SECTION LIAISON
Frederick E. Reed, MD
    Section on Orthopaedics

REFERENCES

1. Kyle SB. *Youth Baseball Protective Equipment Project: Final Report.* Washington, DC: US Consumer Product Safety Commission; 1996
2. Link MS, Wang PJ, Pandian NG, et al. An experimental model of sudden death due to low energy chest wall impact. *N Engl J Med.* 1998;338:1805–1811
3. Little League Baseball Inc. *Official Regulations and Playing Rules.* Williamsport, PA: Little League Baseball Inc; 1999:13–14
4. Congeni J. Treating and preventing little league elbow. *Physician Sportsmed.* 1994;22:54–55, 59–60, 63–64
5. Andrews JR, Fleisig GS. Preventing throwing injuries [editorial]. *J Orthop Sports Phys Ther.* 1998;27:187–188
6. National Operating Committee on Standards for Athletic Equipment Baseball Helmet Task Force. *Standard Method of Impact Test Performance Requirements for Baseball/Softball Batters: Helmets, Baseballs, and Softballs.* Kansas City, MO: National Operating Committee on Standards for Athletic Equipment; 1991
7. Grin TR, Nelson LB, Jeffers JB. Eye injuries in childhood. *Pediatrics.* 1987;80:13–17
8. Caveness LS. Ocular and facial injuries in baseball. *Int Ophthalmol Clin.* 1988;28:238–241
9. Nelson LB, Wilson TW, Jeffers JB. Eye injuries in childhood: demography, etiology, and prevention. *Pediatrics.* 1989;84:438–441
10. American Society for Testing Materials. *Standard Specifications for Face Guards for Youth Baseball.* Philadelphia, PA: American Society for Testing Materials; 1986

AMERICAN ACADEMY OF PEDIATRICS

Committee on Sports Medicine and Fitness

Safety in Youth Ice Hockey: The Effects of Body Checking

ABSTRACT. Ice hockey is a sport enjoyed by many young people. The occurrence of injury can offset what may otherwise be a positive experience. A high proportion of injuries in hockey appear to result from intentional body contact or the practice of checking. The American Academy of Pediatrics recommends limiting checking in hockey players 15 years of age and younger as a means to reduce injuries. Strategies such as the fair play concept can also help decrease injuries that result from penalties or unnecessary contact.

Ice hockey is played by approximately 200 000 children in the United States[1] and a similar number in Canada. It is classified as a collision sport by the American Academy of Pediatrics because of the intentional body contact, called body checking, that occurs. Because collisions in this sport may occur at high speeds, participants are at risk for serious injury. In recent years, an increase in the number of serious head and neck injuries related to body checking has alarmed the hockey community and has led to a reassessment of the role of body checking in the various classifications of youth hockey[2-4]: mite—ages 8 and 9 years; squirt—ages 10 and 11 years; peewee—ages 12 and 13 years; and bantam—ages 14 and 15 years.

In the 1960s, an alarming number of facial injuries in youth hockey players led to the mandatory use of helmets with a face mask.[5] The acceptance and use of the combination helmet–face mask was remarkably successful in virtually eliminating facial trauma. However, shortly after the introduction of the helmet–face mask, an increase in the number of neck and spinal injuries was noted.[4] The improvement in equipment with the helmet–face mask[1,6] was believed to create a false sense of protection from serious injury. A similar situation was observed in football. With additional protection afforded by improved helmets and face masks in the 1950s, there was an increase in cervical spine injuries. The number of spinal injuries did not start decreasing until rule changes in the 1970s prohibited head-first contact. Rule changes instituted in the mid-1970s substantially decreased, but did not eliminate, these tragic injuries. The ice hockey community wanted to learn from the experience in football and avoid a paradoxical increase in injury as a response to wearing protective equipment. This concern led to investigations of the incidence and causes of head, neck, and spine injuries.[7-9]

A Canadian study in 1984[2] revealed 42 spinal injuries in hockey players reported to the Committee on Prevention of Spinal Injuries. The median age of the injured players was 17 years. Of the 42 players, 28 had spinal cord injuries, of which 17 had complete paralysis below the vertebral level of the injury. Being body checked from behind, resulting in a collision with the boards, was the most common mechanism of injury. A 1987 study[7] of high school hockey players revealed that head and neck injuries accounted for 22% of the total number of injuries. The same study showed that body checking was associated with 38% of the total number of injuries. Sixty-six percent of the players surveyed believed that the requirement of a face mask allowed them to be more aggressive in their style of play. The authors of this study recommended rule changes to limit or eliminate body checking to reduce injuries.

A more recent US study reported injuries in youth hockey players 9 to 15 years old.[1] Head and neck injuries accounted for 23% of the total number of injuries. Body checking accounted for 86% of all injuries that occurred during games. Fifty-five percent of the players thought that their helmets and face masks protected them from injuries. Of particular interest is that size differences among players in this series increased with age, with bantam-level players (ages 14 and 15 years) showing the most variation, with reported differences between the smallest and largest players of 53 kg in body weight and 55 cm in height. The bantam-level players sustained the most injuries (54%).

Another Canadian study[10] compared peewee-level players (ages 12 and 13 years) from a league that allowed body checking with another league that did not. Players in the league that allowed body checking had a fracture rate 12 times higher than the rate of the other league. Body checking in combination with substantial differences in size and strength among players was believed to contribute to the high injury rate, with some players being nearly twice as heavy and twice as strong as other players. Players in the same age group could vary significantly in the amount of force they could impart on another player and/or withstand from another player. In 1990, the Canadian Academy of Sports Medicine reported that although the incidence of serious injuries at the mite and squirt level was quite low, serious injuries were noted at the peewee level. Therefore, they recommended banning body checking at the peewee level (ages 12 and 13 years) and below.[11]

PEDIATRICS (ISSN 0031 4005). Copyright © 2000 by the American Academy of Pediatrics.

An innovative, unique concept for improved sportsmanship and injury reduction in youth hockey called fair-play has been introduced recently.[12] The fair-play concept of scoring ice hockey games, seasons, or tournaments was developed in response to the perceived increase in violence in youth hockey. The system rewards teams and individual players with few penalties and punishes teams and players with larger numbers of penalties. The authors of this concept believe that the system decreases penalties, intimidation, and violence during hockey and creates a climate that promotes fun and player development.

The potential benefits for the fair-play concept are demonstrated in a recent study[13] involving a youth hockey tournament. The participants were high school students younger than 20 years old, who played the qualifying rounds of the tournament using fair-play guidelines (points are awarded for playing without excessive penalties) and the championship round following regular rules. When the fair-play and regular rules portions of the tournament were compared, the injury rate was 4 times higher during the regular rules portion of the tournament. A doubling of the number of penalties and injury rate during the championship round occurred when fair-play rules were suspended.

CONCLUSION

Studies have shown that a high proportion of youth hockey injuries are attributable to checking and that limiting checking can reduce injuries. Disparities in size and strength can further increase the risk for serious injury from checking and other collisions. Variations in size and strength are present in all age groups but are most pronounced among the bantam-level players (ages 14 to 15 years). Therefore, minimizing checking and other high-impact collisions in this age group could further reduce injuries.

RECOMMENDATIONS

In the interest of enhancing safety in youth ice hockey, the American Academy of Pediatrics recommends the following.

1. Body checking should not be allowed in youth hockey for children age 15 years or younger.
2. Good sportsmanship programs, such as the fair-play concept, have been shown to reduce injury and penalty rates and should be adopted for all levels of youth hockey.
3. Youth hockey programs need to educate players, coaches, and parents about the importance of knowing and following the rules as well as the dangers of body checking another player from behind.

COMMITTEE ON SPORTS MEDICINE & FITNESS, 1999–2000
Steven J. Anderson, MD, Chairperson
Bernard A. Griesemer, MD
Miriam D. Johnson, MD
Thomas J. Martin, MD
Larry G. McLain, MD
Thomas W. Rowland, MD
Eric Small, MD

LIAISON REPRESENTATIVES
Claire LeBlanc, MD
    Canadian Pediatric Society
Carl Krein, AT, PT
    National Athletic Trainers Association
Robert Malina, PhD
    Institute for the Study of Youth Sports
Judith C. Young, PhD
    National Association for Sport & Physical Education

SECTION LIAISONS
Frederick E. Reed, MD
    Section on Orthopaedics
Reginald L. Washington, MD
    Section on Cardiology

REFERENCES

1. Brust JD, Leonard BJ, Pheley A, Roberts WO. Children's ice hockey injuries. Am J Dis Child. 1992;146:741–747
2. Tator CH, Edmonds VE. National survey of spinal injuries in hockey players. Can Med Assoc J. 1984;130:875–880
3. Tator CH. Neck injuries in ice hockey a recent, unsolved problem with many contributing factors. Clin Sports Med. 1987;6:101–114
4. Tator CH, Edmonds V, Lapczak L. Spinal injuries in ice hockey players 1986–1987. Can Med Assoc J. 1991;34:63–69
5. Reynen PD, Clancy WG. Cervical spine injury, hockey helmets and face masks. Am J Sports Med. 1994;22:167–170
6. Murray TM, Livingston LA. Hockey helmets, face masks and injurious behavior. Pediatrics. 1995;95:419–421
7. Gerberich SG, Finke R, Madden M, Priest JD, Aamoth G, Murray K. An epidemiological study of high school ice hockey injuries. Child Nerv Syst. 1987;3:59–64
8. Bishop PJ, Wells RP. Cervical spine fractures mechanisms, neck loads and methods of prevention. In: Castaldi CR, Hoerner ER, eds. Safety in Ice Hockey. Philadelphia, PA: American Society for Testing and Materials; 1989
9. Blanchard BM, Castaldi CR. Injuries in youth hockey. Phys Sports Med. 1991;19:54–71
10. Regnier G, Bioleau R, Marcotte G, et al. Effects of body-checking in the Pee-Wee (12 and 13 years old) division in the province of Quebec. In: Castaldi CR, Hoerner EF, eds. Safety in Ice Hockey. Philadelphia, PA: American Society for Testing and Materials; 1989:84–103
11. Sullivan P. Sports MDs seek CMA support in bid to make hockey safer. Can Med Assoc J. 1990;142:157–159
12. Marcotte G, Simard D. Fair-play an approach to hockey for the 1990s. In: Castaldi CR, Bishop PJ, Hoerner ER, eds. Safety in Ice Hockey. 2nd ed. Philadelphia, PA: American Society for Testing and Materials; 1993: 103–108
13. Roberts WO, Brust JD, Leonard B, Hebert BJ. Fair-play rules and injury reduction in ice hockey. Arch Pediatr Adolesc Med. 1996;150:140–145

Strength Training by Children and Adolescents

Organizational Principles to Guide and Define the Child Health Care System and/or Improve the Health of All Children

Council on Sports Medicine and Fitness

ABSTRACT

Pediatricians are often asked to give advice on the safety and efficacy of strength-training programs for children and adolescents. This statement, which is a revision of a previous American Academy of Pediatrics policy statement, defines relevant terminology and provides current information on risks and benefits of strength training for children and adolescents.

www.pediatrics.org/cgi/doi/10.1542/peds.2007-3790

doi:10.1542/peds.2007-3790

All policy statements from the American Academy of Pediatrics automatically expire 5 years after publication unless reaffirmed, revised, or retired at or before that time.

Key Words
children, adolescents, strength training, resistance training, Olympic weightlifting

PEDIATRICS (ISSN Numbers: Print, 0031-4005; Online, 1098-4275). Copyright © 2008 by the American Academy of Pediatrics

STRENGTH TRAINING (ALSO known as resistance training) is a common component of sports and physical fitness programs for young people, although some adolescents may use strength training as a means to enhance muscle size for improving appearance. Strength-training programs may include the use of free weights, weight machines, elastic tubing, or an athlete's own body weight. The amount and form of resistance used and the frequency of resistance exercises are determined by specific program goals. Table 1 defines common terms used in strength training.

BENEFITS OF STRENGTH TRAINING

In addition to the obvious goal of getting stronger, strength-training programs may be undertaken to try to improve sports performance and prevent injuries, rehabilitate injuries, and/or enhance long-term health. Similar to other physical activity, strength training has been shown to have a beneficial effect on several measurable health indices, such as cardiovascular fitness, body composition, bone mineral density, blood lipid profiles, and mental health.[1,2] Recent studies have shown some benefit to increased strength, overall function, and mental well-being in children with cerebral palsy.[3,4] Resistance training is being incorporated into weight-control programs for overweight children as an activity to increase the metabolic rate without high impact. Similar to the geriatric population, strength training in youth may stimulate bone mineralization and have a positive effect on bone density.[5,6]

Multiple studies have shown that strength training, with proper technique and strict supervision, can increase strength in preadolescents and adolescents.[7,8] Frequency, mode (type of resistance), intensity, and duration all contribute to a properly structured program. Increases in strength occur with virtually all modes of strength training of at least 8 weeks' duration and can occur with training as little as once a week, although training twice a week may be more beneficial.[7–12] Appropriately supervised programs emphasizing strengthening of the core (focusing on the trunk muscles, eg, the abdominal, low back, and gluteal muscles) are also appropriate for children and theoretically benefit sports-specific skill acquisition and postural control. Unfortunately, gains in strength, muscle size, or power are lost ~6 weeks after resistance training is discontinued.[1,13]

In preadolescents, proper resistance training can enhance strength without concomitant muscle hypertrophy. Such gains in strength can be attributed to a neurologic mechanism whereby training increases the number of motor neurons that are "recruited" to fire with each muscle contraction.[11,14–16] This mechanism accounts for the increase in strength in populations with low androgen concentrations, including female individuals and preadolescent boys. In contrast, strength training augments the muscle growth that normally occurs with puberty in boys and girls by actual muscle hypertrophy.[12,14,17,18]

Strength training is a common practice in sports in which size and strength are desirable. Unfortunately, results are inconsistent regarding the translation of increased strength to enhanced youth athletic performance.[1,14,19,20] Preventive exercise (prehabilitation) refers to strength-training programs that address areas commonly subjected to overuse injuries, such as providing rotator cuff and scapular stabilization exercises preventively to reduce overuse injuries of the shoulder in overhead sports. There is limited evidence to suggest that prehabilitation may help decrease injuries in adolescents, but it is unclear whether it has the same benefit in preadolescent athletes,[1,21,22] and there is no evidence that strength training will reduce the incidence of catastrophic sports-related injuries in youth. Recent research suggested a possible reduction in sports-related anterior cruciate ligament injuries in adolescent girls

TABLE 1 Definition of Terms

Term	Definition
Strength training	The use of resistance methods to increase one's ability to exert or resist force. The training may include use of free weights, the individual's own body weight, machines, and/or other resistance devices to attain this goal.
Core strengthening	Focusing a strengthening program to the muscles that stabilize the trunk of the body. The training emphasizes strengthening of the abdominal, low back, and gluteal muscles as well as flexibility of muscular attachments to the pelvis, such as the quadriceps and hamstring muscles.
Set	A group of repetitions separated by scheduled rest periods (eg, 3 sets of 20 reps).
Reps	Abbreviation for repetitions.
One-rep max (1RM)	The maximum amount of weight that can be displaced in a single repetition.
Concentric contraction	The muscle shortens during contraction (eg, arm curl, leg press).
Eccentric contraction	The muscle lengthens during contraction (eg, lowering a weight).
Isometric contraction	The muscle length is unchanged during contraction (eg, wall sits: athlete holds the position of feet planted flat on ground with knees at a 90° angle and back against the wall).
Isokinetic contraction	The speed of muscle contraction is fixed through the range of motion.
Progressive resistive exercises	An exercise regimen in which the athlete progressively increases the amount of weight lifted and/or the number of repetitions. The more repetitions, the greater the work performed and the greater the endurance development. The more weight lifted, the greater the strength development.
Plyometric exercises	Repeated eccentric and concentric muscle contractions, such as jumping up onto and down from a platform.
Weightlifting	A competitive sport that involves maximum lifting ability. Weightlifting (which is sometimes called Olympic lifting) includes the "snatch" and the "clean and jerk."
Power lifting	A competitive sport that also involves maximum lifting ability. Power lifting includes the "dead lift," the "squat," and the "bench press."
Body building	A competition in which muscle size, symmetry, and definition are judged.

when strength training was combined with specific plyometric exercises.[23] Plyometric exercises enable a muscle to reach maximum strength in a relatively short time span through a combination of eccentric and concentric muscle contractions, such as jumping up onto and down from a platform.

RISKS OF STRENGTH TRAINING

Much of the concern over injuries associated with strength training come from data from the US Consumer Product Safety Commission's National Electronic Injury Surveillance System,[24] which has estimated the number of injuries connected to strength-training equipment. The data from the National Electronic Injury Surveillance System neither specify the cause of injury nor separate recreational from competitive injuries that result from lifting weights. Muscle strains account for 40% to 70% of all strength-training injuries, with the hand, low back, and upper trunk being commonly injured areas.[24,25] Most injuries occur on home equipment with unsafe behavior and unsupervised settings.[24] Injury rates in settings with strict supervision and proper technique are lower than those that occur in other sports or general recess play at school.[26,27]

Appropriate strength-training programs have no apparent adverse effect on linear growth, growth plates, or the cardiovascular system,[1,10,11,28,29] although caution should be used for young athletes with preexisting hypertension, because they may require medical clearance to reduce the potential for additional elevation of blood pressure with strength training if they exhibit poorly controlled blood pressure. Youth who have received chemotherapy with anthracyclines may be at increased risk for cardiac problems because of the cardiotoxic effects of the medications, and resistance training in this population should be approached with caution.[30] Specific anthracyclines that have been associated with acute congestive heart failure include doxorubicin, daunomycin/daunorubicin, idarubicin, and possibly mitoxantrone. Youth with other forms of cardiomyopathy (particularly hypertrophic cardiomyopathy), who are at risk for worsening ventricular hypertrophy and restrictive cardiomyopathy or hemodynamic decompensation secondary to an acute increase in pulmonary hypertension, should be counseled against weight training. Individuals with moderate to severe pulmonary hypertension also should refrain from strenuous weight training, because they are at risk for acute decompensation with a sudden change in hemodynamics.[31] Young people with Marfan syndrome with a dilated aortic root also are counseled against participation in strength-training programs. Young athletes with seizure disorders should be withheld from strength-training programs until clearance is obtained from a physician. Overweight children may appear to be strong because of their size but often are unconditioned with poor strength and would require the same strict supervision and guidance as is necessary with any resistance program.

GUIDELINES FOR STRENGTH TRAINING

A medical evaluation of the child before beginning a formal strength-training program can identify risk factors for injury and provide an opportunity to discuss previous injuries, low-back pain, medical conditions, training goals, motives for wanting to begin such a program, techniques, and expectations from both the child and the parents. Youth should be reminded that strength training is only a small part of an overall fitness or sports program. Although research supports the safety and efficacy of resistance training for children, it is not necessary or appropriate for every child. Youth who are interested in getting bigger and stronger should be discouraged from considering the use of anabolic steroids and other performance-enhancing substances and should be provided with information regarding the risks and health consequences of using such substances. More patient-friendly information on performance-enhancing substances is available at www.aap.org/family/sportsshorts12.pdf. The American Academy of

Pediatrics (AAP) strongly condemns the use of performance-enhancing substances and vigorously endorses efforts to eliminate their use among children and adolescents.[32,33]

Because balance and postural control skills mature to adult levels by ~7 to 8 years of age,[34] it seems logical that strength programs need not start before achievement of those skills. Children also should have advanced to a certain level of skill proficiency in their sport before embarking on a disciplined strength-training program for the strength to have some potential value.

Strength gains can be acquired through various types of strength-training methods and equipment; however, most strength-training machines and gymnasium equipment are designed for adult sizes and have weight increments that are too large for young children. Free weights require better balance control and technique but are small and portable, provide small weight increments, and can be used for strengthening sports-specific movements.

Explosive and rapid lifting of weights during routine strength training is not recommended, because safe technique may be difficult to maintain and body tissues may be stressed too abruptly. This restrictive concept is applied to strength training, as opposed to the competitive sport of weightlifting, which is sometimes referred to as Olympic lifting. The sport of weightlifting is distinct from common strength training, because it involves specific types of rapid lifts, such as the "snatch" and the "clean and jerk."

Prepubertal youngsters are involved in competitive weightlifting, but philosophies often vary between Western nations and Eastern European nations.[35] Limited research on weightlifting as a sport has revealed that children have participated with few injuries,[35–37] and some programs have low rates of injury because they require stringent learning of techniques before adding any weight. As with general strength training, strict supervision and adherence to proper technique are mandatory for reducing the risk for injury. Clearly, this is an area in which more research is necessary to substantiate low injury rates as more youngsters continue to be involved with competitive weightlifting. Because of the limited research regarding prepubertal injury rates in competitive weightlifting, the AAP remains hesitant to support participation by children who are skeletally immature and is opposed to childhood involvement in power lifting, body building, or use of the 1-repetition maximum lift as a way to determine gains in strength.

For the purposes of this policy statement, the research regarding strength gains and the recommendations regarding youth involved in lifting weights apply specifically to the activity of strength training as an adjunct to exercise and sports participation.

When children or adolescents undertake a strength-training program, they should begin with low-resistance exercises until proper technique is perfected. When 8 to 15 repetitions can be performed, it is reasonable to add weight in 10% increments. Increasing the repetitions of lighter resistance may be performed to improve endurance strength of the muscles in preparation for repetitive-motion sports. Exercises should include all muscle groups, including the muscles of the core, and should be performed through the full range of motion at each joint. For achievement of gains in strength, workouts need to be at least 20 to 30 minutes long, take place 2 to 3 times per week, and continue to add weight or repetitions as strength improves. Strength training >4 times per week seems to have no additional benefit and may increase the risk for an overuse injury. Proper technique and strict supervision are mandatory for safety reasons and to reduce the risk for injury. Proper supervision is defined as an instructor-to-student ratio no more than 1:10 and an approved strength-training certification, as discussed in Table 2. Proper 10- to 15-minute warm-up and cool-down periods with appropriate stretching techniques also are recommended. Guidelines have been proposed by the AAP (as follows), the American Orthopaedic Society for Sports Medicine,[38] and the National Strength and Conditioning Association.[39,40]

Young people who want to improve sports performance generally will benefit more from practicing and perfecting the skills of their sport than from strength training alone, although strength training should be part of a multifaceted approach to exercise and fitness. If long-term health benefits are the goal, then strength training should be combined with an aerobic training program.

RECOMMENDATIONS

1. Proper resistance techniques and safety precautions should be followed so that strength-training programs for preadolescents and adolescents are safe and effective. Whether it is necessary or appropriate to start such a program and which level of proficiency the youngster already has attained in his or her sport activity should be determined before a strength-training program is started.

2. Preadolescents and adolescents should avoid power lifting, body building, and maximal lifts until they reach physical and skeletal maturity.

3. As the AAP has stated previously, athletes should not use performance-enhancing substances or anabolic steroids. Athletes who participate in strength-training programs should be educated about the risks associated with the use of such substances.

4. When pediatricians are asked to recommend or evaluate strength-training programs for children and adolescents, the following issues should be considered:

   a. Before beginning a formal strength-training program, a medical evaluation should be performed by a pediatrician or family physician. Youth with uncontrolled hypertension, seizure disorders, or a history of childhood cancer and chemotherapy should be withheld from participation until additional treatment or evaluation. When indicated, a referral may be made to a pediatric or family physician sports medicine specialist who is familiar with various strength-training methods as well as risks and benefits for preadolescents and adolescents.

   b. Children with complex congenital cardiac disease (cardiomyopathy, pulmonary artery hyperten-

TABLE 2 Certification Organizations

Certification	Requirements	Examination Content	Recertification	NCCA	Web Address
National Council on Strength and Fitness Certified Personal Trainer (NCSF-CPT)	18 y of age, high school diploma or equivalent	150 MC questions, 3-h proctored examination	Every 2 y, 10 CEUs	Yes	www.ncsf.org
National Academy of Sports Medicine Certified Personal Trainer (NASM-CPT)	18 y age, CPR certification	120 MC questions, 2-h proctored examination	2.0 NASM CEUs	Yes, 2003	www.nasm.org
National Strength and Conditioning Association Certified Personal Trainer (NSCS-CPT)	18 y of age, high school diploma or equivalent, CPR certification	140 questions, 3-h proctored examination	3 y, 6 CEUs; 2 different categories (conference, research publications, etc)	Yes, 1996	www.nsca-lift.org
National Strength and Conditioning Association Certified Strength and Conditioning Specialist (NSCS-CSCS)	BA/BS degree or chiropractor degree, CPR certification	Scientific 80-question, 1.5-hour proctored examination, practical 110 MC 2.5-hour proctored examination	3 y, 6 CEUs as above	Yes, 1996	www.nsca-lift.org
American Council on Exercise (ACE) Personal Trainer	18 y of age, adult CPR certification	150 MC questions, proctored examination, 2 written simulations	2 y, 2.0-hour ACE approved	Yes, 2003	www.acefitness.org
American Council on Exercise (ACE) Clinical Exercise Specialist	18 y of age, adult CPR certification, 300 h of work experience, current ACE-PT	150 MC questions, proctored examination	2 y, 2.0-hour ACE approved	Yes, 2003	www.acefitness.org
National Federation of Professional Trainers (NFPT)	18 y of age, high school diploma or equivalent, 2 y of experience	120 MC questions, 2-h proctored examination	2 CEC per year	Yes, 2005	www.nfpt.com
American College of Sports Medicine (ACSM) Certified Personal Trainer	High school diploma or equivalent, adult CPR certification	150 MC questions, proctored examination	3 y, CEC 45 h	Yes	www.acsm.org
American College of Sports Medicine (ACSM) Health Fitness Instructor	Associate's or bachelor's degree in health-related field, adult CPR certification	Written examination, 140 MC questions, proctored examination	3 y, CEC 60 h	Yes	www.acsm.org
International Fitness Professional Association (IFPA)	No requirements	105 questions at certification site	2 y, 12 CEC	No	www.ifpa-fitness.com
American Fitness Professional Association (AFPA) Personal Trainer	18 y of age, high school diploma or equivalent, adult CPR certification	Home examination, 90 d to complete	2 y, 16 CEC	No	www.Afpafitness.com
International Sports Science Association (ISSA)	No requirements	Home examination			www.issaonline.com
National Strength Professional Association (NSPA) Personal Trainer	18 y of age, adult CPR certification	Two 10-h lectures, written/practical examination, 50 MC questions, 5 practicals	2 y, 24 NSPA CEC	No	www.nspainc.com

As of 2006, instructor certifications received by the following groups are certified by the National Committee for Certifying Agencies (NCCA): National Strength and Conditioning Association, American College of Sports Medicine, American Council on Exercise, National Council on Sports & Fitness, National Academy of Sports Medicine, and the National Federation of Professional Trainers. CPR indicates cardiopulmonary resuscitation; MC, multiple choice; CEC, continuing education credits; CEU, continuing education unit.

sion, or Marfan syndrome) should have a consultation with a pediatric cardiologist before beginning a strength-training program.

c. Aerobic conditioning should be coupled with resistance training if general health benefits are the goal.

d. Strength-training programs should include a 10- to 15-minute warm-up and cool-down.

e. Athletes should have adequate intake of fluids and proper nutrition, because both are vital in maintenance of muscle energy stores, recovery, and performance.

f. Specific strength-training exercises should be learned initially with no load (no resistance). Once the exercise technique has been mastered, incremental loads can be added using either body weight or other forms of resistance. Strength training should involve 2 to 3 sets of higher repetitions (8 to 15) 2 to 3 times per week and be at least 8 weeks in duration.

g. A general strengthening program should address all major muscle groups, including the core, and exercise through the complete range of motion. More sports-specific areas may be addressed subsequently.

h. Any sign of illness or injury from strength training should be evaluated fully before allowing resumption of the exercise program.

i. Instructors or personal trainers should have certification reflecting specific qualifications in pediatric strength training. See Table 2 for the various avenues of certification and certifying organizations.

j. Proper technique and strict supervision by a qualified instructor are critical safety components in any strength-training program involving preadolescents and adolescents.

COUNCIL ON SPORTS MEDICINE AND FITNESS, 2006–2007
Eric W. Small, MD, Chairperson
*Teri M. McCambridge, MD, Chairperson-elect
Holly J. Benjamin, MD
David T. Bernhardt, MD
Joel S. Brenner, MD, MPH
Charles T. Cappetta, MD
Joseph A. Congeni, MD
Andrew John Maxwell Gregory, MD
Bernard A. Griesemer, MD
Frederick E. Reed, MD
Stephen G. Rice, MD, PhD, MPH

PAST COMMITTEE MEMBERS
Jorge E. Gomez, MD
Douglas B. Gregory, MD
*Paul R. Stricker, MD

LIAISONS
Claire Marie Anne Le Blanc, MD
  Canadian Paediatric Society
James Raynor, MS, ATC
  National Athletic Trainers Association

CONSULTANT
Michael F. Bergeron, PhD

STAFF
Anjie Emanuel, MPH

*Lead authors

REFERENCES

1. Faigenbaum AD. Strength training for children and adolescents. *Clin Sports Med.* 2000;19(4):593–619
2. Stricker PR. Sports training issues for the pediatric athlete. *Pediatr Clin North Am.* 2002;49(4):793–802
3. Blundell SW, Shepherd RB, Dean CM, Adams RD, Cahill BM. Functional strength training in cerebral palsy: a pilot study of a group circuit training class for children aged 4–8 years. *Clin Rehabil.* 2003;17(1):48–57
4. McBurney H, Taylor NF, Dodd KJ, Graham HK. A qualitative analysis of the benefits of strength training for young people with cerebral palsy. *Dev Med Child Neurol.* 2003;45(10):658–663
5. Morris FL, Naughton GA, Gibbs JL, Carlson JS, Wark JD. Prospective ten month exercise intervention in premenarchal girls: positive effects on bone and lean mass. *J Bone Miner Res.* 1997;12(9):1453–1462
6. Blimkie CJ, Rice S, Webber CE, et al. Effects of resistance training on bone mass and density in adolescent females. *Can J Physiol Pharmacol.* 1996;74(9):1025–1033
7. Falk B, Tenenbaum G. The effectiveness of resistance training in children: a meta-analysis. *Sports Med.* 1996;22(3):176–186
8. Payne VG, Morrow JR Jr, Johnson L, Dalton SL. Resistance training in children and youth: a meta-analysis. *Res Q Exerc Sport.* 1997;68(1):80–88
9. Faigenbaum AD, Milliken LA, Loud RL, Burak BT, Doherty CL, Westcott WL. Comparison of 1 and 2 days per week of strength training in children. *Res Q Exerc Sport.* 2002;73(4):416–424
10. Stricker PR, Van Heest JL. Strength training and endurance training for the young athlete. In: Birrer RB, Griesemer BA, Cataletto MB, eds. *Pediatric Sports Medicine for Primary Care.* Philadelphia, PA: Lippincott Williams & Wilkins; 2002:83–94
11. Ramsay JA, Blimkie CJ, Smith K, Garner S, MacDougall JD, Sale DG. Strength training effects in prepubescent boys. *Med Sci Sports Exerc.* 1990;22(5):605–614
12. Blimkie CJ. Resistance training during preadolescence: issues and controversies. *Sports Med.* 1993;15(6):389–407
13. Faigenbaum AD, Westcott WL, Micheli LJ, et al. The effects of strength training and detraining on children. *J Strength Cond Res.* 1996;10(2):109–114
14. Kraemer WJ, Fry AC, Frykman PN, Conroy B, Hoffman J. Resistance training and youth. *Pediatr Exerc Sci.* 1989;1(4):336–350
15. Ozmun JC, Mikesky AE, Surburg PR. Neuromuscular adaptations following prepubescent strength training. *Med Sci Sports Exerc.* 1994;26(4):510–514
16. Guy JA, Micheli LJ. Strength training for children and adolescents. *J Am Acad Orthop Surg.* 2001;9(1):29–36
17. Fleck SJ, Kraemer WJ. *Designing Resistance Training Programs.* 3rd ed. Champaign, IL: Human Kinetics Books; 2004
18. Webb DR. Strength training in children and adolescents. *Pediatr Clin North Am.* 1990;37(5):1187–1210
19. Flanagan SP, Laubach LL, DeMarco GM Jr, et al. Effects of two different strength training modes on motor performance in children. *Res Q Exerc Sport.* 2002;73(3):340–344
20. Häkkinen K, Mero A, Kauhanen H. Specificity of endurance, sprint, and strength training on physical performance capacity in young athletes. *J Sports Med Phys Fitness.* 1989;29(1):27–35

21. Cahill BR, Griffith EH. Effect of preseason conditioning on the incidence and severity of high school football knee injuries. *Am J Sports Med.* 1978;6(4):180–184

22. Hejna WF, Rosenberg A, Buturusis DJ, Krieger A. The prevention of sports injuries in high school students through strength training. *Natl Strength Coaches Assoc J.* 1982;4(1):28–31

23. Hewett TE, Meyer GD, Ford KR. Anterior cruciate ligament injuries in female athletes: part 2—a meta-analysis of neuromuscular interventions aimed at injury prevention. *Am J Sports Med.* 2006;34(3):490–498

24. US Consumer Product Safety Commission. National Electronic Injury Surveillance System [database]. Available at: www.cpsc.gov/library/neiss.html. Accessed March 29, 2007

25. Risser WL, Risser JM, Preston D. Weight-training injuries in adolescents. *Am J Dis Child.* 1990;144(9):1015–1017

26. Risser WL. Weight-training injuries in children and adolescents. *Am Fam Physician.* 1991;44(6):2104–2108

27. Mazur LJ, Yetman RJ, Risser WL. Weight-training injuries. *Sports Med.* 1993;16(1):57–63

28. Weltman A, Janney C, Rians CB, et al. The effects of hydraulic resistance strength training in pre-pubertal males. *Med Sci Sports Exerc.* 1986;18(6):629–638

29. Bailey DA, Martin AD. Physical activity and skeletal health in adolescents. *Pediatr Exerc Sci.* 1994;6(4):330–347

30. Steinherz LJ, Steinherz PG, Tan CT, Heller G, Murphy ML. Cardiac toxicity 4 to 20 years after completing anthracycline therapy. *JAMA.* 1991;266(12):1672–1677

31. Maron BJ, Chaitman BR, Ackerman MJ, et al. Recommendations for physical activity and recreational sports participation for young patients with genetic cardiovascular diseases. *Circulation.* 2004;109(22):2807–2816

32. American Academy of Pediatrics, Committee on Sports Medicine and Fitness. Adolescents and anabolic steroids: a subject review. *Pediatrics.* 1997;99(6):904–908

33. Gomez J, American Academy of Pediatrics, Committee on Sports Medicine and Fitness. Use of performance-enhancing substances. *Pediatrics.* 2005;115(4):1103–1106

34. Harris SS. Readiness to participate in sports. In: Sullivan JA, Anderson SJ, eds. *Care of the Young Athlete.* Elk Grove Village, IL: American Academy of Pediatrics and American Academy of Orthopaedic Surgeons; 2000:19–24

35. Stone MH, Pierce KC, Sands WA, Stone ME. Weightlifting: a brief overview. *Strength Cond J.* 2006;28(1):50–66

36. Byrd R, Pierce K, Reilly L, Brady J. Young weightlifters' performance across time. *Sports Biomech.* 2003;2(1):133–140

37. Hamill BP. Relative safety of weightlifting and weight training. *J Strength Cond Res.* 1994;8(1):53–57

38. Cahill BR, ed. *Proceedings of the Conference on Strength Training and the Prepubescent.* Rosemont, IL: American Orthopaedic Society for Sports Medicine; 1988:1–14

39. Faigenbaum A, Kraemer W, Cahill B, et al. Youth resistance training: position statement paper and literature review. *Strength Cond.* 1996;18(6):62–76

40. National Strength and Conditioning Association. Strength & Conditioning Professional Standards & Guidelines. Colorado Springs, CO: National Strength and Conditioning Association; 2001. Available at: www.nsca-lift.org/Publications/standards.shtml. Accessed March 29, 2007

AMERICAN ACADEMY OF PEDIATRICS

Thomas J. Martin, MD, and the Committee on Sports Medicine and Fitness

Technical Report: Knee Brace Use in the Young Athlete

ABSTRACT. This statement is a revision of a previous statement on prophylactic knee bracing and provides information for pediatricians regarding the use of various types of knee braces, indications for the use of knee braces, and the background knowledge necessary to prescribe the use of knee braces for children.

BACKGROUND

Pediatricians are appropriately becoming more involved in the care of young athletes. The knee is one of the most commonly injured joints in athletes. The correct care of knee injuries is an important part of any sports medicine or general pediatrics practice and may include the use of braces. Therefore, the pediatrician should be knowledgeable about knee bracing. This statement is an update of a previous statement on prophylactic knee bracing[1] and includes information for pediatricians regarding the use of various types of knee braces, indications for the use of knee braces, and the background knowledge necessary to prescribe the use of knee braces for children.

Acute and overuse injuries to the knee are seen as a result of participation in virtually all athletic activities. Injuries to the ligamentous structures of the knee in the young athlete are becoming more common. The medial collateral and anterior cruciate ligaments are prime stabilizers of the knee and can be injured when direct or indirect forces are applied to the knee. In a growing child, the distal femoral physis is subject to these same forces and may also be injured. In the skeletally immature child, acute trauma to the knee is most likely to cause injury to these 2 ligaments and/or to the distal femoral physis. Patella subluxation, dislocation, or tracking abnormalities can occur as a result of mechanical predisposition as well as direct or indirect stress to the knee. Cumulative microtrauma or overuse can lead to patellofemoral disorders or apophysitis of the tibial tuberosity (Osgood-Schlatter disease), which are common in adolescents.

TYPES OF KNEE BRACES

Various types of braces have been designed to provide symptomatic relief and diminish the effects of injury to the knee. The 4 categories of knee braces are knee sleeves, prophylactic knee braces, functional knee braces, and postoperative or rehabilitative knee braces (Table 1).[2,3] Although patients often report benefits from wearing braces,[4,5] these benefits have not been verified by scientific investigation.[2,4]

The ideal knee brace in any of the 4 categories would produce a synergism with the inherent knee stabilizers, both muscular and ligamentous, throughout the normal range of motion. It would increase resistance to injury from valgus, varus, rotational, or anterior-posterior translation forces. The ideal brace would not interfere with normal knee function or increase the risk of injury to other parts of the lower extremity or to other players.

Knee Sleeves

Knee sleeves are expandable, slip-on devices usually made of neoprene with a nylon cover. They increase warmth, provide even compression, and may enhance proprioception.[6] Knee sleeves may provide a feeling of support to the knee. Plain knee sleeves may be used to treat postoperative knee effusions[6] and patellofemoral syndrome.[6] Used in this capacity, the purpose of a knee sleeve is to decrease knee pain.[7,8] When a knee pad is added, it provides protective cushioning to the patella and anterior knee.

The knee sleeve may be modified to include an opening for the patella, 1 or more movable straps, or a buttress. The buttress may be circular, C-shaped, J-shaped, or H-shaped. With these modifications, the knee sleeve is often referred to as an extensor mechanism counterforce brace and is used to treat patellofemoral joint disorders, including patella subluxation, patella dislocation, and patellofemoral syndrome, all of which are very common in athletes.[9] The pathophysiology of patellofemoral syndrome is unclear,[10] but it has been postulated to occur as a result of abnormal tracking of the patella on the femoral trochlear groove.[2,6] The knee sleeve helps compress the tissue and limits patella movement.[6] The extensor mechanism braces are designed to apply a medially directed force to the lateral patella, thereby improving patellofemoral tracking and decreasing the likelihood of lateral patella subluxation or dislocation. Used in this capacity, they may be of benefit in the athlete with an unstable patella.[11] These braces may also contain a lateral hinge that incorporates an extension stop.[2,5,7]

When a strap is placed inferior to the patella, it may be used to treat Osgood-Schlatter disease and patellar tendonitis.[6] This infrapatellar band is used to decrease the traction forces at the tibia tuberosity for patients with Osgood-Schlatter disease and on the patellar tendon for patients with patellar tendonitis.

PEDIATRICS (ISSN 0031 4005). Copyright © 2001 by the American Academy of Pediatrics.

Table 1. Knee Braces and Indications for Use in the Young Athlete*

Brace Category	Indication	Comments
Knee Sleeves†		
Plain sleeve	Postoperative knee effusions; patellofemoral syndrome	Insufficient for treatment of an unstable knee. Should only be worn during sports activities if swelling occurs. Simple to fit and inexpensive.
Sleeve with knee pad	Protection and padding of the anterior knee	
Sleeve with buttress	Patella subluxation, patella dislocation; patellofemoral syndrome	Improves patellofemoral tracking.
Sleeve with strap	Osgood-Schlatter disease; patella tendonitis	Decreases traction forces on the tibia tuberosity and patella tendon.
Knee Braces		
Prophylactic brace	Protect medial collateral ligament and anterior cruciate ligament, especially in contact sports	Insufficient evidence to use in the young athlete.
Functional brace†	Tears of anterior cruciate, posterior cruciate, medial collateral, and lateral collateral ligaments	Intended to prevent reinjury. Not to be used prophylactically.
Postoperative or rehabilitative brace†	Nonsurgical injury to and after surgical repair of anterior cruciate, posterior cruciate, medial collateral, lateral collateral ligaments, medial and lateral meniscus; or nondisplaced epiphyseal fracture	Can be adjusted for swelling, removed for examinations or icing, and adjusted to allow movement in a controlled range.

*Knee brace images reprinted with permission from djOrthopedics, LLC.
†The use of knee sleeves and functional and postoperative or rehabilitative braces has been accepted clinically on the basis of subjective experience and has not been supported by scientific evidence.

It is important to remember that knee sleeves do not provide ligamentous support and, therefore, are insufficient for the treatment of an unstable knee.[11] Knee sleeves can cause swelling by retaining heat around the knee or by obstructing venous and lymphatic return below the sleeve. They should only be worn during sports activities if these complications occur.[11] The use of these sleeves should be combined with quadriceps and hamstring flexibility, stretching, and strengthening exercises as well as correction of biomechanical dysfunction of the hip, ankle, or foot and improved sports technique.[6,7,9] Scientific evidence of benefits of the knee sleeve is lacking[3,10,12–14]; however, patients report benefits that exceed objective effects noticed by researchers.[2–4] Knee sleeves are relatively simple to fit and inexpensive.[6]

Prophylactic Knee Braces

Prophylactic knee braces[15–17] are braces with unilateral or bilateral bars, hinges, and adhesive straps. The deformable metal of these braces can absorb some of the impact and decrease the force applied to the medial collateral ligament by 10% to 30%.

Prophylactic knee braces are intended to protect (prevent or reduce the severity of injury to) the medial collateral ligament from valgus stress applied to the lateral aspects of the extended weight-bearing leg during contact sports. Some studies indicate they may also protect the anterior cruciate ligament from rotational stress in the same situation. In football, offensive linemen, defensive linemen, linebackers, and tight ends most commonly wear lateral knee stabilizers. Despite anecdotal reports of success, scientific studies have not universally shown that prophylactic knee braces significantly reduce knee injuries.[15–18] Thus, there is insufficient evidence to recommend prophylactic knee bracing in the young athlete.[1–3,7,15–18]

Functional Braces

Functional braces are generally made from a metallic plastic composite with medial and lateral vertical hinges and a variable stop to limit hyperextension. There are 2 types of functional braces: the hinge-postshell and hinge-poststrap models. The rigid shell or straps and hinges provide resistance to deformation. Hinges may be polyaxial to mimic the changing center of motion of the flexing knee. The hinge-postshell model theoretically provides improved tibial displacement control, greater rigidity, enhanced durability, and better soft tissue contact.[7] The upright of a functional brace should be the maximum length comfortable to the athlete.[7,19]

A functional brace is designed to enhance the stability of an unstable knee (usually after an anterior cruciate ligament injury with or without other injuries to the menisci, collateral ligaments, or bone contusion) when rotational and anteroposterior forces are applied. They may be used for 6 to 12 months after anterior cruciate ligament reconstruction[19] to reduce the strain on an anterior cruciate ligament graft.[7,20,21] They are intended to reduce the risk of future injuries without significantly impairing function.

Functional braces are most commonly used by the skeletally immature athlete with an anterior cruciate-deficient knee (awaiting skeletal maturation), the anterior cruciate-deficient athlete who is awaiting surgical reconstruction, and the anterior cruciate-deficient athlete who is not a surgical candidate. This type of brace may also be used during the healing phase of a medial or lateral collateral ligament injury or as a supplement to surgery[21] and rehabilitation to prevent reinjury. Functional anterior cruciate ligament braces may prevent hyperextension; however, their control of rotational forces is less efficient,[2,11,21] so the unstable knee is still at risk of subluxation or shifting, which may lead to meniscal or chondral injury.

There is a lack of scientific evidence that these braces are helpful at the level required for athletic participation.[2,7,19,22–25] However, patients report a positive subjective response, claiming an increase in knee stability, pain attenuation, performance enhancement, and confidence during athletics with brace use.[2,7,22–24] There is probably no difference in effectiveness between off-the-shelf models and custom-made braces.[9,18,23,26] Brace wearers have higher energy expenditures than do nonwearers.[22] Current experimental evidence suggests that functional knee braces do not significantly affect performance.[27]

Lower extremity muscle strengthening, flexibility, and ultimately, improvement and refinement of athletic techniques are more important than functional bracing in treating ligamentous knee injuries.[7,20] Functional braces will never substitute for proper rehabilitation and surgical procedures when necessary.[9]

Postoperative or Rehabilitative Braces

The postoperative or rehabilitative knee brace consists of foam liners that surround the calf, thigh, and knee; full-length medial and lateral rigid bars with hinges at the knee that can be adjusted to allow a controlled range of motion; and 6 to 8 nonelastic straps that hold the brace in place. These braces are prefabricated (off-the-shelf) and adjustable in size.

The postoperative or rehabilitative brace can be used to protect injured ligaments and control knee flexion and extension angles during the initial healing period[2] as part of the treatment program for an injured anterior cruciate ligament, posterior cruciate ligament, medial collateral ligament, lateral collateral ligament, or medial or lateral meniscus. These are most often used during crutch-assisted ambulation immediately after meniscal and/or cruciate ligament injury or surgery. They are used for a short period of time (2–8 weeks) after the acute injury or surgery. The value of a rehabilitative brace as opposed to a cast or splint includes the ability to adjust the brace for swelling, the ability to remove the brace for serial examinations or icing, and the ability to allow for movement in a controlled range of motion.

Pediatricians may order a postoperative brace for the treatment of nonsurgical ligamentous injuries or nondisplaced epiphyseal fractures. There are very little data on the clinical performance of rehabilitative braces.[2,20,28–30] They are accepted clinically on the basis of their subjective performance.

PRESCRIBING KNEE BRACES

Prescribing any knee brace requires an accurate diagnosis of the injury, an appreciation and knowledge of the benefits and limitations of a brace, and an understanding of the physical demands and risks of the given sport. Knee sleeves with or without straps and buttresses can be prescribed for problems with patellar instability, patellofemoral pain, patellar tendonitis, or Osgood-Schlatter disease. Because prophylactic knee braces have not been proven to be cost-effective, pediatricians should not prescribe them. Functional braces may help prevent further injuries to a previously injured knee and may help protect a surgically repaired knee. Functional braces are not recommended for prophylaxis. Postoperative or rehabilitative braces are generally used for acute knee ligament or growth plate injuries or after surgical repair of an anterior cruciate ligament or meniscus.

Even when use of a knee brace is indicated, the brace alone is not sufficient to treat or protect the injured knee. The brace is only 1 component of injury rehabilitation, along with therapeutic exercises, such as flexibility, joint mobilization, strengthening, and proprioceptive retraining.

Brace designs will continue to evolve with lighter and stronger materials, more physiologic and durable hinges, and attachment systems that do not excessively compress the musculature or irritate the skin. Better ability to test the effectiveness of these braces will be rewarding.

SUMMARY

When prescribing the use of knee braces, pediatricians should establish an accurate diagnosis of the injury, consider the spectrum of treatment options, and understand the classifications, benefits, limitations, indications, and cost of any brace prescribed.

There is insufficient scientific evidence to recommend the use of prophylactic knee braces for the pediatric athlete, and available studies do not support the prescribing of most knee braces. However, the use of knee sleeves, functional braces, and postoperative braces has been accepted clinically on the basis of subjective performance. If used, knee braces should complement, rather than replace, rehabilitative therapy and required surgery.

COMMITTEE ON SPORTS MEDICINE AND FITNESS, 2000–2001
Reginald L. Washington, MD, Chairperson
David T. Bernhardt, MD
Jorge Gomez, MD
Miriam D. Johnson, MD
Thomas J. Martin, MD
Thomas W. Rowland, MD
Eric Small, MD

LIAISONS
Carl Krein, AT, PT
    National Athletic Trainers Association

Claire LeBlanc, MD
    Canadian Paediatric Society
Robert Malina, PhD
    Institute for the Study of Youth Sports
Judith C. Young, PhD
    National Association for Sport and Physical Education

SECTION LIAISONS
Frederick E. Reed, MD
    Section on Orthopaedics
Reginald L. Washington, MD
    Section on Cardiology

CONSULTANTS
Steven Anderson, MD
Oded Bar-Or, MD

STAFF
Heather Newland

REFERENCES

1. American Academy of Pediatrics, Committee on Sports Medicine. Knee brace use by athletes. *Pediatrics*. 1990;85:228
2. France EP, Paulos LE. Knee bracing. *J Am Acad Orthop Surg*. 1994;2:281–287
3. American Academy of Orthopaedic Surgeons. The use of knee braces. Available at: http://www.aaos.org/wordhtml/papers/position/kneebr.htm. Accessed September 12, 2000
4. Greenwald AE, Bagley AM, France EP, Paulos LE, Greenwald RM. A biomechanical and clinical evaluation of patellofemoral knee brace. *Clin Orthop*. 1996;324:187–195
5. Shellock FG, Mink JH, Deutsch AL, Molnar T. Effect of a newly designed patellar realignment brace on patellofemoral relationships. *Med Sci Sports Exerc*. 1995;27:469–472
6. Paluska SA, McKeag DB, Roberts WO. Using patellofemoral braces for anterior knee pain. *Phys Sportsmed*. 1999;27:81–82
7. Paluska SA, McKeag MD. Knee braces: current evidence and clinical recommendations for their use. *Am Fam Physician*. 2000;61:411–418
8. Arroll B, Ellis-Pegler E, Edmonds A, Sutcliffe G. Patellofemoral pain syndrome: a critical review of the clinical trials on nonoperative therapy. *Am J Sports Med*. 1997;25:207–212
9. Papagelopoulos PJ, Sim FH. Patellofemoral pain syndrome: diagnosis and management. *Orthopedics*. 1997;20:148–159
10. Powers, CM. Rehabilitation of patellofemoral joint disorders: a critical review. *J Orthop Sports Phys Ther*. 1998;5:345–354
11. McGinnis DW, Pasque CB. Knee. In: Anderson SJ, Sullivan JA, eds. *Care of the Young Athlete*. Rosemont, IL: American Academy of Orthopaedic Surgeons and American Academy of Pediatrics; 2000:34
12. BenGal S, Lowe J, Mann G, Finsterbush A, Matan Y. The role of the knee brace in the prevention of anterior knee pain syndrome. *Am J Sports Med*. 1997;25:118–122
13. Powers CM, Shellock FG, Beering TV, Garrido DE, Goldbach RM, Molnar T. Effect of bracing on patellar kinematics in patients with patellofemoral joint pain. *Med Sci Sports Exerc*. 1999;31:1714–1720
14. Muhle C, Brinkman NG, Skaf A, Heller M, Resnick D. Effect of a patellar realignment brace on patients with patellar subluxation and dislocation. Evaluation with kinematic magnetic resonance imaging. *Am J Sports Med*. 1999;27:350–353
15. Teitz CC, Hermanson BK, Kronmal RA, Diehr PH. Evaluation of the use of braces to prevent injury to the knee in collegiate football players. *J Bone Joint Surg Am*. 1987;69:2–9
16. Sitler M, Ryan J, Hopkinson W, et al. The efficacy of a prophylactic knee brace to reduce knee injuries in football. A prospective, randomized study at West Point. *Am J Sports Med*. 1990;18:310–315
17. Rovere GD, Haupt HA, Yates CS. Prophylactic knee bracing in college football. *Am J Sports Med*. 1987;15:111–116
18. Hewson GF Jr, Mendini RA, Wang JB. Prophylactic knee bracing in college football. *Am J Sports Med*. 1986;14:262–266
19. Liu SH, Mirzayan R. Current review. Functional knee bracing. *Clin Orthop*. 1995;317:273–381
20. Risberg MA, Holm I, Steen H, Eriksson J, Ekeland A. The effect of knee

bracing after anterior cruciate ligament reconstruction. A prospective, randomized study with two years' follow-up. *Am J Sports Med.* 1999;27: 76–830

21. Stanitski CL. Anterior cruciate ligament injury in the skeletally immature patient: diagnosis and treatment. *J Am Acad Orthop Surg.* 1995;3: 146–158

22. Kramer JF, Dubowitz T, Fowler P, Schachter C, Birmingham T. Functional knee braces and dynamic performance. A review. *Clin J Sport Med.* 1997;7:32–39

23. Beynnon BD, Pope MH, Wertherimer CM, et al. The effect of functional knee-braces on strain on the anterior cruciate ligament in vivo. *J Bone Joint Surg Am.* 1992;74:1298–1312

24. Cawley PW, France EP, Paulos LE. The current state of functional knee bracing research. A review of the literature. *Am J Sports Med.* 1991;19: 226–233

25. D'Ambrosia R. Knee braces. *Orthopaedics.* 1988;11:1247

26. Marans HJ, Jackson RW, Piccinin J, Silver RL, Kennedy DK. Functional testing of braces for anterior cruciate ligament-deficient knees. *Can J Surg.* 1991;34:167–172

27. Paluska SA, McKeag DB. Prescribing functional braces for knee instability. *Physician Sportsmed.* 1999;27:117–118

28. Harilainen A, Sandelin J, Vanhanen I, Kivinen A. Knee brace after bone-tendon-bone anterior cruciate ligament reconstruction. Randomized, prospective study with 2-year follow-up. *Knee Surg Sports Traumatol Arthrosc.* 1997;5:10–13

29. Kartus J, Stener S, Kohler K, Sernert N, Eriksson BI, Karlson J. Is bracing after anterior cruciate ligament reconstruction necessary? A 2-year follow-up of 78 consecutive patients rehabilitated with or without a brace. *Knee Surg Sports Traumatol Arthrosc.* 1997;5:157–161

30. Muellner T, Alacamlioglu Y, Nikolic A, Schabus R. No benefit of bracing on the early outcome after anterior cruciate ligament reconstruction. *Knee Surg Sports Traumatol Arthrosc.* 1998;6:88–92

ERRATUM

In "Counseling Families Who Choose Complementary and Alternative Medicine for Their Child With Chronic Illness or Disability" by the AAP Committee on Children With Disabilities, Virginia Randall, MD, was omitted from the list of consultants due to an oversight. The statement was published in the March 2001 issue of *Pediatrics*. (*Pediatrics.* 2001;107(3):598–601.)

AMERICAN ACADEMY OF PEDIATRICS

Committee on Injury and Poison Prevention and Committee on Sports Medicine and Fitness

Trampolines at Home, School, and Recreational Centers

ABSTRACT. The latest available data indicate that an estimated 83 400 trampoline-related injuries occurred in 1996 in the United States. This represents an annual rate 140% higher than was reported in 1990. Most injuries were sustained on home trampolines. In addition, 30% of trampoline-related injuries treated in an emergency department were fractures often resulting in hospitalization and surgery. These data support the American Academy of Pediatrics' reaffirmation of its recommendation that trampolines should never be used in the home environment, in routine physical education classes, or in outdoor playgrounds. Design and behavioral recommendations are made for the limited use of trampolines in supervised training programs.

ABBREVIATIONS. CPSC, Consumer Product Safety Commission; NEISS, National Electronic Injury Surveillance System; NPTR, National Pediatric Trauma Registry.

Review of the literature and the previous policy statements by the American Academy of Pediatrics—"Trampolines" and "Trampolines II"—were critical in placing the currently available data on trampoline-related injuries and deaths in perspective.[1,2] Injuries have been reported on trampolines ranging from 3 feet in diameter to running or tumbling trampolines that may be as long as 30 feet.[3] Previous data have shown that injuries are likely to occur equally on large or small trampolines.[4]

Access to accurate longitudinal data about the incidence and severity of injuries resulting from trampoline use is critical in making sound policy recommendations. Although a variety of articles about trampoline-related injuries have been published,[4-16] many lack consistent data sources, overlap in reporting of case series, lack an accurate measure of exposure to trampolines, and often lack detail on the circumstances of injury. Two data sources are available to help guide the present policy statement: 1) the Consumer Product Safety Commission (CPSC) National Electronic Injury Surveillance System (NEISS) and other files of product-related incidents; and 2) the National Pediatric Trauma Registry (NPTR).

TRAMPOLINE INJURIES

In 1996, an estimated 83 400 trampoline-related injuries were treated in US hospital emergency departments, a rate of 31.5 injuries per 100 000 popula-

PEDIATRICS (ISSN 0031 4005). Copyright © 1999 by the American Academy of Pediatrics.

tion (Tables 1 and 2).[3] The figures represent a 140% increase over the 1990 rate of injury (13/100 000). The NEISS data showed that for all years (1991–1996), incidents were about evenly divided between boys and girls. In 1996, more than 66% of victims were ages 5 through 14 years; about 16% were 15 through 24 years; and about 10% were 4 years or younger (Table 2). Children younger than 5 years had the second highest rate of injury. Strain/sprain was the most common diagnosis, and was involved in 40% of the injuries. Fractures accounted for 30% of injuries; contusions/abrasions, 13%; lacerations, 11%; and other, 6%. Of the estimated injuries, 45% occurred to the lower extremity (leg or foot) and 30% to the upper extremity (arm or hand); 14% were head or face injuries. The majority of injuries to the leg or foot were strains or sprains (58%), whereas the majority of injuries to the arm or hand were fractures (58%). Most injuries to the head or face were lacerations (61%). Fractures, concussions, and internal injuries to the head accounted for about 15% of all head injuries. For the most severe injuries resulting in hospitalization, fractures (most frequently to the arm and leg) were diagnosed in almost 90%. Two percent of trampoline-related injuries treated in the emergency department resulted in hospitalization, compared with 4% for other product-related injuries reported to NEISS. Table 1 summarizes the number of cases of trampoline-related injuries, the number of hospitalizations, and the number of head and neck injuries for the years 1991 through 1996. The CPSC data indicate that in 1996, head (excluding face) and neck injuries accounted for 9.8% of trampoline-related injuries, 7.2% of skateboard-related injuries, and 4.9% of in-line skating-related injuries.[3]

Most trampoline-related injuries have occurred on home trampolines (Table 3). The proportion of injuries for which the location was unknown increased from 1991 to 1996 and deserves further study. Review of NEISS 1996 descriptive comments showed that victims were injured when they landed incorrectly while jumping or while performing stunts. Other injuries occurred when the victims fell from the trampoline to the surface below or collided with another person on the equipment. Victims also were injured when they contacted the frame and/or springs while near the edge of the jumping surface. A limited NEISS in-depth study of people in hospital emergency departments in September 1995 revealed that in 57% of cases, the victims were on the trampoline with one or more other persons when they were injured.[3] Many of these multiple-user incidents seemed to result from contact with another user.

TABLE 1.   Trampoline-Related Injuries*

Years	Actual No. of Cases	Estimated No. of Injuries*	Rate per 100 000	Actual No. Hospitalized		No. of Patients With Head and Neck Injuries Hospitalized†
				Total	<15 y	
1991	651	38 800	15.4	19	12	1
1992	780	44 700	17.1	24	16	4
1993	873	46 200	17.9	18	17	4
1994	1065	52 900	20.3	29	20	2
1995	1383	66 200	25.2	25	21	5
1996	1728	83 400	31.5	43	34	2

* From the US Consumer Product Safety Commission, National Electronic Injury Surveillance System, which gives a probability sample. Each injury case has a statistical weight.
† The number of cervical spine injuries in children were 6 for the years 1991–1995.

TABLE 2.   Estimated Injuries and Injury Rates From Trampolines, by Age of Victim (1996)*

Age of Victim, y	Estimated No. of Injuries	Percentage of Total	Rate per 100 000
Total	83 400	100	31.5
0–4	8470	10	43.5
5–14	55 400	66	143.7
15–24	13 270	16	37.0
25–44	5740	7	6.9
45–64	520	<1	1.0
65+	0	—	—

* From the National Electronic Injury Surveillance System; US Census Population Estimates; US Consumer Product Safety Commission.

Most injuries involved relatively new full-size trampolines in residential yards. Most trampolines were at least 2 feet high.

The NPTR is a database of trauma cases treated in a set of pediatric trauma centers or in children's hospitals with a pediatric trauma unit. In October 1996, there were 78 participating hospitals. During the period July 13, 1988, to June 30, 1996, 149 trampoline-related injuries were reported to the NPTR (unpublished data, 1996). About 50% of these patients were transported directly to the operating room. The leading diagnosis was fracture of an extremity. In 16% of cases, the head and neck were involved. One spinal cord lesion without vertebral injury was reported, and one fracture of the vertebral column occurred without spinal cord injury. The majority of head and neck injuries were skull fractures with intracranial injury or concussion.

A recent epidemiologic study of trampoline-related injuries in New Zealand, during a 10-year period 1979 through 1988, revealed an increase in

TABLE 3.   Percentage of Trampoline-Related Injuries by Location of Trampoline*

Year	Location of Trampoline				
	Home	School	Sports	Other	Unknown
1991	65	1	3	1	30
1992	60	1	1	2	36
1993	63	1	2	1	33
1994	58	1	2	<1	38
1995	58	1	3	<1	38
1996	54	<1	3	<1	42

* From the US Consumer Product Safety Commission, National Electronic Injury Surveillance System.

incidence of hospitalization rate from 3.1 to 9.3 per 100 000.[4] Of hospitalized victims, 71% were injured on home trampolines, and in contrast to other studies, 80% fell from the trampoline to the surrounding surface. Fractures were the most common type of injury, and the incidence of severe head and neck injuries was low. Two deaths and 2098 hospitalizations occurred. Most injuries occurred when the victims fell from the trampoline and sustained injury on impact with the surface below.

A recent review of trampoline-related injuries to children in the United States from 1990 through 1995 provided a retrospective analysis of data from the NEISS. The data indicated that an estimated 1400 children, or 2.0 per 100 000, required hospital admission or interhospital transfer because of a trampoline-related injury. This represented 3.3% of all children with a trampoline-related injury.[16]

TRAMPOLINE DEATHS

Since 1990, the CPSC has received reports of six deaths involving trampolines. Victims ranged in age from 3 years through 21 years, although the 21-year-old died 6 years after being injured on a trampoline. Most deaths occurred when victims fell from the trampolines, and most involved the cervical spinal cord.

CONCLUSIONS

The following conclusions may be drawn from the data and literature review:

1. In the United States, the largest proportion of trampoline-related injuries has occurred on home trampolines.
2. Most trampoline-related injuries occur from falls sustained on and off the trampoline.
3. Many trampoline-related injuries occur when there are simultaneous multiple users.
4. The most likely injuries resulting in hospitalization sustained while using a trampoline are fractures to the upper and lower extremities; these injuries may be severe, often resulting in surgery.
5. Catastrophic cervical spine injuries are rare. However, head and neck injuries constitute a notable number of the more serious injuries requiring hospitalization.
6. More data are needed about the incidence, circumstances, and mechanism of catastrophic injuries, such as those to the cervical spine.

RECOMMENDATIONS

Despite all currently available measures to prevent injury, the potential for serious injury while using a trampoline remains. The need for supervision and trained personnel at all times makes home use extremely unwise.

1. The trampoline should not be used at home, inside or outside. During anticipatory guidance, pediatricians should advise parents never to purchase a home trampoline or allow children to use home trampolines.
2. The trampoline should not be part of routine physical education classes in schools.
3. The trampoline has no place in outdoor playgrounds and should never be regarded as play equipment.

The limited use of trampolines under direct supervision of physical therapists, athletic trainers, or other appropriately trained individuals for specific medical conditions, including conditioning and/or rehabilitation of injuries, is not addressed in this statement. The limited use of trampolines in supervised training programs (eg, gymnastics, diving, and other competitive sports), should include the design and behavioral recommendations that follow.

DESIGN

- A safety pad should cover all portions of the steel frame and springs.
- The surface around the trampoline should have an impact-absorbing safety surface material.[17]
- The condition of the trampoline should be regularly checked for tears, rust, and detachments.
- Safety harnesses and spotting belts, when appropriately used, may offer added protection for athletes learning or practicing more challenging skills on the trampoline.
- Setting the trampoline in a pit so the mat is at ground level should be considered.
- Ladders may provide unintended access to the trampoline by small children and should not be used.

BEHAVIOR

- Only one person should use the trampoline at a time.
- In supervised settings, the user of the trampoline should be at the center of the mat. The user of the trampoline should not attempt maneuvers beyond capability or training, thereby putting them at risk for injury.
- Personnel trained in trampoline safety and competent spotters should be present whenever the trampoline is in use.
- Even in supervised training programs, the use of trampolines for children younger than 6 years of age should be prohibited.[18]
- The trampoline must be secured and not accessible when not in use.

COMMITTEE ON INJURY AND POISON PREVENTION, 1998–1999
Murray L. Katcher, MD, PhD, Chairperson
Phyllis Agran, MD, MPH
Danielle Laraque, MD
Susan H. Pollack, MD
Barbara L. Smith, MD
Gary A. Smith, MD, DrPH
Howard R. Spivak, MD
Milton Tenenbein, MD
Susan B. Tully, MD

LIAISON REPRESENTATIVES
Ruth A. Brenner, MD, MPH
    National Institute for Child Health and Development
Stephanie Bryn, MPH
    Maternal and Child Health Bureau
Cheryl Neverman, MS
    National Highway Traffic Safety Administration
Richard A. Schieber, MD, MPH
    Centers for Disease Control and Prevention
Richard Stanwick, MD
    Canadian Paediatric Society
Deborah Tinsworth
    United States Consumer Product Safety Commission
William P. Tully, MD
    Pediatric Orthopaedic Society of North America

SECTION LIAISONS
Marilyn Bull, MD
    Section on Injury and Poison Prevention
Victor Garcia, MD
    Section on Surgery

COMMITTEE ON SPORTS MEDICINE AND FITNESS, 1998–1999
Steven J. Anderson, MD, Chairperson
Bernard A. Griesemer, MD
Miriam D. Johnson, MD
Thomas J. Martin, MD
Larry G. McLain, MD
Thomas W. Rowland, MD
Eric Small, MD

LIAISON REPRESENTATIVES
Claire LeBlanc, MD
    Canadian Paediatric Society
Carl Krein, ATC, PT
    National Athletic Trainers Association
Judith C. Young, PhD
    National Association for Sport and Physical Education

SECTION LIAISONS
Frederick E. Reed, MD
    Section on Orthopaedics
Reginald L. Washington, MD
    Section on Cardiology

REFERENCES

1. American Academy of Pediatrics, Committee on Accident and Poison Prevention. Trampolines. *News and Comment.* September 1977
2. American Academy of Pediatrics, Committee on Accident and Poison Prevention and Committee on Pediatric Aspects of Physical Fitness, Recreation and Sports. Trampolines II. *Pediatrics.* 1981;67:438–439
3. Cassidy SP. United States Consumer Product Safety Commission (US CPSC). Trampolines. Memorandum, May 15, 1996, and National Electronic Injury Surveillance System (NEISS) data, 1991–1995; 1996
4. Chalmers DJ, Hume P, Wilson FD. Trampolines in New Zealand: a decade of injuries. *Br J Sports Med.* 1994;28:234–238
5. Torg JS, Das M. Trampoline-related quadriplegia: review of the literature and reflections on the American Academy of Pediatrics' position

statement. *Pediatrics.* 1984;74:804–812

6. Hume PA, Chalmers DJ, Wilson BD. Trampoline injury in New Zealand: emergency care. *Br J Sports Med.* 1996;30:327–330

7. Torg JS. Trampoline-induced quadriplegia. *Clin Sports Med.* 1987;6: 73–85

8. Torg JS. Epidemiology, pathomechanics, and prevention of athletic injuries to the cervical spine. *Med Sci Sports Exerc.* 1985;17:295–303

9. Silver JR. Spinal injuries in sports in the UK. *Br J Sports Med.* 1993;27: 115–120

10. Woodward GA, Furnival R, Schunk JE. Trampolines revisited: a review of 114 pediatric recreational trampoline injuries. *Pediatrics.* 1992;89: 849–854

11. Larson BJ, Davis JW. Trampoline-related injuries. *J Bone Joint Surg Am.* 1995;77:1174–1178

12. Hammer A, Schwartzbach AL, Paulev PH. Some risk factors in trampolining illustrated by six serious injuries. *Br J Sports Med.* 1982;16:27–32

13. Hammer A, Schwartzbach AL, Paulev PH. Trampoline training injuries: one hundred and ninety-five cases. *Br J Sports Med.* 1981;15:151–158

14. Routley V. Trampoline injuries. *Hazard.* 1992;13:1

15. Clarke KS. A survey of sports-related spinal cord injuries in schools and colleges, 1973–1975. *J Safety Res.* 1977;9:140–146

16. Smith GA. Injuries to children in the United States related to trampolines, 1990–1995: a national epidemic. *Pediatrics.* 1998;101:406–412

17. American Society for Testing and Materials, ASTM Subcommittee F15–29. F1487–95 Standard Consumer Safety Performance Specification for Playground Equipment for Public Use. West Conshohocken, PA; 1997

18. Consumer Product Safety Alert. Trampoline Safety Alert. Washington, DC: US Consumer Product Safety Commission; June 1997

AMERICAN ACADEMY OF PEDIATRICS

POLICY STATEMENT
Organizational Principles to Guide and Define the Child Health Care System and/or Improve the Health of All Children

Committee on Sports Medicine and Fitness

Use of Performance-Enhancing Substances

ABSTRACT. Performance-enhancing substances include dietary supplements, prescription medications, and illicit drugs. Virtually no data are available on the efficacy and safety in children and adolescents of widely used performance-enhancing substances. This statement is intended to provide a generalized but functional definition of performance-enhancing substances. The American Academy of Pediatrics strongly condemns the use of performance-enhancing substances and vigorously endorses efforts to eliminate their use among children and adolescents. *Pediatrics* 2005;115:1103–1106; *ergogenic, anabolic, performance enhancing, banned substance, athlete, adolescent, sport.*

INTRODUCTION

Performance-enhancing substance use in young people is a concern to pediatricians and society because of potential adverse health consequences and the effects that such practices have on moral development of the individual and on fair athletic competition for all. Health care professionals can play a valuable role in counseling the young person using or contemplating use of performance-enhancing substances by conveying factual information about the proven benefits and medical consequences of these substances and providing advice about healthful eating and training. Attempts to discourage use through scare tactics or by dismissing known performance-enhancing effects of these substances may seriously damage the credibility of the physician and do little to diminish use. Efforts to minimize use of performance-enhancing substances require the pediatrician to have an understanding of the incentives for use, a comprehensive definition of performance-enhancing substances, and familiarity with strategies for prevention.

INCENTIVES FOR THE USE OF PERFORMANCE-ENHANCING SUBSTANCES

The temptation for young people to use performance-enhancing substances should be easily understood by anyone who is familiar with high-level sports in our society. Success (that is, winning) is considered by many to be the most important goal of sports. At the level of professional sports, winning is the ultimate goal. This attitude permeates lower

levels of sports as well, down to youth sports. Society rewards success in sports with celebrity, status, and favoritism.

For athletes of all ages, the pursuit of excellence in sports is an endeavor to be admired and encouraged. Success in sports involves obtaining an "edge" over the competition. However, sometimes the drive for success can be so engrossing and so compelling that a young person can easily lose sight of what is fair and right. Some individuals may view the use of performance-enhancing substances as a substitute for hard work. For others, performance-enhancing substances may be considered a necessary adjunct to hard work or part of the price of success. From the user's perspective, the prospects for success in sports often outweigh the prospects for serious medical complications from use of performance-enhancing substances.

For some, winning has a monetary incentive as well. The enormous salaries paid to professional athletes in the United States and elsewhere are powerful inducements for a young person with outstanding athletic talent to try anything to ensure continued athletic success.

Adolescents may be uniquely vulnerable to the lure of performance-enhancing substances. Many adolescents engage in risk-taking behavior and experimentation at a time when they are coping with the developmental tasks of adolescence, including defining their sexual identity, emancipating themselves from their families, achieving a sense of mastery and self-efficacy, and finding a peer group with which they can identify.[1] The adolescent, by nature, feels invincible and often shuns any suggestion that use of a substance for purposes other than legitimate therapy might pose a danger to their health or their eligibility for sports.

Adolescents are also intensely preoccupied with body image. Personal rewards perceived from enhancing size, strength, stamina, or body build can be strong motivators. A significant number of adolescents who are not involved in competitive athletics use performance-enhancing substances.[2]

The child athlete, particularly the adolescent, in today's society is caught in a struggle between ideals highly valued by society but often in direct conflict: the attitude of winning at all costs and the values of fairness and wholesomeness.

doi:10.1542/peds.2005-0085
PEDIATRICS (ISSN 0031 4005). Copyright © 2005 by the American Academy of Pediatrics.

RATIONALE FOR A BROAD-BASED STATEMENT ON PERFORMANCE-ENHANCING SUBSTANCES AND YOUTH

In the last 2 decades, a considerable amount of research has been conducted with performance-enhancing substances such as creatine, amino acids, androstenedione, and dehydroepiandrosterone. Virtually no experimental research on either the ergogenic effects or adverse effects of performance-enhancing substances has been conducted in subjects younger than 18 years. The amount of scientific data from well-designed studies on the effects of these substances in adults continues to accumulate at such a rate that systematic reviews are soon made obsolete.

This statement is not intended to provide a review of currently available data on performance-enhancing substances. A list of resources for detailed information on specific performance-enhancing substances is provided at the end of this statement. Rather, this statement is intended to convey a more general policy on the basis of the following 3 points. First, the intentional use of any substance for performance enhancement is unfair and, therefore, morally and ethically indefensible. Second, use of any substance for the purpose of enhancing sports performance, including over-the-counter supplements, the composition and quality of which are not under federal regulation, may pose a significant health risk to the young person. Third, use and promotion of performance-enhancing substances tends to devalue the principles of a balanced diet, good coaching, and sound physical training.

CURRENT DEFINITIONS OF PERFORMANCE-ENHANCING SUBSTANCES

Limitations of Current Definitions

Traditionally, sports organizations such as the International Olympic Committee and the National Collegiate Athletic Association have defined performance-enhancing substances as substances that create an unfair competitive advantage. These organizations have produced lists of banned or prohibited drugs that include substances with known performance-enhancing effects as well as substances used by athletes that have been associated with adverse health effects. Detection of illegal or banned substances by drug testing is a critical element of the enforcement and efficacy of these policies. However, current definitions of performance-enhancing substances have contextual limitations. If the substance does not have adverse medical consequences, if the substance is not detectable by drug testing, or if testing for the drug is not performed (so that a potentially dangerous substance or unfair practice may go undetected), then the substance in question would not be included in a list of banned substances.

To date, there is no definition of performance-enhancing substances that applies to all potential users. A definition of a performance-enhancing substance that is applicable to the pediatric age group should not exclude any individual who may have a substance-abuse problem or any substance that can-

not be readily detected. With the prohibitive cost of testing and deficiencies associated with a detection-based banned list, widespread drug testing of children and adolescents is unlikely to be effective or practical. A definition of a performance-enhancing substance for the pediatric age group, therefore, must be independent of whether testing of the substance is conducted in that age group. Because new substances for performance enhancement as well as methods for masking the presence of these substances are continually being discovered, a definition of performance-enhancing substances must remain valid in a changing environment.

General Definition of Performance-Enhancing Substances

A performance-enhancing substance is any substance taken in nonpharmacologic doses specifically for the purposes of improving sports performance. A substance should be considered performance enhancing if it benefits sports performance by increasing strength, power, speed, or endurance (ergogenic) or by altering body weight or body composition. Furthermore, substances that improve performance by causing changes in behavior, arousal level, and/or perception of pain should be considered performance enhancing.

Performance-enhancing substances include the following:

- Pharmacologic agents (prescription or nonprescription) taken in doses that exceed the recommended therapeutic dose or taken when the therapeutic indication(s) are not present (eg, using decongestants for stimulant effect, using bronchodilators when exercise-induced bronchospasm is not present, increasing baseline methylphenidate hydrochloride dose for athletic competition)
- Agents used for weight control, including stimulants, diet pills, diuretics, and laxatives, when the user is in a sport that has weight classifications or that rewards leanness
- Agents used for weight gain, including over-the-counter products advertised as promoting increased muscle mass
- Physiologic agents or other strategies used to enhance oxygen-carrying capacity, including erythropoietin and red blood cell transfusions (blood doping)
- Any substance that is used for reasons other than to treat a documented disease state or deficiency
- Any substance that is known to mask adverse effects or detectability of another performance-enhancing substance
- Nutritional supplements taken at supraphysiologic doses or at levels greater than required to replace deficits created by a disease state, training, and/or participation in sports

STRATEGIES FOR PREVENTING USE OF PERFORMANCE-ENHANCING SUBSTANCES

The methods most widely used to prevent use of performance-enhancing substances, namely drug bans and drug testing, are primarily punitive. Drug bans imposed by organizations that regulate and oversee sports programs at various levels, from the International Olympic Committee to the National Collegiate Athletic Association and state high-school sports associations, effectively make the use of such substances "against the rules." Enforcement of drug bans has necessarily involved the use of drug testing, with positive tests carrying stiff penalties or sanctions including loss of playing privileges, removal of awards or championships from the entire team, loss of scholarships, and restrictions on future regular-season and postseason play.[3] Drug testing and legal sanctions are intended to be deterrents but have little effect on most children and adolescents involved in sports.

Neither the use of drug bans nor the implementation of drug testing provides the young athlete with any framework or guidelines for resolving the conflict between the drive to win and the imperative to do the right thing.

A variety of programs educating young athletes about substance abuse in general and targeting specific performance-enhancing drugs such as anabolic steroids have been tested at the international, collegiate, and even high-school levels.[4] It is unfortunate that few evaluations of these programs have included measurement of continued drug use after the intervention, and programs appropriately studied have not been highly successful in curbing use. One program that combined drug education with training in personal skills to resist the social influences that drive the use of performance-enhancing substances was successful in decreasing the intention to use anabolic steroids among adolescent football players.[5]

Little effort has been made to target adults who are responsible for collegiate, high-school, middle-school, and youth sports programs. Permissiveness often has the same effect as active encouragement when it comes to using performance-enhancing substances. A "don't-ask" attitude should be as intolerable to parents as the provision of performance-enhancing substances to athletes by coaches would be.

IDENTIFICATION OF THE YOUNG PERSON USING PERFORMANCE-ENHANCING SUBSTANCES

Data from epidemiologic studies and case descriptions have provided information about users of performance-enhancing substances that can help pediatricians to identify them. Users of anabolic or androgenic compounds are more likely to be male; are more likely to be involved in sports that demand high levels of strength, power, size, and speed; and are likely to use other illegal substances such as tobacco and alcohol.[5-7] Young people who participate in sports that demand leanness are also more likely to use performance-enhancing substances than are those involved in sports in which leanness is not essential. Young men and women who are not competitive athletes but who are obsessed with body image and who train intensely primarily to improve their physique are also more likely to use performance-enhancing substances. Users of certain performance-enhancing substances might be identified by

outward signs such as virilization in females, testicular atrophy in males, and mood changes produced by anabolic steroids. Unfortunately, most young people who use performance-enhancing substances are not readily identified by outward signs. Therefore, it is imperative that all adolescents be asked about use of performance-enhancing substances in the assessment of high-risk behaviors that should be a part of every adolescent health maintenance visit, including sports physicals, camp physicals, and all other scheduled physician-adolescent encounters.

RECOMMENDATIONS

To assist the pediatrician in dealing with users or potential users of performance-enhancing substances, the American Academy of Pediatrics offers the following recommendations:

1. Use of performance-enhancing substances for athletic or other purposes should be strongly discouraged.
2. Parents should take a strong stand against the use of performance-enhancing substances and, whenever possible, demand that coaches be educated about the adverse health effects of performance-enhancing substances.
3. Schools and other sports organizations should be proactive in discouraging the use of performance-enhancing substances, incorporating this message into policy and educational materials for coaches, parents, and athletes.
4. Interventions for encouraging substance-free competition should be developed that are more positive than punitive, such as programs that teach sound nutrition and training practices along with skills to resist the social pressures to use performance-enhancing substances.
5. Colleges, schools, and sports clubs should make use of educational interventions that encourage open and frank discussion of issues related to the use of performance-enhancing substances, with the aim of promoting decisions about personal drug use based on principles of fair competition and character rather than on the fear of getting caught.
6. Coaches at all levels, including youth sports, should encourage wholesome and fair competition by emphasizing healthy nutrition and training practices, taking a strong stand against cheating, and avoiding the "win-at-all-costs" philosophy.
7. Inquiries about the use of performance-enhancing substances should be made in a manner similar to inquiries about use of tobacco, alcohol, or other substances of abuse. Guidelines for patient confidentiality should be followed and explained to the patient.
8. Athletes who admit using performance-enhancing substances should be provided unbiased medical information about benefits, known adverse effects, and other risks. When appropriate, additional testing may be necessary to investigate or rule out adverse medical effects.
9. The pediatric health care professional providing care for an athlete who admits to using a perfor-

mance-enhancing substance should explore the athlete's motivations for using these substances, evaluate other associated high-risk behaviors, and provide counseling on safer, more appropriate alternatives for meeting fitness or sports-performance goals.

10. Nonusers of performance-enhancing substances should have their decisions reinforced while establishing an open channel of communication if questions about performance-enhancing substances arise in the future.

11. Pediatric health care professionals should promote safe physical activity and sports participation by providing or making available sound medical information on exercise physiology, conditioning, nutrition, weight management, and injury prevention and by helping to care for sports-related medical conditions and injuries.

The November 2004 issue of "Sports Shorts" by the American Academy of Pediatrics Section on Sports Medicine and Fitness concerning performance-enhancing substances[8] is available for download and includes guidelines for pediatricians and parents.

COMMITTEE ON SPORTS MEDICINE AND FITNESS, 2002–2003
Reginald L. Washington, MD, Chairperson
David T. Bernhardt, MD
*Jorge Gomez, MD
Miriam D. Johnson, MD
Thomas J. Martin, MD
Frederick E. Reed, MD
Eric Small, MD

LIAISONS
Carl Krein, AT, PT
    National Athletic Trainers Association
Claire LeBlanc, MD
    Canadian Paediatric Society
Judith C. Young, PhD
    National Association for Sport and Physical Education

CONSULTANT
Oded Bar-Or, MD

STAFF
Jeanne Lindros, MPH

*Lead author

REFERENCES

1. Tanner SM, Miller DW, Alongi C. Anabolic steroid use by adolescents: prevalence, motives, and knowledge of risks. *Clin J Sport Med.* 1995;5:108–115
2. Terney R, McLain LG. The use of anabolic steroids in high school students. *Am J Dis Child.* 1990;144:99–103
3. National Collegiate Athletic Association. NCAA enforcement and student-athlete reinstatement. Indianapolis, IN: National Collegiate Athletic Association. Available at: www.ncaa.org/enforcefrontF.html. Accessed January 12, 2005
4. Yesalis CE, Barhke MS. Doping among adolescent athletes. *Baillieres Best Pract Res Clin Endocrinol Metab.* 2000;14:25–35
5. Goldberg L, Elliot D, Clarke GN, et al. Effects of a multidimensional anabolic steroid prevention intervention. The Adolescents Training and Learning to Avoid Steroids (ATLAS) Program. *JAMA.* 1996;276:1555–1562
6. Bahrke MS, Yesalis CE, Kopstein AN, Stephens JA. Risk factors associated with anabolic-androgenic steroid use among adolescents. *Sports Med.* 2000;29:397–405
7. Kindlundh AM, Isacson DG, Berglund L, Nyberg F. Factors associated with adolescent use of doping agents: anabolic-androgenic steroids. *Addiction.* 1999;94:543–553
8. American Academy of Pediatrics, Section on Sports Medicine and Fitness. Sports shorts: performance-enhancing substances. Available at: www.aap.org/family/sportsshorts12.pdf. Accessed January 12, 2005

RESOURCES

United States Anti-Doping Agency. Available at: www.usantidoping.org. Accessed January 6, 2004
National Federation of State High School Associations. Sports medicine. Available at: www.nfhs.org/scriptcontent/va_Custom/VimDisplays/contentpagedisplay.cfm?content_id=203. Accessed January 6, 2004
National Collegiate Athletic Association. Banned drug list. Available at: http://www1.ncaa.org/membership/ed_outreach/health-safety/drug_testing/banned_drug_classes.pdf. Accessed January 6, 2004
American Medical Society for Sports Medicine. Drugs and performance-enhancing agents in sport. *Clin J Sport Med.* 2002;12(theme issue):201–263
Gomez JE. Performance-enhancing substances in adolescent athletes. *Tex Med.* 2002;98(2):41–46
Metzl JD. Performance-enhancing drug use in the young athlete. *Pediatr Ann.* 2002;31:27–32
Ahrendt DM. Ergogenic aids: counseling the athlete. *Am Fam Physician.* 2001;63:913–922

All policy statements from the American Academy of Pediatrics automatically expire 5 years after publication unless reaffirmed, revised, or retired at or before that time.

Index